Essentials of Psychiatric Mental Health Nursing

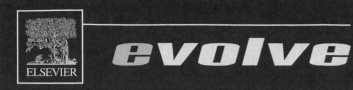

To access your Student Resources, visit:

http://evolve.elsevier.com/Varcarolis/essentials

Evolve® Student Learning Resources for *Varcarolis/Halter: Essentials of Psychiatric Mental Health Nursing,* offers the following features:

- **Chapter Outlines**
  For note-taking in or out of class.

- **Chapter Review Answers**
  Answers, rationales, and textbook page references for the review questions at the end of each chapter.

- **Case Studies and Nursing Care Plans**
  Detailed case studies and care plans for specific psychiatric disorders.

- **Nurse, Patient, and Family Resources**
  Include website addresses, association information, and additional resources for patient teaching material, medication information, and support groups.

- **Concept Map Creator**
  Walks you through the thinking process of creating individualized concept maps.

Essentials of Psychiatric Mental Health Nursing

A Communication Approach to Evidence-Based Care

Elizabeth M. Varcarolis, RN, MA
Professor Emeritus
Formerly Deputy Chairperson, Department of Nursing
Borough of Manhattan Community College;
Associate Fellow
Albert Ellis Institute for Rational Emotional Behavioral Therapy (REBT)
New York, New York

Margaret J. Halter, PhD, PMHCNS-BC
Associate Professor
College of Nursing
University of Akron
Akron, Ohio

SAUNDERS

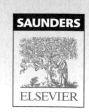

ELSEVIER

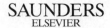

11830 Westline Industrial Drive
St. Louis, Missouri 63146

ESSENTIALS OF PSYCHIATRIC MENTAL HEALTH NURSING: ISBN: 978-1-4160-0051-8
A COMMUNICATION APPROACH TO EVIDENCE-BASED CARE
Copyright © 2009 by Saunders, an imprint of Elsevier Inc.

Library of Congress Cataloging-in-Publication Data

Varcarolis, Elizabeth M.
   Essentials of psychiatric mental health nursing : a communication approach to evidence-based care /
Elizabeth M. Varcarolis, Margaret J. Halter.—1st ed.
     p. ; cm.
   Includes bibliographical references and index.
   ISBN 978-1-4160-0051-8 (pbk. : alk. paper)   1. Psychiatric nursing.   2. Evidence-based medicine.
I. Halter, Margaret J. (Margaret Jordan)   II. Title.
   [DNLM: 1. Mental Disorders—nursing.   2. Evidence-Based Medicine.   3. Psychiatric Nursing—methods. WY 160 V278e 2009]
   RC440.V373 2009
   616.89′0231—dc22
                                          2008029343

Executive Publisher: Tom Wilhelm
Managing Editor: Jill Ferguson
Senior Developmental Editor: Brian Dennison
Associate Developmental Editor: Tiffany Trautwein
Editorial Assistant: Jessica Danziger
Publishing Services Manager: Jeff Patterson
Project Manager: Jeanne Genz
Designer: Kim Denando

Printed in China

Last digit is the print number: 9   8   7   6   5   4   3   2

ACKNOWLEDGMENTS

As is always the case, I owe a huge debt of gratitude to many for their contributions and support.

I am pleased to welcome Dr. Margaret (Peggy) Jordan Halter to this new *Essentials* text. Peggy continues to practice psychiatric nursing and has taught for many years. She has a strong background in research and specializes in stigma and men's mental health. She is committed to evidence-based practice and is a leader in the area of legislation and policy issues that affects psychiatric nursing practice, particularly regarding stigmatizing attitudes.

Peggy and I have worked closely to keep the material current, relevant, and complete. We have added two unique and creative features that are the "gems" of this text. They are as enticing and interesting as they are great learning tools. These two features, "Examining the Evidence" by Peggy Halter and "Applying the Art" by Dawn Scheick, are found in all of the clinical chapters. Of course, there are many other pedagogical features as well that should benefit both the cognitive as well as the visual learner. We hope this text will offer fresh viewpoints for readers studying and engaged in understanding the most essential concepts of psychiatric nursing. Peggy, it has been a joy working with you.

I want to offer special thanks to the amazing authors who have been with me since the earliest editions of *Foundations* and actively contributed their time and expertise once again to our new *Essentials* text. Sincere and profound thanks go to Cherrill Colson, Kathleen Ibrahim, and Penny Brooke. I thank you for sharing your clinical expertise and for sticking with me all these many years. You are all genuine professionals and I am proud to have you as colleagues. I also want to welcome our new contributors, Dorothy Varchol, Dawn Scheick, Ed Herzog, and of course Peggy Halter, who have all brought expanded and creative ideas to this text.

A very special thanks to Teresa Burckhalter and Ann Issacs for their creative work on the instructor ancillaries to accompany the book.

Peggy and I have been fortunate to be part of an amazing dream team. It is always the people who work behind the scenes who are pivotal to the production of any successful text. These are the people who have provided support, kept the project on tract, and solved myriad problems that are inherent in any production. Peggy and I thank you all heartily.

Tom Wilhelm, Executive Publisher: Tom has always supported and provided everything needed to make this new *Essentials* a success, as he has in the past to ensure the success of *Foundations*.

Jill Ferguson, Managing Editor: For most of the writing of this text Jill functioned as Developmental Editor and as always is amazing in her attention to detail, pulling together resources, providing unceasing support, untangling dilemmas, and working tirelessly to support this text in doing whatever was necessary. You are always a star.

Tiffany Trautwein, Associate Developmental Editor: I have Tiffany to thank for the smoothing out and easy flow of much of the manuscript. Thanks Tiffany for making me look good.

Brian Dennison, Senior Developmental Editor, who recently joined our team, has a great eye for detail and good writing skills. We are pleased to work with this new and talented editor and appreciate his willingness to get us what we need to finish first.

Jessica Danziger, Editorial Assistant, handled details too numerous to count and secured all of the permissions for the book.

Jeanne Genz, Project Manager, managed consistency to the minutest detail.

Kim Denando, Book Designer, created a vivid, exciting, and reader-friendly design.

Betsy Varcarolis

CONTRIBUTORS

Penny Simpson Brooke, APRN, MS, JD
Board of Trustees—Intermountain Healthcare, Salt Lake City;
Board of Directors Task Force on Quality,
    Utah Hospitals and Health Systems Association;
The American Association of Nurse-Attorneys (TAANA),
    Past board member and past president of the TAANA
    Foundation;
The Utah State Bar Association—The American Nurses
    Association Foundation;
Intermountain Therapy Animals Board of Advisors
    Chapter 26: Legal and Ethical Basis for Practice

Cherrill W. Colson, MA, CS, EdD
Assistant Professor
Department of Nursing
Hostos Community College
City University of New York, Bronx;
Clinical Specialist
Leake and Watts Children's Services
Yonkers, New York
    Chapter 23: Children and Adolescents

Edward A. Herzog, RN, MSN, APN
Lecturer
College of Nursing
Kent State University
Kent, Ohio
    Chapter 24: Adults

Kathleen Ibrahim, MA, PMHCNS-BC
Assistant Director of Nursing for Staff Development
New York State Psychiatric Institute
New York, New York
    Chapter 11: Eating Disorders

John Raynor, PhD
Professor
Borough of Manhattan Community College
City University of New York
New York, New York
    *Chapter 4: Biological Basis for Understanding
        Psychopharmacology*

Dawn M. Scheick, EdD, PMHCNS-BC
Professor of Nursing and Nurse-Psychotherapist
Department of Nursing
Alderson-Broaddus College;
Circle of Caring, BCHD
Alderson-Broaddus College and Barbour County Health
    Department
Philippi, West Virginia
    Applying the Art

Kathleen Smith-DiJulio, PhD, RN
Visiting Academic Fellow
Institute for Health and Biomedical Innovation
Queensland University of Technology
Brisbane, Australia;
Senior Fellow
Department of Family and Child Nursing
University of Washington
Seattle, Washington
    Chapter 16: Addictive Disorders

Dorothy A. Varchol, MSN, MA, RN-BC
Health Technologies Division
Cincinnati State Technical and Community College
Cincinnati, Ohio
    *Chapter 4: Biological Basis for Understanding
        Psychopharmacology*

Teresa S. Burckhalter, MSN, RN, BC
Nursing Faculty
Technical College of the Lowcountry
Beaufort, South Carolina
    Test Bank

Ann Isaacs, MS, RN
Professor of Nursing
Luzerne County Community College
Nanticoke, Pennsylvania
    Instructor's Manual and PowerPoint Presentations

REVIEWERS

Joseph O. Aina, RN, PhD, FWACN
Associate Professor
Nursing
Western Connecticut State University
Danbury, Connecticut

Nancy A. Craig-Williams, BSN, MS, RN
Professor
Nursing
Greenfield Community College
Greenfield, Massachusetts

Gail Marlene Day, PhD, RN, CNS-PSY/MH, BC
Instructor
Nursing Education
San Antonio College
San Antonio, Texas

Debra Y. Ebaugh, MSN, ARNP
Faculty
Nursing
Edison College
Naples, Florida

Linda W. Edwards, RN, MSN
Assistant Professor
Nursing
Blue Ridge Community College
Weyers Cave, Virginia

Jill M. Espelin, MSN, CNE, RN
Clinical Faculty
Psychiatry, Fundamentals, Capstone, MbEIN
University of Connecticut School of Nursing
Storrs, Connecticut

Laura Meeks Festa, EdD, RN
Division Chair, Health Sciences
Baccalaureate Nursing
University of Charleston
Charleston, West Virginia

Brian Gordon Fonnesbeck, RN, MSN, Certified in Psychiatric Nursing
Associate Professor
Division of Nursing and Health Sciences
Lewis-Clark State College
Lewiston, Idaho

Teresa S. Fox, RN, BSN, AAS
Instructor
Practical Nursing Program, Health Technology Division
Virginia Western Community College
Roanoke, Virginia

Marjorie G. Frazier, MN, APRN-BC
Associate Professor
Nursing
Georgia Highlands College
Rome, Georgia

Jené M. Hurlbut, RN, MSN, MS, CFNP
Assistant Professor of Nursing
Nursing
University of Southern Nevada
Henderson, Nevada

Deborah Kindy, PhD, RN
Professor
Nursing
Sonoma State University
Rohnert Park, California

Barbara Magenheim, RN, EdD, MSN, BSN, CNE
Nursing Faculty
Maricopa Community Colleges Nursing Program
Chandler-Gilbert Community College—Williams
    Campus
Mesa, Arizona

Terran R. Mathers, RN, DNS
Associate Professor
Division of Nursing
Spring Hill College
Mobile, Alabama

Judith M. Pilla, PhD, APRN, BC
President
Health Bridge Associates
Gulph Mills, Pennsylvania

Susan M. Seiboldt, BSN, MSN, RN
Nursing Instructor
Allied Health Department
Carl Sandburg College
Galesburg, Illinois

EXAMINING THE EVIDENCE Combating the Stigma of Mental Illness

During my medical-surgical rotation I was caring for a person with a diagnosis of pneumonia and schizophrenia. The nurse who gave me report said, "Good luck working with Mr. Crazy." I was shocked that a health care provider would talk like that!

This is a real problem, especially because people with psychiatric disorders have enough challenges and we would expect health care professionals (including nurses) to be the most understanding. Although polite people would not dream of using racial slurs or disparaging terms for racial groups or for people with physical handicaps, they seem to accept terms such as crazy, psycho, schizo, mental, nut, and wacko. These result from the stigma that stems from the belief that a person is _____ and that flaw is brought about by such things _____ cter or lack of spiritual strength.

_____ ma be stopped? Research demonstrates that _____ d approaches to dispelling stigma: protest, _____ ntact (Corrigan & Gelb, 2006). Protest _____ rongness or immorality of treating people _____ badly. It can take the form of organized rallies with people carrying signs such as "See the person and not the illness," or

boycotting businesses that use stigmatizing messages in their advertising: "We must be crazy to sell cars at these prices!" Corrigan and associates (2001) caution that this approach may backfire because we aren't really changing people's beliefs; we're just pushing them underground. Yet how we act may truly influence our ch_____ k at the successes of civil and in a bad moo_____ ld be accomplished gay rights pro_____ in mental he_____

Education_____ reducing stigma. This ca_____ debunking myths. This ca_____ of media including the Internet, pub_____ flyers, movies, and educational forums. A sig_____ was undertaken in the United Kingdom to address s_____ which relied heavily on educational strategies (Crisp et al., 2005). This campaign resulted in reductions in stigmatizing attitudes. However, one educational technique in this campaign, the use of fact sheets, did not result in people having kinder attitudes toward those with mental illness (Luty et al.,

Corrigan, P., & Gelb, B. (2006). Three programs that use mass approaches to change attitudes _____
393-398.
Corrigan, P.W., River, P., Lundin, R.K., et al. (2001). Three strategies for changing _____ ed attitudes of people with mental illness. _____
27, 187-195.
Crisp, A., Gelder, M., Goddard, E., & Meltzer, H. (2005) Stigmatisation of people with mental illness. World Psychiatry, 4(2), 106-113.
Minds campaign of the Royal College of Psychiatrists. Effectiveness of Changing Minds campaign factsheets in reducing stig_____
_____ Umoh, O., Sessay, M., & Sarkhel, A. (2007). Effectiveness of Changing _____ al illness. Psychiatric Bulletin, 31, 377-381.

APPLYING THE ART A Person with Schizophrenia

SCENARIO: I noticed Aar_____ standing barefooted in the hallway with both shoes in his outstretched hand. He almost looked like a statue with his blank, unaware demeanor. He deliberately picked up each foot then slowly rubbed the ball of one foot then the other against the carpet.

THERAPEUTIC GOAL: By the end of the present encounter, Aaron will demonstrate increased comfort with the student nurse as evidenced by voluntarily walking together in the hallways of the psychiatric unit.

Student-Patient Interaction

Student: "Aaron, I am _____, one of the nursing students. Aaron, I'm standing next to you, on your right side."
Student's feelings: I'm kind of nervous. How scary and lonely his world _____

_____ "Don't know left, right, right, _____ first one, last one. Can't last _____ oul. Soul train."
_____ nder why he rubs each foot against _____ really needs to feel where the floor is.

Student's feelings: That part, "long lost soul" makes me feel sad. I felt lost when I first arrived here at school without a single friend. When I let myself know what I'm feeling, memories of the losses in my childhood begin to stir.

Student: "Long lost soul. You're feeling kind of lost right now. It's hard to decide what to do next."

Student: "Aaron, it's _____. Come with me and we'll figure out how to help you. I touch his arm to direct him toward the day area.

Aaron: Abruptly tilts his head toward opposite wall. He begins mumbling like he's responding back to an unseen other.
Student's feelings: I'm so upset with myself. I acted without thinking about how threatening my touch would be without asking first. I so want to help him and now I've scared him. I want to say, "I'm sorry" but that's my need. I'll tell him later when he's able to process information. Okay, keep focused. He needs to feel safe more than anything.

Student: "Aaron, I'm here. I'll

Thoughts, Communication Techniques, and Mental Health Nursing Concepts

With schizophrenia it's important to say his name and say my own name to make clear our separateness.

He may have an ego boundary disturbance. He also holds his shoes far away from his body. W_____ ass_____ sho_____

I ne_____ coun_____ That_____ may remember the last words he spoke at some level. I'll then use reflection of feelings.

Maybe he wants to get away on his own "soul train." Is he an elopement risk? Probably not. He's too confused right now to plan anything, though he may follow easily. I'll give some structure to meet safety needs.

The touch violated his precarious ego boundary. He's hallucinating—my touch tipped him from moderate to severe anxiety. I need to speak in short sentences with lots of pause_____ slow this down.

Because many psychiatric nursing courses today are shorter than in the past, and at the same time the information applicable to psychiatric nursing is constantly expanding, many decisions were made on how to present the most important "need to know" information as this book was written. As it was being developed we worked hard to ensure that *Essentials of Psychiatric Mental Health Nursing: A Communication Approach to Evidence-Based Care* presents the essential content for a shorter course without sacrificing either the current research or the nursing and psychotherapeutic interventions necessary to sound practice.

This *Essentials* text provides a comprehensive but concise review of the prominent theorists and all therapeutic modalities in use today, including milieu, group, and family therapies, in Chapter 3, "Theories and Therapies." Within each of the clinical chapters (Chapters 8 through 22) and those that address discrete patient populations across the life span (Chapters 23 through 25), specific therapeutic modalities that have proven effective for each are thoroughly covered.

In addition to the overview of medication groups in Chapter 4, "Biological Basis for Understanding Psychopharmacology," specific medications are covered in full for each of the discrete clinical disorders, including patient and family teaching guidelines. Integrative therapies are also included in each of the clinical chapters where they have proven effective.

In order to present the most essential base of knowledge for a shorter course, the pertinent information on some topics has been incorporated into the clinical chapters where they apply, rather than included in a separate chapter. For example, rather than include a general chapter on culture, each of the clinical chapters incorporates relevant information on cultural aspects of the various clinical disorders, which can also help give the reader a broader cultural perspective.

Forensic issues related to the nursing care of patients is included in specific chapters, especially "Child, Partner, and Elder Abuse" (Chapter 18), and "Sexual Assault" (Chapter 19). This is in addition to Chapter 26, "Legal and Ethical Basis for Practice."

THE SCIENCE AND ART OF PSYCHIATRIC MENTAL HEALTH NURSING

The American Nurses Association's *Psychiatric Mental Health Nursing: Scope and Standards of Practice* begins with the following statement that stresses the importance of both the art and the science employed by nurses caring for patients with mental health problems and psychiatric disorders:

> Psychiatric–mental health nursing, a core mental health profession, employs a purposeful use of self as its art and a wide range of nursing, psychosocial, and neurobiological theories and research evidence as its science.[1]

In *Essentials of Psychiatric Mental Health Nursing: A Communication Approach to Evidence-Based Care*, we integrate and balance these two aspects of nursing care and present all of the essential information on each so that students will be prepared to offer the best possible care when they enter practice.

The Science

Over the past couple decades we have seen remarkable scientific progress in our understanding of the workings of the brain and how abnormalities in the function of the brain are related to mental illness. As confidence in this research grew, the focus on scientific research expanded and led to more scientifically based treatment approaches, and the concept of *evidence-based practice* became a dominant focus of mental health treatment.

While writing this text we made a great effort to provide the most current evidence-based information in the field while at the same time keep the material comprehensible and reader friendly. Relevant information drawn from science is woven throughout the book.

Chapter 1, "Practicing the Science and Art of Psychiatric Nursing," introduces the student to the evolution of evidence-based practice (EBP) and the mechanics of the practice and gives the reader guidelines for where and how to gather information for applying EBP in psychiatric nursing practice.

Perhaps one of the two most unique features of this book is the **Examining the Evidence** feature, which is introduced in Chapter 1 and runs throughout the clinical chapters. Each box poses a question, walks the readers through the process of gathering evidence-based data from a variety of sources, and presents the evidence from different points of view.

[1]American Nurses Association (ANA). (2007). *Psychiatric–mental health nursing: Scope and standards of practice, p. 1.* Silver Spring, MD: ANA.

The Art

In comparison with the medical model, the *recovery model* is a more social, relationship-based model of care. The recovery model began in the addiction field, in which the goal was for individuals to recover from substance abuse and addictions. Today the recovery model is gaining momentum in the larger mental health community. Its focus is on empowering patients by supporting hope, strengthening social ties, developing more effective coping skills, fostering the use of spiritual strength, and more.

By definition, nurses are primed to incorporate the bio-psycho-social and cultural/spiritual approaches to care. Some nursing leaders express concern that the "art" of nursing is becoming marginalized by the emphasis on evidence-based practice. Chapter 1 covers some of these often minimized and uncharted interventions such as the art of caring, the skill of attending, and patient advocacy. However, what also might be minimized and deemphasized are the tools that make nurses unique. Some of these tools include effective communication skills, therapeutic relationships, and how to interview and assess our patients' needs. These areas are stressed in Chapter 6, "Communication Skills: Medium for all Nursing Practice" and Chapter 7, "Therapeutic Relationships and the Clinical Interview." There is also a section in each of the clinical chapters on useful communications techniques for a specific disorder or situation.

The second of the unique features that are also included in the clinical chapters are the **Applying the Art** tables, which depict a clinical scenario demonstrating student-patient interactions (both therapeutic and not therapeutic), the student's perception of the interaction, and the identification of the mental health nursing concepts in play.

ORGANIZATION

Organized into six units, the chapters in the book have been grouped to emphasize the clinical perspective and to facilitate locating information. All clinical chapters are organized in a clear, logical, and consistent format with nursing process as the strong, visible framework. The basic outline for clinical chapters is:

- Prevalence and Comorbidity
  Knowing the comorbid disorders that are often part of the clinical picture of specific disorders helps students as well as clinicians understand how to better assess and treat their patients.
- Theory
- Cultural Considerations
- Clinical Picture
  Includes DSM-IV-TR criteria as appropriate.

- *Application of the Nursing Process*
- Assessment
  Presents appropriate assessment for a specific disorder, including assessment tools and rating scales. The rating scales included help highlight important areas in the assessment of a variety of behaviors or mental conditions. Because many of the answers are subjective, experienced clinicians use these tools as a guide when planning care, in addition to their knowledge of their patients.
- Diagnosis
  Includes the latest NANDA-I terminology.
- Outcomes Identification
- Planning
- Implementation
  Interventions follow the categories set by the ANA Psychiatric–Mental Health Nursing: Scope and Standards of Practice (2007). Various interventions for each of the clinical disorders are chosen based on which of them most fit specific patient needs, including communication guidelines, health teaching and health promotion, milieu therapy, psychotherapy, and pharmacological, biological, and integrative therapies.
- Evaluation

FEATURES

In addition to the **Examining the Evidence** boxes and **Applying the Art** tables described above, the following features are included in the book to inform, heighten understanding, and engage the reader:

- Chapters open with **Objectives** and **Key Terms and Concepts** to orient the reader.
- Numerous **Vignettes** describing psychiatric patients and their disorders grab and hold the readers' interest.
- **Assessment Guidelines** are included in clinical chapters to familiarize readers with methods of assessing patients; also for use in the clinical setting.
- **Potential Nursing Diagnoses** tables give several possible nursing diagnoses for a particular disorder along with the associated signs symptoms.
- *DSM-IV-TR* diagnostic criteria for all major disorders are summarized and simplified in figure format.
- **Nursing Interventions** tables list interventions for a given disorder or clinical situation, along with rationales for each intervention.
- **Key Points to Remember** present the main concepts of each chapter in an easy to comprehend and concise bulleted list.
- **Critical Thinking** questions at the end of all chapters introduce clinical situations in psychiatric nursing and encourage critical thinking processes essential for nursing practice.

- **Chapter Review** questions at the end of each chapter reinforce key concepts. Answers are listed in Appendix C of the book.
- **Glossary** helps readers with unfamiliar terminology.
- Appendices provide the *DSM-IV-TR* **classification** and a list of the latest **NANDA-I diagnoses**.

LEARNING AND TEACHING AIDS

For Students

The Evolve Student Resources for this book include the following:
- *Chapter Outlines* for help with note taking
- *Chapter Review Answers*, including rationales and page references
- *Case Studies* and *Nursing Care Plans* for clinical disorders
- *Nurse, Patient, and Family Resources*, which include web addresses, association information, and additional resources for patient teaching material, medication information, and support groups
- *Concept Map Creator*

The Companion CD features:
- *Audio Glossary* of 150 terms with pronunciations and definitions
- *Interactive Exercises* for independent review, with games such as quiz show and memory match
- *Neurology Review*, with state-of-the-art narrated animations, for a quick review of neurology for a basis of knowledge for psychiatric nursing practice
- *Review Questions* (150) to assist in preparing for the NCLEX® examination

For Instructors

The Evolve Instructor Resources include:
- *Evolve Learning System* is a comprehensive suite of online course communication and organization tools that allows instructors to upload the class calendar and syllabus, post test scores and announcements, and more.
- *Instructor's Manual* featuring a teaching focus, learning objectives, key terms, teaching strategies, and learning activities for each chapter of the text.
- *Test Bank* in Word and ExamView formats, featuring approximately 800 test items, complete with correct answer, rationale, cognitive level, nursing process step, appropriate NCLEX label, and corresponding textbook page references. The ExamView program allows instructors to create new tests; edit, add, and delete test questions; sort questions by NCLEX category, cognitive level, and nursing process step; and administer and grade tests online.
- *PowerPoint Presentations* with more than 600 customizable lecture slides.
- *Audience Response Questions* for i > clicker and other systems with 2 to 5 multiple-answer questions per chapter to stimulate class discussion and assess student understanding of key concepts.
- Access to all Evolve Student Resources (see above).

We are very proud of this new textbook and we hope you, the reader, find that *Essentials of Psychiatric Mental Health Nursing: A Communication Approach to Evidence-Based Care* provides you with the information you need to be successful. We are certain you will find this book interesting and enjoyable to read as well. Good luck to you all.

Betsy Merrill Varcarolis
Peggy Jordan Halter

CONTENTS

Essential Theoretical Concepts for Practice

CHAPTER 1

Practicing the Science and Art of Psychiatric Nursing

Elizabeth M. Varcarolis

Key Terms and Concepts

5 A's, p. 4
attending, p. 8
caring, p. 6
clinical algorithms, p. 5
clinical/critical pathways, p. 5

clinical practice guidelines, p. 5
evidence-based practice (EBP), p. 3
patient advocate, p. 8
psychiatric–mental health nursing, p. 3
recovery model, p. 3

Objectives

1. Contrast and compare the focus and approach of the mental health recovery model to the evidence-based practice (EBP) model.
2. Identify the "5 A's" in the simple multistep process of evidence-based practice and describe what is inherent in each step of this process.
3. Discuss at least three current dilemmas nurses face when they seek the best evidence for their interventions.

4. Identify four resources that nurses can use as guidelines for best evidence interventions.
5. Defend why the concept of "caring" should be a basic ingredient to the practice of nursing and how it is expressed by nurses in the clinical setting.
6. Discuss what is meant by being a patient advocate.

evolve

For additional resources related to the content of this chapter, visit the Evolve website at
http://evolve.elsevier.com/Varcarolis/essentials.

- Chapter Outline
- Chapter Review Answers

- Nurse, Patient, and Family Resources
- Concept Map Creator

Psychiatric nursing is a specialized area of nursing practice. Its focus is the treatment of human responses to mental health problems and psychiatric disorders. "**Psychiatric–mental health nursing**, a core mental health profession, employs a purposeful use of self as its art and a wide range of nursing, psychosocial, and neurobiological theories and research evidence as its science" (ANA, 2007, p. 1).

Starting around the 1990s (the "Decade of the Brain") more funding for brain research became available and remarkable progress was made in our understanding of how to treat illnesses caused by brain dysfunction. The method for using treatment approaches to medical and mental health illness that are scientifically grounded or evidence based became known as **evidence-based practice (EBP)**. In psychiatry, the evidence-based focus extends to treatment approaches in which there is scientific evidence for psychological and sociological treatment approaches, as well as for evidence related to the neurobiology of psychiatric disorders and psychopharmacology.

The mental health **recovery model**, on the other hand, is seen more in terms of a social model of disability than a medical model of disability (Repper & Perkins, 2003). The concept of recovery refers primarily to managing symptoms, reducing psychosocial disability, and improving role performance (Pratt et al., 2006). Recovering from a mental illness is viewed as a personal journey of healing. The goal of recovery is to empower those with mental illness to find meaning and satisfaction in their lives, realize personal potential, and function at their optimum level of independence. It has been found that supportive relationships, social inclusion, acquiring needed coping skills, recovery-oriented services, and sense of hope for the future can lead to a sustainable belief in oneself; a sense of empowerment and self-determination, meaning and satisfaction; and to the highest quality of life within the limitations of the illness. The principles of the recovery model have been adopted by a number of countries and states.

Forchuk (2001), Benner (2004), and other psychiatric nursing leaders stress the importance of psychiatric nursing taking a leadership role in creating patient-centered care that demonstrates how to establish a relationship within a recovery-based model and at the same time understand and incorporate the evidence related to the neurobiology of psychiatric disorders and psychotropic medications.

THE SCIENCE OF NURSING: FINDING THE EVIDENCE FOR THE PRACTICE

Basing nursing and medical practice on a systematic approach to care is not new. In the past century, nursing began with a strong emphasis on practice. McDonald (2001) states that Florence Nightingale (1820-1910), the founder of modern nursing, had a philosophy reflecting an evidence-based framework. Nightingale advocated for the "best possible research, access the best available governmental statistics and expertise . . ." (p. 2). During the 1860 International Statistical Congress held in London, Nightingale made a proposal that was to result in "the first model for systemic collection of hospital data using a uniform classification of diseases and operations and was to form the basis of the *International Statistical Classification of Diseases and Related Health Problems* (ICD) used today world-wide" (Keith, 1988). Mental health professionals in the United States substitute for the mental health section of the ICD the *Diagnostic and Statistical Manual of Mental Disorders (DSM). The DSM* is discussed in more detail in Chapter 2.

Hildegard Peplau (1909-1999), considered the mother of psychiatric nursing, had a passion for clarifying and developing the art and science of professional nursing practice and believed that a scientific approach was essential to the practice of psychiatric nursing (Haber, 2000). Her contributions went far beyond what she brought to the field of psychiatric nursing. She introduced the concept of advanced nursing practice and promoted professional standards and regulation through credentialing among a multitude of other contributions to nursing (Tomey, 2006).

It should be noted that psychiatry was one of the first medical specialties to extensively use randomized controlled trials. One of the founding principles of clinical psychology in the 1950s was that practice should be based on the results of experimental comparisons of treatment methods (Geddes et al., 2004). However, without scientific evidence for practice, much of nursing care has been based on tradition, personal experience, unsystematic trial and error, and the experience of nurses and others who have gone before (Wilson, 2004; Zauszniewski & Suresky, 2003).

The emergence of evidence-based nursing practice in the United States originated from the evidence-based practice movement in the medical community in England and Canada during the 1980s and 1990s (Mick, 2005). During that time there was an increase in research-related journals, the most relevant of which for nurses is the development of the *Evidence-Based Nursing* journal in 1998, which can be accessed online at http://ebn.bmj.com.

The University of Minnesota defines EBP as "the process by which the best available research evidence (from well-designed studies), clinical expertise, and patient preferences are used for making clinical decisions." Melnyk (2004) states there is no magic bullet that provides a formula as to the weight of evidence that patient values and preferences and clinical expertise should take in making clinical decisions. Mantzoukas (2007) warns that although EBP is

TABLE 1-1	Hierarchy of Evidence and Grading of Recommendations

Each recommendation has been allocated a grading that directly reflects the hierarchy of evidence on which it has been based. Please note that the hierarchy of evidence and the recommendation gradings relate to the strength of the literature, not to clinical importance.

Hierarchy of Evidence		**Grading of Recommendations**	
Level	*Type of Evidence*	*Level*	*Type of Evidence*
Ia	Evidence from systematic reviews or meta-analysis of randomized controlled trials	A	Based on hierarchy I evidence
Ib	Evidence from at least one randomized controlled trial		
IIa	Evidence from at least one controlled study without randomization	B	Based on hierarchy II evidence or extrapolated from hierarchy I evidence
IIb	Evidence from at least one other type of quasi-experimental study		
III	Evidence from nonexperimental descriptive studies, such as comparative studies, correlation studies, and case control studies	C	Based on hierarchy III evidence or extrapolated from hierarchy I or II evidence
IV	Evidence from expert committee reports or opinions and/or clinical experience of respected authorities	D	Directly based on hierarchy IV evidence or extrapolated from hierarchy I, II, or III evidence

From Hierarchy of evidence and grading of recommendations. (2004). *Thorax*, *59*(3), 181-272.

equated with effective decision making, avoidance of habitual practice, and enhanced clinical performance, there is a tendency to overlook certain types of knowledge that through reflection can provide useful information for individualized and effective practice.

Numerous definitions delineate the multistep process of integrating EBP into clinical practice. One that is simply put and apt is used at the Children's Mercy Hospital in Kansas City, Missouri (Mick, 2005), referred to as the **5 A's**:

1. *Ask* a question. Identify a problem or need for change for specific patient or situation.
2. *Acquire* literature. Search the literature for scientific studies and articles that address the issue(s) of concern.
3. *Appraise* the literature. Evaluate and synthesize the research evidence as to its validity, relevance, and applicability using criteria of scientific merit.
4. *Apply* the evidence. Choose interventions that are based on the best available evidence with the understanding of the patient's preference and needs.
5. *Assess* the performance. Evaluate the outcomes, using clearly defined criteria, and reports, and document results.

Evaluating the evidence is done through a hierarchical rating system. The strongest evidence on which to base clinical practice is randomized control studies and evidence-based clinical practice guidelines. In a randomized control trial (RCT) patients are chosen at random (by chance) to receive one of several clinical interventions. One intervention would be the one under study, and another might be

the standard intervention or a placebo. The weakest level is from expert committee reports, opinions, clinical experience, or descriptive studies. Table 1-1 presents a hierarchy of evidence and grading for each level.

The first Surgeon General's report published on the topic of mental health was in 1999 (USDHHS, 1999). This landmark document was based on an extensive review of the scientific literature and in consultation with mental health providers and consumers (Zauszniewski & Suresky, 2003). The document concluded that there are numerous effective psychopharmacological and psychosocial treatments for most mental disorders. However, it raised some questions for psychiatric nurses, including (Stuart, 2001):

- Are psychiatric nurses aware of the efficacy of the treatment and interventions they provide?
- Are they truly practicing evidence-based care?
- Is there documentation of the nature and outcomes of the care they provide?

There is no question that emphasis on evidence-based practice in medicine and mental health is expanding. Interventions based on the best research evidence combined with clinical expertise seem an ideal approach. However, this approach will not provide easy answers, and much discussion and questions are raised regarding the practice of evidence-based mental health nursing. For one, who interprets "best evidence"?

Second, not all nursing problems are able to be reduced to a clear issue solvable by scientific experiments (White, 1997). White continues to stress that many problems are addressed by using "artistry" to find solutions.

Third, relatively few studies backed by rigorous quantitative research are available from which to select nursing interventions and to guide psychiatric nursing care practices. Out of 227 databased studies published between 2000 and 2003, only 52 (23%) included nurses, student nurses, or other mental health care professionals. Of these 52 studies, only 11 (21%) involved examining psychiatric nursing interventions. Promoting EBP in psychiatric nursing will require increasing the number of studies by researchers who possess clinical knowledge and research expertise (Zauszniewski & Suresky, 2003).

And fourth, a question: How do nurses who are practicing in an environment of reduced staffing, increased complexity, and stress on issues of cost effectiveness find time to research the literature, evaluate numerous studies, if indeed they are available, and make decisions on "best evidence"? This question still needs a definitive answer; however, some of the following provide valuable guidelines for practice at present:

1. *Internet mental health resources.* A number of sites provide mental health resources online for information, treatment provisions, and the results of recent clinical studies. There are self-tests for people to see if they may be experiencing, at least in part, a specific syndrome or disorder (e.g., depression, elation, attention deficit hyperactivity disorder [ADHD]). There are also resources for acquiring support and treatment. Box 1-1 provides a short list of popular mental health sites. It is best to focus on sites that are maintained by professional societies, professional librarians, or other organizations whose quality is

evidence based in order to cut down on uncensored information of low quality.

2. *Clinical practice guidelines.* **Clinical practice guidelines** are systematically developed statements that identify, appraise, and summarize the best evidence about prevention, diagnosis, prognosis, therapy, and other knowledge necessary to make informed decisions about specific health problems. They are based on literature review (scientific research in the form of randomized, controlled clinical trials; reports of series, or case studies; or "expert clinical experience" [AAPMR, 2006]). The development and use of practice guidelines can increase quality and consistency of care and facilitate outcome research. Essentially, they (1) identify practice questions and explicitly identify all the decision options and outcomes; (2) identify the "best evidence" about prevention, diagnosis, prognosis, therapy, harm, and cost-effectiveness; and (3) identify the decision points at which this "best evidence" needs to be integrated with individual clinical experience and patients' needs and goals in deciding on a course of action. The American Psychiatric Association's (APA) Clinical Practice Guidelines and the National Quality Measures Clearinghouse offer such guidelines. The U.S. Department of Health and Human Services sponsors a National Guidelines Clearinghouse of evidence-based guidelines pertaining to a wide range of medical and mental health conditions (www.guidelines.gov).

3. *Clinical algorithms.* **Clinical algorithms** are step-by-step guidelines prepared in a flowchart format. Alternative diagnostic and treatment approaches are described based on decisional points using a large database relevant for the symptoms, diagnosis or treatment modalities. Algorithms are especially helpful in deciding what medication to use considering a wide variety of variables related to the patient's personal situation (e.g., age, sex, current medications, ethnic origin, allergies). Figure 1-1 depicts a clinical algorithm for the suspicion of suicide risk.

4. *Clinical/critical pathways.* **Clinical/critical pathways** are usually specific to the institution using them. They are most often used in relation to hospitalized patients targeting a specific population (e.g., suicidal patient, bipolar patient—manic, a depressed patient, an individual with schizophrenia, and so forth). These clinical pathways serve as a "map" for specified treatments and interventions to occur within a specific time frame, often days. For example, the clinical guide may state for the day of admission certain goals are to be reached and specific interventions are to be

BOX 1-1

Mental Health Web Resources

- American Association of Pastoral Counselors: www.aapc.org
- American Psychiatric Association: www.psych.org
- American Psychological Association: www.apa.org
- American Psychiatric Nurses Association: www.apna.org
- Brain Technologies: www.braintechnologies.com
- Centre for Addiction and Mental Health: www.camh.net
- National Institute of Mental Health: www.nimh.nih.gov
- National Institute of Nursing Research: www.ninr.nih.gov
- U.S. Department of Health and Human Services: National Guideline Clearinghouse: www.guidelines.gov

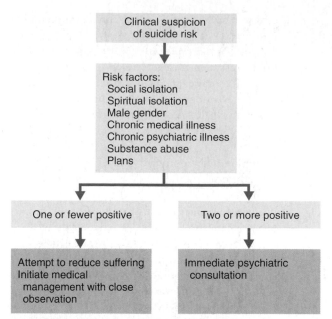

Figure 1-1 ■ Clinical algorithm for the suspicion of suicide risk. (Modified from Goldman, L., & Ausiello, D. [2008]. *Cecil medicine* [23rd ed.]. Philadelphia: Saunders.)

carried out by different members of the health team (e.g., physicians, nurses, social workers, dietitians). The interventions include preadmission workup, tests, diet, health teaching, medication, and observation of effectiveness or adverse effects, through discharge plans and follow-up care. Each pathway spells out the expected outcomes using a measurable, time-limited format, and documentation is ongoing. Some institutions computerize these clinical pathways within the patient's chart. Clinical/critical pathways and maps offer a great opportunity for the integration of research into clinical practice when the interventions are evidence based.

The Research-Practice Gap

Unfortunately, there is a wide gap between the best evidence treatments and their effective delivery into practice. The need for continued research on how best to apply the findings of clinically relevant issues and their delivery into clinical practice have been the emphasis of the Institute of Medicine (IOM) (2006): ". . . research that has identified the efficacy of specific treatments under rigorously controlled conditions has been accompanied by almost no research identifying how to make these same treatments effective when delivered in usual settings of care . . . when administered by service providers without specialized education in the therapy" (p. 350).

Research needs to be reported in language that is understandable and free of statistical and research jargon (Zauszniewski & Suresky, 2003), and appropriate dissemination of findings needs to reach nursing practitioners. However, there is no mistaking, despite the complexities and concerns that need to be addressed, evidence-based nursing practice is here to stay.

To help the reader understand how best evidence is identified and applied to nursing interventions, this text contains a feature titled "Examining the Evidence." It is hoped that this feature, presented in each of the clinical chapters, will underscore the importance of sound scientific inquiry and ignite the reader's interest in research.

THE ART OF NURSING: DEVELOPING THE SKILLS FOR THE PRACTICE

Contemporary nursing relies on a high level of scientific thought in its theories, research, and knowledge base. However, there is an "art" to nursing as well. Even the best evidence-based guidelines may not be sufficient for the patient who stands in front of you with a very individualized set of problems and capacities. Such individuality is complex, demanding that nurses use intuition, interpersonal skills, and the therapeutic use of self. These "arts" complement nursing's scientific base and are indispensable for treating any patient effectively. As Williams and Garner (2002, p. 8) conclude, "Too great an emphasis on evidence-based medicine oversimplifies the complex and interpersonal nature of clinical care."

What components are integral to nursing as an art as well as a science? Benner (2004) suggests that many of the attributes of nursing that fall under the "art of nursing" are invisible, intangible, rarely charted, and almost never suggested in a nursing care plan. Consequently these attributes are often marginalized, undervalued, and demeaned. Three areas inherent in the "art" of nursing that addressed here are (1) caring, (2) attending, and (3) patient advocacy.

Caring

Kari Martinsen (b.1943) a psychiatric nurse and philosopher from Norway, believed that "caring involves how we relate to each other, how we show concern for each other in our daily life. **Caring** is the most natural and the most fundamental aspect of human existence" (Alvsvåg, 2006, p. 173). A survey by Schoenhofer and colleagues (1998) used a group process method (13 groups of three to five people each) to synthesize what was meant by caring to the par-

EXAMINING THE EVIDENCE   The Importance of Evidence-Based Research in Practice

Nursing Mental Diseases is a textbook written by a registered nurse, Harriet Bailey, in 1934. It is fascinating, informative, and well written yet clearly dated. Let's try to answer a hypothetical question based on information presented in this textbook of common nursing measures used during this period.

Nursing measures to improve a patient's mood include all of the following *except:*

1. Hosing them down alternately with hot and cold water
2. Providing a diet that consists exclusively of milk for several days
3. Encouraging social support and family involvement
4. Putting the patient to bed for 4 to 10 weeks

Incorrect answers: 1. Hydrotherapy was commonly used as a "nerve stimulant" to improve mood. 2. A milk diet was followed by a sudden introduction of a full diet (no rationale given; your guess is as good as mine). 4. Bed rest was seen as a treatment for mental illness.

Correct answer: 3. The patient was removed from family and friends who may have sympathized or criticized too much; after 4 to 10 weeks patients were permitted to receive a letter from home on a test basis.

Psychiatric nurses today do not hose down patients, provide milk diets, or enforce prolonged bed rest. They do encourage patients to interact with others and promote family involvement when possible. Although sophistication in psychiatric nursing interventions has improved drastically in the past century, it is certain that some currently accepted treatments and nursing interventions will one day be abandoned and replaced with ones that are more effective.

Formal decisions to adopt practice protocols or guidelines (innovation) or abandon old ones (exnovation) are not typically based on a single study, but are made after a comprehensive review of information. Evidence-based practice includes not only evaluating research but also integrating it with input from experts and patients (Polit & Beck, 2006).

While the vast majority of nurses—professionals charged with decisions about lives and even life and death issues—do not conduct extensive literature reviews, it is essential to consider your education a continual endeavor. Reading professional journals and keeping abreast of current research play an essential role in this education.

In each of this text's clinical chapters, an interesting question (which is how *any* research project initially starts: with a question) about mental health, psychiatric disorders, and treatment that you might actually ask yourself is presented. Literature and expert opinions are provided that explore possible responses and opposing positions to the question. You are encouraged to read these boxes and evaluate the evidence. What is your opinion? What other information would you need to draw a conclusion? How can researchers best approach this question?

We hope that these boxes will not only make you think but also increase your appreciation for research and explain why it is necessary.

Bailey, H. (1934). *Mental health nursing* (2nd ed.). New York: Macmillan.
Polit, D.F., & Beck, C.T. (2006). *Essentials of nursing research: Method, appraisal, and utilization* (6th ed.). Philadelphia: Lippincott.

ticipants. The following three themes emerged from the shared narratives:

1. Caring is evidenced by empathic understanding, actions, and patience on another's behalf.
2. Caring for one another by actions, words, and being there leads to happiness and touches the heart.
3. Caring is giving of self while preserving the importance of self.

The caring nurse is first and foremost a competent nurse (Cooper & Powell, 1998). Indeed, Locsin (1995) expanded the concept of caring in the theory of technological competence as caring in critical care nursing. Without knowledge and competence, the demonstration of compassion and caring alone is powerless to help those under our care. Without a base of knowledge and skills, care alone cannot eliminate another person's confusion, grief, or pain, but a response of care can transform fear, pain, and suffering into a tolerable, shared experience (Cooper, 2001).

However, a nurse may be at a level of competence but unable to demonstrate caring. The absence of caring can leave memorable scars and make patients feel distrustful, disconnected, uneasy, and discouraged (Halldorsdottir & Hamrin, 1997). Using communications that are destructive or devalue a patient's worth can have lasting negative effects. Examples of uncaring behaviors include denying patients' feelings, responding with indifference to patients' concerns, and failing to check to see if medications given to relieve discomfort or distress are working. These are examples of behaviors that violate a patient's integrity and dignity and are never justified (Cooper, 2001).

Comforting can also be assumed under the mantle of caring. Benner (2004) states that comforting includes providing social, emotional, physical, and spiritual support for a patient that is consistent with the holistic approach to nursing care. The provision of comfort measures can even be lifesaving in fragile patients, and is a basic component to good care.

Unfortunately there are many impediments to practicing "caring" in our present health care system that are driven by economic considerations (Cooper, 2001). We continue to be in a period of nursing shortage, which puts a greater burden on nurses while working with greater workloads and sicker patients. However, as Cooper aptly points out, caring is both an attitude that one communicates, a way of being with a patient, as well as a set of skills that can be learned and developed. Both require nurturing and practice. Cooper goes on to say that while it does take time to listen to patients, "in time you will be able to do the tasks of nursing while attending to the patient, and get to know the patient as you are doing an assessment or intervention" (p. 95).

Attending

Attending refers to an *intensity of presence,* being there for and in tune with the patient. The experience of emotional or physical suffering can be isolating. When patients perceive that the nurse is there for them, a human connection is made and the patient's sense of isolation is minimized or eliminated (Cooper, 2001). Being present requires entering the patient's experience. Attending behaviors may include listening, touching, or giving attentive physical care (Cooper, 2001). It is through active listening skills and the use of effective communication skills that we can fully understand another person's immediate experience and distressing fears, perceptions, and concerns. Attending behaviors are learned and are inherent in a true therapeutic relationship. Chapter 7 discusses attending behaviors more fully within the context of the nurse-patient relationship.

Patient Advocacy

An advocate is essentially one who speaks up for another's cause, who helps another by defending and comforting him or her, especially when the other lacks the knowledge, skills, ability, or standing to speak up for themselves. Lawyers are often viewed as advocates for their clients; however, in nursing, being a **patient advocate** is not a legal role but rather an ethical one. Ethics is an integral part of the foundation of nursing. You, no doubt, have had a class that includes the ethical code for nurses. However, the role of patient advocate bears mentioning here. The term *patient advocate* was first placed in the 1976 ANA Code of Ethics revision, and remains essentially unchanged up to the present. It reads:

> The nurse must be alert to and take appropriate action regarding any instances of incompetent, unethical, illegal, or impaired practices(s) by any member of the health team or the health care system itself, or any action on the part of others that places the rights or best interest of the patient in jeopardy. (ANA Code of Ethics, 2001, 3.5)

And, yes, sometimes it takes a great deal of courage to advocate for our patients when we witness behaviors or actions of other health care professionals that could have serious consequences for the patient.

Advocacy in nursing includes a commitment to patients' health, well-being, and safety across the life span, and the alleviation of suffering and promoting a peaceful, comfortable, and dignified death (ANA, 2001). Nurses advocate for patients when they advise patients of their rights, provide accurate and current information so patients can make informed decisions, and support those decisions (Mallik, 1997). Advocating for the patient demonstrates respect for human life (the patient's as well as our own) and validates the belief in the value of human life, whether it is to save a life or to bring comfort to those who are dying. Psychiatric mental health nurses function as advocates when they engage in public speaking, write articles for the popular press, and lobby congressional representatives to help improve and expand mental health care for everyone (APA, 2007).

Throughout the text a special feature titled *Applying the Art* gives the reader a glimpse of a nurse-patient interaction and the nurse's thought processes while attending to the patient's immediate concern.

KEY POINTS TO REMEMBER

- Evidence-based practice (EBP) is a process by which the best available research evidence, clinical expertise, and patient preferences are used for making clinical decisions.
- The "5 A's" process to delineate the multistep process of integrating best evidence into clinical practice includes (1) asking, (2) acquiring, (3) appraising, (4) applying, and (5) assessing.
- The mental health recovery model is one of helping people with psychiatric disabilities effectively manage their symp-

toms, reduce psychosocial disability, and find a meaningful life in a community of their choosing.
- Some sources for obtaining research findings are (1) Internet mental health resources, (2) clinical practice guidelines, (3) clinical algorithms, and (4) clinical/critical pathways.
- A sound body of knowledge of effective psychiatric nursing interventions is available and in use today. However, a great deal more observations and study need to be done to ascer-

KEY POINTS TO REMEMBER—cont'd

tain whether we are using best-evidence interventions in our clinical practice.
- Best evidence for appropriate medication and therapies for use in patients with specific mental health

conditions has been more readily studied and documented.
- Three specific areas are inherent within the art of nursing: (1) caring, (2) attending, and (3) patient advocacy.

CRITICAL THINKING

1. A friend of yours has recently come back from the war in Iraq. You are startled when you see him on the street in a disheveled state. He appears frightened, seems to be talking to himself, and jumps a mile when a car backfires nearby. You are astounded because he was always so smart, well liked, thought of as kind and personable, and had a good career ahead of him as a computer programmer. When you approach him he backs away in a protective manner.
   A. How would the contribution of evidence-based practice (EBP) be helpful to his recovery? Give examples.
   B. What might be some specific needs that could be met under the recovery model?
   C. Discuss how nurses can incorporate both EBP and the recovery model in their practice.
   D. Explain which model might be the most useful during the acute phase of his recovery, and which model might be more effective in the continuation period of his recovery.
2. A friend of yours says that he heard about a new practitioner in the area that is going to teach alcoholics how to safely drink in moderation. You are thinking of two of your friends who are now in recovery, one of whom nearly died from an alcoholic event. You state that from all you have read, and from your friends' experience, that "controlled drinking isn't thought to be an acceptable practice." Your friend says, sure

there is good evidence, "This professional has lots of stories and affidavits from people who are alcoholics whom he has treated with success to drink in a controlled manner." You tell him that that is not good evidence for such a claim.
   A. How would you, as a nurse, evaluate this claim? Explain the five steps you would take to find the strength of this claim.
   B. Using Table 1-1, what would you say about the quality of the evidence given above?
   C. If your friend were in recovery and thinking of trying this treatment, what would you say to him that would make a strong argument against such a decision?
3. You are a new nursing student and a friend of yours says, "What the devil is the 'art of nursing'? Isn't that from the middle ages?"
   A. Discuss three components that might be considered under the art of nursing.
   B. Give your friend an example of how nurses demonstrate "caring" in the clinical area.
   C. Explain why patients need to have nurses act as their advocate. Can you think of an example from your clinical experience?
4. Go to the Centre for Evidence-Based Mental Health at www.cebmh.com and check out at least one of the available clinical trials.

CHAPTER REVIEW

Choose the most appropriate answer(s).
1. Evidence-based practice (EBP) depends on a combination of which of the following sources of information and knowledge? Select all that apply.
   1. Clinical expertise
   2. Randomized controlled *trials*
   3. Theories of ethical decision making
   4. Patient preferences
2. A student nurse receives her final course evaluation for her clinical practicum in psychiatry, which took place at an urban mental health clinic. Her professor reported that she demonstrated competent and knowledgeable practice but gave her a grade of "C." The student is disbelieving and

confused. Which of the following is the most likely rationale of the professor?
   1. The student was reported to be anxious about patients' reactions during the first week.
   2. The student was reported to lack a compassionate attitude toward patients.
   3. The student was unable to delineate the differences between symptoms of bipolar disorder and manic depression.
   4. The student did not conduct a comprehensive review of psychiatric nursing literature during her semester.

CHAPTER REVIEW—cont'd

3. Which of the following defines "clinical practice guideline"?
   1. A step-by-step flowchart representing alternative diagnostic and treatment approaches
   2. A compilation of interventions that should occur within a specific timeframe
   3. A systematically developed summary of the best available evidence used to make informed decisions about specific health problems
   4. A list of expected outcomes using a measurable format

4. Which of the following provides the strongest evidence on which to base clinical nursing practice?
   1. A randomized, controlled study
   2. A nurse's clinical experience in a direct patient care setting
   3. A descriptive clinical study
   4. A report from a practice guidance committee

5. When an experienced psychiatric nurse listens carefully to a patient's detailed recounting of a traumatic emotional experience, the nurse is:
   1. acting as a patient advocate.
   2. using an attending behavior.
   3. interpreting "best evidence."
   4. using a systematic approach to care.

REFERENCES

Alvsvåg, H. (2006). Philosophy of caring. In A.M. Tomey & M.R. Alligood (Eds.), *Nursing theorists and their work.* St. Louis: Mosby.

American Academy of Physical Medicine and Rehabilitation (AAPMR). (2006). *Practice guidelines committee develops definitions of term.* Retrieved August 24, 2006, from www.aapmr.org/hpl/pracguide/terms.htm.

American Nurses Association. (2007). *Psychiatric–mental health nursing: Scope and standards of practice.* Silver Spring, MD: the Association.

American Nurses Association (ANA) Code of Ethics with Interpretive Statements. (2001). American Nurses Association.

Benner, P. (2004). Relational ethics of comfort, touch, and solace endangered arts? *American Journal of Critical Care, 13,* 346-349.

Cooper, C. (2001). *The art of nursing: A practical introduction.* Philadelphia: Saunders.

Cooper, C., & Powell, E. (1998). Technology and care in a bone marrow transplant unit: Creating and assuaging vulnerability. *Holistic Nursing Practice, 12,* 57-68.

Forchuk, C. (2001). Evidence-based psychiatric/mental health nursing. *Evidence-Based Mental Health, 4*(2), 39-40.

Geddes, J., Reynolds, S., Streiner, D., & Szatmari, P. (2004). *Evidence based practice in mental health.* Centre for Evidence-Based Medicine. www.cebm.utoronto.ca/syllabi/men/intro.htm.

Haber, J. (2000). Hildegard Peplau: The psychiatric nursing legacy of a legend. *Journal of the American Psychiatric Nurses Association 6*(2), 56-62.

Halldorsdottir, S., & Hamrin, E. (1997). Caring and uncaring encounters in nursing and health care from the cancer patient's perspective. *Cancer Nursing, 20,* 120-128.

Institute of Medicine (IOM). (2006). *Improving the quality of health care for mental and substance-use conditions.* Institute of Medicine of the National Academies. Washington, DC: National Academies Press.

Keith, J.M. (1988). Florence Nightingale: Statistician and consultant epidemiologist. *International Nursing Review, 35,* 147-150.

Locsin, R.C. (1995). Machine technologies and caring in nursing. *Image: Journal of Nursing Scholarship, 27*(3), 201-203.

Mallik, M. (1997). Advocacy in nursing: a review of the literature. *Journal of Advanced Nursing, 23,* 130-138.

Mantzoukas, S. (2007). A review of evidence-based practice, nursing research and reflection: leveling the hierarchy. *Journal of Clinical Nursing, 17*(2), 214-223.

McDonald, L. (2001). Florence Nightingale and the early origins of evidence-based nursing. *Evidence-Based Nursing, 4,* 68-69.

Melnyk, B.M. (2004). Integrating levels of evidence into clinical decision making. *Pediatric Nursing, 30*(4), 323-324.

Mick, K. (2005). *Evidence-based nursing practice: Putting the pieces together.* Retrieved July 18, 2006, from www.apon.org.

Pratt, C., Gill, K., Barrett, N., & Roberts, M. (2006). *Psychiatric rehabilitation* (2nd ed.). San Diego: Academic Press.

Repper, J., & Perkins, R. (2003). *Social inclusion and recovery: A model for mental health practice.* United Kingdom: Baillière Tindall.

Schoenhofer, S., Bingham, V., & Hutchins, G. (1998). Giving of oneself on another's behalf: the phenomenology of everyday caring. *International Journal of Human Caring, 2*(2), 32-29.

Stuart, G.W. (2001). Evidence-based psychiatric nursing practice: Rhetoric or reality. *Journal of the American Psychiatric Nurses Association, 7*(4), 103-114.

Tomey, A.M. (2006). Nursing theorists of historical significance. In A. M. Tomey & M.R. Alligood (Eds.), *Nursing theorists and their work* (6th ed.). St. Louis: Mosby.

U.S. Department of Health and Human Services (1999). *Mental health: A report from the surgeon general.* Rockville, MD: National Institute of Mental Health.

White, S.I. (1997). Evidence-based practice and nursing: the new panacea? *British Journal of Nursing, 6*(3), 175-178.

Williams, D.D.R., & Garner, J. (2002). The case against "the evidence": A different perspective on evidence-based medicine. *British Journal of Psychiatry, 180,* 8-12.

Wilson, H.S. (2004). Evidence-based practice in psychiatric-metal health nursing. In C.R. Kneisl, H.S. Wilson, & E. Trigoboff (Eds.), *Contemporary psychiatric-mental health nursing.* Upper Saddle River, NJ: Pearson Prentice-Hall.

Zauszniewski, J.A., & Sureksy, J. (2003). Evidence for psychiatric nursing practice: An analysis of three years of published research. *Online Journal of Issues in Nursing, 9*(1). Retrieved July 18, 2006, from http://nursingworld.org/ojin/hirsh/topic4/tpc4_1.htm.

CHAPTER 2

Mental Health and Mental Illness

Elizabeth M. Varcarolis and Julius Trubowitz

Key Terms and Concepts

biologically based mental illness, p. 16
culture-related syndromes, p. 20
Diagnostic and Statistical Manual of Mental Disorders (DSM-IV-TR), p. 12
epidemiology, p. 13
mental disorders, p. 12
mental health, p. 12

mental illness, p. 12
myths and misconceptions, p. 12
prevalence rate, p. 13
psychiatry's definition of normal mental health, p. 12
psychobiological disorder, p. 16
resiliency, p. 12

Objectives

1. Assess mental health using the seven signs of mental health identified in this chapter (Table 2-1 and Figure 2-1).
2. Summarize factors that can affect the mental health of an individual and the ways that these factors influence conducting a holistic nursing assessment.
3. Discuss some dynamic factors (including social climate, politics, myths, and biases) that contribute to making a clear-cut definition of mental health elusive.

4. Demonstrate how the *DSM-IV-TR* multiaxial system can influence a clinician to consider a broad range of information before making a *DSM-IV-TR* diagnosis.
5. Compare and contrast a *DSM-IV-TR* diagnosis with a nursing diagnosis.
6. Give examples of how consideration of norms and other cultural influences can affect making an accurate *DSM-IV-TR* diagnosis.

evolve

For additional resources related to the content of this chapter, visit the Evolve website at http://evolve.elsevier.com/Varcarolis/essentials.

- Chapter Outline
- Chapter Review Answers

- Nurse, Patient, and Family Resources
- Concept Map Creator

Mental health is defined as successful performance of mental functions, resulting in the ability to engage in productive activities, enjoy fulfilling relationships, and change or cope with adversity. Mental health provides people with the capacity for rational thinking, communication skills, learning, emotional growth, resilience, and self-esteem (USDHHS, 1999). **Mental illness** is considered a clinically significant behavioral or psychological syndrome experienced by a person and marked by distress, disability, or the risk of suffering disability or loss of freedom (APA, 2000). Basically, mental illness can be seen as the result of a chain of events that include flawed biological, psychological, social, and cultural processes (Favazza, 2004).

This chapter discusses concepts of mental health and mental illness. The reader will be introduced to the concept of **mental disorders** as medical diseases. You will come to understand how mental disorders are categorized using the *Diagnostic and Statistical Manual of Mental Disorders (DSM-IV-TR)* (APA, 2000). The *DSM* is a manual that classifies mental disorders. The *DSM-IV-TR* (fourth edition, text revision) focuses on research and clinical observation when constructing diagnostic categories for a discrete mental disorder. This chapter describes how nursing diagnoses can be used to ensure appropriate care. The need to assess a person's ethnic background and culture before a valid diagnosis can be made is emphasized.

CONCEPTS OF MENTAL HEALTH AND ILLNESS

Our understanding of mental illness is plagued by a host of **myths and misconceptions**. One myth is that to be mentally ill is to be different and odd. Another misconception is that to be mentally healthy, a person must be logical and rational. All of us dream "irrational" dreams at night, and "irrational" emotions are not only universal human experiences but also essential to a fulfilling life. There are people who show extremely abnormal behavior and are characterized as mentally ill who are far more like the rest of us than different from us. There is no obvious and consistent line between mental illness and mental health. In fact, all human behavior lies somewhere along a continuum of mental health and mental illness.

Psychiatry's definition of normal mental health changes over time and reflects changes in cultural norms, society's expectations and values, professional biases, individual differences, (Sadock & Sadock, 2007), and even the political climate of the time. For example, criticisms have come from various groups who believe that they were or are stereotyped in the psychiatric community. Their concerns include the way in which the psychiatric community places an emphasis on the group's psychopathology rather than on health attributes. The psychology of women and the issues surrounding homosexuality are two very important examples but are by no means the only ones. This topic is discussed in more detail in the section on the *DSM-IV-TR* axis system later in this chapter.

We are taught to evaluate our patients with mental health issues to identify their strengths and their areas of high functioning. You will find many attributes of mental health in some of your patients with mental health issues. It is these strengths that we build on and encourage. By the same token, those who are "normal" or "mentally healthy" may have several areas of dysfunction at different times in their lives. We are all different, have different backgrounds, and reflect different cultural influences even within the same subculture. We grow at different rates intellectually and emotionally, make different decisions at different times in our lives, choose or choose not to evaluate our behaviors and grow within ourselves, have deep-seated spiritual beliefs or not, and so on. Understandably, then, there can be no one definition of mental health that fits all. However, there are some traits that mentally healthy people share and that contribute to a better quality of life. Some of these traits are depicted in Figure 2-1.

A characteristic of mental health that is increasingly being promoted is the concept of resiliency. **Resiliency** is the ability to recover from or adjust easily to misfortune and change. Resiliency is closely associated with the process of adapting and helps people facing tragedy, loss, trauma, and severe stress (APA, 2004). Research has demonstrated that this ability to bounce back from painful experiences and difficult events is not an unusual quality, but is a trait possessed by many people, and can be developed in most everyone. Disasters, such as the attack on the World Trade towers in 2001 and the devastation of Hurricane Katrina, in which people pulled together to help one another and carried on despite horrendous loss, illustrate resilience. Being resilient does not mean that people are unaffected by stressors. It means that rather than falling victim to the negative emotions, resilient people recognize the feelings, readily deal with them, and learn from the experience.

Table 2-1 compares some important aspects of mental health with those of specific mental disorders. These aspects include degree of (1) happiness, (2) control over behavior, (3) appraisal of reality, (4) effectiveness in work, (5) healthy self-concept, (6) satisfying relationships, and (7) effective coping strategies.

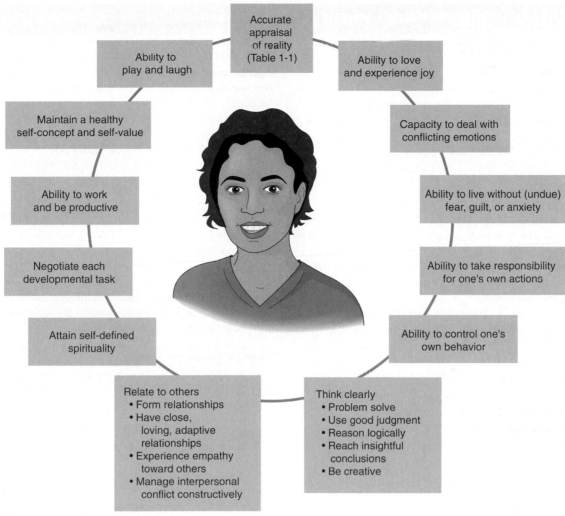

Figure 2-1 ■ Some attributes of mental health.

EPIDEMIOLOGY AND PREVALENCE OF MENTAL DISORDERS

Epidemiology is the quantitative study of the distribution of mental disorders in human populations. Once the distribution of mental disorders has been determined quantitatively, epidemiologists can identify high-risk groups and high-risk factors. Study of these high-risk factors may lead to important clues about the etiology of various mental disorders.

Clinical epidemiology is a broad field that addresses what happens to people with illnesses who are seen by providers of clinical care. Studies use traditional epidemiological methods and are conducted in groups that are usually defined by illness or symptoms, or by diagnostic procedures or treatments given for the illness or symptoms.

Results of epidemiological studies are now routinely included in the *DSM-IV-TR* to describe the frequency of mental disorders. Analysis of epidemiological studies can assess the frequency with which symptoms appear together. For example, epidemiological studies demonstrate the significance of depression as a risk factor for death in people with cardiovascular disease and for premature death in people with breast cancer.

The **prevalence rate** is the proportion of a population with a mental disorder at a given time. Kessler and colleagues (2005) published an updated study of the Lifetime Prevalence of Mental Disorders and concluded in their

TABLE 2-1	Mental Health Versus Mental Illness

Signs of Mental Health	Signs of Mental Illness
Happiness	**Major Depressive Episode**
Finds life enjoyable	Loses interest or pleasure in all or almost all usual activities and pastimes
Can see in objects, people, and activities the possibilities for meeting his or her needs	Describes mood as depressed, sad, hopeless, discouraged, "down in the dumps"
Control Over Behavior	**Control Disorder: Undersocialized, Aggressive**
Can recognize and act on cues to existing limits	Shows repetitive and persistent pattern of aggressive conduct in which the basic rights of others are violated
Can respond to the rules, routines, and customs of any group to which he or she belongs	
Appraisal of Reality	**Schizophrenic Disorder**
Accurate picture of what is happening around the individual	Shows bizarre delusions, such as delusions of being controlled
Good sense of the consequences, both good and bad, that will follow his or her acts	Has auditory hallucinations
Can see the difference between the "as if" and "for real" in situations	Manifests delusions with persecutory or jealous content
Effectiveness in Work	**Adjustment Disorder with Work (or Academic) Inhibition**
Within limits set by abilities, can do well in tasks attempted	Shows inhibition in work or academic functioning in which previously there was adequate performance
When meeting mild failure, persists until determines whether he or she can do the job	
A Healthy Self-Concept	**Dependent Personality Disorder**
Sees self as approaching individual ideals, as capable of meeting demands	Passively allows others to assume responsibility for major areas of life because of inability to function independently
Has reasonable degree of self-confidence that helps in being resourceful under stress	Lacks self-confidence (i.e., sees self as helpless, stupid)
Satisfying Relationships	**Borderline Personality Disorder**
Experiences satisfaction and stability in relationships	Shows pattern of unstable and intense interpersonal relationships
Socially integrated and can rely on social supports	Has chronic feelings of emptiness
Effective Coping Strategies	**Substance Dependencies**
Uses stress reduction strategies that address the problem, issue, threat (e.g., problem solving, cognitive restructuring)	Repeatedly self-administers substances despite significant substance-related problems (e.g., threat to job, family, social relationships)
Uses coping strategies in a healthy way that does not cause harm to self or others	

Modified from Redl, F., & Wattenberg, W. (1959). *Mental hygiene in teaching* (pp. 198-201). New York: Harcourt, Brace & World; American Psychiatric Association. (2000). *Diagnostic and statistical manual of mental disorders* (4th ed., text rev.). Washington, DC: Author; Farber, E.W., & Kaslow, F.W. (2003). Social psychology: Theory, research, and mental health implications. In A. Tasman, J. Kay, & J. A. Lieberman (Eds.), *Psychiatry* (2nd ed.). West Sussex, England: Wiley.

survey that about half of Americans will meet the criteria for a *DSM* disorder sometime in their life, with the first onset in childhood or adolescence. It is important to note that many individuals have more than one mental disorder at a time. For example, some people diagnosed with a depressive disorder may also have a coexisting anxiety disorder. Therefore some people have dual diagnoses.

Table 2-2 shows the prevalence rates and includes the epidemiology of some psychiatric disorders in the United States.

MENTAL ILLNESS AND POLICY ISSUES

Many factors can affect the severity and progress of a mental illness, biologically based or otherwise, and these same factors can affect a "normal" person's mental health as well. Some of these factors include available support systems, family influences, developmental events, cultural or subcultural beliefs and values, health practices, and negative influences impinging on an individual's life. If possible,

TABLE 2-2	Prevalence and Epidemiology of Psychiatric Disorders in the United States		
Disorder	Prevalence Over 12 Months (%)	Estimated Number of People Affected by Disorder in the United States	Epidemiology
Schizophrenia	1.1	2.2 million	Affects men and women equally; may appear earlier in men than in women
Any affective (mood) disorder; includes major depression, dysthymic disorder, and bipolar disorder	9.5	18.8 million	Women affected twice as much as men (12.4 million women; 6.4 million men); depressive disorders may appear earlier in life in those born in recent decades compared with past; often co-occurs with anxiety and substance abuse
Major depressive disorder	5	9.9 million	Leading cause of disability in United States and established economies worldwide; nearly twice as many women (6.5%) as men (3.3%) suffer from major depressive disorder every year
Bipolar affective disorder	1.2	2.3 million	Affects men and women equally
Anxiety disorders; includes panic disorder, obsessive-compulsive disorder, posttraumatic stress disorder (PTSD), generalized anxiety disorder, and phobias	13.3	19.1 million	Anxiety disorders frequently co-occur with depressive disorders, eating disorders, and/or substance abuse
Panic disorder	1.7	2.4 million	Typically develops in adolescence or early adulthood; about one in three people with panic disorder develops agoraphobia
Obsessive-compulsive disorder	2.3	3.3 million	First symptoms begin in childhood or adolescence
PTSD	3.6	5.2 million	Can develop at any time; approximately 30% of Vietnam veterans experienced PTSD after the war; percentage high among first responders to 9/11/01 terrorist attacks on the United States
Generalized anxiety disorder	2.8	4 million	Can begin across life cycle; risk is highest between childhood and middle age
Social phobia	3.7	5.3 million	Typically begins in childhood or adolescence
Agoraphobia	2.2	3.2 million	
Specific phobia	4.4	6.3 million	
Any substance abuse	11.3		
Alcohol dependence	7.2		

Data from National Institute of Mental Health. (2004). *The numbers count: Mental disorders in America* (NIH Publication No. 01-4584). Retrieved August 1, 2004, from www.nimh.nih.gov/publicat/numbers.cfm.

these influences need to be evaluated and factored into an individual's plan of care. Figure 2-2 identifies some influences that can have an effect on a person's mental health.

In 1996, the Mental Health Parity Act was passed by Congress. This legislation required insurers that provide mental health coverage to offer benefits at the same level provided for medical and surgical coverage. In 2000, the Government Accounting Office found that although 86% of health plans complied with the 1996 law, 87% of health plans that complied with the law imposed new limits on mental health coverage. On April 29, 2002, President George W. Bush endorsed parity and established a new mental health commission. In February 2003, the Senator Paul Wellstone Mental Health Equitable Treatment Act was introduced into the Senate and the House of Representatives. In July 2003, the President's New Freedom Commission on Mental Health also endorsed parity.

Since 1996 the limited federal law has been kept in place through a series of 1-year extensions, and stronger bills have repeatedly been introduced and voted down (NMHA, 2004). State bills were proposed to close the federal loopholes, and as of 2006, 34 states had adopted laws. However, many require full insurance parity for only a limited number of psychiatric diagnoses. One method many states use to determine coverage is by making a distinction of whether the problem is a **biologically based mental illness**, that is, a mental disorder caused by neurotransmitter dysfunction, abnormal brain structure, inherited genetic factors, or other biological causes. Another term for such an illness is **psychobiological disorder**. These biologically influenced illnesses include the following:

- Schizophrenia
- Bipolar disorder
- Major depression
- Obsessive-compulsive and panic disorders
- Posttraumatic stress disorder
- Autism

Other severe and disabling mental disorders include the following:

- Anorexia nervosa
- Attention deficit hyperactivity disorder

Many of the most prevalent and disabling mental disorders have been found to have strong biological influences; therefore, we can look at these disorders as "diseases."

The *DSM-IV-TR* cautions that the emphasis on the term *mental disorder* implies a distinction between "mental" disorder and "physical" disorder, which is an outdated concept, and stresses mind-body dualism: "There is much 'physical' in 'mental' disorders and much 'mental' in 'physical' disorders" (APA, 2000).

MEDICAL DIAGNOSIS AND NURSING DIAGNOSIS OF MENTAL ILLNESS

To carry out their professional responsibilities, clinicians and researchers need clear and accurate guidelines for identifying and categorizing mental illness. Such guidelines help clinicians plan and evaluate treatment for their patients. A necessary element for categorization includes agreement regarding which behaviors constitute a mental illness.

Medical Diagnoses and the *DSM-IV-TR*

In the *DSM-IV-TR*, each of the mental disorders is conceptualized as a clinically significant behavioral or psychological syndrome or pattern that occurs in an individual and is associated with present **distress** (e.g., a painful symptom) or **disability** (i.e., impairment in one or more important areas of functioning) or with a significantly increased risk of suffering death, pain, disability, or an important loss of freedom (APA, 2000). This syndrome or pattern must not be merely an expected and culturally sanctioned response to a particular event, such as the death of a loved one. Whatever the original cause, it must currently be considered a manifestation of a behavioral, psychological, or biological dysfunction in the individual. Deviant behavior (e.g., political, religious, or sexual) and conflicts between the individual and society are not considered mental disorders unless the deviance or conflict is a symptom of a dysfunction in the individual.

A common misconception is that a classification of mental disorders classifies *people* when actually the *DSM-IV-TR* classifies disorders that people have. For this reason, the text of the *DSM-IV-TR* avoids the use of expressions such as "a schizophrenic" or "an alcoholic" and instead uses the more accurate terms "an individual with schizophrenia" or "an individual with alcohol dependence." Since the third edition of the *DSM* appeared in 1980, the criteria for classification of mental disorders have been sufficiently detailed for clinical, teaching, and research purposes.

The *DSM-IV-TR* in Culturally Diverse Populations

Special efforts have been made in the *DSM-IV-TR* to incorporate an awareness that the manual is used in culturally diverse populations in the United States and internationally. Clinicians evaluate individuals from numerous ethnic groups and cultural backgrounds (including many who are recent immigrants). Diagnostic assessment can be especially challenging when a clinician from one ethnic or cultural

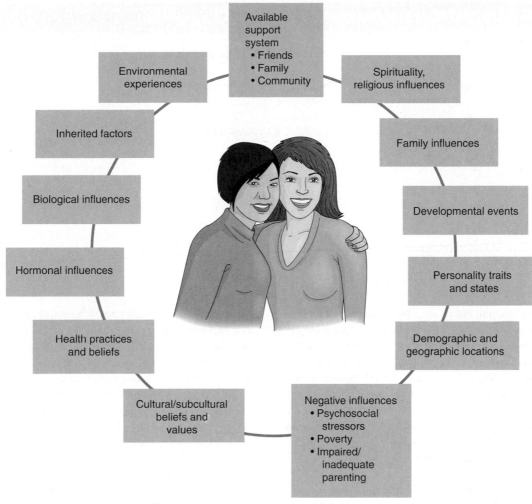

Figure 2-2 ■ Influences that can have an effect on an individual's mental health.

group uses the *DSM-IV-TR* classification to evaluate an individual from a different ethnic or cultural group. For example, among certain cultural groups, particular religious practices or beliefs (e.g., hearing or seeing a deceased relative during bereavement) may be misdiagnosed as manifestations of a psychotic disorder; furthermore, a syndrome often takes different superficial forms in different cultures. Also, people from minority or migrant populations may have good reason to be distrustful, and it should not be assumed that these patients are suffering from paranoia or paranoid schizophrenia. The *DSM-V*, scheduled to publish in 2011, will further emphasize the importance of culture in psychopathology.

The *DSM-IV-TR* Multiaxial System

The *DSM-IV-TR* axis system forces the diagnostician to consider a broad range of information by requiring judgments to be made on each of five axes (Table 2-3).

Axis I refers to the collection of signs and symptoms that together constitute a particular disorder, for example, schizophrenia, or a condition that may be a focus of treatment. (Refer to Appendix A for a list of all the mental disorders catalogued in the *DSM-IV-TR*.) Axis II refers to the personality disorders and mental retardation. Thus, Axes I and II constitute the classification of abnormal behavior. Axes I and II were separated to ensure that the possible presence of long-term disturbance is considered when attention is directed to the current one. For example, a heroin addict would be diagnosed on Axis I as having a substance-related disorder; this patient might also have a long-standing antisocial personality disorder, which would be noted on Axis II. This is another example of a person having more than one mental disorder at the same time. This phenomenon of coexisting disorders is often termed *comorbidity* or *dual diagnosis*.

Axis	Example
I Clinical disorders Other conditions that may be a focus of clinical attention	Major depressive disorder
II Personality disorders Mental retardation	Dependent personality disorder
III General medical conditions	Diabetes
IV Psychosocial and environmental problems	Divorce 3 months previously
V Global Assessment of Functioning (GAF) (see Box 2-1)	31 years old and unable to work or respond to family and friends

TABLE 2-3   *DSM-IV-TR* Multiaxial System of Evaluation

Adapted from American Psychiatric Association. (2000). *Diagnostic and statistical manual of mental disorders (DSM-IV-TR)* (4th ed., text rev.). Washington, DC: Author.

Although the remaining three axes are not needed to make the actual diagnosis, their inclusion in the *DSM-IV-TR* indicates the recognition that factors other than a person's symptoms should be considered in an assessment. On Axis III the clinician indicates any general medical conditions believed to be relevant to the mental disorder in question. In some individuals, a physical disorder (e.g., a neurological dysfunction) may be the cause of the abnormal behavior, whereas in others, it may be an important factor in the individual's overall condition (e.g., diabetes in a child with a conduct disorder).

Axis IV is for reporting psychosocial and environmental problems that may affect the diagnosis, treatment, and prognosis of a mental disorder. These may include occupational problems, educational problems, economic problems, interpersonal difficulties with family members, and a variety of problems in other life areas. Often a psychosocial assessment will uncover these (see Chapter 5).

Finally, Axis V, called Global Assessment of Functioning (GAF), gives an indication of the person's best level of psychological, social, and occupational functioning during the preceding year, rated on a scale of 1 to 100 (1 indicates persistent danger of severely hurting oneself or others, and 100 indicates superior functioning in a variety of activities at the time of the evaluation, as well as the highest level of functioning for at least a few months during the past year). Box 2-1 presents the GAF scale. Table 2-4 illustrates how the multiaxial system of classification might be applied to a hypothetical case.

Caution must be exercised to avoid labeling or stereotyping when a medical diagnosis or a nursing diagnosis is being formulated. Anthropologists, historians, and students of cross-cultural society have long observed that every society has its own view of health and illness and its own classification of diseases (Klerman, 1986). The process of psychiatric labeling or stereotyping can have harmful effects on an individual and family, especially if the diagnosis is made on insufficient evidence and proves faulty.

An example of the influence of cultural and social bias on psychiatric diagnosis is the inclusion of homosexuality as a psychiatric disease in both the first and second editions of the *DSM*. All research consistently failed to demonstrate that people with a homosexual orientation were any more maladjusted than heterosexuals, but despite the research data, change occurred in the medical community only when gay rights activists advocated an end to discrimination against lesbians and gay men. No longer is homosexuality classified as a mental disorder.

Instances of bias may involve many other minority groups, including African Americans, older adults, children, and women. These biases are often reflected in our power structures and political systems. Awareness of the cultural bias and dangers in labeling and stereotyping has enormous implications for nursing practice, especially in the field of mental health, because nurses often take their cues from the medical structure.

Nursing Diagnoses and NANDA International

Psychiatric mental health nursing includes the diagnosis and treatment of human responses to actual or potential mental health problems. The NANDA International (NANDA-I) describes a nursing diagnosis as a clinical judgment about individual, family, or community responses to actual or potential health problems and life processes.

BOX 2-1

Global Assessment of Functioning (GAF) Scale

Consider psychological, social, and occupational functioning on a hypothetical continuum of mental health–mental illness. Do not include impairment in functioning that is a result of physical (or environmental) limitations. *Note:* Use intermediate codes when appropriate (e.g., 45, 68, 72).

Code

100 **Superior functioning in a wide range of activities, life's problems never seem to get out of hand, is sought out by**
↓   **others because of his or her many positive qualities. No symptoms.**
91

90 **Absent or minimal symptoms** (e.g., mild anxiety before an exam), **good functioning in all areas, interested and**
↓   **involved in a wide range of activities, socially effective, generally satisfied with life, no more than everyday**
81   **problems or concerns** (e.g., an occasional argument with family members).

80 **If symptoms are present, they are transient and expected reactions to psychosocial stressors** (e.g., difficulty
↓   concentrating after family argument); **no more than slight impairment in social, occupational, or school**
71   **functioning** (e.g., temporarily falling behind in schoolwork).

70 **Some mild symptoms** (e.g., depressed mood and mild insomnia) **OR some difficulty in social, occupational, or**
↓   **school functioning** (e.g., occasional truancy, or theft within the household), **but generally functioning pretty well,**
61   **has some meaningful interpersonal relationships.**

60 **Moderate symptoms** (e.g., flat affect and circumstantial speech, occasional panic attacks) **OR moderate difficulty in**
↓   **social, occupational, or school functioning** (e.g., few friends, conflicts with peers or co-workers).
51

50 **Serious symptoms** (e.g., suicidal ideation, severe obsessional rituals, frequent shoplifting) **OR any serious impairment**
↓   **in social, occupational, or school functioning** (e.g., no friends, unable to keep a job).
41

40 **Some impairment in reality testing or communication** (e.g., speech is at times illogical, obscure, or irrelevant) **OR**
↓   **major impairment in several areas, such as work or school, family relations, judgment, thinking, or mood** (e.g.,
31   depressed man avoids friends, neglects family, and is unable to work; child frequently beats up younger children, is
      defiant at home, and is failing at school).

30 **Behavior is considerably influenced by delusions or hallucinations OR serious impairment in communication or**
↓   **judgment** (e.g., sometimes incoherent, acts grossly inappropriately, suicidal preoccupation) **OR inability to function**
21   **in almost all areas** (e.g., stays in bed all day; no job, home, or friends).

20 **Some danger of hurting self or others** (e.g., suicide attempts without clear expectation of death; frequently violent;
↓   manic excitement) **OR occasionally fails to maintain minimal personal hygiene** (e.g., smears feces) **OR gross**
11   **impairment in communication** (e.g., largely incoherent or mute).

10 **Persistent danger of severely hurting self or others** (e.g., recurrent violence) **OR persistent inability to maintain**
↓   **minimal personal hygiene OR serious suicidal act with clear expectation of death.**
1

0   **Inadequate information.**

From American Psychiatric Association. (2000). *Diagnostic and statistical manual of mental disorders (DSM-IV-TR)* (4th ed., text rev.). Washington, DC: Author.

The rating of overall psychological functioning on a scale of 0 to 100 was operationalized by Luborsky (1962) in the Health-Sickness Rating Scale. Spitzer and colleagues developed a revision of the Health-Sickness Rating Scale called the Global Assessment Scale (GAS) (Endicott et al., 1976). A modified version of the GAS was included in the *Diagnostic and Statistical Manual of Mental Disorders,* third edition, revised (American Psychiatric Association, 1987) as the Global Assessment of Functioning scale.

This rating scale highlights important areas in the assessment of functioning. Because many of the judgments are subjective, experienced clinicians use this tool as a guide when planning care, and draw on their knowledge of their patients.

Therefore, the *DSM-IV-TR* is used to diagnose a psychiatric disorder, whereas a well-defined nursing diagnosis provides the framework for identifying appropriate nursing interventions for dealing with the phenomena a patient with a mental health disorder is experiencing (e.g., hallucinations, self-esteem issues, impaired ability to function [in job and family], etc.). See Chapter 5 for more on the formulation of nursing diagnosis in psychiatric nursing.

Appendix B lists NANDA-I–approved nursing diagnoses. The individual clinical chapters offer suggestions for

TABLE 2-4	Clinical Example Demonstrating *DSM-IV-TR* Axes
Clinical Example	**Diagnoses According to *DSM-IV-TR* Axes**
For the past 9 months, Michael, a 33-year-old sales representative, has suffered delusions of grandeur and persecution. Believing himself to be a genius, he became convinced that another salesman in his firm was trying to kill him because the other man could not tolerate Michael's superiority. In the past 2 weeks, Michael has become certain that this other man has had a pale green gas pumped into his office through the air-conditioning ducts, but there is no objective evidence of such gas or any other malfunction of the air-conditioning system.	I: Schizophrenic disorder, paranoid
Michael has always tended to be suspicious and distrustful of people. He looks constantly for evidence that others are trying to get the better of him or to harm him, and his manner is guarded. He has trouble relaxing, and others see him as cold and unemotional. He has no close friends and is considered a loner. He was extremely jealous of his wife, from whom he is now separated, and often accused her, falsely, of having affairs with other men.	II: Paranoid traits; no personality disorder
Michael sees a flare-up of his colitis (inflammation of the colon) as evidence that the salesman is poisoning him, even though Michael has had the same symptoms many times before.	III: Colitis
Michael left his wife 10 months ago. Two months ago the president of Michael's firm reassigned one of Michael's important accounts to the salesman Michael now suspects of hostile intent. Michael thinks this was maneuvered by the other salesman, but in fact the president acted because the quality of Michael's work was deteriorating. His work had slowed visibly, and co-workers complained that they could not perform their work properly when he was present.	IV: Psychosocial and environmental problems – Marital separation – Loss of work responsibility Rated severe
Michael's functioning was adequate until he separated from his wife. At that point he began to withdraw further from friends and acquaintances. He appeared to concentrate more on his job but actually spent his time checking and rechecking his work. When the firm's president reassigned his major account, Michael's work deteriorated further, and Michael began to air some of his suspicions about the partner who took over the account. When his colitis flared up 2 weeks ago, he requested an appointment with the president and accused the partner openly. Michael was fired.	V: Highest level of adaptive functioning in last year (GAF): serious symptoms 45-50 Rated moderate to serious

GAF, Global Assessment of Functioning.
Adapted from Altrocchi, J. (1980). *Abnormal behavior*. New York: Harcourt Brace Jovanovich; American Psychiatric Association. (2000). *Diagnostic and statistical manual of mental disorders (DSM-IV-TR)* (4th ed., text rev.). Washington, DC: Author.

potential nursing diagnoses for the behaviors and phenomena often encountered in association with specific disorders.

INTRODUCTION TO CULTURE AND MENTAL ILLNESS

As stated, we must consider the norms and influence of culture in determining the mental health or mental illness of the individual. Throughout history, people have interpreted health or sickness according to their own cultural views. People in the Middle Ages, for example, regarded bizarre behavior as a sign that the disturbed person was possessed by a demon. To exorcise the demon, priests resorted to prescribed religious rituals. During the 1880s, when the "germ theory" of illness was popular, physicians interpreted bizarre behavior as stemming from attacks by biological agents.

Cultures differ not only in their views regarding mental illness but also in the types of behavior categorized as mental illness. For example, the content of people's delusions, hallucinations, obsessional thoughts, and phobias often reflect what is important in an individual's culture.

A number of **culture-related syndromes** appear to be more influenced by culture alone and are not seen in all areas of the world. For example, one form of mental illness recognized in parts of Southeast Asia is **running amok,** in which someone (usually a male) runs around engaging in furious, almost indiscriminate violent behavior.

Pibloktoq is an uncontrollable desire to tear off one's clothing and expose oneself to severe winter weather; it is a recognized form of psychological disorder in parts of Greenland, Alaska, and the Arctic regions of Canada. In our own society, we recognize **anorexia nervosa** as a psychobiological disorder that entails voluntary starvation. That disorder is well known in Europe, North America, and Australia, but unheard of in many other parts of the world.

What is to be made of the fact that certain disorders occur in some cultures but are absent in others? One interpretation is that the conditions necessary for causing a particular disorder occur in some places but are absent in other places. Another interpretation is that people learn certain kinds of abnormal behavior by imitation. However, the fact that some disorders may be culturally determined does not prove that all mental illnesses are so determined. The best evidence suggests that schizophrenia and bipolar affective disorders are found throughout the world. The symptom patterns of schizophrenia have been observed among indigenous Greenlanders and West African villagers, as well as in our own Western culture.

The *DSM-IV-TR* includes information specifically related to culture in three areas:

1. A discussion of cultural variations for each of the clinical disorders
2. A description of culture-bound syndromes
3. An outline designed to assist the clinician in evaluating and reporting the impact of the individual's cultural context

KEY POINTS TO REMEMBER

- Mental illness is difficult to define, and people hold many myths regarding mental illness.
- There are many important aspects of mental health (e.g., happiness, control over behavior, appraisal of reality, effectiveness in work, a healthy self-concept, presence of satisfying relationships, and effective coping strategies). Some components of mental health are identified in Figure 2-1.
- The study of epidemiology can help identify high-risk groups and behaviors. In turn, this can lead to a better understanding of the causes of some disorders. Prevalence rates help us identify the proportion of a population who has a mental disorder at a given time.
- With the current recognition that many common mental disorders are biologically based, it is easier to see how these biologically based disorders can be classified as medical diseases as well.
- Clinicians use the five axes of the *DSM-IV-TR* and the GAF scale as a guide for diagnosing and categorizing mental disorders, allowing for a more holistic approach to the assessment. Medical condition, psychosocial and environmental influences, and present and past levels of functioning are considered.
- Factors that may influence the intensity or cause of a mental illness are illustrated in Figure 2-2. Using well-thought-out nursing diagnoses helps target the symptoms and needs of patients so that ideally they may achieve a higher level of functioning and a better quality of life.
- The influence of culture on behavior and the way in which symptoms present may reflect a person's cultural patterns. Symptoms need to be understood in terms of a person's cultural background.
- Caution is recommended for all health care professionals concerning the damage and disservice that stereotyping can cause for medical and mental health patients. Lack of cultural knowledge can result in improper care or delivery of inappropriate services to those under our care.

CRITICAL THINKING

1. Timothy Harris is a college sophomore with a grade point average of 3.4. He was brought to the emergency department after a suicide attempt. He has been extremely depressed since the death of his girlfriend 5 months previously when the car he was driving careened out of control and crashed. Timothy's parents have been very distraught since the accident. To compound things, the parents' religious beliefs include the conviction that taking one's own life will prevent a person from going to heaven. Timothy has epilepsy and has had increased seizures since the accident; he refuses help because he says he should be punished for his carelessness and doesn't care what happens to him. He has not been to school and has not shown up for his part-time job of tutoring younger children in reading.

    A. Questions regarding Timothy and the use of the *DSM-IV-TR* multiaxial system:

    (1) What might be a possible *DSM-IV-TR* diagnosis for Axis I?
    (2) What information should be included on Axis III?
    (3) What should be included on Axis IV?
    (4) What score (range) might you give to Timothy on the GAF scale?

CRITICAL THINKING—cont'd

B. Questions regarding mental health and mental illness:
   (1) What are some factors that you would like to assess regarding aspects of Timothy's overall mental health and other influences that can affect mental health before you plan your care?
   (2) If an antidepressant medication could help him with his depression, explain why this alone would not meet his multiple needs. What issues do you think have to be addressed if Timothy is to receive a holistic approach to care?

   (3) Formulate at least two potential nursing diagnoses for Timothy.
   (4) Would Timothy's parents' religious beliefs factor into your plan of care? If so, how?
2. Using Table 2-1, evaluate yourself and one of your patients in terms of mental health.
3. In a small study group, share experiences you have had with others from unfamiliar cultural, ethnic, or racial backgrounds and identify two positive learning experiences from these encounters.

CHAPTER REVIEW

Choose the most appropriate answer.

1. Which statement about mental illness is true?
   1. Mental illness is a matter of individual nonconformity with societal norms.
   2. Mental illness is present when individual irrational and illogical behavior occurs.
   3. Mental illness is defined in relation to the culture, time in history, political system, and group in which it occurs.
   4. Mental illness is evaluated solely by considering individual control over behavior and appraisal of reality.
2. A nursing student new to psychiatric nursing asks a peer what resource he or she can use to figure out which symptoms are part of the picture of a specific psychiatric disorder. The best answer would be:
   1. Nursing Interventions Classification (NIC).
   2. Nursing Outcomes Classification (NOC).
   3. NANDA-I nursing diagnoses.
   4. *DSM-IV-TR.*
3. Why is it important for a nurse to be aware of the multiple factors that can influence an individual's mental health?
   1. Rates of illness differ among various groups.
   2. The *DSM-IV-TR* cannot be used without information on multiple factors.
   3. The nurse diagnoses and treats human responses, which are influenced by many factors.

   4. The nurse must contribute these data for epidemiological research.
4. Epidemiological studies contribute to improvements in care for individuals with mental disorders by:
   1. providing information about effective nursing techniques.
   2. identifying risk factors that contribute to the development of a disorder.
   3. identifying who in the general population will develop a specific disorder.
   4. identifying which individuals will respond favorably to a specific treatment.
5. Which statement best describes a major difference between a *DSM-IV-TR* diagnosis and a nursing diagnosis?
   1. There is no functional difference between the two. Both serve to identify a human deviance.
   2. The *DSM-IV-TR* diagnosis disregards culture, whereas the nursing diagnosis takes culture into account.
   3. The *DSM-IV-TR* is associated with present distress or disability, whereas a nursing diagnosis considers past and present responses to actual mental health problems.
   4. The *DSM-IV-TR* diagnosis distinguishes a person's specific psychiatric disorder, whereas a nursing diagnosis offers a framework for identifying interventions for phenomena a patient is experiencing.

REFERENCES

Altrocchi, J. (1980). *Abnormal behavior.* New York: Harcourt Brace Jovanovich.

American Psychiatric Association. (2000). *Diagnostic and statistical manual of mental disorders (DSM-IV-TR)* (4th ed., text rev.). Washington, DC: Author.

American Psychological Association (2004). *The road to resilience.* Washington DC: American Psychological Association.

Endicott, J., Spitzer, R.L., Fleiss, J.L., et al. (1976). The global assessment scale: A procedure for measuring overall severity of psychiatric disturbance. *Archives of General Psychiatry, 33,* 766-771.

Favazza, A. (2004). The psychiatric scientist and psychoanalyst. In B.J. Sadock & V.A. Sadock (Eds.), *Kaplan and Sadock's comprehensive textbook of psychiatry* (8th ed., vol. 1, pp. 598-562). Philadelphia: Lippincott Williams & Wilkins.

Kessler, R.C., Berglund, P., Demler, O.L., et al. (2005). Lifetime prevalence and age-of-onset distribution of DSM-IV disorders in the national comorbidity survey replication. *Archives of General Psychiatry 62,* 593-602.

Klerman, G.L. (1986). *Contemporary directions in psychopathology: Toward the DSM-IV.* New York: Guilford Press.

Luborsky, L. (1962). Clinician's judgments of mental health. *Archives of General Psychiatry, 7,* 407-417.

National Institute of Mental Health. (2004). *The numbers count: Mental disorders in America* (NIH Publication No. 01-4584). Retrieved August 1, 2004, from www.nimh.nih.gov/publicat/numbers.cfm.

National Mental Health Association. (2004). *Congress must pass mental health parity now.* Retrieved July 31, 2004, from www.nmha.org/federal/parity/parityfactsheet.cfm.

Sadock, B.J., & Sadock, V.A. (2007). *Kaplan and Sadock's synopsis of psychiatry* (10th ed.). Philadelphia: Lippincott Williams & Wilkins.

U.S. Department of Health and Human Services. (1999). *Mental health: A report of the surgeon general.* Rockville, MD: U.S. Department of Health and Human Services, Center for Mental Health Services, National Institutes of Health.

CHAPTER 3

Theories and Therapies

Margaret Jordan Halter

Key Terms and Concepts

automatic thoughts, p. 30
boundaries, p. 41
cognitive distortions, p. 30
conscious, p. 25
conservation, p. 32
countertransference, p. 26
curative factors, p. 39
ego, p. 25
group content, p. 37

group process, p. 37
id, p. 25
object permanence, p. 32
operations, p. 32
preconscious, p. 25
schemata, p. 31
superego, p. 25
transference, p. 26
unconscious, p. 25

Objectives

1. Describe major theories relevant to psychiatric and mental health nursing care.
2. Identify the origins and progression of dominant theories and treatment modalities.
3. Discuss the relevance of these theories and treatments to the provision of psychiatric and mental health care.
4. Identify some of the components from Peplau's theoretical base that are beneficial to nursing practice in all settings.
5. Articulate a rationale for employing different theoretical models of mental health care in specific circumstances.
6. Distinguish models of care used in clinical settings, and cite benefits and limitations of these models.

evolve

For additional resources related to the content of this chapter, visit the Evolve website at http://evolve.elsevier.com/Varcarolis/essentials.

- Chapter Outline
- Chapter Review Answers
- Nurse, Patient, and Family Resources
- Concept Map Creator

We expect ourselves and others to behave in certain ways, and we seek explanations for behavior that deviates from what we believe to be normal. What causes excessive sadness or extreme happiness? Can we explain mistrust, anxiety, confusion, or apathy—degrees of which may range from mildly disturbing to intensely incapacitating? It is by understanding a problem that we can begin to devise solutions to treat or eradicate it. Mental illness has long defied explanation, even as other so-called physical illnesses were being quantified and often controlled.

It wasn't until the late 1800s that psychological models and theories were conceived, developed, and disseminated into mainstream thinking. They provided structure for considering developmental processes and possible explanations about how we think, feel, and behave. The theorists believed if complex workings of the mind could be understood, they also could be treated, and from these models and theories, therapies evolved.

Early practitioners used various forms of talk therapy, or **psychotherapy,** focusing on the complexity and inner workings of the mind and emphasizing environmental influences on its development and its stability. Beginning in the early twentieth century, biological explanations for mental alterations began to grow in acceptance. Currently the dominant and common belief is that mental health and illness are based on both psychological and biological factors and that there is a dynamic interplay between the two.

Mental health professionals continue to rely on theoretical models as a basis for understanding and treating psychiatric alterations and mental health issues. No single model fully explains psychiatric illness and pathology. This chapter provides an overview of developmental theories, psychotherapeutic models, and related treatments and discusses the potential connection between them and the provision of psychiatric nursing care. Table 3-1 provides a brief overview of the major theories.

PROMINENT THEORIES AND THERAPEUTIC MODELS
Psychoanalytic Theory

Sigmund Freud (1856-1939), an Austrian neurologist, is considered the "father of psychiatry." His work was based on psychoanalytic theory, in which Freud claims that most psychological disturbances are the result of early trauma or incidents that are often not remembered or recognized.

Freud (1961) identified three layers of mental activity: the **conscious**, the **preconscious**, and the **unconscious** mind. The conscious mind is your current awareness—thoughts, beliefs, and feelings. However, most of the mind's activity occurs outside of this conscious awareness, like an iceberg with its bulk hidden underwater. The preconscious mind contains what is lying immediately below the surface, not currently the subject of our attention, but accessible. The biggest chunk of the iceberg is the unconscious mind; it is here where our primitive feelings, drives, and memories reside, especially those that are unbearable and traumatic. The conscious mind is then influenced by the preconscious and unconscious mind (Figure 3-1).

One of Freud's later and widely known constructs concerns the intrapsychic struggle that occurs within the brain among the **id**, the **ego**, and the **superego**. The id is the primitive, pleasure-seeking part (particularly sexual pleasure) of our personalities that lurks in the unconscious mind.

TABLE 3-1	Major Theories of Psychiatric Care		
Theory	**Theorist**	**Tenets**	**Therapeutic Model**
Psychoanalytic	Freud	Unconscious thoughts; psychosexual development	Psychoanalysis to learn unconscious thoughts; therapist is nondirective and interprets meaning
Interpersonal	Sullivan	Relationships as basis for mental health or illness	Therapy focuses on here and now and emphasizes relationships; therapist is an active participant
Behavioral	Pavlov Watson-Skinner	Behavior is learned through conditioning	Behavioral modification addresses maladaptive behaviors by rewarding adaptive behavior
Cognitive	Beck	Negative and self-critical thinking causes depression	Cognitive behavioral therapists assist in identifying negative thoughts patterns and replace them with rational ones
Biological	Many	Psychiatric disorders are the result of physical (brain) alterations	Neurochemical imbalances are corrected through medication and talk therapy

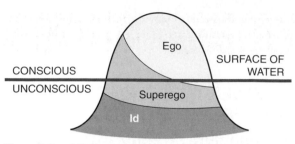

Figure 3-1 ■ Mind as an iceberg.

The ego is our sense of self and acts as intermediary between the id and the world by using ego defense mechanisms, such as repression, denial, and rationalization (see Chapter 8).

The superego is our conscience and is greatly influenced by our parents' or caregivers' moral and ethical stances. In healthy individuals, the ego is able to realistically evaluate situations, limit the id's primitive impulses, and keep the superego from becoming too rigid and obsessive.

Freud's theory of development focused on sexual urges and has been criticized for being sexist; perhaps his harshest criticism stems from the notion of "penis envy" in which girls suffer from feelings of inferiority for not having male genitalia. Freud describes each developmental stage in terms of the id's focus of an erogenous zone of the body. Fixation, typically as the result of childhood sexual abuse, at any given point results in pathology and personality disorders. Table 3-2 provides a comparison of Freud's, Sullivan's, and Erikson's developmental stages.

Therapeutic Model

Psychoanalytic therapy was Freud's answer for a scientific method to relieve emotional disturbances by knowing the unconscious mind. An often time-consuming (sometimes daily), expensive, and emotionally painful process, the goal of this therapy is to know and understand what is happening at the unconscious level in order to uncover the truth. The analyst uses *free association*, to search for forgotten and repressed memories by encouraging the patient to say anything comes to mind. For example, "What do you think of when I say 'water'?" The patient may respond with, "Warm . . . June . . . darkness . . . can't breathe," which may reveal a long-forgotten, but traumatic near-drowning incident.

The analyst is nondirective, but does make interpretations of symbols, thoughts, and dreams. *Psychodynamic therapy* is theoretically related to psychoanalytic therapy and views the mind in essentially the same way. It tends to be shorter, on average 23 sessions (Leichsenring & Leibing, 2003) and the therapist takes a more active role because the therapeutic relationship is part of the healing process.

Transference occurs as the patient projects intense feelings onto the therapist related to unfinished work from previous relationships; safe expression of these feelings is crucial to successful therapy. Psychodynamic therapists recognize that they, too, have unconscious emotional responses to the patient, or **countertransference,** that must be scrutinized in order to prevent damage to the therapeutic relationship.

Interpersonal Theory

Whereas psychoanalytic theory focuses on what goes on in the mind, interpersonal theory focuses on what goes on between people. Harry Stack Sullivan (1892-1949), an American psychiatrist, believed that personality dynamics and disorders were caused primarily by social forces and interpersonal situations. Human beings are driven by the need for interaction; indeed, Sullivan (1953) viewed loneliness as the most painful human experience. He emphasized the early relationship with the *significant other* (primary parenting figure) as crucial for personality development, and believed that healthy relationships were necessary for a healthy personality. Anxiety is an interpersonal phenomenon that is transmitted empathically from the significant other to the child, and also by perceived degrees of approval or disapproval felt by the child. According to Sullivan, all behavior is aimed at avoiding anxiety and threats to self-esteem.

One of the ways that we avoid anxiety is by focusing on our positive attributes or the *good me* (I'm a good skier, I have a nice car), and hiding the negative aspects of ourselves from others and maybe even ourselves, or the *bad me* (I failed an exam; I hoard food in my room). The most drastic attempt we use to prevent anxiety is through the *not me.* This part of us represents things that we find so objectionable that we cannot even imagine them being part of us. The not-me is pushed deeply into the unconscious. An example of this is an adolescent in a strict and conservative family who begins to feel stirrings of attraction, yet firmly maintains (and believes) that she is not interested in boys.

Sullivan's theory of development echoes that of Freud's in that personalities are influenced by the social environment as children, particularly as adolescents. He believed that personality is most influenced by the mother, but that personality could be molded even as adults. Stages occur in a stepwise fashion that is environmentally influenced (see Table 3-2).

Therapeutic Model

Interpersonal therapy (IPT) is a hands-on system in which therapists actively guide and challenge maladaptive behaviors and distorted views. The focus is on the here and now

TABLE 3-2   Development of Personality According to Freud, Sullivan, and Erikson

Freud	Sullivan	Erikson
Oral—birth to 1½ years **Pleasure-pain principle** **Id,** the instinctive and primitive mind, is dominant Demanding, impulsive, irrational, asocial, selfish, trustful, omnipotent, and dependent Primary thought processes Unconscious instincts—source-energy-aim-object Mouth—primary source of pleasure Immediate release of tension/anxiety and immediate gratification through oral gratification Task—Develop a sense of trust that needs will be met	**Infancy**—birth to 1½ years Mothering object relieves tension through empathic intervention and tenderness, leading to decreased anxiety and increased satisfaction and security. Mother becomes symbolized "good mother." Goal is biological satisfaction and psychological security. Denial of tension relief creates anxiety, and mother becomes symbolized as "bad mother." Anxiety in mother yields anxiety and fear in child via empathy. These states are experienced by the child in diffuse-undifferentiated manner Task—Learn to count on others for satisfaction and security to trust.	**Infancy**—birth to 1½ years **Trust vs. Mistrust** Egocentric Danger: During second half of first year, an abrupt and prolonged separation may intensify the natural sense of loss and may lead to a sense of mistrust that may last through life. Task—Develop a basic sense of trust that leads to hope. Trust requires a feeling of physical comfort and a minimal experience of fear or uncertainty. If this occurs, the child will extend trust to the world and self.

Anal—1½ to 3 years
Reality principle—postpone immediate discharge of energy and seek actual object to satisfy needs.
Learning to defer pleasure.
Gaining satisfaction from tolerating some tension-mastering impulses.
Focus on toilet training—retaining/letting go; power struggle
Ego development—functions of the ego include problem-solving skills, perception, ability to mediate id impulses.
Task—Delay immediate gratification
	Childhood—1½ to 6 years
	Muscular maturation and learning to communicate verbally.
	Learning social skills through consensual validation.
	Beginning to develop self system via reflected appraisals:
	  Good me
	  Bad me
	  Not me
	  Levels of awareness
	  Aware
	  Selective inattention
	  Dissociation
	Task—Learn to delay satisfaction of wishes with relative comfort.
		Early Childhood—1½ to 3 years
		Autonomy vs.
		Shame/Doubt
		Develop confidence in physical and mental abilities that leads to the development an autonomous will.
		Danger: Development of a deep sense of shame/doubt if child is deprived of the opportunity to rebel. Learns to expect defeat in any battle of wills with those who are bigger and stronger.
		Task—Gain self-control of and independence within the environment.

Phallic—3 to 7 years **Superego develops** via incorporating moral values, ideals, and judgments of right and wrong that are held by parents. Superego is primarily unconscious and functions on the **reward and punishment principle** (sexual identity attained via resolving oedipal conflict). Conflict differs for boy and girl masturbatory activity. Task—Develop sexual identity through identification with same sex parent.		**Play**—3 to 6 years **Initiative vs. Guilt** Interest in socially appropriate goals leads to a sense of purpose. Imagination is greatly expanded because of increased ability to move around freely and increased ability to communicate. Intrusive activity and curiosity and consuming fantasies, which lead to feelings of guilt and anxiety. Establishment of conscience. Danger: May develop a deep-seated conviction that he or she is essentially bad, with a resultant stifling of initiative or a conversion of moralism to vindictiveness. Task—Achieve a sense of purpose and develop a sense of mastery over tasks.

Continued

TABLE 3-2	Development of Personality According to Freud, Sullivan, and Erikson—cont'd		
Freud	**Sullivan**	**Erikson**	
Latency—7 to 12 years De-sexualization. Libido diffused. Involved in learning social skills, exploring, building, collecting, accomplishing, and hero worship. Peer group loyalty begins. Gang and scout behavior. Growing independence from family. Task—Sexuality is repressed during this time; learn to form close relationship(s) with same sex peers.	**Juvenile**—6 to 9 years Absorbed in learning to deal with ever widening outside world, peers, and other adults. Reflections and revisions of self-image and parental images. Task—Develop satisfying interpersonal relationships with peers that involve competition and compromise.	**School Age**—6 to 12 years **Industry vs. Inferiority** Develops a healthy competitive drive that leads to confidence. In learning to accept instruction and to win recognition by producing "things," the child opens the way for the capacity of work enjoyment. Danger: The development of a sense of inadequacy and inferiority in a child who does not receive recognition. Task—Gain a sense of self-confidence and recognition through learning, competing, and performing successfully.	
	Preadolescence—9 to 12 years Develops intimate interpersonal relationship with person of same sex who is perceived to be much like oneself in interests, feelings, and mutual collaboration. Task—Learn to care for others of same sex who are outside the family. Sullivan called this the "normal homosexual phase."		
Genital Phase (Adolescence)—13 to 20 years Fluctuation regarding emotion stability and physical maturation. Very ambivalent and labile, seeking life goals and emancipation from parents. Dependence vs. independence reappraisal of parents and self; intense peer loyalty. Task—Form close relationships and with members of the opposite sex based on genuine caring and pleasure in the interaction.	**Adolescence**—12 to 20 years *Early Adolescence—12-14 years* Establishing satisfying relationships with opposite sex. *Late Adolescence—14 to 20 years* Interdependent and establishing durable sexual relations with a select member of the opposite sex. Task—Form intimate and long-lasting relationships with the opposite sex and develop a sense of identity.	**Adolescence**—12 to 20 years **Identity vs. Identity** Diffusion Differentiation from parents leads to fidelity (sense of self). The physiological revolution that comes with puberty (rapid body growth and sexual maturity) forces the young person to question beliefs and to re-fight many of the earlier battles. Danger: Temporary identity diffusion (instability) may result in a permanent inability to integrate a personal identity. Task—Integrate all the tasks previously mastered into a secure sense of self. **Young Adulthood**—20 to 30 years **Intimacy vs. Isolation** Maturity and social responsibility results in the ability to love and be loved. As people feel more secure in their identity, they are able to establish intimacy with themselves (their inner life) and with others, eventually in a love-based satisfying sexual relationship with a member of the opposite sex.	

TABLE 3-2	Development of Personality According to Freud, Sullivan, and Erikson—cont'd	
Freud	**Sullivan**	**Erikson**
		Danger: Fear of losing identity may prevent intimate relationship and result in a deep sense of isolation.
		Task—Form intense long-term relationships and commit to another person, cause, institution, or creative effort.
		Adulthood—30 to 65 years
		Generativity vs. Self-absorption
		Interest in nurturing subsequent generations creates a sense of caring, contributing, and generativity.
		Danger: Lack of generativity results in self-absorption and stagnation.
		Task—Achieve life goals and obtain concern and awareness of future generations.
		Senescence—65 years to death
		Integrity vs. Despair
		Acceptance of mortality and satisfaction with life leads to wisdom.
		Satisfying intimacy with other human beings and adaptive response to triumphs and disappointments.
		Marked by a sense of what life is, was, and its place in the flow of history.
		Danger—Without this "accrued ego integration," there is despair, usually marked by a display of displeasure and distrust.
		Task—Derive meaning from one's whole life and obtain/maintain a sense of self-worth.

Developed from original sources by Freud, Sullivan, and Erikson.

with an emphasis on the patient's life and relationships at home, at work, and in the social realm. The therapist becomes a "participant observer" and reflects the patient's interpersonal behavior, including responses to the therapist. The premise for this work is that if people are aware of their dysfunctional patterns and unrealistic expectations, they can modify them.

Behavioral Theories

As the psychoanalytic movement was developing in the twentieth century, so, too, was the behaviorist school of thought. Ivan Pavlov (1927) is famous for investigating *classical conditioning* in which involuntary behavior or reflexes could be conditioned to respond to neutral stimuli. Pavlov's experimental dogs became accustomed to receiving food after a bell was rung; later these dogs salivated in response to the ring of the bell alone. Researchers today can actually measure the dramatic neuronal responses associated with neutral stimuli (Thompson, 2005). For human beings, classical conditioning can occur under such circumstances as when a baby's crying induces a milk let-down reflex, or when a rape victim begins to hyperventilate and gets sweaty palms when she hears footsteps behind her.

John B. Watson (1930) rejected psychoanalysis and was seeking an objective therapy that did not focus on unconscious motivations. He contended that personality traits and responses, adaptive and maladaptive, were learned. In a famous (but terrible) experiment, Watson conditioned Little Albert, a 9-month-old, to be terrified at the sight of white fur or hair. He concluded that through behavioral techniques anyone could be trained to be anything, from a beggar to a merchant.

B.F. Skinner (1938) conducted research on operant conditioning in which voluntary behaviors are learned through consequences of reinforcement (a consequence that causes the behavior to occur more frequently) or negative reinforcement or punishment (a consequence that causes the behavior to occur less frequently). Studying hard results in good grades and increases the chances that studying will continue to occur; driving too fast may result in a speeding ticket and in mature and healthy individuals, decreases the chances that speeding will occur.

Therapeutic Models

Behavioral therapy, or **behavior modification,** uses basic tenets from each of the behaviorists described previously. It attempts to correct or eliminate maladaptive behaviors or responses by rewarding and reinforcing adaptive behavior.

Systematic desensitization is based on classical conditioning. The premise is that learned responses can be reversed by first promoting relaxation and then gradually facing a particular anxiety-provoking stimulus. This method has been particularly successful in extinguishing phobias. Agoraphobia, the fear of open places, can be treated initially by visualizing trips outdoors while using relaxation techniques to reduce the accompanying anxiety and increase coping mechanisms. Later, the individual can practice increasingly more challenging excursions, which should result in eliminating or reducing agoraphobia.

Aversion therapy is based on both classical and operant conditioning and is used to eradicate unwanted habits by associating unpleasant consequences with them. A pharmacologically based aversion therapy is a regimen of disulfiram (Antabuse); people who take this medication and then ingest alcohol become extremely ill. Aversion therapy also has been used with sex offenders who may, for example, receive electric shocks in response to arousal from child pornography.

Biofeedback is a technique in which individuals learn to control physiological responses such as breathing rates, heart rates, blood pressure, brain waves, and skin temperature. This control is achieved by providing visual or auditory biofeedback of the physiological response and then using relaxation techniques such as slow, deep breathing or meditation.

Cognitive Theory

When Aaron T. Beck developed a cognitive therapy approach with depressed patients, he became convinced that depressed people generally had standard patterns of negative and self-critical thinking (Beck, 1963). Cognitive appraisals of events therefore lead to emotional responses—it is not the stimulus itself that causes the response, but one's evaluation of the stimulus. An example of the stimulus-appraisal-response comes from a woman whose sister had been depressed since their tumultuous and unsteady childhoods. In response to a question about how she and her sibling handled their parents' divorce and subsequent move to a small apartment, one of the siblings observed, "My sister fell apart. She retreated, barely talked. Mom asked me how I was doing. I told her I was excited to get a new bedroom and make new friends. And I was telling the truth."

Therapeutic Model

Cognitive behavioral therapy (CBT) is a commonly used effective and well-researched therapeutic tool. It is based on both cognitive and behavioral theory and seeks to modify negative thoughts that lead to dysfunctional emotions and actions. Several concepts underlie this therapy. One is that we all have *schemas,* or unique assumptions about ourselves, others, and the world around us. For example, if someone has a schema that no one can be trusted but themselves, this person will question everyone else's motives and expect others to lie and eventually hurt them. Other negative schemas include incompetence, abandonment, evilness, and vulnerability.

Typically, people are unaware of their basic assumptions; however, their beliefs and attitudes will make them apparent. Rapid, unthinking responses based on these schemas are known as **automatic thoughts**. These responses are particularly intense and frequent in psychiatric disorders such as depression and anxiety. Often these automatic thoughts, or **cognitive distortions**, are irrational because people make false assumptions and misinterpretations. Common cognitive distortions are listed in Table 3-3.

The goal of CBT is first to identify the negative patterns of thought that lead to negative emotions. Once the maladaptive patterns of thought are identified, they can be replaced with rational thoughts. A particularly useful technique in CBT is to use a four-column format to record the precipitating event or situation, the resulting automatic thought, the proceeding feeling(s) and behavior(s), and finally, a challenge to the negative thoughts based on rational evidence and thoughts. This is sometimes referred to as the ABCs of Irrational Beliefs and is a good exercise for nursing students to try for themselves (Box 3-1).

TABLE 3-3   Examples of Cognitive Distortions

Distortion	Definition	Example
All-or-nothing thinking	Thinking in black and white, reducing complex outcomes into absolutes	Cheryl got second-highest score in the cheerleading competition. She considers herself a loser.
Overgeneralization	Using a bad outcome (or a few bad outcomes) as evidence that nothing will ever go right again	Marty had a traffic accident. She refuses to drive and says, "I shouldn't be allowed on the road."
Labeling	A form of generalization where a characteristic or event becomes definitive and results in an overly harsh label for self or others	"Because I failed the advanced statistics exam, I am a failure. I might as well give up."
Mental filter	Focusing on a negative detail or bad event and allowing it to taint everything else	Anne's boss evaluated her work as exemplary and gave her a few suggestions for improvement. She obsessed about the suggestions and ignored the rest.
Disqualifying the positive	Maintaining a negative view by rejecting information that supports a positive view as being irrelevant, inaccurate, or accidental	"I've just been offered the job I've always wanted. No one else must have applied."
Jumping to conclusions	Making a negative interpretation despite the fact that there is little or no supporting evidence	"My fiancé, Mike, didn't call me for 3 hours; therefore, he doesn't love me."
a. Mind reading	Inferring negative thoughts, responses, and motives of others	The grocery store clerk was grouchy and barely made eye contact. "I must have done something wrong."
b. Fortune-telling error	Anticipating that things will turn out badly as an established fact	"I'll ask her out, but I know she won't have a good time."
Magnification or minimization	Exaggerating the importance of something (such a personal failure or the success of others) or reducing the importance of something (such as a personal success or the failure of others)	"I'm alone on a Saturday night because no one likes me. When other people are alone, it's because they want to be."
a. Catastrophizing	Catastrophizing is an extreme form of magnification in which the very worst is assumed to be a probable outcome.	"If I don't make a good impression on the boss at the company picnic, she will fire me."
Emotional reasoning	Drawing a conclusion based on an emotional state	"I'm nervous about the exam. I must not be prepared. If I were, I wouldn't be afraid."
"Should" and "must" statements	Rigid self-directives that presume an unrealistic amount of control over external events	"My patient is worse today. I should give better care so that she will get better."
Personalization	Assuming responsibility for an external event or situation that was likely out of personal control	"I'm sorry that your party wasn't more fun. It's probably because I was there."

Adapted from Burns, D.D. (1980). *Feeling good: The new mood therapy.* New York: William Morrow.

OTHER MAJOR THEORIES
Cognitive Development

Jean Piaget (1896-1980), was a Swiss psychologist and researcher (Smith, 1997). While working at a boys' school run by Alfred Binet, developer of the Binet Intelligence Test, Piaget helped to score the intelligence tests. He became fascinated by the fact that young children consistently gave wrong answers on intelligence tests, wrong answers that revealed a discernible pattern of cognitive processing that was different from that of older children and adults. He later studied his own three children's cognitive development. Ultimately he described cognitive development as a dynamic progression from primitive awareness and simple reflexes to complex thought and responses (Piaget & Inhelder, 1969). According to Piaget, our mental representations of the world, or **schemata**, depend on the cognitive stage we have reached.

An understanding of cognitive development can assist nurses to tailor their care to suit the cognitive level of the patient. For example, the concept of dying is difficult for the 5-year-old who has lost a parent to grasp; support for this child will require a different set of skills than would be necessary for a 10-year-old who can understand the permanence of death. Whereas each of the cognitive stages describes a child, Piaget's theory can be useful in understanding cognitive ability in people with problems such as developmental delay and mental retardation:

BOX 3-1

Example of ABCs of Irrational Beliefs

Activating Event
Trent has been in counseling for depression. His therapist's secretary called and canceled this week's appointment.

Belief
My therapist is disgusted with me and wants to avoid me.

Consequence
Sadness, rejection, and hopelessness. Decides to call off work and return to bed.

Reframing
There is no evidence to believe that I disgust my therapist. Why would he have rescheduled if he really didn't want to see me?

- *Sensorimotor stage (0 to 2 years).* This stage begins with basic reflexes and culminates with purposeful movement, spatial abilities, and hand-eye coordination. Physical interaction with the environment provides the child with a basic understanding of the world. By about 9 months of age, **object permanence** is achieved and the child can conceptualize objects that are no longer visible. Part of the delight of the game of peek-a-boo can be explained by this emerging skill as the child begins to anticipate the face hidden behind the hands.
- *Preoperational stage (2 to 7 years).* **Operations** is a term for thinking about objects. During this stage children are not yet able to think abstractly or generalize qualities in the absence of specific objects, but rather think in a concrete fashion. Egocentric thinking is demonstrated through a tendency to expect others to view the world as they do. A hallmark of the preoperational stage is the inability to conserve mass, volume, or number. An example of this is thinking that a tall, thin glass holds more liquid than a short, wide glass.
- *Concrete operational stage (7 to 11 years).* As interaction with the world increases, logical thought appears, and abstract problem solving is possible. The child is able to see a situation from another's point of view and can take into account a variety of solutions to a problem. **Conservation** is possible, and two small cups of liquid can be seen to equal a tall glass. At this stage, children are able to classify based on discrete characteristics, order objects in a pattern, and understand the concept of reversibility.

- *Formal operational stage (11 years to adulthood).* Conceptual reasoning commences at roughly the same time as does puberty. At this stage the child's basic abilities to think abstractly and problem solve mirror those of an adult.

Theory of Psychosocial Development

Erik Erikson (1902-1994) was a German-born American child psychoanalyst. Erikson (1963) described development as occurring in eight predetermined life stages, stages whose success are related to the proceeding stage (see Table 3-2). These stages are characterized by developmental tasks that ideally result in a successful resolution. One of the stages, for example, occurs from the ages of 7 to 12. During that time, the child's task is to gain a sense of his or her own abilities and competence, and expand relationships beyond the immediate family to include peers. The attainment of this task *(industry)* brings with it the virtue of confidence. If children fail to navigate this stage successfully, are unable to gain a mastery of age-appropriate tasks, and cannot make a connection with their peers, they will feel like failures *(inferiority)*.

It is important to note that the resolution of each stage does not depend completely on integrating the positive characteristic and completing eschewing the negative. Ideally, harmony is achieved between the two characteristics. For example, we would not want a child to be 100% trusting—a child who trusted everyone would be totally vulnerable; a degree of mistrust is essential to survival. Additionally, Erikson did not say that developmental tasks had to be mastered within the prescribed time period, but he did believe that some tasks are naturally easier at certain junctures. For example, the first task in life is to learn to trust. If, for example, a male infant had inconsistent and abusive parenting, he may grow into a mistrustful adult. However, by experiencing corrective, dependable, and positive relationships later in life, he could become an appropriately trusting adult.

Humanistic Theory

Humanistic psychologists rejected the psychoanalysts' focus on unconscious conflicts and the behaviorists' focus on learning (much of which was based on observations of animal behavior). They sought a psychological science concerned with the human potential for development, knowledge attainment, motivation, and understanding. Carl Rogers (1961) developed patient-centered psychotherapy, a technique that emphasized the role of the patient in understanding one's own problems;

the role of the therapist is that of facilitator rather than director.

Abraham Maslow (1970) is known for developing a theory of personality and motivation based on a hierarchy of needs. He placed these needs conceptually on a pyramid, with the most basic and important needs placed on the lower level (Figure 3-2). The higher levels, the more distinctly human needs, occupy the top sections of the pyramid. According to Maslow, when lower level needs are met, higher needs are able to emerge.

- *Physiological needs.* The most basic needs are the physiological drives, including the need for food, oxygen, water, sleep, sex, and a constant body temperature. If all the needs were deprived, this level would take priority.
- *Safety needs.* Once physiological needs are met, the safety needs emerge. They include security, protection, freedom from fear/anxiety/chaos, and the need for law, order, and limits. Adults in a stable society usually feel safe. They may feel threatened by debt, job insecurity, and lack of insurance. It is during times of crisis such as war, disasters, assaults, and social breakdown that safety needs really take precedence. Children, who are more vulnerable and dependent, respond far more readily and intensely to safety threats.
- *Belongingness and love needs.* People have a need for an intimate relationship, love, affection, and belonging and will seek to overcome feelings of aloneness and alienation. Maslow stresses the importance of having a family, a home, and being part of identifiable groups.
- *Esteem needs.* People need to have a high self-regard and have it reflected to them from others. If self-esteem needs are met, we feel confident, valued, and valuable. When self-esteem is compromised, we feel inferior, worthless, and helpless.
- *Self-actualization.* We are preset to strive to be everything that we are capable of becoming. Maslow said, "What a man *can* be, he *must* be." What we are capable of becoming is highly individual—an artist must paint, a writer must write, and a healer must heal. The drive to satisfy this need is felt as a sort of restlessness, a sense that something is missing. It is up

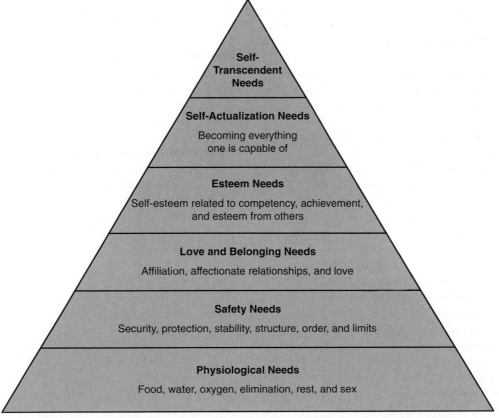

Figure 3-2 ■ Maslow's hierarchy of needs. (Adapted from Maslow, A.H. [1972]. *The farther reaches of human nature.* New York: Viking.)

to each person to choose a path that will bring about inner peace and fulfillment.

Although Maslow's early work included only five levels of needs, he later took into account two additional factors, (1) cognitive needs (the desire to know and understand), and (2) aesthetic needs (Maslow, 1970). He describes the acquisition of knowledge (first) and the need to understand (second) as being hard-wired and essential. Furthermore, he identified aesthetic needs as a craving for beauty and symmetry as universal.

Theory of Object Relations

The theory of object relations was developed by interpersonal theorists who emphasize past relationships in influencing a person's sense of self as well as the nature and quality of relationships in the present. The term *object* refers to another person, particularly a significant person.

Margaret Mahler (1895-1985), was a Hungarian-born child psychologist who worked with emotionally disturbed children. She developed a framework for looking at how an infant goes from complete self-absorption with an inability to itself as separate from its mother, to a physically and psychologically differentiated toddler. Mahler believed that psychological problems were largely the result of a disruption of this separation. Her most famous work is *The Psychological Birth of the Human Infant: Symbiosis and Individuation*, in which she describes the process of psychological separation between mother and child (Mahler et al., 1975).

Mahler emphasized the role of the significant other (traditionally the mother) in providing a secure, psychic base of support that promotes enough confidence for the child to separate. This base of support is achieved by a balance of holding (emotionally and physically) a child enough for the child to feel safe, while at the same time fostering and encouraging independence and natural exploration. The overlapping phases of separation-individuation occur during the first 3 years.

Problems may arise in this separation-individuation. If a toddler leaves his or her mother on the park bench and wanders off to the sandbox, the action ideally should be accompanied by two things. First, the child should be encouraged to set off into the world with smiles and reassurance, "Go on honey, it's safe to go away a little." Second, the mother needs to be reliably present when the toddler returns, thereby rewarding his or her efforts. Clearly parents are not perfect and are sometimes distracted and short tempered. Mahler notes that raising healthy children does not require that parents never make mistakes, and that "good enough parenting" will promote successful separation-individuation.

Theories of Moral Development
Stages of Moral Development

Lawrence Kohlberg (1927-1987) was an American psychologist whose work reflected and expanded on Piaget's by applying his theory to moral development, a development that coincided with cognitive development (Crain, 1985). While visiting Israel, Kohlberg became convinced that children living in a kibbutz had advanced moral development, and he believed that the atmosphere of trust, respect, and self-governance nurtured this development. On returning to the United States, he created schools, or "just communities" that were based on these concepts. Based on interviews with youths, Kohlberg developed a theory of how people progressively develop a sense of morality (Kohlberg & Turiel, 1971).

He viewed moral development in terms of three levels and six stages that continue throughout the life span. His theory provides a framework for understanding the progression from black-and-white thinking about right and wrong to a complex, variable, and context-dependent decision-making process regarding the rightness or wrongness of action.

Pre-Conventional Level
Stage 1: Obedience and Punishment. The hallmarks of this stage are a focus on rules and on listening to authority. People at this stage believe that obedience is the method to avoid punishment.

Stage 2: Individualism and Exchange. Individuals become aware that not everyone thinks the way that they do, and that rules are seen differently by different people. If they or others decide to break the rules, they are risking punishment.

Conventional Level
Stage 3: Good Interpersonal Relationships. At this stage people begin to view rightness or wrongness as related to motivations, personality, or the goodness or badness of the person. Generally speaking, people should get along and have similar values.

Stage 4: Maintaining the Social Order. At this stage, a "rules are rules" mindset returns. However, the reasoning behind it is not simply to avoid punishment, it is because the person has begun to adopt a broader view of society. Listening to authority maintains the social order; bureau-

TABLE 3-4	Gilligan's Stages of Moral Development	
Stage	**Goal**	**Action**
Pre-conventional	Goal is individual survival—selfishness	Caring for self
Conventional	Self sacrifice is goodness—responsibility to others	Caring for others
Post-conventional	Principle of nonviolence—do not hurt others or self	Balancing caring for self with caring for others

cracies and big government agencies often seem to operate with this tenet.

Post-Conventional Level

Stage 5: Social Contract and Individual Rights. As an extension of the previous stage, people in stage 5 still believe that the social order is important, but the social order must be *good*. For example, if the social order is corrupt, then rules should be changed and it is a duty to protect the rights of others.

Stage 6: Universal Ethical Principles. Actions should create justice for everyone involved. We are obliged to break unjust laws.

Ethics of Care Theory

Carol Gilligan (b. 1936) is an American psychologist, ethicist, and feminist who inspired the normative ethics of care theory. She worked with Kohlberg as he developed his theory of moral development and later criticized his work for being based on a sample of boys and men. Additionally, she believed that he used a scoring method that favored males' methods of reasoning, resulting in a finding that girls reach lower levels of moral development than do boys. Based on Gilligan's critique, Kohlberg later revised his scoring methods, which resulted in girls' and boys' scores evening out.

Gilligan's 1982 book, *In a Different Voice: Psychological Theory and Women's Development,* suggests that a morality of care should replace Kohlberg's "justice view" of morality, which holds that we should do what is right no matter the personal cost or the cost to those we love. Gilligan's "care view" emphasizes the importance of relationships, banding together, and putting the needs of those for whom we care above the needs of strangers. Gilligan asserts that a female approach to ethics has always been in existence but has been trivialized due to women's traditional positions of limited power and influence. Like Kohlberg, Gilligan asserts that moral development progresses through three major divisions: pre-conventional, conventional, and

post-conventional. These transitions are not dictated by cognitive ability, but rather through personal development and changes in a sense of self (Table 3-4).

MODELS, THEORIES, AND THERAPIES IN CURRENT PRACTICE

Biological Model

The dominant model for psychiatric care is the biological model, in which mental disorders are believed to have physical causes; therefore, mental disorders will respond to physical treatment. Interestingly, Sigmund Freud himself researched neurological causes for mental illness and considered cocaine a possible treatment. (He abandoned this research because of its obvious downside, and focused on talk therapy.)

In the 1950s a surgeon noticed that patients waiting for surgery were calmed by the administration of chlorpromazine (Thorazine); it soon became widely used for the treatment of schizophrenia and dramatically reduced the use of restraint and seclusion. This discovery spurred the development of other drug-based treatments and the adoption of a chemical imbalance theory of mental disorders.

If chemical imbalances exist, how do they come about? Research through twin studies has been useful to support the genetic transmission of certain disorders. Whereas only 1% of the population has schizophrenia, among identical twins the concordance rate (the percent of the time that both twins will be affected) is 40% to 65% (Cardno & Gottesman, 2000). Although this indicates genetic involvement, it can't be the whole story. If it were, the concordance rate of schizophrenia in identical twins would be 100%. It is likely that the environment exerts an influence on the developing embryo or child. Research has shown that toxins, viruses, hostile environments, and brain traumas have been proposed as catalysts for the development of psychiatric disorders (see Chapter 4).

Biological Therapy

Psychopharmacology is the primary biological treatment for mental disorders. (Refer to Chapter 4 for a full discussion of the biological basis for understanding psychopharmacology.) Major classifications of medications are antidepressants, antipsychotics, antianxiety agents, mood stabilizers, and psychostimulants. Clinicians recognize the importance of optimizing other biological variables, such as correcting hormone levels (as in hypothyroidism), regulating nutritionally deficient diets, and balancing inadequate sleep patterns. (Refer to Chapters 8 through 16 for relevant uses of psychopharmacology.)

Electroconvulsive therapy (ECT) has proven to be an effective treatment for severe depression and other psychiatric conditions. ECT is a procedure that uses electrical current to induce a seizure, and is thought to work by affecting neurotransmitters and neuroreceptors (see Chapter 12 for more discussion regarding ECT).

Most mental health professionals make use of talk therapy in conjunction with biological approaches. Research indicates that the combination of medication and cognitive behavioral therapy is an extremely effective treatment for many psychiatric disorders, especially major depression (Keller et al., 2000). If a hostile environment can bring about negative brain chemistry or transmission, then a positive environment may reverse and improve the process.

Nursing Model

The name most commonly associated with psychiatric nursing is Hildegard Peplau (1909-1999). Her seminal work, *Interpersonal Relationships in Nursing*, was first published in 1952 and has served as a foundation for understanding and conducting therapeutic nursing relationships ever since. Peplau based her work on Sullivan's interpersonal theory and emphasized that the nature of the nurse-patient relationship strongly influenced the outcome for the patient.

Peplau made an extremely useful contribution to understanding anxiety by conceptualizing the four levels still in use today:

1. Mild anxiety is day-to-day, "I'm awake and taking care of business" alertness. Stimuli in the environment are perceived and understood, and learning can easily take place.
2. Moderate anxiety is felt as a heightened sense of awareness, such as when you're about to take an exam. The perceptual field is narrowed and an individual hears, sees, and understands less. Learning can still take place, although it may require more direction.
3. Severe anxiety interferes with clear thinking and the perceptual field is greatly diminished. Nearly all behavior is directed at reducing the anxiety. An example of this is your response to skidding on wet pavement.
4. Panic anxiety is overwhelming and results in either paralysis or dangerous hyperactivity. An individual cannot communicate, function, or follow direction. This is the sort of anxiety that is associated with the terror of panic attacks.

Refer to Chapter 8 for application of these levels to the nursing process.

One of the most useful constructs of Peplau's theory is in providing structure for how we view the therapeutic relationship, which she divided into four phases. Each of these overlapping and interlocking phases includes tasks, the expression of needs by the patient, and the interventions facilitated by the nurse.

Preinteraction Phase

This phase occurs before the patient and nurse meet. Perhaps you have received your shift assignment, heard report, and read the chart. You find that your patient is recovering from a drug overdose and hasn't been paying child support for three small children. It is important to be aware of your own biases and preconceived notions. If, for example, your own father was an alcoholic who neglected your family, you need to recognize your feeling and seek to respond objectively to the patient as a unique person and not as an extension of your father.

Orientation (Introductory) Phase

During this phase, the patient and nurse meet and determine what the other would like to be called, and contract for time (how often to meet, length of meetings, and termination). This phase is accompanied by anxiety for both the patient and nurse. The patient commonly tests the nurse's strength and integrity. Ideally, trust and unconditional positive regard, or rapport, are beginning to be established. The nurse assesses the patient's strengths and weaknesses, formulates nursing diagnoses, and together with the patient, establishes goals.

Working Phase
Identification Subphase

During the first part of the working phase, the patient begins to identify with the nurse, and trust and rapport are maintained. The patient is able to identify problems, but may resist working on them, particularly if it requires abandoning comfortable old defenses. If the nurse is able to facilitate the safe expression of feelings, then it is possible for the patient to grow from the experience of illness.

Exploitation Subphase

The patient is encouraged to exploit (or make use of) all available services, depending on the level of need. Growth is evident as the patient becomes more independent and tests newfound skills in communicating.

Termination (Resolution) Phase

The final phase of the nurse-patient relationship is accompanied by some feelings of loss and anxiety. These feelings are explored and accepted. Goals have been achieved, and the patient is stronger and able to stand alone without the need for identification with "helping persons" (Peplau, 1992). Together, the nurse and patient review the patient's progress. The patient is able to reject some maladaptive patterns and aspires to new goals. Plans should be made for sources of support and coping methods (see Chapter 7).

Historical Influences

Although it is clear that Peplau's work is relevant to psychiatric nursing, the other theories and therapies presented earlier in this chapter also are relevant. Nurses constantly borrow concepts and carry out interventions that are supported by these models. Some examples of how they may be used are as follows:

- **Behavioral:** Promoting adaptive behaviors through reinforcement can be valuable and important in working with patients, especially when working with a pediatric population. These patients look forward to positive reinforcement for good behavior and will work hard for gold stars or privileges to go off the unit.
- **Cognitive:** Helping patients identify negative thought patterns is a worthwhile intervention in promoting healthy functioning and improving neurochemistry. Workbooks are available to aid in the process of identifying these cognitive distortions.
- **Psychosocial development:** Erikson's theory provides structure for understanding critical junctures in development. The older adult gentleman who has suffered a stroke may be depressed and despairing because he can no longer take care of his house. In this case the nurse and patient could explore ways of optimizing the patient's remaining strengths and talents, such as in nurturing and tutoring young people and developing attainable and progressive goals like working toward walking well enough to get the mail, and then to take out the trash, and so forth.
- **Hierarchy of needs:** Maslow's work is useful in prioritizing nursing care. When working with an actively suicidal patient, students sometimes think it is rude to ask if the patient is thinking about killing him- or

herself. However, safety supersedes this potential threat to self-esteem. Although the "must do's" in nursing begin with physical care, tending to the most important aspects such as medicating and hydrating through IV fluids, the goal should be to also include the higher levels by listening, observing, through touch, and collaboration with the patient in the development of the plan of care.

Therapies for Specific Populations

Group Therapy

We live and work in groups every day including our families, friends, and colleagues. Group therapy provides a formal setting for this influence to occur. This therapeutic method is commonly derived from interpersonal theory and operates under the assumption that interaction among participants can provide support or bring about desired change among individual participants.

"A **group** is defined as (a) a gathering of two or more individuals (b) who share a common purpose and (c) meet over a substantial time period (d) in face-to-face interaction (e) to achieve an identifiable goal" (Arnold & Boggs, 2007, p. 261). The ideal size of the group varies from expert to expert, but it is usually somewhere from 6 to 10 members. A group that is too small will limit diversity of opinion and put pressure on members to participate. Overly large groups reduce the members' ability to share, especially if some members dominate the group.

Setting

Settings for groups are important. The room should be private, and the seating should be comfortable. Because it is important for people to see one another, a circle is the preferred arrangement. Using tables is discouraged because they can be psychological barriers between group members. One of the worst arrangements for discussion is the traditional "classroom seating" with everyone facing a central speaker, thereby limiting free interaction among participants.

Groups possess both content and process dimensions. **Group content** refers to the actual dialogue between members or the type of information that can be transcribed (written down) in minutes of meetings. **Group process** includes all the other elements of human interaction, such as nonverbal communication, adaptive and maladaptive roles, energy flow, power plays, conflict, hidden agendas, and silences. Although the content is essential to the group's work, it is the process that becomes the real challenge for leaders as well as participants.

Group development tends to follow a sequential pattern of growth and requires less leadership with time. Under-

TABLE 3-5	**Tuckman's Stages of Group Development and Comparable Life Phase**

Stage	Comparable Life Phase	Description
Forming	Infancy	The task and/or purpose of the group is defined. Connecting with others, desiring acceptance, and avoiding conflict define early groups. Members gather commonalities and differences as they attempt to know one another. The leader is the main connection and necessary for direction.
Storming	Adolescence	Important issues are being addressed, and conflict begins to surface. Personal relations may interfere with the task at hand. Some members will dominate, and some will be silent. Rules and structure are helpful. Members may challenge the role of the leader who has the opportunity to model adaptive behavior.
Norming	Early adulthood	Members know one another, and rules of engagement (norms) are evident. There is a sense of group identity and cohesion. Members resist change, which could lead to a group breakup or a return to the discomfort of storming. Leadership is shared.
Performing	Mature adulthood	Groups who reach this stage are characterized by loyalty, flexibility, interdependence, and productivity. There is a balance between focus on work and focus on the welfare of group members.
Adjourning (mourning)	Older adult years	Groups in this stage are ready to disband, tasks are terminated, and relationships are disengaged. Accomplishments are recognized and members are pleased to have been part of the group. A sense of loss is an inevitable consequence.

From Tuckman, B.W., & Jensen, M.A. (1977). Stages of small-group development revisited. *Group & Organization Management, 2,* 419-427.

standing this pattern is especially helpful to the leader in order to anticipate distinct phases and provide guidance and interventions that are most effective. Tuckman (1965) proposed a model of group development composed of four stages: forming, storming, norming, and performing. A fifth stage, adjourning (mourning), was later added (Tuckman & Jensen, 1977). These stages are comparable to human development from infancy into old age, accompanied by varying levels of maturity, confidence, and need for direction (Table 3-5).

Roles of Group Members

Studies of group dynamics have identified informal roles of members that are necessary to develop a successful group. The most common descriptive categories for these roles are task, maintenance, and individual roles (Buffum & Madrid, 2003). Task roles serve to keep the group focused and see to the business at hand. Maintenance roles function to keep the group together and provide interpersonal support. There are also individual roles that can interfere with the group's functioning because they are not related to the group goals, but rather to specific personalities. Table 3-6 describes roles of group members.

Roles of the Group Leader

The group leader has multiple responsibilities in starting, maintaining, and terminating a group. In the initial phase, the leader defines the structure, size, composition, purpose, and timing for the group. Task and maintenance functions may be discussed and demonstrated. To maintain the group, the leader facilitates communication and ensures that meetings start and end on time. In the termination phase, the leader ensures that each member summarizes individual accomplishments and gives positive and negative feedback regarding the group experience.

Leadership style depends on group type (Jacobs et al., 2005). A leader selects the style that is best suited to the therapeutic needs of a particular group. The **autocratic leader** exerts control over the group and does not encourage much interaction among members. In contrast, the **democratic leader** supports extensive group interaction in the process of problem solving. A **laissez-faire leader** allows the group members to behave in any way that they choose and does not attempt to control the direction of the group. For example, staff leading a community meeting with a fixed, time-limited agenda may tend to be more autocratic. In a psychoeducational group, the leader

TABLE 3-6   Roles of Group Members

Role	Function
Task Roles	
Coordinator	Connects various ideas and suggestions
Initiator-contributor	Offers new ideas or a new outlook on an issue
Elaborator	Gives examples and follows up meaning of ideas
Energizer	Encourages the group to make decisions or take action
Evaluator	Measures the group's work against a standard
Information/Opinion giver	Shares opinions, especially to influence group values
Orienter	Notes the progress of the group toward goals
Maintenance Roles	
Compromiser	In a conflict, yields to preserve group harmony
Encourager	Praises and seeks input from others; warm and accepting
Follower	Attentive listener and integral to the group
Gatekeeper	Ensures participation, encourages participation, points out commonality of thought
Harmonizer	Mediates conflicts constructively among members
Standard setter	Assesses explicit and implicit standards for the group
Individual Roles	
Aggressor	Criticizes and attacks others' ideas and feelings
Blocker	Disagrees with group issues, opposes others, stalls the process
Help seeker	Asks for sympathy of group excessively, self-deprecating
Playboy/Playgirl	Distracts others from the task; jokes, introduces irrelevant topics
Recognition seeker	Seeks attention by boasting and discussing achievements
Monopolizer	Dominates the conversation, thereby preventing equal input
Special interest pleader	Advocates for a special group, usually with own prejudice or bias

Data from Benne, K., & Sheats, P. (1948). Functional roles of group members. *Journal of Social Issues*, *4*(2), 41.

may be more democratic to encourage members to share their experiences. In a creative group such as an art or horticulture group, the leader may choose a laissez-faire style, giving minimal direction to allow for a variety of responses.

Types of Groups

Education groups form for the purpose of imparting information and require active expert leadership and careful planning. Task groups are typically time limited and have a common goal, and the role of the leader is to facilitate team building and cooperation. Support groups bring together people with common concerns and may be facilitated by a supportive leader or by group members. Therapy groups are led by professional group therapists whose styles may range from a directive and confrontational approach to a more hands-off, let the group members learn from each other, approach.

Benefits of Group Therapy

One of the commonly cited benefits of group therapy as compared to individual therapy is that the former is more efficient, both pragmatically and financially, because many people can engage in therapy at once. However, it is the nature of the interaction between people with common concerns and frames of references that seems to provide the greatest benefit. Yalom (1985) identified 11 benefits, or **curative factors**, of group membership (Table 3-7).

Roles of Nurses

Psychiatric mental health nurses are involved in a variety of therapeutic groups in acute care and long-term treatment settings. For all group leaders, a clear theoretical framework is necessary to provide a structure to understand the group interaction. Co-leadership of groups is a common practice and has several benefits: it provides training for less experienced staff; it allows for immediate feedback between the leaders after each session; and it gives two role models for teaching communication skills to members.

Basic level registered nurses have biopsychosocial educational backgrounds and are ideally suited to teach a variety of health subjects. *Psychoeducational groups* are set up to teach about a specific somatic or psychological subject;

TABLE 3-7	Yalom's Curative Factors of Group Membership	
Curative Factor	**Definition**	**Example**
Altruism	Giving appropriate help to other members	"We've spent all this time talking about me. Lou needs to talk about his visit with his dad. Let's focus on him."
Cohesiveness	Feeling connected to other members and belonging to the group	"People in our group always listen to each other. We've been polite since the first day."
Interpersonal learning	Learning from other members	"Sammi said it takes 2 weeks for Prozac to really work. I should give it more time."
Guidance	Receiving help and advice	"I've also have had that feeling where I just had to have a drink, Don. Just pick up the phone and call me next time it happens."
Catharsis	Releasing feelings and emotions	A new mother of twins begins to cry and says, "It sounds terrible, but sometimes I wish I'd never had children."
Identification	Modeling after member or leader	David notices that the leader projects confidence by speaking clearly, making good eye contact, and sitting up straight. David does the same.
Family reenactment	Testing new behaviors in a safe environment	"I learned to always smile and agree so Dad wouldn't go off on me. I don't have to be cheery and I can speak my mind here."
Self-understanding	Gaining personal insights	Dale realizes that his negativity has kept him from getting the friends he wants.
Instillation of hope	Feeling hopeful about one's life	"Sue has managed to stay sober for 2 years. I think I can do this."
Universality	Feeling that one is not alone	Aaron, a quiet group member finally comments, "My son has schizophrenia, too, and it helps to hear that other people have the same worries I do."
Existential factors	Coming to understand what life is about	"I guess I've been obsessing about being a perfect housekeeper and haven't noticed that my children are growing up without me."

From Yalom, I.D. (1985). *The theory and practice of group psychotherapy.* New York: Basic Books.

they also allow members to communicate about emotional concerns. These groups may be time limited or may be supportive for long-term treatment. Generally, written handouts or audiovisual aids are used to focus on specific teaching points. The following psychoeducational groups are commonly led by nurses:

- **Medication education groups** allow patients to hear the experiences of others who have taken medication and have an opportunity to ask questions without the fear that they will go against the prescriber's recommendations.
- **Dual-diagnosis groups** focus on co-occurring psychiatric illness and substance abuse. The RN may co-lead this group with a dual-diagnosis specialist (master's level clinician). The goal is to engage patients in treatment and to decrease their use of substances in a step-by-step process.
- **Multifamily groups** have evidence-based support as an effective method within the severely mentally ill

population (Dyck et al., 2002). The focus is on education about the mental illness and strategies for the family to cope with long-term disability.

- **Symptom management groups** are designed for patients with a common problem such as anger or psychosis to share coping skills. Self-control is improved and relapse is reduced by helping patients to develop a plan for action at the first sign of losing control.
- **Stress management groups** teach members about various relaxation techniques, including deep breathing, exercise, music, and spirituality.
- **Self-care groups** focus on basic hygiene issues such as bathing and grooming.

Advanced practice registered nurses (APRNs) may lead any of the groups described earlier as well as psychotherapy groups. Psychotherapy groups require specialized training in techniques that allow for deep disclosure, sharing, confrontation, and healing among participants.

Therapeutic Milieu

A therapeutic milieu, or healthy environment combined with a healthy social structure, within an inpatient setting or structured outpatient clinic such as partial hospitalization, is essential to supporting and treating those with mental illness. Within these small versions of society at large, people are safe to try out new behaviors and increase their ability to interact adaptively within the outside community.

Community meetings usually include all patients and the treatment team, which meets frequently to discuss common goals. Functions include orienting new members to the unit, encouraging patients to engage in treatment, and evaluating the treatment program. Nursing staff are the largest group of providers and give valuable feedback to the team about group interactions. Goal-setting meetings may be conducted in inpatient settings and partial hospitalization programs to plan daily goals for each patient to achieve.

Other therapeutic milieu groups aim to help increase patients' self-esteem, decrease social isolation, encourage appropriate social behaviors, and educate patients in basic living skills. These groups are often led by occupational or recreational therapists, although nurses frequently co-lead them. Examples of therapeutic milieu groups are recreational groups, physical activity groups, creative arts groups, and storytelling groups.

Family Therapy

Family therapy is a relatively new development that came about in the mid-twentieth century as an adjunct to individual treatment and refers to the treatment of the family as a whole. Family therapists use a wide variety of theoretical philosophies and techniques to bring about change in dysfunctional patterns of behavior and interaction. Some therapists may focus on the here and now, whereas others may rely more heavily on the family's history and reports of what happened between sessions. Most family therapists use an eclectic approach, drawing on a variety of techniques to fit the particular personality and strengths of the family (Box 3-2).

Although different therapists may adhere to different theories and use a wide variety of methods, the goals of family therapy are basically the same. These goals include the following (Nichols, 2004):

- To reduce dysfunctional behavior of individual family members
- To resolve or reduce intrafamily relationship conflicts
- To mobilize family resources and encourage adaptive family problem-solving behaviors
- To improve family communication skills

BOX 3-2

Central Concepts to Family Therapy

- **Boundaries: Clear boundaries** maintain distinctions between individuals within the family and between the family and the outside world. Clear boundaries allow for balanced flow of energy between members. **Diffuse** or **enmeshed boundaries** are those in which there is a blending of the roles, thoughts, and feelings of the individuals so that clear distinctions among family members fail to emerge. **Rigid** or **disengaged boundaries** are those in which the rules and roles are adhered to no matter what.
- **Triangulation:** The tendency, when two-person relationships are stressful and unstable, to draw in a third person to stabilize the system through formation of a coalition in which two members are pitted against a third.
- **Scapegoating:** A form of displacement in which a family member (usually the least powerful) is blamed for another family member's distress. The purpose is to keep the focus off the painful issues and the problems of the blamers.
- **Double bind:** A double bind is a no-win situation in which you are "darned if you do, darned if you don't."
- **Hierarchy:** The function of power and its structures in families, differentiating parental and sibling roles and generational boundaries.
- **Differentiation:** The ability to develop a strong identity and sense of self while maintaining an emotional connectedness with one's family of origin.
- **Sociocultural context:** The framework for viewing the family in terms of the influence of gender, race, ethnicity, religion, economic class, and sexual orientation.
- **Multigenerational issues:** The continuation and persistence from generation to generation of certain emotional interactive family patterns (e.g., reenactment of fairly predictable patterns; repetition of themes or toxic issues; and repetition of reciprocal patterns such as those of overfunctioner and underfunctioner).

- To heighten awareness and sensitivity to other family members' emotional needs and help family members meet their needs
- To strengthen the family's ability to cope with major life stressors and traumatic events, including chronic physical or psychiatric illness
- To improve integration of the family system into the societal system (e.g., school, medical facilities, workplace, and especially the extended family)

KEY POINTS TO REMEMBER

- Theoretical models and therapeutic strategies provide a useful framework for the delivery of psychiatric nursing care.
- The psychoanalytic model is based on unconscious motivations and the dynamic interplay between the primitive brain (id), the sense of self (ego), and the conscience (superego). The focus of psychoanalytic theory is on understanding the unconscious mind.
- The behavioral model suggests that because behavior is learned, behavioral therapy should improve behavior through rewards and reinforcement of adaptive behavior.
- The cognitive model posits that disorders, especially depression, are the result of faulty thinking. Cognitive behavioral therapy is effective and empirically supported and focuses on helping people recognize distorted thinking and replace it with more accurate and positive thoughts.
- The humanistic model is based on the notion of human potential, and therapy is aimed at maximizing this potential. Abraham Maslow, a humanist, developed a theory of personality that is based on the hierarchical satisfaction of needs.
- The interpersonal model maintains that the personality and disorders are created by social forces and interpersonal experiences. Interpersonal therapy aims to provide positive and repairing interpersonal experiences.

- The biological model is currently the dominant model and focuses on physical causation for personality problems and psychiatric disorders. Medication is the primary biological therapy.
- Developmental theories provide general guidelines for expected progression throughout the life span. Major developmental theories focus on stage-specific tasks, the attainment of a separate sense of self, cognitive maturation, and moral maturity.
- Hildegard Peplau developed an interpersonal theory for providing nursing care that has particular relevance for the provision of psychiatric nursing care.
- Group therapy offers the patient significant interpersonal feedback from multiple people.
- Groups develop through predictable stages, benefit from therapeutic factors, and are characterized by members filling specific roles.
- Psychoeducational groups and milieu groups are often led by nurses and provide significant treatment as part of the multidisciplinary treatment plan.
- Family therapy is based on various theoretical models and aims to decrease emotional reactivity among family members and encourage differentiation among individual family members.

CRITICAL THINKING

1. What influences can or do the theorists discussed in this chapter have on your practice of nursing? Specifically:
   A. How do Freud's concepts of the conscious, preconscious, and unconscious affect your understanding of patients' behaviors?
   B. Are Erikson's psychosocial stages a sound basis for identifying disruptions in stages of development in some of your patients? Can you give a clinical example?
   C. What are the implications of Sullivan's focus on the importance of interpersonal relationships for your interactions with patients?
   D. Peplau believed that nurses must exercise self-awareness within the nurse-patient relationship. Describe situations in your student experience in which this self-awareness played a vital role in your relationship(s) with patient(s).
   E. Can you think of anyone who seems to be self-actualized? What is your reason for this conclusion? What characteristics does this person have that make you think he or she is a self-actualized individual? How do you make use of Maslow's hierarchy of needs in your nursing practice?
   F. What do you think about the behaviorist point of view that to change behaviors is to change personality?
2. Which of the therapies described here do you think can be the most helpful to you in your nursing practice? What are your reasons for this choice?

CHAPTER REVIEW

Choose the most appropriate answer.

1. Which of the following contributions to modern psychiatric nursing practice was made by Freud?
    1. The theory of personality structure and levels of awareness
    2. The concept of a "self-actualized personality"
    3. The thesis that culture and society exert significant influence on personality
    4. Provision of a developmental model that includes the entire life span
2. The theory of interpersonal relationships developed by Hildegard Peplau is based on the foundation provided by which of the following early theorists?
    1. Freud
    2. Piaget
    3. Sullivan
    4. Maslow
3. The concepts at the heart of Sullivan's theory of personality are:

1. needs and anxiety.
2. basic needs and meta-needs.
3. schemata, assimilation, and accommodation.
4. developmental tasks and psychosocial crises.

4. The premise that an individual's behavior and affect are largely determined by the attitudes and assumptions the person has developed about the world underlies:
    1. modeling.
    2. milieu therapy.
    3. cognitive therapy.
    4. psychoanalytic psychotherapy.
5. Providing a safe environment for patients with impaired cognition, referring an abused spouse to a "safe house," and conducting a community meeting are nursing interventions that address aspects of:
    1. milieu therapy.
    2. cognitive therapy.
    3. behavioral therapy.
    4. interpersonal psychotherapy.

REFERENCES

Arnold, E., & Boggs, K.U. (2007). *Interpersonal relationships: Professional communication skills for nurses* (5th ed.). St. Louis: Saunders.

Beck, A.T. (1963). Thinking and depression. *Archives of General Psychiatry, 9,* 324-333.

Benne, K., & Sheats, P. (1948). Functional roles of group members. *Journal of Social Issues, 4*(2), 41.

Buffum, M., & Madrid, E. (2003). Group therapy. In D. Antai-Otong (Ed.), *Psychiatric nursing: Biological & behavioral concepts.* New York: Thomson Delmar Learning.

Burns, D.D. (1989). *The feeling good handbook.* New York: William Morrow.

Cardno, A.G., & Gottesman, II. (2000). Twin studies of schizophrenia: From bow-and-arrow concordances to star wars Mx and functional genomics. *American Journal of Medical Genetics, 97*(1), 12-7.

Crain, W.C. (1985). *Theories of development* (2nd ed.). Englewood Cliffs, NJ: Prentice-Hall.

Dyck, D.G., Hendryx, M.S., Short, R.A., et al. (2002). Service use among patients with schizophrenia in psycho-educational multiple-family group treatment. *Psychiatric Services, 53,* 749-754.

Erikson, E. (1963). *Childhood and society.* New York: Norton.

Freud, S. (1961). The ego and id. In J. Strachey (Ed. and Trans.), *The standard edition of the complete psychological works of Sigmund Freud* (vol. 19, pp. 3-66). London: Hogarth Press. (Original work published 1923.)

Gilligan, C. (1982). *In a different voice: Psychological theory and women's development.* Cambridge: Harvard University Press.

Jacobs, E. E., Masson, R.L., & Harvill, R.L. (2005). *Group counseling: Strategies and skills.* Pacific Grove, CA: Brooks/Cole.

Keller, M.B., McCullough, J.P., Klein, D.N., et al. (2000). A comparison of nefazodone, the cognitive behavioral-analysis system of psychotherapy, and their combination for the treatment of chronic depression. *New England Journal of Medicine, 342,* 1462-1470.

Kohlberg, L., & Turiel, E. (1971). Moral development and moral education. In G. S. Lesser (Ed.), *Psychology and educational practice.* Glenview, IL: Scott Foresman.

Leichsenring, F, & Leibing, E. (2003). The effectiveness of psychodynamic therapy and cognitive behavior therapy in the treatment of personality disorders: A meta-analysis. *American Journal of Psychiatry, 160,* 1223-1232.

Mahler, M.S., Pine, F., & Bergman, A. (1975). *The psychological birth of the human infant.* New York: Basic Books.

Maslow, A.H. (1970). *Motivation and personality* (2nd ed.). New York: Harper and Row.

Nichols, M.P. (2004). *Family therapy: Concepts and methods* (6th ed.). New York: Pearson Education.

Pavlov, I.P. (1927). *Conditioned reflexes.* London: Routledge and Kegan Paul.

Peplau, H.E. (1992). *Interpersonal relations in nursing.* New York: Putnam.

Piaget, J., & Inhelder, B. (1969). *The psychology of a child.* New York: Basic Books.

Rogers, C.R. (1961). *On becoming a person: A therapist's view of psychotherapy.* Boston: Houghton Mifflin.

Skinner, B.F. (1938) *The behavior of organisms.* New York: Appleton-Century-Crofts.

Smith, L. (1997). Jean Piaget. In N. Sheehy, A. Chapman, & W. Conroy (Eds.), *Biographical dictionary of psychology.* London: Routledge.

Sullivan, H.S. (1953). *The interpersonal theory of psychiatry.* New York: Norton.

Thompson, R.F. (2005). In search of memory traces. *Annual Review of Psychology, 56,* 1-23.

Tuckman, B.W. (1965). Developmental sequence in small groups. *Psychological Bulletin, 63,* 384-399.

Tuckman, B.W., & Jensen, M.A. (1977). Stages of small-group development revisited. *Group & Organization Studies, 2,* 419-427.

Watson, J.B. (1930). *Behaviorism* (rev. ed.). Chicago: University of Chicago Press.

Yalom, I.D. (1985). *The theory and practice of group psychotherapy.* New York: Basic Books.

CHAPTER 4

Biological Basis for Understanding Psychopharmacology

Dorothy A. Varchol and John Raynor

Key Terms and Concepts

Objectives

1. Identify three major brain structures and three major brain functions that can be altered by mental illness and psychotropic medications.
2. Describe how neuroimaging techniques are used to identify brain structure and function.
3. Explain the basic process of neurotransmission.
4. Briefly identify the main neurotransmitters affected by the various psychotropic drugs (e.g., antipsychotics, antidepressants, and anxiolytics).
5. Compare and contrast the side effect profiles of the standard antipsychotic drugs with the side effect profiles of the atypical antipsychotic drugs.
6. Explain why a person taking a monoamine oxidase inhibitor would have dietary and drug restrictions.
7. Describe how genes and culture affect an individual's response to psychotropic medication.

continued

Whether conscious or unconscious, focused on the logical or filled with fantasy, all mental activity has its locus in the brain. Implied in the biological approach to psychiatric illness is the idea that although the origin of a psychiatric illness may be related to any number of factors (e.g., genetics, neurodevelopment factors, drugs, infections, psychosocial experience), there will eventually be an alteration in cerebral function that accounts for the disturbances in the patient's behavior and mental experience.

A primary goal of psychiatric mental health nursing is to understand the biological basis of both normal and abnormal brain function and apply this understanding to the care of individuals treated with drugs referred to as **psychotropic.** Because all brain functions are carried out by similar mechanisms (interactions of neurons), often in similar locations, it is not surprising that mental disturbances are frequently associated with alterations in other brain functions and that the drugs used to treat mental disturbances can also interfere with other activities of the brain. Box 4-1 summarizes some major activities for which the brain is responsible.

BOX 4-1

Functions of the Brain

- Monitor changes in the external world
- Monitor the composition of body fluids
- Regulate the contractions of the skeletal muscles
- Regulate the internal organs
- Initiate and regulate the basic drives: hunger, thirst, sex, aggressive self-protection
- Mediate conscious sensation
- Store and retrieve memories
- Regulate mood (affect) and emotions
- Think and perform intellectual functions
- Regulate the sleep cycle
- Produce and interpret language
- Process visual and auditory data

BRAIN STRUCTURES AND FUNCTIONS

The brain is composed of a vast network of interconnected and specialized nerve cells. These neurons and their supporting cells function to integrate the many and varied activities of the brain.

Cerebrum

The outermost, deeply convoluted covering of the cerebral hemispheres, the cerebral cortex, has four major lobes (Figure 4-1). The cerebrum is responsible for mental activities, conscious sense of being, conscious perception of the external world, emotional status, memory, and control of the skeletal muscles that allow the willful direction of movement. The cerebrum is also responsible for language and the ability to communicate.

Frontal Lobe

There are four subdivisions of the large **frontal** lobe. The first three—the motor strip, the supplemental motor area, and Broca's area—play a part in voluntary movement and language production. The fourth, the **prefrontal cortex (PFC),** is connected to all other brain regions to execute goal-directed activity. When circuitry in the PFC is impaired by a mental disorder, such as schizophrenia, there is a decrease in executive function, attention, impulse control, socialization, regulation of drives (e.g., sex), and emotions.

Newer atypical antipsychotic agents have been shown to improve an important aspect of executive function called working memory, and researchers continue to look for new drugs to improve attention so that tasks can be completed when the PFC network is disrupted. However, older typical, or traditional, antipsychotic agents and some atypicals may result in extrapyramidal side effects that necessitate treatment with anticholinergic medication, such as benztropine (Cogentin). Anticholinergics themselves can impair working

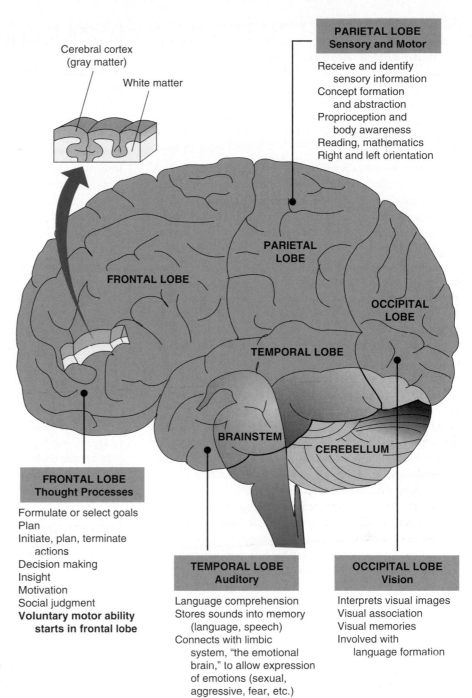

Figure 4-1 ■ The functions of the cerebral lobes: frontal, parietal, temporal, and occipital.

memory (Erickson et al., 2007), illustrating how both mental illness and pharmacotherapy may disrupt executive function.

Parietal Lobe

Individuals with working memory deficits have also demonstrated abnormal **parietal** cortex activation (Barch & Csernansky, 2007). Containing the primary sensory area

for touch, pressure, pain, and temperature, the parietal lobe is also involved in attention, spatial orientation, and language development. Both the frontal and parietal lobes are important for good decision making.

Occipital Lobe

At the back of the skull, the **occipital** lobe borders the parietal and temporal lobes. The occipital lobe contains the primary visual cortex and is mainly responsible for visual reception. It also contains association areas that help in the recognition of shapes and colors. The visual cortex is influenced by attentional and emotional modulation, which occurs in other brain regions such as the parietal or frontal regions or the amygdala (Vuilleumier & Driver, 2007).

Temporal Lobes

Below the frontal and parietal lobes, the **temporal** lobe is primarily concerned with sensory experience, but it also plays a role in memory processing and in emotion. The **hippocampus,** a curved sheet of cortex folded in the medial temporal lobe, interacts with the prefrontal areas in memory and learning. The hippocampus fails to develop adequately in schizophrenia and atrophies in recurrent unipolar or bipolar depression and in severe stress disorders such as posttraumatic stress disorder (PTSD). It also is damaged by the toxicity of alcohol addiction or Alzheimer's dementia (Nasrallah, 2007).

Stress management, as well as the use of antidepressants and atypical antipsychotic agents, is believed to increase the growth of neurons (neurogenesis) in the hippocampus by inducing **neurotrophic growth factors**, a diverse group of protein molecules released by postsynaptic cells that promote the growth or **plasticity** of presynaptic neurons. Nerve growth factor (NGF) and brain-derived neurotrophic factor (BDNF) are examples of neurotrophic growth factors that may help to prevent stress-induced suppression of neurogenesis in the hippocampus.

To achieve an appropriate level of hippocampal activity, another structure in the temporal lobe, the **amygdala,** plays a major role in memory and in processing fear and anxiety. The amygdala is hyperactive in excessive fearfulness, whereas loss of connection to the amygdala results in difficulty responding to a potential threat. The amygdala also sends signals that are reward related as occurs with the reinforcing effects of many drugs of abuse, including alcohol (Zhu et al., 2007).

The amygdala and hippocampus, along with the hypothalamus and thalamus, are part of a circle of structures called the **limbic system** or "emotional brain." Linking the frontal cortex, **basal ganglia**, and upper brainstem, the limbic system appears to house the emotional association areas and is implicated in what is termed the "four F's" of motivation: fighting, fleeing, feeding, and "sexual behavior" (Pinel, 2005). Processing of emotional signals in limbic brain regions can influence perception, attention, and memory. Emotional modulation can arise when emotionally significant stimuli, rather than strictly visual properties, influence the visual cortex (Vuillemier & Driver, 2007). Thus the limbic system is connected to higher brain regions in a highly integrated way. Antianxiety drugs (anxiolytics) slow the limbic system.

Subcortical Structures

In addition to the four lobes of the cerebrum, subcortical structures also affect brain function.

Basal Ganglia

The four subcortical basal ganglia that lie deep within the cerebrum are the striatum, the pallidum, the substantia nigra, and the subthalamic nucleus. This group of gray matter nuclei allows for a smooth integration of emotions, thoughts, and physical movement. The basal ganglia play a major role in motor responses via the extrapyramidal motor system, which relies on the neurotransmitter dopamine to maintain proper muscle tone and motor stability. It is important to remember that movement is regulated by the basal ganglia, including the diaphragm—essential for breathing—and the muscles of the throat, tongue, and mouth—essential for speech. Thus, drugs that affect brain function can stimulate or depress respiration or lead to slurred speech.

Thalamus

The **thalamus** is the major sensory relay station to the cortex. Abnormalities of the thalamus and changes in the gray matter bridge connecting the two thalamic lobes are thought to be central to the pathophysiology of schizophrenia (Ettinger et al., 2007).

Hypothalamus

The **hypothalamus** maintains homeostasis. It regulates temperature, blood pressure, perspiration, sexual drive, hunger, thirst, and **circadian rhythms**, such as sleep and wakefulness. Hypothalamic **neurohormones,** often called releasing hormones, direct the secretion of hormones from the anterior pituitary gland. For example, corticotropin-releasing hormone (CRH) is involved in the stress response. It stimulates the pituitary to release corticotropin, which in turn stimulates the cortex of each adrenal gland to secrete cortisol. This system is disrupted in mood disorders, PTSD, and dementia of the Alzheimer's type, but abnormalities in the system may be reversed by successful treatment with antidepressant medications (Sadock & Sadock, 2007).

The thyrotropin-releasing hormone (TRH) results in pituitary secretion of thyrotropin (thyroid-stimulation hormone or TSH), which in turn stimulates the thyroid gland release of thyroid hormones, thyroxine (T_4), and triiodothyronine (T_3). The hypothalamic-pituitary-thyroid

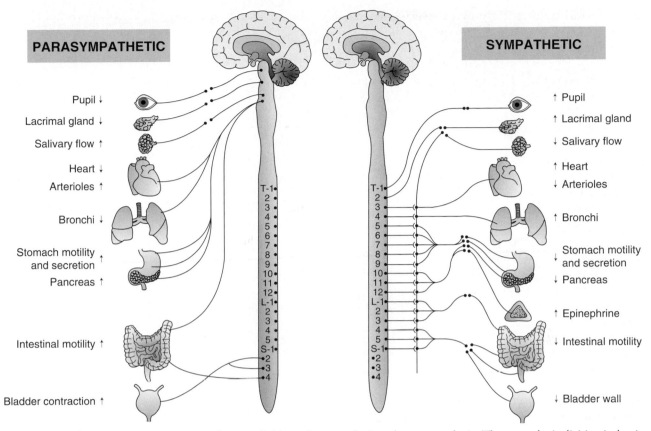

PARASYMPATHETIC

Pupil ↓
Lacrimal gland ↓
Salivary flow ↑
Heart ↓
Arterioles ↑
Bronchi ↓
Stomach motility and secretion ↑
Pancreas ↑
Intestinal motility ↑
Bladder contraction ↑

SYMPATHETIC

↑ Pupil
↑ Lacrimal gland
↓ Salivary flow
↑ Heart
↓ Arterioles
↑ Bronchi
↓ Stomach motility and secretion
↓ Pancreas
↑ Epinephrine
↓ Intestinal motility
↓ Bladder wall

Figure 4-2 ■ The autonomic nervous system has two divisions: the sympathetic and parasympathetic. The sympathetic division is dominant in stress situations, such as fear and anger—known as the fight-or-flight response.

axis is involved in the regulation of nearly every organ system because all major hormones and catecholamines (e.g., cortisol, gonadal hormones, insulin) depend on thyroid status. Thyroid hormones are used to treat people with depression or rapid cycling bipolar I disorder. They are also used as replacement therapy for people who developed a hypothyroid state from lithium treatment (Sadock & Sadock, 2007).

The hypothalamic regulation of prolactin secretion from the pituitary is different from the hypothalamic regulation of other pituitary hormones because the hypothalamic neurohormone, dopamine, primarily inhibits rather than stimulates the release of prolactin. When too much dopamine is blocked by standard antipsychotic drugs, blood prolactin levels increase (hyperprolactinemia) with subsequent amenorrhea, galactorrhea (milk flow), or gynecomastia (development of breast tissue).

In addition to working with the endocrine system to affect the function of internal organs, the hypothalamus sends instructions to the **autonomic nervous system,** divided into the **sympathetic and parasympathetic**

systems (Figure 4-2). The sympathetic system usually increases heart rate, respirations, and blood pressure to prepare for fight or flight, whereas the parasympathetic system slows the heart rate and begins the process of digestion. The sympathetic system is highly activated by sympathomimetic drugs, such as amphetamine and cocaine, as well as by withdrawal from sedating drugs, such as alcohol, benzodiazepines, and opioids (Sadock & Sadock, 2007).

Brainstem

Basic vital life functions occur through the brainstem, made up of the midbrain, pons, and medulla (Figure 4-3). Through projections called the **reticular activating system (RAS),** the brainstem sets the level of consciousness and regulates the cycle of sleep and wakefulness. Unfortunately, drugs used to treat psychiatric problems may interfere with the regulation of sleep and alertness, thus the warning to use caution while driving or to take sedating drugs at bedtime.

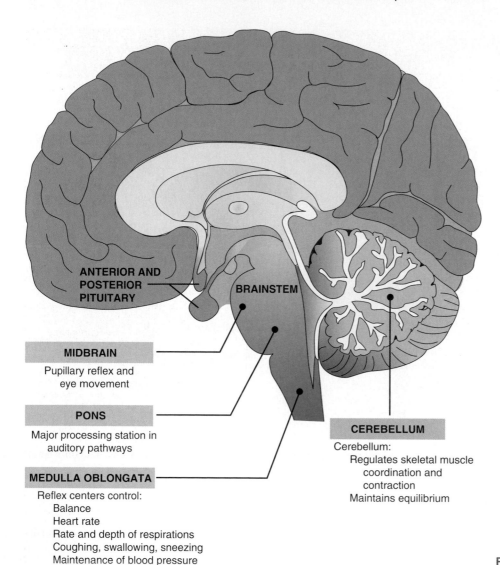

ANTERIOR AND POSTERIOR PITUITARY

BRAINSTEM

MIDBRAIN
Pupillary reflex and
eye movement

PONS
Major processing station in
auditory pathways

MEDULLA OBLONGATA
Reflex centers control:
    Balance
    Heart rate
    Rate and depth of respirations
    Coughing, swallowing, sneezing
    Maintenance of blood pressure
    Vomiting

CEREBELLUM
Cerebellum:
    Regulates skeletal muscle
        coordination and
        contraction
Maintains equilibrium

Figure 4-3 ■ The functions of the brainstem and cerebellum.

Cerebellum

Located posteriorly to the brainstem, the cerebellum (Figure 4-3) is primarily involved in balance and smooth muscle movement.

NEUROIMAGING OF BRAIN STRUCTURE AND FUNCTION

Table 4-1 identifies some **neuroimaging** techniques that measure structure, function, and chemistry in the brain. Structural imaging techniques are computed tomography (CT) and magnetic resonance imaging (MRI). CT scans use a series of x-rays to view brain structure, whereas MRI scans use a strong magnetic field and radio waves, distinguishing gray and white matter better than CT scans do.

In the past, research primarily focused on gray matter, where the neuronal cell bodies, dendrites, and synapses are located. Only recently has attention been given to white matter in schizophrenia.

The newer functional MRI (fMRI) shows brain function without contrast injections or invasive tests. However, functional neuroimaging with positron-emission tomography (PET), and the less expensive single photon emission computed tomography (SPECT), use radioactive material to assess regional brain glucose metabolism and to secure

TABLE 4-1	Common Brain Imaging Techniques		
Technique	**Description**	**Uses**	**Clinical Research Examples**
Structural: Show Gross Anatomical Details of Brain Structures			
Computed tomography (CT)	A series of x-rays of the head is taken, and a computer estimates how much x-ray is absorbed in a small cross section of the brain.	Most useful in early stages of brain injury to detect clots, hemorrhages, swelling	**Schizophrenia** Cortical atrophy Compensatory enlargement of the lateral and third ventricles
Magnetic resonance imaging (MRI)	Uses a magnetic field and radio waves rather than x-rays to produce cross-sectional images.	Most useful in later stages of recovery from brain injury when the patient is more stable and can remain motionless for up to 20 minutes	MRI measures same structures as CT, but has higher resolution and can visualize smaller brain lesions
Functional: Show Some Activity of the Brain			
Positron-emission tomography (PET)	Radioactive substance is injected, travels to the brain, and shows up as bright spots on a scan. Data relayed to a computer produce three-dimensional (3-D) images.	Looks directly at blood flow and indirectly at activity or metabolism in the working brain. Identifies which brain receptors are being activated by neurotransmitters and by drugs.	PET and SPECT: **Schizophrenia** Decreased metabolic activity in the frontal lobes, especially during tasks that require the prefrontal cortex (PFC) Dopamine system dysregulation
Single photon emission computed tomography (SPECT)	Radioactive substance is injected and is taken up by certain receptor sites in the brain, where a special gamma camera rotates around the patient and secures images of brain function.	Use is similar to PET. SPECT tracers are more limited in the kinds of brain activities they can monitor, but longer-lasting brain functions can be measured. SPECT is less costly, but resolution is poorer.	Blockade of dopamine receptors with antipsychotic medications **Depression** Loss of monoamines Blockade of serotonin transporter receptors with antidepressant medications Alzheimer's disease Reduction in nicotinic receptor subtype
Functional magnetic resonance imaging (fMRI)	Relies on magnetic properties to see images of blood flow in the brain as it occurs. Needs no radioactive materials and produces images at a higher resolution than PET.	Uses are similar to PET scans.	

images of brain function. PET scans have provided evidence of decreased metabolism in the frontal lobes of unmedicated individuals with depression or schizophrenia and increased metabolism in obsessive-compulsive disorder (Figure 4-4). PET and SPECT also have shown dopamine system dysregulation in schizophrenia and loss of monoamines in depression.

Antipsychotic medications are now prescribed at a fraction of the dosages that were considered standard only a decade ago, in large part because imaging studies illustrated how low dosages of antipsychotics bonded to dopamine type 2 (D_2) receptors to a degree that is expected with a therapeutic response (Zipursky et al., 2007). SPECT is currently used to examine nicotine receptors to which the neurotransmitter acetylcholine binds (Hashikawa, 2006), and it may be used in the future for clinical trials involving neuroprotective drugs for Alzheimer's disease (Mueller et al., 2006).

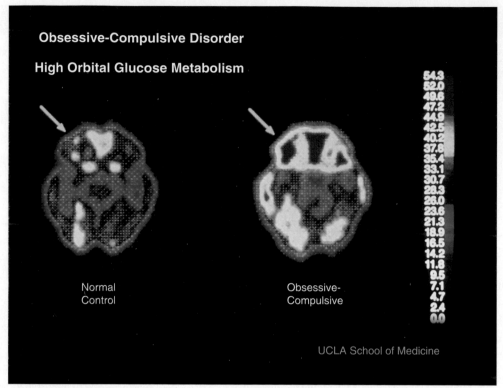

Figure 4-4 ▪ Positron emission tomographic scans show increased brain metabolism *(brighter colors)*, particularly in the frontal cortex, in a patient with obsessive-compulsive disorder (OCD), compared with a normal control. This suggests altered brain function in OCD. (From Lewis Baxter, MD, University of Alabama, courtesy National Institute of Mental Health.)

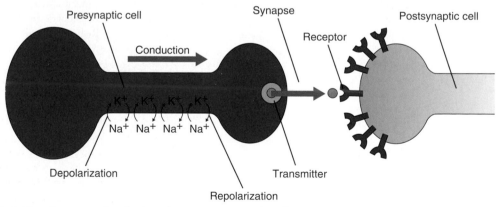

Figure 4-5 ▪ Activities of neurons. Conduction along a neuron involves the inward movement of sodium ions (Na^+) followed by the outward movement of potassium ions (K^+). When the current reaches the end of the cell, a neurotransmitter is released. The transmitter crosses the synapse and attaches to a receptor on the postsynaptic cell. The attachment of transmitter to receptor either stimulates or inhibits the postsynaptic cell.

CELLULAR COMPOSITION OF THE BRAIN

Neurons

The brain is composed of approximately 100 billion nerve cells (**neurons**) and the supporting cells that surround these neurons. An essential feature of neurons is their ability to conduct an electrical impulse from one end of the cell to the other, called **neurotransmission** (Figure 4-5). Electrical signals within neurons are then converted at synapses into chemical signals through the release of molecules called **neurotransmitters**, which then elicit electrical signals on

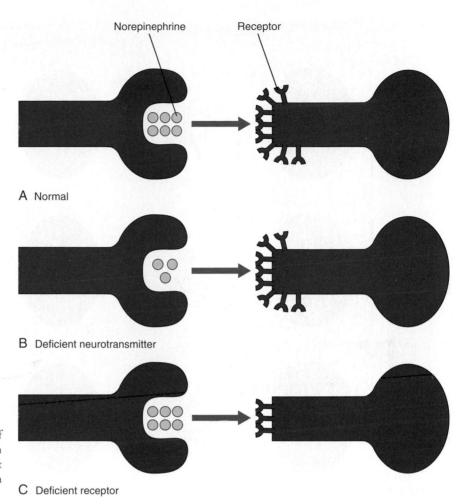

Figure 4-6 ▪ Normal transmission of neurotransmitters **(A).** Deficiency in transmission may be caused by a deficient release of transmitter, as shown in **B,** or a reduction in receptors, as shown in **C.**

the other side of the synapse. Together, these two signaling mechanisms (action potentials and synaptic signals) enable information processing in the brain.

Once an electrical impulse reaches the end of a neuron, the neurotransmitter is released from the axon terminal at the presynaptic neuron. This transmitter then diffuses across a narrow space, or **synapse,** to an adjacent postsynaptic neuron, where it attaches to specialized **receptors** on the cell surface and either inhibits or excites the postsynaptic neuron. It is the interaction between transmitter and receptor that is a major target of psychotropic drugs. Figure 4-6 shows how an insufficient degree of transmission may be caused by a deficient release of transmitters by the presynaptic cell or to a decrease in receptors. Figure 4-7 illustrates how excessive transmission may be due to excessive release of a transmitter or to increased receptor responsiveness as occurs in schizophrenia.

After attaching to a receptor and exerting its influence on the postsynaptic cell, the transmitter separates from the receptor and is destroyed. Some transmitters (e.g., acetyl-

choline) are destroyed by specific enzymes (e.g., acetylcholinesterase) at the postsynaptic cell. In the case of monoamine transmitters (e.g., norepinephrine, dopamine, serotonin), the destructive enzyme is monoamine oxidase (MAO).

Other transmitters (e.g., norepinephrine) are taken back into the cell from which they were originally released by a process called cellular **reuptake.** On return to these cells, the transmitters are either reused or destroyed by intracellular enzymes. The two basic mechanisms of destruction are described in Box 4-2.

Neurotransmission not only transmits current information but also alters subsequent neurotransmission.

Neurotransmitters

A **neurotransmitter** is a chemical messenger between neurons by which one neuron triggers another. Four major groups of neurotransmitters in the brain are monoamines (biogenic amines), amino acids, peptides, and cholinergics (acetylcholine). Monoamine neurotransmitters **(dopamine,**

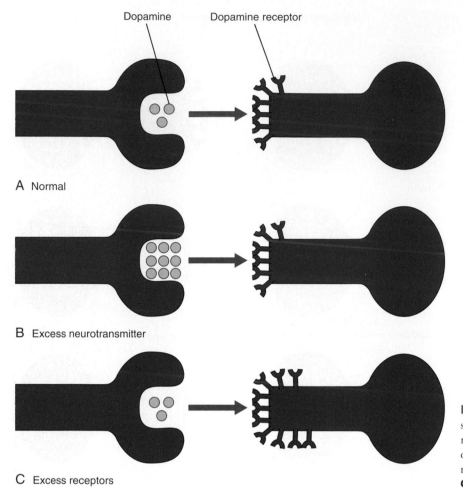

A Normal

B Excess neurotransmitter

C Excess receptors

Figure 4-7 ■ Causes of excess transmission of neurotransmitters. Excess transmission may be caused by excess release of transmitter, as shown in **B,** or excess responsiveness of receptors, as shown in **C.**

BOX 4-2

Destruction of Neurotransmitters

A full explanation of the various ways in which psychotropic drugs alter neuronal activity requires a brief review of the manner in which neurotransmitters are destroyed after attaching to the receptors. To avoid continuous and prolonged action on the postsynaptic cell, the neurotransmitter is released shortly after attaching to the postsynaptic receptor. Once released, the transmitter is destroyed in one of two ways.

One way is the immediate inactivation of the transmitter at the postsynaptic membrane. An example of this method of destruction is the action of the enzyme acetylcholinesterase on the neurotransmitter acetylcholine. Acetylcholinesterase is present at the postsynaptic membrane and destroys acetylcholine shortly after it attaches to nicotinic or muscarinic receptors on the postsynaptic cell.

A *second* method of neurotransmitter inactivation is a little more complex. After interacting with the postsynaptic

receptor, the transmitter is released and taken back into the presynaptic cell, the cell from which it was released. This process, referred to as the reuptake of neurotransmitter, is a common target for drug action. Once inside the presynaptic cell, the transmitter is either recycled or inactivated by an enzyme within the cell. The monoamine transmitters norepinephrine, dopamine, and serotonin are all inactivated in this manner by the enzyme monoamine oxidase.

In looking at this second method, one might naturally ask what prevents the enzyme from destroying the transmitter before its release. The answer is that before release the transmitter is stored within a membrane and is thus protected from the degradative enzyme. After release and reuptake, the transmitter is either destroyed by the enzyme or reenters the membrane to be used again.

norepinephrine, serotonin) and **acetylcholine** are implicated in a variety of neuropsychiatric disorders.

Amino acid neurotransmitters, such as the inhibitory γ-aminobutyric acid (GABA) and the excitatory **glutamate,** balance brain activity. Peptide neurotransmitters such as hypothalamic CRH can be thought of as modulating or adjusting general brain function. Table 4-2 lists important neurotransmitters, types of receptors to which they attach, and mental disorders that are associated with an increase or decrease in them.

HOW THE PSYCHOTROPICS WORK

Interaction of Neurons, Neurotransmitters, and Receptors

Most psychotropic drugs produce effects through alteration of synaptic concentrations of dopamine, acetylcholine, norepinephrine, serotonin, histamine, GABA, or glutamate. These changes are thought to result from receptor **antago-**

TABLE 4-2	**Transmitters and Receptors**		
Transmitters	**Receptors**	**Functions**	**Clinical Relevance**
Monoamines			
Dopamine (DA)	D_1, D_2, D_3, D_4, D_5	**Excitatory:** Fine muscle movement Integration of emotions and thoughts Decision making Stimulates hypothalamus to release hormones (sex, thyroid, adrenal)	**Increase:** Schizophrenia Mania **Decrease:** Parkinson's disease Depression

Norepinephrine (NE) (noradrenaline)	α_1, α_2, β_1, β_2	**Excitatory:**
		Mood
		Attention and arousal
		Stimulates sympathetic branch of
		  autonomic nervous system for "fight or
		  flight" in response to stress
			Increase:
			Mania
			Anxiety
			Schizophrenia
			Decrease:
			Depression

Serotonin (5-HT)	5-HT, 5-HT_2, 5-HT_3, 5-HT_4	**Excitatory:** Mood Sleep regulation Hunger Pain perception Aggression Hormonal activity	**Increase:** Anxiety (high levels) **Decrease:** Depression
Histamine	H_1, H_2	**Excitatory:** Alertness Inflammatory response Stimulates gastric secretion	**Increase:** Hyperactivity Compulsivity Suicidal depression **Decrease:** Sedation Weight gain Hypotension
Amino Acids			
γ-aminobutyric acid (GABA)	GABA_A, GABA_B	**Inhibitory:** Reduces anxiety, excitation, aggression May play a role in pain perception Anticonvulsant and muscle-relaxing properties	**Increase:** Reduction of anxiety **Decrease:** Mania Anxiety Schizophrenia

Continued

TABLE 4-2	Transmitters and Receptors—cont'd		
Transmitters	**Receptors**	**Functions**	**Clinical Relevance**
Glutamate	NMDA, AMPA	**Excitatory:** AMPA plays a role in learning and memory	**Increased NMDA:** Prolonged activation kills neurons **Decreased NMDA:** Psychosis
Cholinergics Acetylcholine (ACh)	Nicotinic, muscarinic (M_1, M_2, M_3)	Plays a role in learning, memory Regulates mood: mania, sexual aggression Affects sexual and aggressive behavior Stimulates parasympathetic nervous system	**Decrease:** Alzheimer's disease Huntington's chorea Parkinson's disease **Increase:** Depression
Peptides (Neuromodulators) Substance P (SP)	SP	Centrally active SP antagonist has antidepressant and antianxiety effects in depression Promotes and reinforces memory Enhances sensitivity to pain receptors to activate	Involved in regulation of mood and anxiety Role in pain management
Somatostatin (SRIF)	SRIF	Altered levels associated with cognitive disease	**Decrease:** Alzheimer's disease Decreased levels of SRIF found in spinal fluid of some depressed patients **Increase:** Huntington's chorea
Neurotensin (NT)	NT	Endogenous antipsychotic-like properties	Decreased levels found in spinal fluid of schizophrenic patients

AMPA, α-Amino-3-hydroxy-5-methyl-4-isoxazolepropionic acid; *NMDA*, N-methyl-D-aspartate.

nists (interfering with an action) or **agonists** (mimicking an action), interference with neurotransmitter reuptake, enhancement of neurotransmitter release, or inhibition of enzymes (Sadock & Sadock, 2007).

Dopamine

The monoamine **dopamine** stimulates the heart; increases blood flow to the liver, spleen, kidneys, and other visceral organs; and controls muscle movements and motor coordination. Abnormally low levels of dopamine are associated with tremors, muscle rigidity, and low blood pressure. The dopamine hypothesis of schizophrenia grew from the observations that drugs that block dopamine receptors (e.g., haloperidol) have antipsychotic activity and drugs that stimulate dopamine activity (e.g., amphetamines) can induce psychotic symptoms (Sadock & Sadock, 2007).

Antipsychotic drugs, to varying degrees, block or antagonize dopamine receptors, specifically the D_2 receptors in

the basal ganglia. This produces two kinds of movement disturbances: (1) acute **extrapyramidal symptoms (EPS),** which develop early in treatment and (2) tardive dyskinesia, which occurs much later (Julien, 2005). Although blockade of D_2 receptors and subsequent EPS occur most frequently with standard antipsychotic drugs, high doses of the atypical agent risperidone (Risperdal) also may cause EPS and an uncomfortable feeling called dysphoria (Mizrahi et al., 2007). Evidence for altered dopamine system activity also exists for depression, bipolar disorder, substance abuse, and attention deficit disorder (Cohen & Carlezon, 2007; Scholes et al., 2007).

Acetylcholine

Dopamine is balanced by the neurotransmitter **acetylcholine.** Neurons that release acetylcholine are said to be cholinergic and are thought to be involved in cognitive functions, especially memory. Because acetylcholine is deficient in Alzheimer's disease, attempts have been made to enhance the function of neurons that secrete acetylcholine with drugs that inhibit the enzyme that degrades acetylcholine. Therefore, acetylcholinesterase (AChE) inhibitors such as donepezil (Aricept), galantamine HBR (Razadyne), and rivastigmine (Exelon) are given to delay cognitive decline in Alzheimer's disease.

Although all acetylcholine receptors respond to acetylcholine, they also respond to other molecules. For example, nicotinic acetylcholine receptors are particularly responsive to nicotine. Thus nicotine, a cholinergic receptor agonist, might delay the onset of some of the cognitive deficits in Alzheimer's disease (Julien, 2005). It is well known that people with schizophrenia and attention problems are more likely to smoke, perhaps as a way of unconsciously self-medicating. Because these individuals are also more likely to suffer adverse effects, scientists are trying to develop drugs that target the nicotine receptors without the carcinogenic, cardiovascular, and addictive effects. A nicotine nasal spray tested in patient populations has shown that it increased attention as well as computational abilities (Myers et al., 2007).

Norepinephrine

Neurons that release the monoamine **norepinephrine (NE)** are called noradrenergic. NE and serotonin play a major role in regulating mood. A deficiency of one or both of these monoamines within the limbic system is thought to underlie depression, whereas an excess has been associated with mania. Many of the standard first-generation antipsychotic drugs act as antagonists at the α_1 receptors for NE. Blockage of these receptors can bring about vasodilation and a consequent drop in blood pressure or orthostatic hypotension. The α_1 receptors are also found on the vas deferens and are responsible for the propulsive contractions leading to ejaculation. Blockage of these receptors can lead to a failure to ejaculate.

Serotonin

The monoamine **serotonin,** found in the brain and spinal cord, helps regulate attention, behavior, and body temperature. Drugs that block the enzyme that metabolizes monoamines are called monoamine oxidase inhibitors (MAOIs) and may, on occasion, be used to increase serotonin and norepinephrine in intractable depression. However, selective serotonin reuptake inhibitors (SSRIs) and serotonin-norepinephrine reuptake inhibitors (SNRIs) are more commonly used antidepressants.

When some antidepressants are combined with other drugs or supplements that increase serotonin (e.g., St. John's wort or over-the-counter cough and cold medications containing dextromethorphan), the **serotonin syn-**

drome may occur. Symptoms of high levels of serotonin range from restlessness to muscle rigidity and seizures. These symptoms can be alleviated by muscle relaxants and drugs that block serotonin production (MayoClinic.com, 2007). Current research focuses on serotonin dysfunction in impulsive aggression and suicide (Cardish, 2007).

Histamine

Many standard antipsychotic agents, as well as a variety of other psychiatric drugs, block the H_1 receptors for **histamine.** Two significant side effects of blocking these receptors are sedation and substantial weight gain. Sedation may be beneficial in severely agitated patients, but weight gain can lead to disturbances in glucose and lipid metabolism and insulin resistance.

γ-Aminobutyric Acid (GABA)

The major inhibitory neurotransmitter, **γ-aminobutyric acid (GABA)**, modulates neuronal excitability. Not surprisingly, most antianxiety (anxiolytic) drugs act by increasing the effectiveness of this transmitter, primarily by increasing receptor responsiveness. Now researchers are examining an antipsychotic drug to simultaneously target dopamine hyperactivity and GABA hypoactivity, thereby reducing anxiety and improving cognitive function in schizophrenic individuals (Davidson, 2007).

Glutamate

Glutamate is an excitability neurotransmitter that activates *N*-methyl-D-asparate (NMDA) receptors. Reduction in NMDA receptor activity causes psychotic symptoms as seen with the street drug, phencyclidine (PCP). Overstimulation of NMDA receptors is thought to be toxic to neurons. The purpose of using an NMDA receptor antagonist, such as memantine (Namenda), is to treat this neurotoxicity and limit further deterioration in moderate to severe Alzheimer's disease (Julien, 2005).

ANTIPSYCHOTIC DRUGS
Standard Antipsychotics

The **standard antipsychotic drugs** (i.e., typical, traditional antipsychotics) were once called **neuroleptics** because they caused significant neurological effects. They are also referred to as **dopamine receptor antagonists (DRAs)** because they bind to D_2 receptors and reduce dopamine transmission as illustrated in Figure 4-8.

D_2 blockade achieves the therapeutic effect of decreasing positive symptoms in schizophrenia, but it also causes adverse effects. Because dopamine plays a major role in the basal ganglia to regulate movement, D_2 blockade can lead

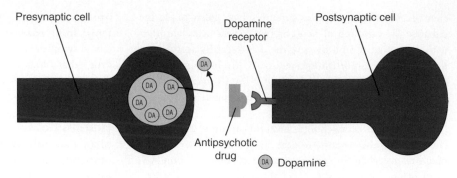

Figure 4-8 ■ How the standard (first-generation) antipsychotics block dopamine receptors.

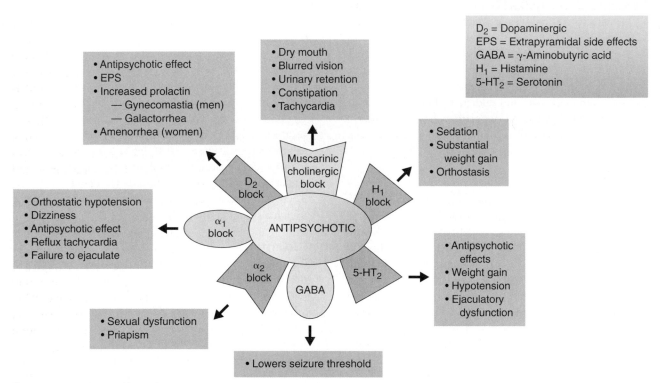

Figure 4-9 ■ Adverse effects of receptor blockage of antipsychotic agents. (From Varcarolis, E. [2006]. *Manual of psychiatric nursing care plans* [3rd ed.]. St. Louis: Saunders.)

to motor abnormalities (**extrapyramidal side effects**) such as dystonia, akathisia, tardive dyskinesia (TD), and drug-induced parkinsonism. D_2 blockade also may lead to a rare but life-threatening complication called **neuroleptic malignant syndrome (NMS)** involving autonomic, motor, and behavioral symptoms.

In addition, DRAs cause adverse effects by blocking other receptors. For example, blocking muscarinic receptors for acetylcholine can result in blurred vision, dry mouth, constipation, and urinary hesitancy. Antagonism of the **histamine** receptors provides sedation in acute psychosis,

but it is problematic afterward when one must carry out daily activities. Figure 4-9 identifies side effects experienced when specific neurotransmitters are blocked or bound.

evolve

For a more detailed description of how the antipsychotic drugs block specific receptors, visit the Evolve website at http://evolve.elsevier.com/Varcarolis/essentials.

Standard antipsychotics have been divided into two groups: high potency and low potency. Low-potency neuroleptics such as **chlorpromazine** (Thorazine) are used less frequently than high-potency neuroleptic medications because of problems with orthostatic hypotension. Their sedative effect can also be obtained by using lorazepam (Ativan) with a high-potency drug, such as **haloperidol** (Haldol). The combination of lorazepam and haloperidol is very effective in controlling aggression in violent patients.

Another high-potency neuroleptic is **fluphenazine** (Prolixin). Although these high-potency drugs have less sedation and fewer anticholinergic effects, they cause more EPS than low-potency agents. Deep intramuscular (depot) treatment with haloperidol or fluphenazine is common in maintenance therapy for schizophrenia. Dystonia (muscle stiffness), akathisia (restlessness), and Parkinson-like symptoms should be evaluated with any antipsychotic, but an acute dystonic reaction (ADR) is more likely to occur early in treatment with a high-potency neuroleptic, especially if the patient uses cocaine. Severe muscle rigidity with confusion, agitation, increased temperature, pulse, and blood pressure suggest a serious condition—neuroleptic malignant syndrome (NMS)—in which the drug should be stopped immediately and appropriate treatment instituted.

Atypical Antipsychotics

The **atypical antipsychotic drugs** are known as serotonin-dopamine antagonists (SDAs) because they have a higher ratio of serotonin type 2 (5-HT$_2$) to D$_2$ receptor blockade than the older, standard DRAs (Sadock & Sadock, 2007). Because of their different receptor-binding profile, atypical agents have fewer motor side effects, and they target the negative as well as the positive symptoms of schizophrenia. There is also some evidence that atypicals may improve cognitive function. Because each episode of schizophrenia may be considered neurotoxic, researchers are investigating the use of atypicals even in the prodromal stage to reduce or delay the transition to psychosis (Parker & Lewis, 2006).

Clozapine

Clozapine (Clozaril), the first of the atypicals, is a relatively weak blocker of D$_2$ receptors and a strong blocker of serotonin 5-HT$_2$ receptors. Clozapine is relatively free of motor side effects, and it is indicated for severely ill schizophrenic individuals who have failed to respond to standard therapy. Clozapine is not used as a first-line treatment because it may suppress bone marrow, resulting in a rare but serious drop in granulated white blood cells (WBCs) called **agran-**

ulocytosis. The risk of neutropenia and agranulocytosis is highest in the first few months of treatment.

Olanzapine

Olanzapine (Zyprexa), a derivative of clozapine, has a higher affinity for 5-HT$_2$ serotonin receptors than D$_2$ receptors. Both olanzapine and clozapine cause significant weight gain, perhaps by antagonizing serotonin and histamine receptors. Also, both atypical agents are thought to interfere with glucose metabolism and may lead to insulin resistance, hyperlipidemia, and changes in the coronary arteries (DeLeon & Diaz, 2007).

Metabolic monitoring for patients on all atypical antipsychotics is recommended, although risperidone (Risperdal) and quetiapine (Seroquel) have a lower weight gain, and ziprasidone (Geodon) and aripiprazole (Abilify) are considered weight neutral. Metabolic monitoring usually includes weight, body mass index (BMI), waist circumference, fasting plasma glucose, and fasting lipid profile. When there is concern about weight gain and metabolic effects of atypical antipsychotic agents, metformin—a medication used to regulate blood glucose—has been shown to halt weight gain, decrease measures of insulin resistance, and possibly increase adherence (Klein et al., 2006).

Although weight gain and metabolic effects are unhealthy, these adverse effects were more tolerable in the Clinical Antipsychotic Trials of Intervention Effectiveness (CATIE) study than the neurological adverse effects of standard antipsychotics (Lieberman, 2006). Because olanzapine is sedating due to antagonism of H$_1$ receptors, it is common practice to administer the medication at bedtime. Also, olanzapine is available as Zydis tablets, which dissolve in the mouth, thereby increasing successful administration with "cheekers" or those with swallowing difficulty.

Risperidone

Risperidone (Risperdal) exhibits high levels of D$_2$ receptor blockade and a very high affinity for 5-HT$_2$ receptors (Julien, 2005). EPS may occur if the dosage is only slightly higher than that which is effective. The patient should be carefully monitored for motor difficulties if the dosage exceeds 4 mg/day. Because risperidone blocks α_1 and H$_1$ receptors, it can cause orthostatic hypotension and sedation, which can lead to falls—a serious problem for older adults. Weight gain, sedation, and sexual dysfunction also are adverse effects that may affect adherence with the medication regimen.

Risperidone is the first atypical antipsychotic available as a long-acting injectable. This aqueous solution, Risperdal Consta, is considered advantageous because its slow release into the bloodstream does not have the peaks of oral antipsychotics, and it ensures a steady state, maintaining remission and avoiding rehospitalization. When long-acting antipsychotic therapy is initiated, oral risperidone is given with the first injection and continued for 3 weeks to ensure adequate plasma concentration.

Paliperidone is the principal active metabolite of risperidone in the new **INVEGA Extended Release Tablets** (FDA, 2006). It is delivered at a controlled rate through osmotic pressure, thereby avoiding high peak blood concentrations and enabling a smoother drug concentration over 24 hours. This suggests better tolerability and possibly greater adherence.

Quetiapine

Quetiapine (Seroquel) has a broad receptor-binding profile, but only D_2 and serotonin 5-HT_2 receptor binding is responsible for its therapeutic activity in schizophrenia. It has been used to treat depression and bipolar disorder, but it is only FDA approved for the acute treatment of mania. Most people fail to stay on their prescribed antipsychotic medication after 1 year, but the risk of discontinuation of all atypical antipsychotics is highest with quetiapine (Mullins et al., 2008), perhaps in part because of its effect on H_1 receptors. Orthostatic hypotension is explained by antagonism of adrenergic α_1 and α_2 receptors. The FDA approved once-daily Seroquel XR tablets in 2007, thereby decreasing the number of tablets taken daily. It is expected that the simplicity of the dosing routine will increase adherence to treatment.

Ziprasidone

Ziprasidone (Geodon) is a serotonin-norepinephrine reuptake inhibitor that also binds to multiple receptors (e.g., 5-HT_2, D_2, α, and H_1). The main side effects are hypotension and sedation. One major safety concern with ziprasidone, as well as the atypicals listed earlier, is prolongation of the QT_c interval, which can be fatal if the patient has a history of cardiac dysrhythmias. Thus a baseline electrocardiogram and blood chemistry testing for magnesium and potassium are recommended before treatment. Food increases its absorption, so a light meal is recommended. It is unlikely to cause significant interactions with drugs metabolized by cytochrome P450. Ziprasidone may be given intramuscularly for acute agitation, but it is important to note that it is not a long-acting preparation.

Aripiprazole

Aripiprazole (Abilify) is a unique atypical known as a dopamine system stabilizer. In areas of the brain with excess dopamine, it lowers the dopamine level by acting as a receptor antagonist; however, in regions with low dopamine, it stimulates receptors to raise the dopamine level, acting as a dopamine agonist. It is also an antagonist at serotonin 5-

HT_2 receptors and a partial agonist at 5-HT_1A receptors (Julien, 2005). Aripiprazole is available in a ready-to-use vial for intramuscular injection and control of agitation in schizophrenia or bipolar disorder.

Refer to Chapter 14 for more information on adverse and toxic effects, nursing considerations, and patient and family teaching of the antipsychotics.

MOOD STABILIZERS

Lithium

Although **lithium** (Eskalith, Lithobid) has been used for many years to control or prevent mania in bipolar illness, its **mood-stabilizing** effects are only vaguely understood. As a positively charged ion, similar in structure to sodium and potassium, lithium may act by stabilizing electrical activity in neurons. If the alteration of electrical currents is not responsible for its beneficial effects, it certainly explains some adverse effects. The foremost danger is inducing cardiac dysrhythmias. Extreme alteration of cerebral conductivity can lead to seizures. Alteration in nerve and muscle conduction can lead to tremors or more extreme motor dysfunction.

Primarily because of its effects on electrical conductivity, lithium has the lowest **therapeutic index** of all psychiatric drugs. The therapeutic index represents the ratio of the lethal dose to the effective dose. So it is important to monitor blood lithium levels on a regular basis to be sure that the drug is not accumulating and rising to dangerous levels. The strong role that sodium and potassium play in regulating fluid balance explains the side effects of polyuria (the output of large volumes of urine) and edema (the accumulation of fluid in the interstitial space). There is evidence that long-term use of lithium increases the risk of kidney and thyroid disease.

Chapter 13 considers lithium treatment in more detail. Used as adjuncts to lithium, benzodiazepines can rapidly calm a person in an acute manic episode and increase the time between mood cycles (Sadock & Sadock, 2007).

Anticonvulsants

Divalproex sodium (Depakote) is recommended in bipolar disorder for mixed episodes and rapid cycling. It is very effective in managing impulsive aggression. When lithium is not tolerated, divalproex sodium may be used for long-term maintenance therapy. Its action in bipolar illness is unknown, but it may be related to increased bioavailability of the inhibitory neurotransmitter GABA. Baseline laboratory work includes liver function tests and complete blood count (CBC). Therapeutic blood levels generally range from 50 to 100 mcg/mL.

Carbamazepine (Tegretol), in a controlled-release formula, is used to treat acute mania. A CBC must be done periodically because of rare but serious blood dyscrasias (e.g., aplastic anemia, agranulocytosis). Unlike carbamazepine, the newer **oxcarbazepine** (Trileptal) does not require blood tests before or during its use. However, it does interact with oral contraceptives and its usefulness in treating mania or other psychiatric disorders has not been established in controlled trials (Sadock & Sadock, 2007).

Lamotrigine (Lamictal), approved for maintenance treatment of bipolar disorder, modulates the release of glutamate and aspartate and is most effective in preventing depressive episodes. The most common adverse effects are usually mild, but about 8% of patients started on lamotrigine develop a benign rash during the first 4 months of treatment. If this occurs, the drug should be stopped. Although the rash is usually benign, there is a concern that it is an early manifestation of a toxic epidermal necrolysis called Stevens-Johnson syndrome (Sadock & Sadock, 2007).

Gabapentin (Neurontin), structurally related to GABA, offers some promise for people with comorbid bipolar disorder with chronic pain and insomnia, thus preventing mania relapse.

Topiramate (Topamax) enhances GABA and blocks glutamate. The cognitive depressant effects are greater than those of gabapentin or lamotrigine, but topiramate may be appropriate for some patients when weight loss is desirable.

Refer to Chapter 12 for nursing considerations and patient and family teaching for the mood stabilizing drugs.

ANTIDEPRESSANT DRUGS

One third of patients with depression do not respond to an initial trial of antidepressant medication treatment, possibly as a result of variations in the serotonin receptor (Levin et al., 2007). Antidepressant drugs may take as long as 4 to 6 weeks to have a significant effect.

Monoamine Oxidase Inhibitors

To understand the action of these drugs, keep in mind the following definitions:

- **Monoamines**: a type of organic compound, including the neurotransmitters norepinephrine, epinephrine, dopamine, and serotonin and many different drugs and food substances
- **Monoamine oxidase (MAO)**: an enzyme that destroys monoamines
- **Monoamine oxidase inhibitors (MAOIs)**: drugs that prevent the destruction of monoamines by inhibiting the action of MAO

The monoamine neurotransmitters, as well as any monoamine food substance or drugs, are degraded (destroyed) by the enzyme MAO. Antidepressant drugs, such as isocarboxazid (Marplan), phenelzine (Nardil), and tranylcypromine (Parnate) are MAOIs that inhibit the enzyme and interfere with destruction of monoamines. This in turn increases the synaptic level of the transmitters and makes possible the antidepressant effects of these drugs (Figure 4-10).

Normally, the monoamine tyramine is destroyed by MAO as it passes through the liver before entering the general blood circulation. If allowed to circulate freely in

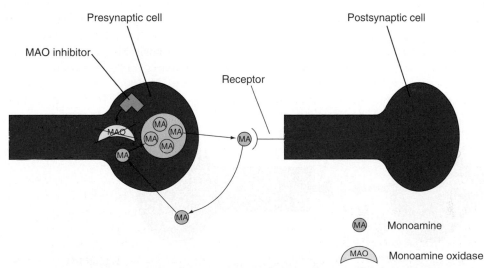

Figure 4-10 ▪ Blocking of monoamine oxidase (MAO) by inhibiting agents (MAOIs), which prevents the breakdown of monoamine by MAO.

the blood, tyramine produces intense vasoconstriction, and thus an elevation in blood pressure. Inhibition of hepatic MAO by MAOIs might result in a hypertensive crisis if the patient does not avoid foods high in tyramine (e.g., aged cheese) and drugs (e.g., cough medicines) while using the MAOI and for 2 weeks after discontinuing its use.

EMSAM (selegiline transdermal system) is the first antidepressant patch. Chapter 12 discusses the treatment of depression, contains a list of foods and beverages to avoid while taking MAOIs, and gives nursing measures and instructions for patient teaching on MAOIs.

> **evolve**
>
> For a more detailed description of how MAOIs work, visit the Evolve website at http://evolve. elsevier.com/Varcarolis/essentials.

Tricyclic Antidepressants (TCAs)

TCAs, such as amitriptyline (Elavil) and nortriptyline (Pamelor), act primarily by blocking the reuptake of norepinephrine and, to a lesser degree, serotonin (Figure 4-11). This blocking prevents norepinephrine from coming into contact with its degrading enzyme, MAO, and thus increases the level of norepinephrine at the synapse.

Strong binding at adrenergic receptors causes dizziness and hypotension, thereby increasing the risk for falls. Slow cardiac conduction may explain fatality in TCA overdose. To varying degrees, many TCAs also block the muscarinic receptors that normally bind acetylcholine, leading to typical anticholinergic effects. Again to varying degrees, TCAs can block H_1 receptors, causing sedation and weight gain.

> **evolve**
>
> For a more detailed description of how TCAs work, visit the Evolve website at http://evolve.elsevier. com/Varcarolis/essentials.

Selective Serotonin Reuptake Inhibitors (SSRIs)

As the name implies, the **selective serotonin reuptake inhibitors (SSRIs)**, such as fluoxetine (Prozac), sertraline (Zoloft), paroxetine (Paxil), citalopram (Celexa), and escitalopram (Lexapro), preferentially block the reuptake and thus, the destruction of serotonin with little or no effect on other monoamine transmitters. Roughly one third of patients do not respond to an initial trial of antidepressants, possibly as a result of structural variations in the $5\text{-HT}/_1\text{A}$ receptor (Levin et al., 2007). Refer to Figure 4-12 for an explanation of how the SSRIs work.

> **evolve**
>
> For a more detailed description of how SSRIs work, visit the Evolve website at http://evolve. elsevier.com/Varcarolis/essentials.

Symptoms of depression begin to improve by the end of the first week of use, and the improvement continues for at least 6 weeks (Taylor et al, 2006). It may take several weeks to see improvement because it takes time for the autoreceptors to downregulate (Levin et al., 2007). As a result of their more selective action, SSRIs show comparable efficacy to TCAs but do not elicit the anticholinergic and sedating side effects that limit patient adherence. Also, the activating SSRIs are less likely to be hoarded and used for overdose than the sedating TCAs, and they are less lethal.

However, too much serotonin in certain neural circuits can produce other negative effects such as *anxiety, insomnia, sexual dysfunction, and gastrointestinal disturbances.* Symptoms of the "SSRI stimulant syndrome" range from mild irritability to severe mania and violence. The patient may describe seemingly bizarre feelings as "electrical impulses down my nerves" or "skin crawling."

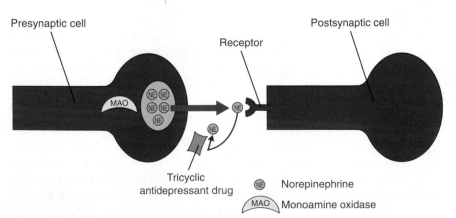

Presynaptic cell   Postsynaptic cell   Receptor

Tricyclic antidepressant drug

NE Norepinephrine

MAO Monoamine oxidase

Figure 4-11 ■ How the tricyclic antidepressant drugs block the reuptake of norepinephrine.

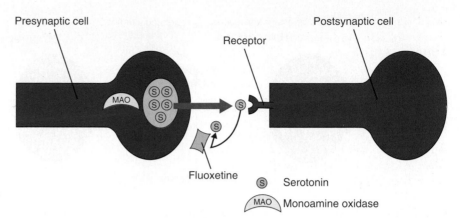

Figure 4-12 ■ How the selective serotonin reuptake inhibitors (SSRIs) work.

Because SSRIs may activate impulsive or aggressive behaviors, the individual treated with SSRIs should be assessed for suicidal and homicidal thoughts. It is especially important to closely monitor all individuals, especially children and adolescents, when they start taking SSRIs or whenever a change is noted in their behavior. Slow tapering over several weeks is advisable when discontinuing SSRIs because a withdrawal reaction may occur if there is intermittent nonadherence or abrupt cessation. The discontinuation syndrome is most likely to occur with SSRIs or SNRIs having a short half-life. Thus it is more common with paroxetine (Paxil) than with fluoxetine (Prozac).

Atypical or Novel Antidepressants

Atypical antidepressants differ structurally and seem to work by mechanisms less clearly defined than those of the MAOIs, TCAs, and SSRIs. **SNRIs** block the reuptake of serotonin and norepinephrine. **Duloxetine** (Cymbalta), available as a delayed-release capsule, is used for major depressive disorder and management of pain associated with diabetic neuropathy. It also improves sphincter function in stress incontinence. **Mirtazapine** (Remeron) is a sedating antidepressant often used to treat people with anxiety and sleep disturbances. **Venlafaxine** (Effexor) has the unusual effect of becoming an SNRI rather than SSRI at higher doses.

Unlike other currently used antidepressants, **bupropion** (Wellbutrin), does not act on the serotonin system; it is a norepinephrine-dopamine reuptake inhibitor (NDRI). It also inhibits nicotinic acetylcholine receptors to reduce the addictive action of nicotine. Thus it is an effective antidepressant and a first-line agent for smoking cessation. **Trazodone** (Desyrel) is not a first choice for antidepressant treatment, but it is often given along with another agent because somnolence, one of its side effects, helps with sleep disturbance.

Refer to Chapter 12 for more information on the antidepressant medications, nursing considerations, and patient and family teaching.

ANTIDEPRESSION TREATMENT OF CONDITIONS ASSOCIATED WITH ANXIETY

The sedative effects of antidepressants may be useful in the short term in some cases of depression accompanied by anxiety, agitation, or sleep impairment (Moncrieff, 2007). For example, SSRIs and SNRIs are considered first-line treatments for panic disorder. However, *anxiety or agitation* may occur when an SSRI or SNRI is first started. Use of a benzodiazepine, either on a regular or prn basis, may alleviate side effects and reduce the risk of medication discontinuation at the start of treatment (Vanelli, 2005).

ANTIANXIETY OR ANXIOLYTIC DRUGS

The neurotransmitter GABA has an inhibitory effect on neurons in many parts of the brain. Drugs that enhance this effect tend to reduce anxiety and exert a sedative-hypnotic action. The most commonly used **antianxiety or anxiolytic drugs** are the **benzodiazepines (BZs),** such as diazepam (Valium), clonazepam (Klonopin), and alprazolam (Xanax). Figure 4-13 shows that benzodiazepines bind to specific receptors adjacent to the GABA receptors. Because of their ability to bind benzodiazepines, these receptors are called benzodiazepine receptors. Binding of benzodiazepines to these receptors at the same time that GABA binds to its receptors allows GABA to inhibit more forcefully than it would if binding alone.

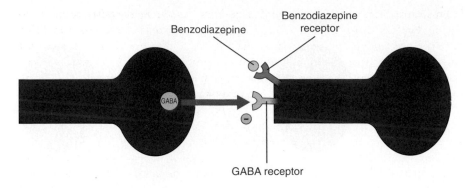

Figure 4-13 ▪ Action of the benzodiazepines. Drugs in this group attach to receptors adjacent to the receptors for the neurotransmitter γ-aminobutyric acid (GABA). Drug attachment to these receptors results in a strengthening of the inhibitory effects of GABA. In the absence of GABA, there is no inhibitory effect of benzodiazepines.

The fact that benzodiazepines do not inhibit neurons in the absence of GABA limits the potential toxicity of these drugs. However, benzodiazepines have the potential for tolerance and withdrawal reactions to develop. Tolerance involves a decreased effect or an increased need for larger doses, and withdrawal is brought on by the elimination of benzodiazepines from the body when the individual is physically dependent on it. People with a personal or family history of alcohol or other substance abuse are at risk for developing a dependence on these drugs; thus the benzodiazepines are not appropriate for these individuals (Preston et al., 2005).

Some of the various benzodiazepines, such as flurazepam (Dalmane) and triazolam (Halcion), have a predominantly **hypnotic** (sleep-inducing) effect, whereas others, such as lorazepam (Ativan) and alprazolam (Xanax), reduce anxiety without being as **soporific** (sleep producing). Currently, there is no clear explanation for the differential effects of the various benzodiazepines. There seems to be some evidence that there are subtypes of the benzodiazepine receptors in different areas of the brain, and these subtypes differ in their ability to bind the different drugs.

The fact that the benzodiazepines potentiate the ability of GABA to inhibit neurons probably accounts for their efficacy as anticonvulsants and for their ability to reduce the neuronal overexcitement of alcohol withdrawal. When used alone, even at high dosages, these drugs rarely inhibit the brain to the degree that respiratory depression, coma, and death result. However, when combined with other central nervous system (CNS) depressants, such as alcohol, opiates, or TCAs, the inhibitory actions of the benzodiazepines can lead to life-threatening respiratory depression.

Any drug that inhibits electrical activity in the brain can interfere with motor ability, attention, and judgment. A patient taking benzodiazepines must be cautioned about engaging in activities that could be dangerous if reflexes and attention are impaired. These include specialized activities, such as working in construction on a tall building and more common activities such as driving a car. In older adults, benzodiazepines increase the risk for falls and hip fractures,

and they may worsen conditions such as emphysema, urinary incontinence, and depression (NIMH, 2007).

Buspirone (BuSpar) is a drug that reduces anxiety without having strong sedative-hypnotic properties. Its mechanism of action is unknown, but it has a high affinity for serotonin receptors. The end result is an increased synaptic level of serotonin that presumably accounts for the beneficial action of this drug. Because this agent does not leave the patient sleepy or sluggish, it is often much better tolerated than the benzodiazepines. It is not a CNS depressant and thus does not have as great a danger of interaction with other CNS depressants such as alcohol. Also there is not the potential for addiction that exists with benzodiazepines.

PHARMACOGENOMICS AND PHARMACOGENETICS

Pharmacogenomics and **pharmacogenetics** are terms that have been used interchangeably for the study of how one's genes affect the body's response to drugs. Technically, pharmacogenomics refers to the general study of the many different genes that determine drug behavior, whereas pharmacogenetics is the study of inherited differences (variation) in drug metabolism and response (Ito & Demers, 2004).

Cultural Considerations

Cultural and ethnic beliefs surrounding mental illness and pharmacotherapy affect a person's perception of the need for treatment, adherence, reporting of adverse events, and the preference for alternative or complementary therapies. Also, drugs can have different effects among those in diverse cultural and ethnic groups.

Genetic variations that affect specific neurotransmitter functions could explain why some patients respond to some drugs but not to others. Depressed patients who have abnormally low levels of serotonin respond to SSRIs; others with abnormal levels of norepinephrine or dopamine may not respond to SSRIs. In the future, it may be possible to biologically personalize treatments through a simple blood test that characterizes a patient's unique genetic profile, determining what biological type of depression the patient has, and which antidepressant is likely to work best (Friedman, 2007).

Studies have shown a genetic variation favoring a response to citalopram (Celexa) was six times more prevalent in whites than in African Americans (McMahon et al., 2006). Another study determined that 20% to 30% of whites may not respond to fluoxetine (Prozac) or other SSRIs because they have a *BDNF* genetic mutation (Chen et al., 2006). And Korean individuals with two copies of a specific gene mutation had more than an 80% likelihood of responding to norepinephrine reuptake inhibitors (NRIs) but those with only one copy of the gene mutation were only 39% likely to respond to NRIs (Kim et al., 2006).

To predict patients' responses, scientists continue to search for variants in genes that code for drug-metabolizing enzymes in the liver that influence those enzymes that handle psychotropic medications. Most attention has focused on the enzyme cytochrome P4502D6 (CYP2D6), important for metabolizing drugs. In addition, many pharmaceutical companies screen their chemical compounds to see how well they are broken down by variant forms of CYP enzymes (HGP, 2006).

Research is ongoing to personalize doses required for individuals who are poor or ultra-rapid metabolizers, and gene-based tests may soon individualize treatment to meet each person's needs. At present, treatment focuses on specific symptoms of mental disorders. In the future, genetic research might enable treatment of the genetic flaw or underlying causes of these disorders.

KEY POINTS TO REMEMBER

- All actions of the brain—sensory, motor, intellectual—are carried out physiologically through the interactions of nerve cells. These interactions involve impulse conduction, transmitter release, and receptor response. Alterations in these basic processes can lead to mental disturbances and physical manifestations.
- In particular, it seems that excess activity of dopamine, among other factors, is involved in the thought disturbances of schizophrenia.
- Deficiencies of norepinephrine or serotonin or both underlie the mood disturbances of depression.
- Insufficient activity of GABA seems to play a role in anxiety.
- Pharmacological treatment of mental disturbances is directed at the suspected transmitter receptor problem. Thus, antipsychotic drugs block dopamine receptors, antidepressant drugs increase synaptic levels of norepinephrine or serotonin, and antianxiety drugs increase the effectiveness of GABA.

- Because the immediate target activity of a drug can result in many downstream alterations in neuronal activity, it has been found that drugs with a variety of chemical actions may show efficacy in treating the same clinical condition. Thus, in the treatment of schizophrenia, depression, and anxiety, newer drugs with novel mechanisms of action are being brought into use. This often makes understanding the pharmacology of mental disease more, rather than less, difficult.
- Unfortunately, as is the case for almost all pharmacological agents, the agents used to treat mental disease can cause various undesired effects. Prominent among these can be sedation or excitement, motor disturbances, muscarinic blockage, alpha adrenergic (norepinephrine) antagonism, lowering of mood, sexual dysfunction, and weight gain. There is a continuing effort on the part of pharmacologists to develop new drugs that are effective as well as safe and comfortable for people suffering from emotional disorders.

CRITICAL THINKING

1. No matter where you practice nursing, many individuals under your care will be taking one psychotropic drug or another. How important is it for you in your nursing practice to understand normal brain structure and function as they relate to mental disturbances and psychotropic drugs? Include the following in your answer:
   - Ways nurses can use the knowledge about how normal brain function (control of skeletal muscles, the autonomic nervous system, hormones, and circadian rhythms) can be affected by either psychotropic drugs or psychiatric illness
   - Ways brain imaging can help in understanding and treating people with mental disorders

   - Ways your understanding of how neurotransmitters work may affect your ability to assess your patients' responses to specific medications
2. What specific information could you include in your medication teaching for your patient based on your understanding of what symptoms may occur with alterations of the following neurotransmitters?
   - Dopamine D_2
   - Blockage of muscarinic receptors
   - α_1 receptors
   - Histamine
   - MAO
   - GABA

CHAPTER REVIEW

Choose the most appropriate answer(s).

1. A nurse administering a benzodiazepine should understand that the therapeutic effect results from the benzodiazepine binding to receptors adjacent to receptors for the neurotransmitter:
   1. GABA.
   2. dopamine.
   3. serotonin.
   4. acetylcholine.
2. Fluoxetine (an SSRI) exerts its antidepressant effect by blocking the reuptake of:
   1. GABA.
   2. dopamine.
   3. serotonin.
   4. norepinephrine.
3. A psychiatric nurse routinely administers the following drugs to patients in the community mental health center. The patients who should be most carefully assessed for untoward cardiac side effects are those receiving:
   1. lithium.
   2. clozapine.
   3. diazepam.
   4. sertraline.
4. Which of the following classes of psychotropic medications could trigger the development of parkinsonian movement disorders among individuals who take therapeutic doses?
   1. SSRIs
   2. DRAs
   3. Benzodiazepines
   4. Tricyclic antidepressants
5. Atypical antipsychotic medications have which of the following effects? Select all that apply.
   1. Reduction of positive symptoms of schizophrenia
   2. Reduction of negative symptoms of schizophrenia
   3. Reduction of body mass
   4. Possible improvement in cognitive function

REFERENCES

Barch, D.M., & Csernansky, J.G. (2007). Abnormal parietal cortex activation during working memory in schizophrenia: Verbal phonological coding disturbances versus domain-general executive dysfunction. *American Journal of Psychiatry, 164,* 1090-1098.

Cardish, R.J. (2007). Psychopharmacologic management of suicidality in personality disorders. *Canadian Journal of Psychiatry, 52*(6 Suppl 1), 115S-127S.

Chen, Z.Y., Jing, D., Bath, K.G., et al. (2006). Genetic variant BDNF (Val66Met) polymorphism alters anxiety-related behavior. *Science, 314*(5796), 140-143.

Cohen, B.M., & Carlezon, W.A. (2007). Can't get enough of that dopamine. *American Journal of Psychiatry, 164,* 543-546.

Davidson, M. (2007). *First antipsychotic targeting GABA to enter phase II trials.* Schizophrenia.com. Retrieved February 14, 2007, from http://www.schizophrenia.com/sznews/archives/004647.html

DeLeon, J., & Diaz, F.J. (2007). Planning for the optimal design of studies to personalize antipsychotic prescriptions in the post-CATIE era. *Schizophrenia Research, 96*(1-3), 185-197.

Erickson, S.K., Ciccone, J.R., Schwarzkopf, S.B., et al. (2007). Legal fallacies of antipsychotic drugs. *Journal of the American Academy of Psychiatry and the Law, 35*(2), 235-246.

Ettinger, U., Picchioni, M.M., Landau, S., et al. (2007). Magnetic resonance imaging of the thalamus and adhesio interthalamica in twins with schizophrenia. *Archives of General Psychiatry, 64*(4), 401-409.

FDA (Food and Drug Administration) news release (2006). *FDA approves new drug for schizophrenia.* Retrieved February 8, 2007, from www.fda.gov/bbs/topics/NEWS/2006/NEW01534.html.

Friedman, R.A. (2007, June 19). On the horizon, personalized depression drugs. *New York Times.* Retrieved from www.nytimes.com/2007/06/19/health/psychology/19beha.html?fta=y.

Hashikawa, K. (2006). Nicotinic acetylcholine receptor imaging for dementia. *International Congress Series, 1290,* 144-149.

Human Genome Project (HGP) information: Pharmacogenetics, 2006. available at www.ornl.gov/sci/techresources/Human_Genome/medicine/pharma.shtml.

Invega.com. (2006). New INVEGA™ approved by FDA as new treatment for schizophrenia. Retrieved December 20, 2006, from www.invega.com/invega/news.html.

Ito, R.K., & Demers, L.M. (2004). Pharmacogenomics and pharmacogenetics: Future role of molecular diagnostics in the clinical diagnostic laboratory. *Clinical Chemistry, 50,* 1526-1527. Julien, R.M. (2005). *A primer of drug action* (10th ed.). New York: Worth.

Kim, H., Lim, S.W., Kim, S., et al. (2006). Monoamine transporter gene polymorphisms and antidepressant response in Koreans with late-life depression. *Journal of the American Medical Association, 296*(13), 1609-1618.

Klein, D.J., Cottingham, E.M., Sorter, M., et al. (2006). A randomized, double-blind, placebo-controlled trial of metformin treatment of weight gain associated with initiation of atypical antipsychotic therapy in children and adolescents. *American Journal of Psychiatry, 163,* 2072-2079.

Levin, Gary M., Bowles, Toya M., Ehret, Megan J., Langaee, Taimour, Tan, Jennifer Y, Johnson, Julie A, & Millard, William J. (2007). Assessment of human serotonin 1A receptor polymorphisms and SSRI responsiveness. *Molecular Diagnosis & Therapy, 11*(3):155-160.

Lieberman, J.A. (2006). *The significance of CATIE: An Expert Interview with Jeffrey A. Lieberman, MD.* Retrieved July 10, 2007, from www.medscape.com/viewarticle/525641.

MayoClinic.com. *Serotonin syndrome.* Retrieved July 5, 2007, from http://mayoclinic.com/health/serotonin-syndrome/DS00860.

McMahon, F.J., Buervenich, S., Charney, D., et al. (2006). Variation in the gene encoding the serotonin 2A receptor is associated with outcome of antidepressant treatment. The *American Journal of Human Genetics, 78*(5), 804-814.

Mizrahi, R., Rusjan, P., Ofer, A., et al. (2007). Adverse subjective experience with antipsychotics and its relationship to striatal and extra striatal D$_2$ receptors: A PET study in schizophrenia. *American Journal of Psychiatry, 164,* 630-637.

Moncrieff, J. (2007). Are antidepressants as effective as claimed? *Canadian Journal of Psychiatry, 52,* 96-97.

Mueller, S.G., Schuff, N., & Weiner, M.W. (2006). Evaluation of treatment effects in Alzheimer's and other neurodegenerative diseases with MRI and MRS. *NMR in Biomedicine 19*(6): 655-668.

Mullins, C.D., Obeidat, C.D., Cuffel, B.J., et al. (2008). Risk of discontinuation of atypical antipsychotic agents in the treatment of schizophrenia. *Schizophrenia Research, 98*(1-3), 8-15.

Myers, C.S., Taylor, R.C., Moolchan, E.T., & Heishman, S.J. (2007). Dose-related enhancement of mood and cognition in smokers administered nicotine nasal spray. *Neuropsychopharmacology, 33*(3), 588-598.

Nasrallah, H.A. (2007). Remember the hippocampus! You can protect the brain's regeneration center. *Current Psychiatry, 6*(10), 17-18.

NIMH (National Institute of Mental Health). (2007) New study will examine effects of excluding anti-anxiety medications in Medicare part D coverage. *Science News.* Retrieved July 5, 2007, from www.nimh.nih.gov/science-news/2007/new-study-will-examine-effects-of-excluding-anti-anxiety-medications-in-medicare-part-d-coverage.shtml.

Parker, S., & Lewis, S. (2006). Identification of young people at risk of psychosis. *Advances in Psychiatric Treatment, 12,* 249-255.

Pinel, J.P.J. (2005). *Biopsychology* (6th ed.). Pearson Education. Boston: Allyn & Bacon.

Preston, J.D., O'Neal, J., & Talaga, M.C. (2005). *Handbook of clinical psychopharmacology for therapists* (4th ed.). Oakland: New Harbinger Publications.

Sadock, B.J., & Sadock, V.A. (2007). *Synopsis of psychiatry: behavioral sciences/clinical psychiatry* (10th ed.). Philadelphia: Lippincott Williams & Wilkins.

Scholes, K.E., Harrison, B.J., O'Neil, B.V., et al. (2007). Acute serotonin and dopamine depletion improves attentional control: Findings from the stroop task. *Neuropsychopharmacology, 32,* 1600-1610.

Taylor, M.J., Freemantle, N., Geddes, M.D., et al. (2006). Early onset of selective serotonin reuptake inhibitor antidepressant action. *Archives of General Psychiatry, 63,* 1217-1223.

Vanelli, M. (2005). Improving treatment responses in panic disorder. *Primary Psychiatry, 12*(11), 68-73.

Vuilleumier, P., & Driver, J. (2007). Modulation of visual processing by attention and emotional windows on causal interactions between human brain regions. *Philosophical Transactions of The Royal Society, 362,* 837-855.

Zhu, W., Bie, B., & Pan, Z. (2007). Involvement of non-NMDA glutamate receptors in central amygdala in synaptic actions of ethanol and ethanol-induced reward behavior. *Journal of Neuroscience, 27*(2), 289-298.

Zipursky, R.B., Meyer, J.H., & Verhoeff, N.P. (2007). PET and SPECT imaging in psychiatric disorders. *Canadian Journal of Psychiatry, 52,* 146-157.

Tools for Practice of the Art

CHAPTER 5

Nursing Process: The Foundation for Safe and Effective Care

Elizabeth M. Varcarolis

Key Terms and Concepts

evidence-based practice (EBP), p. 80
health teaching, p. 82
mental status examination (MSE), p. 73
milieu therapy, p. 82
Nursing Interventions Classification (NIC),
   p. 81

Nursing Outcomes Classification (NOC), p. 78
outcomes criteria, p. 78
Psychiatric Mental Health Nursing Standards
   of Practice, p. 71
psychosocial assessment, p. 75
self-care activities, p. 82

Objectives

1. Conduct a mental status examination.
2. Perform a psychosocial assessment including cultural and spiritual components.
3. Explain three principles a nurse follows in planning actions to reach agreed-upon outcome criteria.
4. Construct a plan of care for a patient with a mental or emotional health problem.
5. Identify three advanced practice psychiatric nursing interventions.
6. Demonstrate basic nursing interventions and evaluation of care using the Standards of Practice (ANA, 2007).
7. Compare and contrast the Nursing Interventions Classification, Nursing Outcomes Classification, and evidence-based nursing practice.

evolve

For additional resources related to the content of this chapter, visit the Evolve website at
http://evolve.elsevier.com/Varcarolis/essentials.

- Chapter Outline
- Chapter Review Answers
- Nurse, Patient, and Family Resources
- Concept Map Creator

The nursing process continues to be the basic framework for all significant action taken by nurses in providing developmentally and culturally relevant psychiatric mental health care to all patients. The nursing process is integral to *Psychiatric–Mental Health Nursing: Scope and Standards of Practice* as defined by the American Nurses Association (ANA, 2007). The **Psychiatric Mental Health Nursing Standards of Practice** are the bases for the following:

- Criteria for certification
- Legal definition of nursing, as reflected in many states' nurse practice acts
- National Council of State Boards of Nursing Licensure Examination (NCLEX-RN®)

The nursing process is a six-step problem-solving approach intended to facilitate and identify appropriate safe and quality care for patients. A patient may be an individual, a family, a group, or a community. Psychiatric mental health nursing practice bases nursing judgments and behaviors on an accepted theoretical framework. Whenever possible, interventions are supported by evidence-based research. The importance of a theoretical framework has been supported by *Psychiatric–Mental Health Nursing: Scope and Standards of Practice* (ANA, 2007). Figure 5-1 depicts the nursing process in psychiatric mental health nursing.

STANDARD 1: ASSESSMENT

A view of the individual as a complex blend of many parts is consistent with nurses' **holistic approach to care.** Nurses who care for people with physical illnesses ideally maintain a holistic view that involves an awareness of psychological, social, cultural, and spiritual issues. Likewise, nurses who work in the mental health field need to assess or have access to past and present medical history, a recent physical examination, and any physical complaints a patient is experiencing, as well as document any observable physical conditions or behaviors (e.g., unsteady gait, abnormal breathing patterns, wincing as if in pain, doubling over to relieve discomfort).

Assessments are conducted by a variety of professionals including nurses, psychiatrists, social workers, dietitians, and other therapists. Every patient should have a thorough and formal nursing assessment on entering treatment to develop a basis for the plan of care in preparation for discharge. Subsequent to the formal assessment, data are collected continually and systematically as the patient's condition changes, and, it is hoped, improves. Perhaps the patient came into treatment actively suicidal, and the initial focus of care was on protection from injury; through regular assessment it may be determined that although suicidal ideation has diminished, negative self-evaluation is still certainly a problem.

Virtually all facilities have standardized nursing assessment forms to aid in organization and consistency among reviewers. These forms may be paper or computerized versions according to the resources and preferences of the institution. The time required for the nursing interview varies, depending on the assessment form and on the patient's response pattern (e.g., a lengthy or rambling historian, prone to tangential thought, having memory disturbances, or markedly slowed responses). In emergency situations, immediate intervention is often based on a minimal amount of data. Refer to Chapter 7 for sound guidelines for setting up and conducting a clinical interview.

The nurse's *primary source* for data collection is the patient; however, there may be times when it is necessary to supplement or rely completely on another for the assessment information. These *secondary sources* can be invaluable when caring for a patient experiencing psychosis, muteness, agitation, or catatonia. Such secondary sources include members of the family, friends, neighbors, police, health care workers, and medical records.

Age Considerations
Assessment of Children
When assessing children it is important to gather data from a variety of sources. Although the child is the best source in determining inner feelings and emotions, it is the caregivers (parents or guardians) who can often best describe the behavior, performance, and conduct of the child. Caregivers also are often helpful in interpreting the child's words and responses. However, a separate interview is advisable when an older child is reluctant to share information, especially in cases of suspected abuse (Arnold & Boggs, 2007).

Developmental levels should be considered in the evaluation of children. One of the hallmarks of psychiatric disorders in children is the tendency to regress, that is, return to a previous level of development. Although it is developmentally appropriate for toddlers to suck their thumbs, such a gesture is unusual in an older child.

Assessment of children should be accomplished by a combination of interview and observation. Watching children at play provides important clues to their functioning. Storytelling, dolls, drawing, and games can be useful as assessment tools when determining critical concerns and painful issues a child may have difficulty expressing. Usually, a clinician with special training in child and adolescent psychiatry works with young children. Refer to Chapter 23 for more on assessment of children.

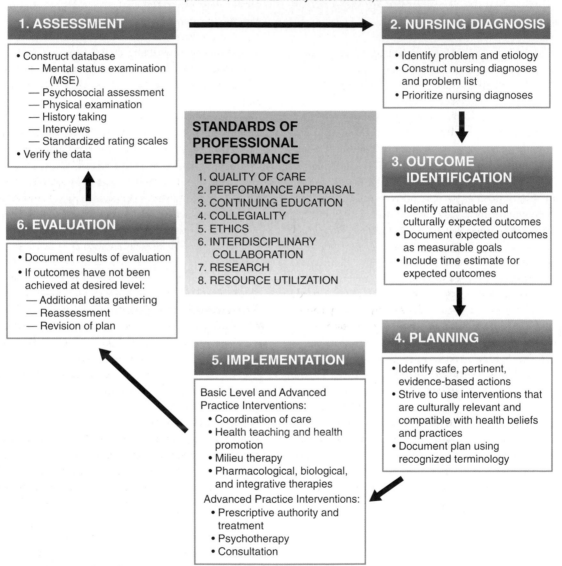

NURSING ASSESSMENT

The assessment interview requires culturally effective communication skills and encompasses a large database (e.g., significant support system; family; cultural and community system; spiritual and philosophical values, strengths, and health beliefs and practices; as well as many other factors).

1. ASSESSMENT

- Construct database
  — Mental status examination (MSE)
  — Psychosocial assessment
  — Physical examination
  — History taking
  — Interviews
  — Standardized rating scales
- Verify the data

2. NURSING DIAGNOSIS

- Identify problem and etiology
- Construct nursing diagnoses and problem list
- Prioritize nursing diagnoses

STANDARDS OF PROFESSIONAL PERFORMANCE

1. QUALITY OF CARE
2. PERFORMANCE APPRAISAL
3. CONTINUING EDUCATION
4. COLLEGIALITY
5. ETHICS
6. INTERDISCIPLINARY COLLABORATION
7. RESEARCH
8. RESOURCE UTILIZATION

3. OUTCOME IDENTIFICATION

- Identify attainable and culturally expected outcomes
- Document expected outcomes as measurable goals
- Include time estimate for expected outcomes

6. EVALUATION

- Document results of evaluation
- If outcomes have not been achieved at desired level:
  — Additional data gathering
  — Reassessment
  — Revision of plan

4. PLANNING

- Identify safe, pertinent, evidence-based actions
- Strive to use interventions that are culturally relevant and compatible with health beliefs and practices
- Document plan using recognized terminology

5. IMPLEMENTATION

Basic Level and Advanced Practice Interventions:
- Coordination of care
- Health teaching and health promotion
- Milieu therapy
- Pharmacological, biological, and integrative therapies

Advanced Practice Interventions:
- Prescriptive authority and treatment
- Psychotherapy
- Consultation

Figure 5-1 ▪ The nursing process in psychiatric mental health nursing.

Assessment of Adolescents

All patients are concerned with confidentiality. This is especially true for adolescents. Adolescents may fear that anything they say to the nurse will be repeated to their parents. Adolescents need to know that their records are private and should receive an explanation as to how information will be shared among the treatment team. Questions related to substance abuse, sexual abuse, and so on demand confidentiality (Arnold & Boggs, 2007). However, threats of suicide, homicide, use of illegal drugs, or issues of abuse have to be shared with other professionals as well as with the parents. Because identifying risk factors is one of the key objectives

BOX 5-1

The HEADSSS Psychosocial Interview Technique

H Home environment (e.g., relations with parents and siblings)

E Education and employment (e.g., school performance)

A Activities (e.g., sports participation, afterschool activities, peer relations)

D Drug, alcohol, or tobacco use

S Sexuality (e.g., whether the patient is sexually active, practices safe sex, or uses contraception)

S Suicide risk or symptoms of depression or other mental disorder

S "Savagery" (e.g., violence or abuse in home environment or in neighborhood)

---

when assessing adolescents, it is helpful to use a brief structured interview technique called the HEADSSS interview (Box 5-1). Refer to Chapter 23 for more on assessment of adolescents.

Assessment of the Older Adult

Older adults often need special attention. The nurse needs to be aware of any physical limitations—any sensory condition (difficulty seeing or hearing), motor condition (difficulty walking or maintaining balance), or medical condition (cardiac or refractory)—that could cause increased anxiety, stress, or physical discomfort for the patient while attempting to assess mental and emotional needs.

It is wise to identify any physical deficits the patient may have at the onset of the assessment and make accommodations for them. For example, if the patient is hard of hearing, speak a little more slowly and in clear, louder tones (but not too loud) and seat the patient close to you without invading his or her personal space. Refer to Chapter 25 for more on communicating with the older adult.

Psychiatric Nursing Assessment

The purpose of the psychiatric nursing assessment is to:

- Establish rapport.
- Obtain an understanding of the current problem or chief complaint.
- Review physical status and obtain baseline vital signs.
- Assess for risk factors affecting the safety of the patient or others.
- Perform a mental status examination (MSE).
- Assess psychosocial status.
- Identify mutual goals for treatment.
- Formulate a plan of care.

Gathering Data

Review of Systems

The mind-body connection is significant in the understanding and treatment of psychiatric disorders. Many patients who are admitted for treatment of psychiatric conditions also are given a thorough physical examination by a primary care provider. Likewise, most nursing assessments include a physical component that includes obtaining a baseline set of vital statistics, a historical and current review of body systems, and a documentation of allergic responses.

People with certain physical conditions may be more prone to psychiatric disorders such as depression. It is believed, for example, that the disease process of multiple sclerosis itself may actually bring about depression. Other medical diseases that are typically associated with depression are coronary artery disease, diabetes, and stroke. Individuals need to be evaluated for any medical origins of their depression or anxiety.

There is a long list of medical conditions that may mimic psychiatric illnesses (Box 5-2). By the same token, often when depression is secondary to a known medical condition, it goes unrecognized and thus untreated. Conversely, psychiatric disorders can result in physical or somatic symptoms such as stomachaches, headaches, lethargy, insomnia, intense fatigue, and even pain. Therefore, all patients who come into the health care system need to have both a medical and mental health evaluation to ensure a correct diagnosis and appropriate care.

Laboratory Data

Disorders such as hypothyroidism may have the clinical appearance of depression, and hyperthyroidism may appear to be a manic phase of bipolar disorder; a simple blood test can usually differentiate between depression and thyroid problems. Abnormal liver enzyme levels can explain irritability, depression, and lethargy. People who have chronic renal disease often suffer from the same symptoms when their blood urea nitrogen and electrolyte levels are abnormal. Results of a toxicology screen for the presence of either prescription or illegal drugs also may provide useful information.

Mental Status Examination

Fundamental to the assessment is a **mental status examination (MSE).** In fact, an MSE is part of the assessment in all areas of medicine. The MSE in psychiatry is analogous to the physical examination in general medicine. The purpose of the MSE is to evaluate an individual's current

BOX 5-2

Some Medical Conditions That May Mimic Psychiatric Illness

Depression

Neurological disorders:
- Cerebrovascular accident (stroke)
- Alzheimer's disease
- Brain tumor
- Huntington's disease
- Epilepsy (seizure disorder)
- Multiple sclerosis
- Parkinson's disease
- Cancer

Infections:
- Mononucleosis
- Encephalitis
- Hepatitis
- Tertiary syphilis
- Human immunodeficiency virus (HIV) infection

Endocrine disorders:
- Hypothyroidism and hyperthyroidism
- Cushing's syndrome
- Addison's disease
- Parathyroid disease

Gastrointestinal disorders:
- Liver cirrhosis
- Pancreatitis

Cardiovascular disorders:
- Hypoxia
- Congestive heart failure

Respiratory disorders:
- Sleep apnea

Nutritional disorders:
- Thiamine deficiency
- Protein deficiency
- B_{12} deficiency
- B_6 deficiency
- Folate deficiency

Collagen vascular diseases:
- Lupus erythematosus
- Rheumatoid arthritis

Anxiety

Neurological disorders:
- Alzheimer's disease
- Brain tumor
- Stroke
- Huntington's disease

Infections:
- Encephalitis
- Meningitis

- Neurosyphilis
- Septicemia

Endocrine disorders:
- Hypothyroidism and hyperthyroidism
- Hypoparathyroidism
- Hypoglycemia
- Pheochromocytoma
- Carcinoid

Metabolic disorders:
- Low calcium
- Low potassium
- Acute intermittent porphyria
- Liver failure

Cardiovascular disorders:
- Angina
- Congestive heart failure
- Pulmonary embolus

Respiratory disorders:
- Pneumothorax
- Acute asthma
- Emphysema

Drug effects:
- Stimulants
- Sedatives (withdrawal)

Lead, mercury poisoning

Psychosis

Medical conditions:
- Temporal lobe epilepsy
- Migraine headaches
- Temporal arteritis
- Occipital tumors
- Narcolepsy
- Encephalitis
- Hypothyroidism
- Addison's disease
- HIV infection

Drug effects:
- Hallucinogens (e.g., LSD)
- Phencyclidine
- Alcohol withdrawal
- Stimulants
- Cocaine
- Corticosteroids

BOX 5-3

Mental Status Examination

Personal Information
Age
Sex
Marital status
Religious preference
Race
Ethnic background
Employment
Living arrangements

Appearance
Grooming and dress
Level of hygiene
Pupil dilation or constriction
Facial expression
Height, weight, nutritional status
Presence of body piercing or tattoos, scars, other
Relationship between appearance and age

Behavior
Excessive or reduced body movements
Peculiar body movements (e.g., scanning of the environment, odd or repetitive gestures, level of consciousness, balance and gait)
Abnormal movements (e.g., tardive dyskinesia, tremors)
Level of eye contact (keep cultural differences in mind)

Speech
Rate: slow, rapid, normal
Volume: loud, soft, normal
Disturbances (e.g., articulation problems, slurring, stuttering, mumbling)
Cluttering (e.g., rapid, disorganized, tongue-tied speech)

Affect and Mood
Affect: flat, bland, animated, angry, withdrawn, appropriate to context
Mood: sad, labile, euphoric

Thought
Thought process (e.g., disorganized, coherent, flight of ideas, neologisms, thought blocking, circumstantiality)
Thought content (e.g., delusions, obsessions, suicidal thought)

Perceptual Disturbances
Hallucinations (e.g., auditory, visual)
Illusions

Cognition
Orientation: time, place, person
Level of consciousness (e.g., alert, confused, clouded, stuporous, unconscious, comatose)
Memory: remote, recent, immediate
Fund of knowledge
Attention: performance on serial sevens, digit span tests
Abstraction: performance on tests involving similarities, proverbs
Insight
Judgment

cognitive processes. For acutely disturbed patients it is not unusual for the mental health clinician to administer MSEs every day. Sommers-Flanagan and Sommers-Flanagan (2003) advise anyone seeking employment in the medical–mental health field to be competent in communicating with other professionals via MSE reports. Box 5-3 lists the elements of a basic MSE. An example of a mental status examination is printed on the inside back cover of this text.

The MSE, by and large, aids in collecting and organizing *objective data*. The nurse observes the patient's physical behavior, nonverbal communication, appearance, speech patterns, mood and affect, thought content, perceptions, cognitive ability, and insight and judgment.

Psychosocial Assessment

A **psychosocial assessment** provides additional information from which to develop a plan of care beyond the MSE. It includes obtaining the following information about the patient:

- Central or chief complaint (in the patient's own words)
- History of violent, suicidal, or self-mutilating behaviors
- Alcohol and/or substance abuse
- Family psychiatric history
- Personal psychiatric treatment including medications and complementary therapies
- Stressors and coping methods
- Quality of activities of daily living
- Personal background
- Social background including support system
- Weaknesses, strengths, and goals for treatment
- Racial, ethnic, and cultural beliefs and practices
- Spiritual beliefs or religious practices

The patient's psychosocial history is most often the *subjective* part of the assessment. The focus of the history is the patient's perceptions and recollections of current lifestyle, and life in general (family, friends, education, work experience, coping styles, and spiritual and cultural beliefs).

BOX 5-4

Psychosocial Assessment

A. Previous hospitalizations
B. Educational background
C. Occupational background
   1. Employed? Where? What length of time?
   2. Special skills
D. Social patterns
   1. Describe family.
   2. Describe friends.
   3. With whom does the patient live?
   4. To whom does the patient go in time of crisis?
   5. Describe a typical day.
E. Sexual patterns
   1. Sexually active? Practices safe sex? Practices birth control?
   2. Sexual orientation
   3. Sexual difficulties
F. Interests and abilities
   1. What does the patient do in his or her spare time?
   2. What sport, hobby, or leisure activity is the patient good at?
   3. What gives the patient pleasure?
G. Substance use and abuse
   1. What medications does the patient take? How often? How much?
   2. What herbal or over-the-counter drugs does the patient take? How often? How much?

3. What psychotropic drugs does the patient take? How often? How much?
4. How many drinks of alcohol does the patient take per day? Per week?
5. What recreational drugs does the patient take? How often? How much?
6. Does the patient identify the use of drugs as a problem?
H. Coping abilities
   1. What does the patient do when he or she gets upset?
   2. To whom can the patient talk?
   3. What usually helps to relieve stress?
   4. What did the patient try this time?
I. Spiritual assessment
   1. What importance does religion or spirituality have in the patient's life?
   2. Do the patient's religious or spiritual beliefs relate to the way the patient takes care of himself or herself or of the patient's illness? How?
   3. Does the patient's faith help the patient in stressful situations?
   4. Whom does the patient see when he or she is medically ill? Mentally upset?
   5. Are there special health care practices within the patient's culture that address his or her particular mental problem?

A psychosocial assessment elicits information about the systems in which a person operates. To conduct such an assessment, the nurse should have fundamental knowledge of growth and development and of basic cultural and religious practices, as well as of pathophysiology, psychopathology, and pharmacology. Box 5-4 provides a basic psychosocial assessment tool.

Spiritual or Religious Assessment

The importance of spirituality and religious beliefs to the health of the American public has been increasingly highlighted by the media, opinion polls, and empirical studies (Koenig et al., 2001). Spiritual values and skills are becoming recognized as necessary aspects of clinical care to be more openly discussed and taught (Culliford, 2002; Swinton, 2001). Carson and Koenig (2004) stress the importance of a spiritual and religious assessment as integral to a holistic nursing assessment. Spirituality and religious beliefs have the potential to exert an influence on people's view of themselves and how they interact with and respond to others (Mackenzie et al., 2000).

A comprehensive analysis of empirical research covering more than 1200 studies and 400 reviews examined relations between religion or spirituality and many physical and mental conditions. The analysis found that there was a 60% to 80% relationship between better health and religion or spiritual beliefs. The studies covered a variety of physical conditions such as heart disease, hypertension, immunological dysfunction, cancer, pain, and other conditions. Psychiatric phenomena include depression, anxiety, suicide, and more (Koenig et al., 2001).

Spirituality and religion are, however, quite different in their influences. Spirituality is an internal phenomenon. It is the part of us that seeks to understand life (Koenig, 2001) and may or may not be connected with the community or religious rituals. Spirituality has been found to increase healthy behaviors, social support, and a sense of meaning, which are linked to decreased overall mental and physical illness (George et al., 2000). Spiritual assessment should focus on what gives meaning to a person's life.

In contrast, religion is an external system that includes beliefs, patterns of worship, and symbols (Koenig, 2001). Religious affiliation is a choice to connect personal spiritual beliefs with a larger organized group or institution and typically involves rituals. Belonging to a religious community can provide support during difficult times. For some patients prayer is a source of hope, comfort, and support in healing.

The following questions help with a spiritual or religious assessment:

- Who or what supplies you with strength and hope?
- Do you have a religious affiliation?
- Do you participate in any religious activities?
- What role does religion play in your life?
- Does your faith help you in stressful situations?
- Do you pray or meditate?
- Has your illness affected your religious practices?
- Would you like to have someone from your church/synagogue/temple or from our facility visit?

Cultural and Social Assessment

Because nurses are increasingly faced with caring for culturally diverse populations, there is a growing need for nursing assessment, nursing diagnoses, and subsequent care to be planned around unique cultural health care beliefs, values, and practices. Kavanaugh (2003) advocates that mental health nurses have a thorough understanding of the complexity of the cultural and social factors that influence health and illness. Awareness of individual cultural beliefs and health care practices can help nurses minimize labeling of patients.

For patients who have difficulty with the English language or have language difficulties, federal law maintains the use of a trained interpreter (Arnold & Boggs, 2007). Some questions we can ask to help with a cultural and social assessment are the following:

- What is your primary language? Would you like an interpreter?
- How would you describe your cultural background?
- To whom are you close?
- Who do you seek in times of crisis?
- With whom do you live?
- Who do you seek when you are medically ill? Mentally upset or concerned?
- What do you do to get better when you are medically ill? Mentally or emotionally ill?
- What are the attitudes toward mental illness in your culture?
- How is your mental health problem viewed by your culture? Is it seen as a problem that can be fixed? A disease? A taboo? A fault or curse?
- Are there special foods that you eat?
- Are there special health care practices within your culture that address your particular mental or emotional health problem?
- Are there any special cultural beliefs about your illness that might help me give you better care?
- How do you pay for your health care needs?

After the assessment it is useful to summarize pertinent data with the patient. This summary provides patients with reassurance that they have been heard, and it gives them the opportunity to clarify any misinformation. The patient should be told what will happen next. For example, if the initial assessment takes place in the hospital, you should tell the patient who else he or she will be seeing. If the initial assessment was conducted by a psychiatric nurse in a mental health clinic, the patient should be told when and how often he or she will meet with the nurse to work on the patient's problems. If you believe a referral is necessary, this should be discussed with the patient.

Validating the Assessment

In order to gain an even clearer picture of your patient, it is helpful to look to outside sources. Emergency department records can be a valuable resource in understanding an individual's presenting behavior and problems. Police reports may be available in cases in which hostility and legal altercations occurred. Old charts and medical records, most now computer accessible, are a great help in validating information you already have or adding new information to your database. If the patient was admitted to a psychiatric unit in the past, information about the patient's previous level of functioning and behavior gives you a baseline for making clinical judgments. Occasionally consent forms may need to be signed by the patient or other appropriate relative, in order to obtain access to records.

Using Rating Scales

A number of standardized rating scales are useful for psychiatric evaluation and monitoring. Rating scales are often administered by a clinician, but many are self-administered. Table 5-1 lists some of the common ones in use. Many of the clinical chapters in this book include a rating scale.

STANDARD 2: DIAGNOSIS
Formulating a Nursing Diagnosis

A nursing diagnosis is a clinical judgment about a patient's response, needs, actual and potential psychiatric disorders, mental health problems, and potential comorbid physical illnesses. A well-chosen and well-stated nursing diagnosis is the basis for selecting therapeutic outcomes and interventions (NANDA-I, 2007). Refer to Appendix B for list of NANDA-approved nursing diagnoses.

A nursing diagnosis has three structural components:

1. Problem (unmet need)
2. Etiology (probable cause)
3. Supporting data (signs and symptoms)

TABLE 5-1	Standardized Rating Scales*
Use	**Scale**
Depression	Beck Inventory
	Geriatric Depression Scale (GDS)
	Hamilton Depression Scale
	Zung Self-Report Inventory
	Patient Health Questionnaire (PHQ-9)
Anxiety	Modified Spielberger State Anxiety Scale
	Hamilton Anxiety Scale
Substance use disorders	Addiction Severity Index (ASI)
	Recovery Attitude and Treatment Evaluator (RAATE)
	Brief Drug Abuse Screen Test (B-DAST)
Obsessive-compulsive behavior	Yale-Brown Obsessive-Compulsive Scale (Y-BOCS)
Mania	Mania Rating Scale
Schizophrenia	Scale for Assessment of Negative Symptoms (SANS)
	Brief Psychiatric Rating Scale (BPRS)
Abnormal movements	Abnormal Involuntary Movement Scale (AIMS)
	Simpson Neurological Rating Scale
General psychiatric assessment	Brief Psychiatric Rating Scale (BPRS)
	Global Assessment of Functioning Scale (GAF)
Cognitive function	Mini-Mental State Examination (MMSE)
	Cognitive Capacity Screening Examination (CCSE)
	Alzheimer's Disease Rating Scale (ADRS)
	Memory and Behavior Problem Checklist
	Functional Assessment Screening Tool (FAST)
	Global Deterioration Scale (GDS)
Family assessment	McMaster Family Assessment Device
Eating disorders	Eating Disorders Inventory (EDI)
	Body Attitude Test
	Diagnostic Survey for Eating Disorders

*These rating scales highlight important areas in psychiatric assessment. Because many of the answers are subjective, experienced clinicians use these tools as a guide when planning care and also draw on their knowledge of their patients.

The *problem,* or unmet need, describes the state of the patient at present. Problems that are within the nurse's domain to prescribe for and treat are termed *nursing diagnoses.* The nursing diagnostic title states what should change. For example: *Hopelessness.*

Etiology, or probable cause, is linked to the diagnostic title with the words "related to." Stating the etiology or probable cause tells what needs to be addressed to effect the change and identifies causes that the nurse can treat through nursing interventions. For example: *Hopelessness* related to multiple losses.

Supporting data, or signs and symptoms, state what the condition is like at present. It may be linked to the diagnosis and etiology with the words "as evidenced by." Supporting data (defining characteristics) that validate the diagnosis include the following:

- Patient's statement (e.g., "It's no use; nothing will change.")
- Lack of involvement with family and friends
- Lack of motivation to care for self or environment

The complete nursing diagnosis might be *Hopelessness* related to multiple losses as evidenced by lack of motivation to care for self and the statement, "It's no use, nothing will change."

STANDARD 3: OUTCOMES IDENTIFICATION
Determining Outcomes

Outcomes criteria are the hoped-for outcomes that reflect the maximal level of patient health that can realistically be achieved through nursing interventions. Whereas nursing diagnoses identify nursing problems, outcomes reflect the desired change. The expected outcomes provide direction for continuity of care (ANA, 2007). Outcomes need to take into account the patient's culture, values, and ethical beliefs. *Specifically, outcomes are stated in attainable and measurable terms and include a time estimate for attainment (ANA, 2007).* Therefore outcomes criteria are patient centered, geared to each individual, and documented as obtainable goals.

Moorhead and colleagues (2008) have compiled a standardized list of nursing outcomes in **Nursing Outcomes Classification (NOC).** NOC includes a total of 385 standardized outcomes that provide a mechanism for communicating the effect of nursing interventions on the well-being of patients, families, and communities. Each outcome has an associated group of indicators that is used to determine patient status in relation to the outcome. Table 5-2 provides suggested NOC indicators for the outcome of Suicide

TABLE 5-2	Suicide Self-Restraint (NOC)

Definition:
Personal actions to refrain from gestures and attempts at killing self
Outcome Target Rating:
Maintain at _____. Increase to _____.

Suicide Self-Restraint Overall Rating	Never Demonstrated 1	Rarely Demonstrated 2	Sometimes Demonstrated 3	Often Demonstrated 4	Consistently Demonstrated 5	
Indicators						
Expresses feelings	1	2	3	4	5	NA
Expresses sense of hope	1	2	3	4	5	NA
Maintains connectedness in relationships	1	2	3	4	5	NA
Obtains assistance as needed	1	2	3	4	5	NA
Seeks help when feeling self-destructive	1	2	3	4	5	NA
Verbalizes suicidal ideas	1	2	3	4	5	NA
Controls impulses	1	2	3	4	5	NA
Refrains from gathering means for suicide	1	2	3	4	5	NA
Refrains from giving away possessions	1	2	3	4	5	NA
Refrains from inflicting serious injury	1	2	3	4	5	NA
Refrains from using non-prescribed mood-altering substance(s)	1	2	3	4	5	NA
Discloses plan for suicide if present	1	2	3	4	5	NA
Upholds suicide contract	1	2	3	4	5	NA
Maintains self-control without supervision	1	2	3	4	5	NA
Refrains from attempting suicide	1	2	3	4	5	NA
Obtains treatment for depression	1	2	3	4	5	NA
Obtains treatment for substance abuse	1	2	3	4	5	NA
Reports adequate pain control for chronic pain	1	2	3	4	5	NA
Uses suicide prevention resources	1	2	3	4	5	NA
Uses social support group	1	2	3	4	5	NA
Uses available mental health services	1	2	3	4	5	NA
Plans for future	1	2	3	4	5	NA

From Moorhead, S., Johnson, M., Maas, M.L. & Swanson, E. (2008). *Nursing outcomes classification (NOC)* (4th ed.). St. Louis: Mosby.

TABLE 5-3	Examples of Long- and Short-Term Goals for a Suicidal Patient
Long-Term Goals or Outcomes	**Short-Term Goals or Outcomes**
1. Patient will remain free from injury throughout the hospital stay.	a. Patient will state he or she understands the rationale and procedure of the unit's protocol for suicide precautions. b. Patient will sign a "no-suicide" contract for the next 24 hours, renewable at the end of every 24-hour period. c. Patient will seek out staff when feeling overwhelmed or self-destructive during hospitalization.
2. By discharge, patient will state he or she no longer wishes to die and has at least two people to contact if thoughts arise.	a. Patient will meet with the nurse twice a day for 15 minutes to problem-solve alternatives to the situation throughout the hospital stay. b. Patient will meet with social worker to find supportive resources in his community on discharge. c. By discharge, patient will state the purpose of medication, time and dose, adverse effects, and who to call for questions or concerns.

Self-Restraint along with the Likert scale that quantifies the achievement on each indicator from 1 (never demonstrated) to 5 (consistently demonstrated).

However, NOC does not distinguish between short- and long-term outcomes. It is helpful when assessing the effectiveness of nursing interventions to use long- and short-term outcomes, often stated as goals. The use of long- and short-term outcomes or goals is particularly helpful for teaching and learning purposes. It is also valuable for providing guidelines for appropriate interventions. The use of goals guides nurses in building incremental steps toward meeting the desired outcome. All outcomes (goals) are written in positive terms following the criteria set out by the Standards of Practice. Table 5-3 shows how a specific outcome criterion might be stated for a suicidal individual with a nursing diagnosis of *Risk for suicide* related to depression and suicide attempt.

STANDARD 4: PLANNING

More and more inpatient and community-based facilities are using standardized care plans or clinical pathways for patients with specific diagnoses. Standardizing pathways or plans of care allow for inclusion of evidence-based practice and newly tested interventions as they become available. They are more time efficient, although less focused on the specific individual patient needs. Other health care facilities continue to devise individual plans of care. Whatever the care planning procedures in a specific institution, the nurse considers the following specific principles when planning care:

- *Safe.* They must be safe for the patient as well as for other patients, staff, and family.
- *Appropriate.* They must be compatible with other therapies and with the patient's personal goals and cultural values, as well as with institutional rules.
- *Individualized.* They should be realistic (1) within the patient's capabilities given the patient's age, physical strength, condition, and willingness to change; (2) based on the number of staff available; (3) reflective of the actual available community resources; and (4) within the student's or nurse's capabilities.
- *Evidence based.* They should be based on scientific principles when available.

Using best-evidence interventions and treatments as they become available is being stressed in all areas of medical and mental health care (as discussed in detail in Chapter 1). David Sackett, one of the founders of evidence-based medicine, has defined it as "the conscientious, explicit, and judicious use of current best evidence in making decisions about the care of individual patients" (Sackett et al., 2000). **Evidence-based practice (EBP)** for nurses is a combination of clinical skill and the use of clinically relevant research in the delivery of effective patient-centered care. Therefore the use of best available research, coupled with patient preferences and sound clinical judgment and skills, makes for an optimal patient-centered nurse-patient relationship (Sackett et al., 2000). Box 5-5 lists several websites available for nurses to use as resources on evidence-based practice. Keep in mind that whatever interventions are decided on, they need to be acceptable and appropriate to the individual patient.

BOX 5-5

Useful Evidence-Based Practice Websites

- Academic Center for Evidence-Based Nursing (ACE): www.acestar.uthscsa.edu
- Center for Research and Evidence-Based Practice (CREP): www.son.rochester.edu/son/research/centers/research-evidenced-based-practice
- Centre for Evidence-Based Mental Health: www.cebmh.com
- The Cochrane Collaboration: www.cochrane.org
- The Joanna Briggs Institute: www.joannabriggs.edu.au
- The Sarah Cole Hirsch Institute for Best Nursing Practice Based on Evidence: http://fpb.case.edu/HirshInstitute/index.shtm
- University of Iowa, Evidence-Based Practice Guidelines: www.nursing.uiowa.edu/products_services/evidence_based.htm
- University of Minnesota Evidence-Based Health Care Project: http://evidence.ahc.umn.edu/ebn.htm

Interventions Planning

The **Nursing Interventions Classification (NIC)** (Bulechek et al., 2008) is a research-based standardized listing of 542 interventions that the nurse can use to plan care, and reflects current clinical practice. Nurses in all settings can use NIC to support quality patient care and incorporate evidence-based nursing actions. Although many safe and appropriate interventions may not be included in NIC, it is a useful guide for standardized care, but individualizing interventions to meet a patient's special needs should always be part of the planning.

When choosing nursing interventions from NIC or other sources, the nurse uses not just those that fit the nursing diagnosis (e.g., *Risk for suicide*) but interventions that match the defining data. Although the outcome criteria (NOC) might be similar or the same (e.g., Suicide Self-Restraint), the safe and appropriate interventions may be totally different because of the defining data. For example, consider the nursing diagnosis *Risk for suicide* related to feelings of despair as evidenced by two recent suicide attempts and repeated statements that "I want to die."

The planning of appropriate nursing interventions might include the following:

- Initiate suicide precautions (e.g., ongoing observations and monitoring of the patient, provision of a protective environment) for the person who is at serious risk for suicide.
- Search the newly hospitalized patient and personal belongings for weapons or potential weapons during inpatient admission procedure, as appropriate.
- Use protective interventions (e.g., area restriction seclusion, physical restraints) if the patient lacks the restraint to refrain from harming self, as needed.
- Assign hospitalized patient to a room located near the nursing station for ease in observations, as appropriate.

However, if the defining data are different, so will be the appropriate interventions. For example: *Risk for suicide* related to loss of spouse as evidenced by lack of self-care and statements evidencing loneliness.

The nurse might choose the following interventions for this patient's plan of care:

- Determine the presence and degree of suicidal risk.
- Facilitate support of the patient by family and friends.
- Consider strategies to decrease isolation and opportunity to act on harmful thoughts.
- Assist the patient in identifying a network of supportive personnel and resources within the community (e.g., support groups, clergy, care providers).
- Provide information about available community resources and outreach programs.

Chapter 20 addresses assessment of and intervention for suicidal patient in more depth.

STANDARD 5: IMPLEMENTATION

Psychiatric–Mental Health Nursing: Scope and Standards of Practice (ANA, 2007) identifies seven areas for intervention. Recent graduates and practitioners new to the psychiatric setting will participate in many of these activities with the guidance and support of more experienced health care professionals. The following four interventions identified in psychiatric mental health nurse (PMHN) practice guidelines (ANA, 2007) are performed by both the psychiatric mental health nurse (basic education) as well as the advanced practice psychiatric mental health nurse (master's prepared).

The basic level for the psychiatric mental health registered nurse is accomplished through the nurse-patient relationship and therapeutic intervention skills. The nurse implements the plan using evidence-based interventions whenever possible, using community resources, and collaborating with nursing colleagues.

Basic Level and Advanced Practice Interventions
Coordination of Care

The psychiatric mental health nurse coordinates the implementation of the plan and provides documentation.

Health Teaching and Health Promotion

Psychiatric mental health nurses use a variety of health teaching methods adaptive to the patient's needs (e.g., age, culture, ability to learn, readiness, etc.), integrating current knowledge and research and seeking opportunities for feedback and effectiveness of care. **Health teaching** includes identifying the health education needs of the patient and teaching basic principles of physical and mental health, such as giving information about coping, interpersonal relationships, social skills, mental disorders, the treatments for such illnesses and their effects on daily living, relapse prevention, problem-solving skills, stress management, crisis intervention, and self-care activities. The last of these, **self-care activities**, assists the patient in assuming personal responsibility for activities of daily living (ADL) and is aimed at improving the patient's mental and physical well-being.

Milieu Therapy

Milieu therapy is an extremely important consideration for the nurse working with a patient who should feel comfortable and safe. Milieu management includes orienting patients to their rights and responsibilities, selecting specific activities that meet patients' physical and mental health needs, and ensuring that patients are maintained in the least restrictive environment. Among other things, it also includes that patients are informed in a culturally competent manner about the need for limits and the conditions necessary to remove them.

Pharmacological, Biological, and Integrative Therapies

Nurses need to know the intended action, therapeutic dosage, adverse reactions, and safe blood levels of medications being administered. The nurse also must monitor these when appropriate (e.g., blood levels for lithium). The nurse is expected to discuss and provide medication teaching tools to the patient and family regarding drug action, adverse side effects, dietary restrictions, and drug interactions, and to provide time for questions. The nurse's assessment of the patient's response to psychobiological interventions is communicated to other members of the mental health team. Interventions are also aimed at alleviating untoward effects of medication.

Advanced Practice Interventions Only

The following three interventions are carried out by the advanced practice registered nurse in psychiatric mental health (APRN-PMH) nursing.

Prescriptive Authority and Treatment

The APRN-PMH is educated and clinically prepared to prescribe psychopharmacological agents for patients with mental health or psychiatric disorders in accordance with state and federal laws and regulations. Such prescriptions take into account the individual variables such as culture, ethnicity, gender, religious beliefs, age, and physical health.

Psychotherapy

The APRN-PMH is educationally and clinically prepared to conduct individual, couples, group, and family psychotherapy using evidence-based psychotherapeutic frameworks and nurse-patient therapeutic relationships (ANA, 2007).

Consultation

The APRN-PMH works with other clinicians to provide consultation, influence the identified plan, enhance the ability of other clinicians, provide services for patients, and effect change.

STANDARD 6: EVALUATION

Unfortunately, evaluation of patient outcomes is often the most neglected part of the nursing process. Evaluation of the individual's response to treatment should be systematic, ongoing, and criterion-based. Supporting data are included to clarify the evaluation. Ongoing assessment of data allows for revisions of nursing diagnoses, changes to more realistic outcomes, or identification of more appropriate interventions when outcomes are not met.

DOCUMENTATION

Documentation could be considered the seventh step in the nursing process. Keep in mind that patient records are legal documents and may be used in a court of law (see Chapter 26). Besides the evaluation of stated outcomes, the chart should record changes in patient condition, informed consents (for medications and treatments), reaction to medication, documentation of symptoms (verbatim when appropriate), concerns of the patient, and any untoward incidents in the health care setting. Documentation of patient progress is the responsibility of the entire mental health team.

Although communication among team members and coordination of services are the primary goals when choosing a system for charting, practitioners in all settings must also consider professional standards, legal issues, requirements for reimbursement by insurers, and accreditation by regulatory agencies.

Information also must be in a format that is retrievable for quality assurance monitoring, utilization management, peer review, and research. Documentation, using the nursing process as a guide, is reflected in many of the different formats that are commonly used in health care settings (Table 5-4). Computerized clinical documentation is increasingly seen in inpatient as well as outpatient settings today. Whatever documentation format is used by a health care facility, it needs to be focused, organized, and pertinent and must conform to certain legal and other generally accepted principles (Box 5-6).

BOX 5-6

Legal Considerations for Documentation of Care

Do's

- Chart in a timely manner all pertinent and factual information.
- Be familiar with the nursing documentation policy in your facility and make your charting conform to this standard. The policy generally states the method, frequency, and pertinent assessments, interventions, and outcomes to be recorded. If your agency's policies and procedures do not encourage or allow for quality documentation, bring the need for change to the administration's attention.
- Chart legibly in ink.
- Chart facts fully, descriptively, and accurately.
- Chart what you see, hear, feel, and smell.
- Chart pertinent observations: psychosocial observations, physical symptoms pertinent to the medical diagnosis, and behaviors pertinent to the nursing diagnosis.
- Chart follow-up care provided when a problem has been identified in earlier documentation. For example, if a patient has fallen and injured a leg, describe how the wound is healing.
- Chart fully the facts surrounding unusual occurrences and incidents.
- Chart all nursing interventions, treatments, and outcomes (including teaching efforts and patient responses), and safety and patient protection interventions.
- Chart the patient's expressed subjective feelings.
- Chart each time you notify a physician and record the reason for notification, the information that was communicated, the accurate time, the physician's instructions or orders, and the follow-up activity.
- Chart physicians' visits and treatments.
- Chart discharge medications and instructions given for use, as well as all discharge teaching performed, and note which family members were included in the process.

Don'ts

- Do *not* chart opinions that are not supported by the facts.
- Do *not* defame patients by calling them names or by making derogatory statements about them (e.g., "an unlikable patient who is demanding unnecessary attention").
- Do *not* chart before an event occurs.
- Do *not* chart generalizations, suppositions, or pat phrases (e.g., "patient in good spirits").
- Do *not* obliterate, erase, alter, or destroy a record. If an error is made, draw one line through the error, write "mistaken entry" or "error," and initial. Follow your agency's guidelines closely.
- Do *not* leave blank spaces for chronological notes. If you must chart out of sequence, chart "late entry." Identify the time and date of the entry and the time and date of the occurrence.
- If an incident report is filed, *do not note in the chart that one was filed.* This form is generally a privileged communication between the hospital and the hospital's attorney. Describing it in the chart may destroy the privileged nature of the communication.

TABLE 5-4 **Narrative Versus Problem-Oriented Charting**	
Narrative Charting	**Problem-Oriented Charting: SOAPIE**
Characteristics	
A descriptive statement of patient status written in chronological order throughout a shift. Used to support assessment finding from a flow sheet. In charting by exception, narrative notes are used to indicate significant symptoms, behaviors, or events that are exceptions to norms identified on an assessment flow sheet.	Developed in the 1960s for physicians to reduce inefficient documentation. Intended to be accompanied by a problem list. Originally SOAP, with IE added later. The emphasis is on problem identification, process, and outcome. **S:** Subjective data (patient statement) **O:** Objective data (nurse observations) **A:** Assessment (nurse interprets S and O and describes either a problem or a nursing diagnosis) **P:** Plan (proposed intervention) **I:** Interventions (nurse's response to problem) **E:** Evaluation (patient outcome)
Example	
Date/time/discipline. Patient was agitated in the morning and pacing in the hallway. Blinked eyes, muttered to self, and looked off to the side. Stated heard voices. Verbally hostile to another patient. Offered 2 mg haloperidol (Haldol) prn and sat with staff in quiet area for 20 minutes. Patient returned to community lounge and was able to sit and watch television.	Date/time/discipline. **S:** "I'm so stupid. Get away, get away." "I hear the devil telling me bad things." **O:** Patient paced the hall, mumbling to self and looking off to the side. Shouted derogatory comments when approached by another patient. Watched walls and ceiling closely. **A:** Patient was having auditory hallucinations and increased agitation. **P:** Offered patient haloperidol prn. Redirected patient to less stimulating environment. **I:** Patient received 2 mg haloperidol PO prn. Sat with patient in quiet room for 20 minutes. **E:** Patient calmer. Returned to community lounge, sat and watched television.
Advantages	
Uses a common form of expression (narrative writing). Can address any event or behavior. Explains flow sheet findings. Provides multidisciplinary ease of use.	Structured. Provides consistent organization of data. Facilitates retrieval of data for quality assurance and utilization management. Contains all elements of the nursing process. Minimizes inclusion of unnecessary data. Provides multidisciplinary ease of use.
Disadvantages	
Unstructured. May result in different organization of information from note to note. Makes it difficult to retrieve quality assurance and utilization management data. Frequently leads to omission of elements of the nursing process. Commonly results in inclusion of unnecessary and subjective information.	Requires time and effort to structure the information. Limits entries to problems. May result in loss of data about progress. Not chronological. Carries negative connotation.

KEY POINTS TO REMEMBER

- The nursing process is a six-step problem-solving approach to patient care.
- The *primary source* of assessment is the patient. *Secondary sources* of information include the family, neighbors, friends, police, and other members of the health team.
- The assessment interview includes gathering objective data (mental or emotional status) and subjective data (psychosocial assessment).
- Medical examination, history, and systems review round out a complete assessment.
- Assessment tools and standardized rating scales may be used to evaluate and monitor a patient's progress.
- Determination of the nursing diagnosis (NANDA) defines the practice of nursing, improves communication between staff members, and assists in accountability for care.
- A nursing diagnosis consists of (1) an unmet need or problem, (2) an etiology or probable cause, and (3) supporting data.
- Outcomes are variable, measurable, and stated in terms that reflect a patient's actual state. NOC provides 330 standardized outcomes. Planning involves determining desired outcomes.
- Behavioral goals support outcomes. Goals are measurable, indicate the desired patient behavior(s), include a set time for achievement, and are short and specific.
- Planning nursing actions (NIC or other sources) to achieve the outcomes includes the use of specific principles: the plan should be (1) safe, (2) evidence based whenever possible, (3) realistic, and (4) compatible with other therapies. NIC provides nurses with standardized nursing interventions that are applicable for use in all settings.
- Practice in psychiatric nursing encompasses four basic level interventions: coordination of care, health teaching and health promotion, milieu therapy, and pharmacological, biological, and integrative therapies.
- Advanced practice interventions are carried out by a nurse who is educated at the master's level or higher. Nurses certified for advanced practice psychiatric mental health nursing can practice psychotherapy, prescribe certain medications, and perform consulting work.
- The evaluation of care is a continual process of determining to what extent the outcome criteria have been achieved. The plan of care may be revised based on the evaluation.
- Documentation of patient progress through evaluation of the outcome criteria is crucial. The chart is a legal document and should accurately reflect the patient's condition, medications, treatment, tests, responses, and any untoward incidents.

CRITICAL THINKING

1. Pedro Gonzales, a 37-year-old Hispanic, arrived by ambulance from a supermarket, where he had fallen. He remains lethargic. On his arrival to the emergency department (ED), his breath smelled "fruity." He appears confused and anxious, saying that "they put the 'evil eye' on me, they want me to die, they are drying out my body . . . it's draining me dry . . . they are yelling, they are yelling . . . no, no I'm not bad . . . oh God don't let them get me." When his mother arrives in the ED, she tells the staff through the use of an interpreter, that Pedro is a severe diabetic, has a diagnosis of paranoid schizophrenia, and this happens when he doesn't take his medications. In a group or in collaboration with a classmate respond to the following:
    1. A number of nursing diagnoses are possible in this scenario. Formulate in writing at least two nursing diagnoses (problems) given the above information, and include "related to" and "as evidenced by."

2. For each of your nursing diagnoses, write out one long-term outcome (the problem, what should change, etc.). Include a time frame, desired change, and three criteria that will help you evaluate if the outcome has been met, not met, or partially met.
3. For each long-term outcome, write two short-term outcomes (goals) (the steps that need to be taken in order for the goal to be accomplished), including time frame, desired outcomes, and evaluation criteria.
4. What are the four basic principles for planning nursing interventions?
5. What specific needs might you take into account when planning nursing care for Mr. Gonzales?
6. Using the SOAPIE format in Table 5-4, formulate an initial nurse's note for Mr. Gonzalez.

CHAPTER REVIEW

Choose the most appropriate answer.

1. Which statement by a nurse suggests an undesirable outcome of a psychiatric assessment interview conducted by the psychiatric nurse?
   1. "I think I was able to establish good rapport with the patient."
   2. "I believe the patient understands that my values differ from his."
   3. "I was able to obtain a good understanding of the patient's current problem."
   4. "I was able to perform a complete assessment of the patient's level of psychological functioning."

2. Assessment of an older adult patient will be facilitated if the nurse:
   1. identifies and accommodates patient physical needs early.
   2. pledges complete confidentiality of all topics to the patient.
   3. adheres strictly to the order of questions on the standardized assessment tool.
   4. interprets data without regard to the patient's spiritual and cultural beliefs and practices.

3. A nurse tells a peer, "I place greatest weight on the subjective data I obtain during patient assessment." From this the peer can infer that the nurse depends more on:
   1. data obtained from secondary sources than data obtained from the primary source.
   2. the patient's perceptions of the presenting problem than on data obtained from the mental status examination.
   3. data obtained from the mental status examination than on information elicited during history taking.
   4. gut-level hunches about patient strengths and weaknesses than on data obtained from rating scales.

4. Which statement about a nursing diagnosis is correct?
   1. A nursing diagnosis has three structural components: a problem, the etiology of the problem, and supporting data that validate the diagnosis.
   2. A nursing diagnosis is complete when the problem statement reflects an unmet need and the etiology given reflects a probable cause.
   3. An accurate nursing diagnosis requires a problem statement that identifies causes the nurse can treat via nursing interventions.
   4. A nursing diagnosis always must be based on objective data measured by the nurse; subjective data may be used only as supporting data to validate the diagnosis.

5. What is the relationship between evidence-based practice and clinically relevant research?
   1. Evidence-based practice reflects realistic processes for achieving patient progress, whereas clinical research suggests best nursing practices.
   2. Evidence-based practice is a set of guidelines for meeting nursing standards and does not relate directly to clinical research.
   3. Evidence-based practice is accomplished partly by using clinically relevant research.
   4. Evidence-based practice is required as part of interdisciplinary treatment plans, whereas clinically relevant research is specific to the discipline of nursing.

REFERENCES

American Nurses Association (ANA), American Psychiatric Nurses Association, & International Society of Psychiatric–Mental Health Nurses. (2007). *Psychiatric–mental health nursing: Scope and standards of practice.* Washington, DC: Nursesbooks.org.

Arnold, E.C., & Boggs K.U. (2007). *Interpersonal relationships: Professional communication skills for nurses* (5th ed.). St. Louis: Saunders.

Bulechek, G.M., Butcher, H.K., & Dochterman, J.M. (2008). *Nursing interventions classification (NIC)* (5th ed.). St. Louis: Mosby.

Carson, V.B., & Koenig, H.G. (2004). *Spiritual caregiving as a ministry.* Philadelphia: Templeton.

Culliford, L.D. (2002). Spiritual care and psychiatric treatment—An introduction. *Advanced Psychiatric Treatment, 8,* 249-260.

George, L.K., Larson, D.B., Koenig, H.G., & McCullough, M.E. (2000). Spirituality and health: What we know, what we need to know. *Journal of Social and Clinical Psychology, 19*(1), 102-116.

Kavanaugh, K.H. (2003). Transcultural perspectives in mental health nursing. In M. Andrews & J. Boyle (Eds.), *Transcultural concepts in nursing care.* Philadelphia: Lippincott Williams & Wilkins.

Koenig, H.G. (2001). *Handbook of religion and mental health.* New York: Oxford Press.

Koenig, H.G., McCullough, M., & Larson, D.B. (2001). *Handbook of religion and health.* New York: Oxford University Press.

Mackenzie, E., Rajagopal, D., Meibohm, M., & Lavizzo-Mourey, R. (2000). Spiritual support and psychological well-being: Older adults' perceptions of the religion and health connection. *Alternative Therapies in Health and Medicine, 6*(6), 37-45.

Moorhead, S., Johnson, M., Maas, M.L. & Swanson, E. (2008). *Nursing outcomes classification (NOC)* (4th ed.). St. Louis: Mosby.

North American Nursing Diagnosis Association International (NANDA-I). (2007-2008). *NANDA nursing diagnoses: Definitions and classification 2007-2008.* Philadelphia: Author.

Sackett, D. L., Straus, S., Richardson, W., et al. (2000). *Evidence-based medicine: How to practice and teach EBMB.* London: Churchill Livingstone.

Sommers-Flanagan J., & Sommers-Flanagan, R. (2003). *Clinical interviewing* (3rd ed.). Hoboken, NJ: Wiley.

Swinton, J. (2001). *Spirituality and mental health care: Rediscovering a forgotten dimension.* London: Jessica Kingsley.

CHAPTER 6

Communication Skills: Medium for All Nursing Practice

Elizabeth M. Varcarolis

Key Terms and Concepts

cultural filters, p. 100
double messages, p. 91
double-bind messages, p. 91
feedback, p. 88
nonverbal communication, p. 90

nontherapeutic techniques, p. 92
therapeutic communication, p. 88
therapeutic techniques, p. 92
verbal communication, p. 90

Objectives

1. Identify three personal and two environmental factors that can impede accurate communication.
2. Discuss the differences between verbal and nonverbal communication and identify five areas of nonverbal communication.
3. Identify two attending behaviors that the nurse might focus on to increase communication skills.
4. Relate problems that can arise when nurses are insensitive to cultural differences in patients' communication styles.

5. Compare and contrast the range of verbal and nonverbal communication of different cultural groups in the areas of (a) communication style, (b) eye contact, and (c) touch. Give examples.
6. Demonstrate the use of four techniques that can enhance communication, highlighting what makes them effective.
7. Demonstrate the use of four techniques that can obstruct communication, highlighting what makes them ineffective.

evolve

For additional resources related to the content of this chapter, visit the Evolve website at http://evolve.elsevier.com/Varcarolis/essentials.

- Chapter Outline
- Chapter Review Answers

- Nurse, Patient, and Family Resources
- Concept Map Creator

Our advanced ability to communicate is a fundamental aspect of being human; in fact, all of our actions, words, and expressions convey meaning to others. It's even said that we cannot *not* communicate. Silence, for example, can communicate acceptance, anger, or thoughtfulness. In the provision of nursing care, communication takes on a new emphasis. Just as social relationships are different from therapeutic relationships, basic communication is different from a professional, goal-directed, and scientifically based communication we call **therapeutic communication**.

COMMUNICATION

Therapeutic communication is essential in nursing care regardless of the setting. Developing the skill to determine levels of pain in the postoperative patient, to listen as parents express feelings of fear concerning their child's diagnosis, or to understand, without hearing the words, the needs of the intubated voiceless patient in the intensive care unit is essential in the provision of quality nursing care. In psychiatric nursing communication skills take on a different and new emphasis because psychiatric disorders cause not only physical symptoms such as fatigue, loss of appetite, and insomnia, but also emotional symptoms such as sadness, anger, hopelessness, and euphoria that affect a person's very ability to relate to others.

It is often in the psychiatric rotation that students discover the utility of therapeutic communication and begin to rely on techniques they once considered artificial. With continued practice, you will develop your own style and rhythm, and eventually these techniques will become a part of the way you communicate with others.

Beginning psychiatric practitioners are often concerned that they may say the wrong thing, especially when learning to apply therapeutic techniques. Will you say the wrong thing? The answer is, yes, you probably will. That is how we all learn to find more useful and effective ways of helping individuals reach their goals. The challenge is to recover from your mistakes and use them for learning and growth (Sommers-Flanagan & Sommers-Flanagan, 2003).

Will saying the wrong thing be harmful to the patient? This is doubtful, especially if your intent is honest, your approach is respectful, and you have a genuine concern for the patient. Communication can be 90% nonverbal, and individuals pay attention to the intent as is discussed in greater detail later in this chapter. Scientific investigations have identified special skills and methods that can aid people in becoming more effective helpers. However, knowledge of skills and techniques is not enough. Being an effective communicator, whether in nursing or any other area of life, is not just a matter of knowing what techniques to use. Genuine respect for the individual, the ability to listen and to understand the person's concerns, and a desire to work with the individual to help his or her situation are also key factors.

The Communication Process

Communication is the process of sending and receiving messages. One way of thinking about the process of communication is to use a basic communication model that identifies the parts of an interaction (Berlo, 1960). Very simply put then, the basic format is the following:

1. One person has a need to communicate with another **(stimulus).** For example, the stimulus for communication can be a need for information, comfort, or advice.
2. The person sending the message **(sender)** initiates interpersonal contact.
3. The **message** is the information sent or expressed to another. The clearest messages are those that are well organized and expressed in a manner familiar to the receiver.
4. The message can be sent through a variety of **media,** including auditory (hearing), visual (seeing), tactile (touch), smell, or any combination of these.
5. The person receiving the message **(receiver)** then interprets the message and responds to the sender by providing **feedback.** The nature of the feedback often indicates whether the meaning of the message sent has been correctly interpreted by the receiver. Validating the accuracy of the sender's message is extremely important. An accuracy check may be obtained by simply asking the sender, "Is this what you mean?" or "I notice you turn away when we talk about your going back to college. Is there a conflict there?"

Figure 6-1 shows this simple model of communication along with some of the many factors that affect it.

Effective communication in helping relationships depends on nurses' knowing what they are trying to convey (the purpose of the message), communicating what is really meant to the patient, and comprehending the meaning of what the patient is intentionally or unintentionally conveying (Arnold & Boggs, 2007). Fundamental to all of this is determining where the person is coming from so that the nurse and patient can start on common ground. Peplau (1952) identified two main principles that can guide the communication process during the nurse-patient interview: (1) **clarity,** which ensures that the meaning of the message

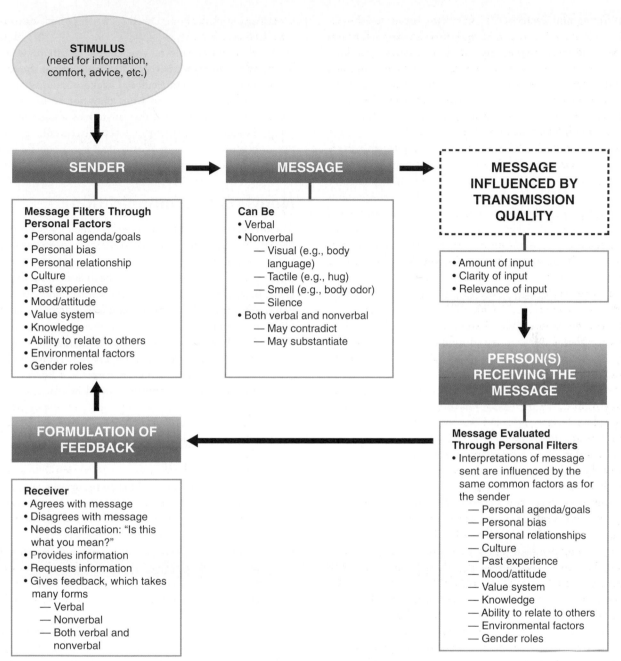

Figure 6-1 ■ Operational definition of communication. (Data from Ellis, R., & McClintock, A. [1990]. *If you take my meaning.* London: Arnold.)

is accurately understood by both parties "as the result of joint and sustained effort of all parties concerned," and (2) **continuity,** which promotes connections among ideas "and the feelings, events, or themes conveyed in those ideas" (p. 290).

Communication is complex and involves a variety of personal and environmental factors that can distort both the sending and receiving of messages.

Factors That Affect Communication
Personal Factors

Personal factors that can impede accurate transmission or interpretation of messages include emotional factors (e.g., mood, responses to stress, personal bias), social factors (e.g., previous experience, cultural differences, language differences), and cognitive factors (e.g., problem-solving ability, knowledge level, language use).

Environmental Factors

Environmental factors that may affect communication include physical factors (e.g., background noise, lack of privacy, uncomfortable accommodations) and societal determinants (e.g., sociopolitical, historical, and economic factors, the presence of others, expectations of others).

Relationship Factors

Relationship factors refer to whether the participants are equal or unequal. When the two participants are equal, such as friends or colleagues, the relationship is said to be **symmetrical.** However, when there is a difference in status or power, such as between nurse and patient or teacher and student, the relationship is characterized by inequality (one participant is "superior" to the other) and is called a **complementary** relationship (Ellis et al., 2003).

Verbal Communication

Verbal communication consists of all words a person speaks. We live in a society of symbols, and our supreme social symbols are words. Talking is our most common activity—our public link with one another, the primary instrument of instruction, a need, an art, and one of the most personal aspects of our private lives. When we speak, we:

- Communicate our beliefs and values.
- Communicate perceptions and meanings.
- Convey interest and understanding *or* insult and judgment.
- Convey messages clearly *or* convey conflicting or implied messages.

- Convey clear, honest feelings *or* disguised, distorted feelings.

Words are often culturally perceived. Clarifying what is meant by certain words is very important. Even if the nurse and patient have the same cultural background, the mental image they have of a given word may not be exactly the same. Although they believe they are talking about the same thing, the nurse and patient may actually be talking about two quite different things. Words are the symbols for emotions as well as mental images.

Nonverbal Communication

The tone of voice and the manner in which a person paces speech are examples of **nonverbal communication**. Other common examples of nonverbal communication (often called **cues**) are physical appearance, facial expressions, body posture, amount of eye contact, eye cast (i.e., emotion expressed in the eyes), hand gestures, sighs, fidgeting, and yawning. Table 6-1 identifies key components of nonverbal behaviors. Nonverbal behaviors need to be observed and interpreted in light of a person's culture, class, gender, age, sexual orientation, and spiritual norms. Cultural influences on communication will be discussed later in this chapter.

Interaction of Verbal and Nonverbal Communication

Communication consists of verbal and nonverbal elements. Although we tend to think of communication primarily in terms of what is said, Shea (1998), a nationally renowned

TABLE 6-1	Nonverbal Behaviors	
Behavior	**Possible Nonverbal Cues**	**Example**
Body behaviors	Posture, body movements, gestures, gait	The patient is slumped in a chair, puts her face in her hands, and occasionally taps her right foot.
Facial expressions	Frowns, smiles, grimaces, raised eyebrows, pursed lips, licking of lips, tongue movements	The patient grimaces when speaking to the nurse; when alone, he smiles and giggles to himself.
Eye cast	Angry, suspicious, and accusatory looks	The patient's eyes harden with suspicion.
Voice-related behaviors	Tone, pitch, level, intensity, inflection, stuttering, pauses, silences, fluency	The patient talks in a loud sing-song voice.
Observable autonomic physiological responses	Increase in respirations, diaphoresis, pupil dilation, blushing, paleness	When the patient mentions discharge, she becomes pale, her respirations increase, and her face becomes diaphoretic.
Personal appearance	Grooming, dress, hygiene	The patient is dressed in a wrinkled shirt and his pants are stained; his socks are dirty and he is unshaven.
Physical characteristics	Height, weight, physique, complexion	The patient appears grossly overweight and his muscles appear flabby.

psychiatrist and communication workshop leader, indicates that communication is roughly 10% verbal and 90% nonverbal. Rankin (2001) believes that nonverbal behaviors comprise from 65% to 95% of a sent message. Both sets of statistics point to the surprising degree to which nonverbal behaviors and cues influence communication. Effective communicators pay attention to verbal as well as nonverbal cues.

Communication thus involves two radically different but interdependent kinds of symbols. The first type is the **spoken word,** which represents our public selves. Verbal assertions can be straightforward comments or skillfully can be used to distort, conceal, deny, and generally disguise true feelings. The second type, **nonverbal behaviors,** covers a wide range of human activities, from body movements to responses to the messages of others. How a person listens and uses silence and sense of touch may also convey important information about the private self that is not available from conversation alone, especially when viewed from a cultural perspective.

Some elements of nonverbal communication, such as facial expressions, seem to be inborn and are similar across cultures. Dee (1991) cited studies that found a high degree of agreement in spontaneous facial expressions or emotions across 10 different cultures. In public, however, some cultural groups (e.g., Japanese) may control their facial expressions when observers are present. Other types of nonverbal behaviors, such as how close people stand to each other when speaking, depend on cultural conventions. Some nonverbal communication is formalized and has specific meanings (e.g., the military salute, the Japanese bow).

Messages are not always simple and can appear to be one thing when in fact they are another (Ellis et al., 2003). An interaction consists of verbal and nonverbal messages. Often, people have more conscious awareness of their verbal messages and less awareness of their nonverbal behaviors. The verbal message is sometimes referred to as the **content** of the message, and the nonverbal behavior is called the **process** of the message.

When the content is congruent with the process, the communication is more clearly understood and is considered healthy. For example, if a student says, "It's important that I get good grades in this class," that is *content*. If the student has bought the books, takes good notes, and has a study buddy, that is *process*. Therefore the content and process are congruent and straightforward, and there is a "healthy" message. If, however, the verbal message is not reinforced or is in fact contradicted by the nonverbal behavior, the message is confusing. For example, if the student does not have the books, skips several classes, and does not study, that is *process*. Here the student is sending out two different messages.

Conflicting messages are known as **double messages** or *mixed messages*. Dee (1991) suggested that one way a nurse can respond to verbal and nonverbal incongruity is to reflect and validate the patient's feelings. "You say you are upset that you did not pass this semester, but I notice that you look more relaxed and less conflicted than you have all term. What do you see as some of the pros and cons of not passing the course this semester?"

Bateson and colleagues (1956) coined the term **double-bind messages.** Messages are sent to create meaning but also can be used defensively to hide what is actually going on, create confusion, and attack relatedness (Ellis et al., 2003). A double-bind message is a mix of content (what is said) and process (what is going on picked up nonverbally) that has both nurturing and hurtful aspects. For example:

VIGNETTE

A 17-year-old female who lives at home with her mother wants to go out for an evening with her friends. She is told by her chronically ill but not helpless mother: "Oh, go ahead, have fun. I'll just sit here by myself, and I can always call 911 if I don't feel well, but you go ahead and have fun." The mother says this while looking sad, eyes cast down, slumped in her chair, and letting her cane drop to the floor.

The recipient of this double-bind message is caught inside contradictory statements so that she cannot do the right thing. If she goes, the implication is that she is being selfish by leaving her sick mother alone, but if she stays, the mother could say, "I told you to go have fun." If she does go, the chances are she won't have much fun. No matter what the daughter does, she just can't win.

With experience, nurses become increasingly aware of a patient's verbal and nonverbal communication. Nurses can compare patients' dialogue with their nonverbal communication to gain important clues about the real message. What individuals do may either express and reinforce, or contradict, what they say. As in the saying "Actions speak louder than words," actions often reveal the true meaning of a person's intent, whether it is conscious or unconscious.

EFFECTIVE COMMUNICATION SKILLS FOR NURSES

The art of communication was emphasized by Peplau to highlight the importance of nursing interventions in facilitating achievement of quality patient care and quality of life (Haber, 2000). Therefore, as stated, the goals of the nurse in the mental health setting are to help the patient:

- Feel understood and comfortable
- Identify and explore problems relating to others
- Discover healthy ways of meeting emotional needs
- Experience satisfying interpersonal relationships

The goal for the nurse is to establish and maintain a therapeutic relationship in which the patient will feel safe and hopeful that positive change is possible.

Once specific needs and problems have been identified, the nurse can work with the patient on increasing problem-solving skills, learning new coping behaviors, and experiencing more appropriate and satisfying ways of relating to others. To do this the nurse needs to have a sound knowledge of communication skills. Therefore nurses must become more aware of their own interpersonal methods, eliminating obstructive **nontherapeutic techniques** and developing additional responses that maximize nurse-patient interactions and increase the use of helpful **therapeutic techniques**.

Useful tools for nurses when communicating with their patients are (1) silence, (2) active listening, and (3) clarifying techniques.

Use of Silence

Silence can frighten interviewers as well as patients (Sommers-Flanagan & Sommers-Flanagan, 2003). In our society, and in nursing, there is an emphasis on action. In communication we tend to expect a high level of verbal activity. Many students and practicing nurses find that when the flow of words stops, they become uncomfortable. **Silence** is not the absence of communication; it is a specific channel for transmitting and receiving messages. The practitioner needs to understand that silence is a significant means of influencing and being influenced by others.

In the initial interview the patient may be reluctant to speak because of the newness of the situation, the fact that the nurse is a stranger, self-consciousness, embarrassment, or shyness. Talking is highly individualized; some find the telephone a nuisance, whereas others believe they cannot live without their cell phones. The nurse must recognize and respect individual differences in styles and tempos of responding. People who are quiet, those who have a language barrier or speech impediment, older adults, and those who lack confidence in their ability to express themselves may communicate a need for support and encouragement through their silence (Collins, 1983).

Although there is no universal rule concerning how much silence is too much, silence has been said to be worthwhile only as long as it is serving some function and not frightening the patient. Knowing when to speak during the interview largely depends on the nurse's perception about what is being conveyed through the silence. Icy silence may be an expression of anger and hostility. Being ignored or given the silent treatment is recognized as an insult and is a particularly hurtful form of communication. Silence among some African American patients may relate to anger, insulted feelings, or acknowledgment of a nurse's lack of cultural sensitivity (Smedley et al., 2002).

Silence may provide meaningful moments of reflection for both participants. It gives each an opportunity to contemplate thoughtfully what has been said and felt, weigh alternatives, formulate new ideas, and gain a new perspective on the matter under discussion. If the nurse waits to speak and allows the patient to break the silence, the patient may share thoughts and feelings that would otherwise have been withheld. Nurses who feel compelled to fill every void with words often do so because of their own anxiety, self-consciousness, and embarrassment. When this occurs, the nurse's need for comfort tends to take priority over the needs of the patient.

Conversely, prolonged and frequent silences by the nurse may hinder an interview that requires verbal articulation. Although the untalkative nurse may be comfortable with silence, this mode of communication may make the patient feel like a fountain of information to be drained dry. Moreover, without feedback, patients have no way of knowing whether what they said was understood.

Active Listening

People want more than just physical presence in human communication. Most people want the other person to be there for them psychologically, socially, and emotionally (Egan, 2001). **Active listening** includes the following:

- Observing the patient's nonverbal behaviors
- Listening to and understanding the patient's verbal message
- Listening to and understanding the person in the context of the social setting of his or her life
- Listening for "false notes" (i.e., inconsistencies or things the patient says that need more clarification)
- Providing the patient with feedback about himself or herself of which the patient might not be aware

Effective interviewers must become accustomed to silence, but it is just as important for effective interviewers to learn to become active listeners when the patient is talking, as well as when the patient becomes silent. During active listening nurses carefully note what the patient is saying verbally and nonverbally, as well as monitor their own nonverbal responses. Using silence effectively and learning to listen on a deeper, more significant level—to the patient as well as to your own thoughts and reaction—are both key ingredients in effective communication. Both skills take time to develop but can be learned; you will become more proficient with guidance and practice.

Some principles important to active listening include the following (Mohl, 2003):

- The answer is always inside the patient.
- Objective truth is never as simple as it seems.
- Everything you hear is modified by the patient's filters.
- Everything you hear is modified by your own filters.
- It is okay to feel confused and uncertain.
- Listen to yourself, too.

Active listening helps strengthen the patient's ability to solve problems. By giving the patient undivided attention, the nurse communicates that the patient is not alone. This kind of intervention enhances self-esteem and encourages the patient to direct energy toward finding ways to deal with problems. Serving as a sounding board, the nurse listens as the patient tests thoughts by voicing them aloud. This form of interpersonal interaction often enables the patient to clarify thinking, link ideas, and tentatively decide what should be done and how best to do it (Collins, 1983). Alderman (2000) refers to active listening as an art.

Clarifying Techniques

Understanding depends on clear communication, which is aided by verifying with a patient the nurse's interpretation of the patient's messages. The nurse must request feedback on the accuracy of the message received from verbal as well as nonverbal cues. The use of **clarifying techniques** helps both participants identify major differences in their frame of reference, giving them the opportunity to correct misperceptions before these cause any serious misunderstandings. The patient who is asked to elaborate on or to clarify vague or ambiguous messages needs to know that the purpose is to promote mutual understanding.

Paraphrasing

For clarity, the nurse might use **paraphrasing,** which means restating in different (often fewer) words the basic content of a patient's message. Using simple, precise, and culturally relevant terms, the nurse may readily confirm interpretation of the patient's previous message before the interview proceeds. By prefacing statements with a phrase such as "I'm not sure I understand" or "In other words, you seem to be saying . . . ," the nurse helps the patient form a clearer perception of what may be a bewildering mass of details. After paraphrasing, the nurse must validate the accuracy of the restatement and its helpfulness to the discussion. The

patient may confirm or deny the perceptions through nonverbal cues or by direct response to a question such as, "Was I correct in saying . . .?" As a result, the patient is made aware that the interviewer is actively involved in the search for understanding.

Restating

In **restating,** the nurse mirrors the patient's overt and covert messages; thus this technique may be used to echo feeling as well as content. Restating differs from paraphrasing in that it involves repeating the same key words the patient has just spoken. If a patient remarks, "My life is empty . . . it has no meaning," additional information may be gained by restating, "Your life has no meaning?" The purpose of this technique is to explore more thoroughly subjects that may be significant. However, too frequent and indiscriminate use of restating might be interpreted by patients as inattention, disinterest, or worse.

It is easy to overuse this tool so that its application becomes mechanical. Parroting or mimicking what another has said may be perceived as poking fun at the person, so that use of this nondirective approach can become a definite barrier to communication. To avoid overuse of restating, the nurse can combine restatements with direct questions that encourage descriptions: "What does your life lack?" "What kind of meaning is missing?" "Describe one day in your life that appears empty to you."

Reflecting

Reflection is a means of assisting people to better understand their own thoughts and feelings. **Reflecting** may take the form of a question or a simple statement that conveys the nurse's observations of the patient when sensitive issues are being discussed. The nurse might then describe briefly to the patient the apparent meaning of the emotional tone of the patient's verbal and nonverbal behavior. For example, to reflect a patient's feelings about his or her life, a good beginning might be, "You sound as if you have had many disappointments."

Sharing observations with a patient shows acceptance. The nurse helps make the patient aware of inner feelings and encourages the patient to own them. For example, the nurse may tell a patient, "You look sad." Perceiving the nurse's concern may allow a patient spontaneously to share feelings. The use of a question in response to the patient's question is another reflective technique (Arnold & Boggs, 2007). For example:

Patient: "Nurse, do you think I really need to be hospitalized?"
Nurse: "What do you think, Jane?"
Patient: "I don't know; that's why I'm asking you."

Nurse: "I'll be willing to share my impression with you at the end of this first session. However, you've probably thought about hospitalization and have some feelings about it. I wonder what they are."

Exploring

A technique that enables the nurse to examine important ideas, experiences, or relationships more fully is **exploring.** For example, if a patient tells the nurse that he does not get along well with his wife, the nurse will want to further explore this area. Possible openers include the following:

- *"Tell me* more about your relationship with your wife."
- *"Describe* your relationship with your wife."
- *"Give me an example* of how you and your wife don't get along."

Asking for an example can greatly clarify a vague or generic statement made by a patient.

Patient: "No one likes me."

Nurse: "Give me an example of one person who doesn't like you."

or

Patient: "Everything I do is wrong."

Nurse: "Give me an example of one thing you do that you think is wrong."

Table 6-2 lists more examples of techniques that enhance communication.

NONTHERAPEUTIC TECHNIQUES

Although people may use nontherapeutic techniques in their daily lives, they can become problematic when one is working with patients. Table 6-3 offers samples of nontherapeutic techniques and suggestions for more helpful responses.

Asking Excessive Questions

Excessive questioning, or asking multiple questions at the same time, especially closed-ended questions, casts the nurse in the role of interrogator, raising a demand for information without respect for the patient's willingness or readiness to respond. This approach conveys lack of respect for and sensitivity to the patient's needs. Excessive questioning or asking multiple questions at the same time controls the range and nature of the response and can easily result in a therapeutic stall or shut down an interview. It is a controlling tactic and may reflect the interviewer's lack of security in letting the patient tell his or her own story. It is

better to ask more open-ended questions and follow the patient's lead. For example:

Excessive questioning: "Why did you leave your wife? Did you feel angry at her? What did she do to you? Are you going back to her?"

More therapeutic approach: "Tell me about the situation between you and your wife."

Giving Approval or Disapproval

"You look great in that dress." "I'm proud of the way you controlled your temper at lunch." "That's a great quilt you made." What could be bad about giving someone a pat on the back once in a while? Nothing, if it is done without carrying a judgment (positive or negative) by the nurse. We often give our friends and family approval when they do something well. However, in a nurse-patient situation, **giving approval** often becomes much more complex. A patient may be feeling overwhelmed, experiencing low self-esteem, feeling unsure of where his or her life is going, and very needy for recognition, approval, and attention. Yet, when people are feeling vulnerable, a value comment might be misinterpreted. For example:

Giving approval: "You did a great job in group telling John just what you thought about how rudely he treated you."

Implied in this message is that the nurse was pleased by the manner in which the patient talked to John. The patient then sees such a response as a way to please the nurse by doing the right thing. To continue to please the nurse (and get approval), the patient may continue the behavior. The behavior might be useful for the patient, but when a behavior is being done to please another person, it is not coming from the individual's own volition or conviction.

Also when the other person whom the patient needs to please is not around, the motivation for the new behavior might not be there either. Thus the new response really is not a change in behavior as much as a ploy to win approval and acceptance from another person. Giving approval also cuts off further communication. It is a statement of the observer's (nurse's) judgment about another person's (patient's) behavior. A more useful comment would be the following:

More therapeutic approach: "I noticed that you spoke up to John in group yesterday about his rude behavior. How did it feel to be more assertive?"

This opens the way for finding out if the patient was scared, comfortable, wants to work more on assertiveness, or something else. It also suggests that this was a self-choice the patient made. The patient is given recognition for the change in behavior, and the topic is also opened for further discussion.

TABLE 6-2	Techniques That Enhance Communication	
Technique	**Discussion**	**Examples**
Using silence	Gives the person time to collect thoughts or think through a point.	Encouraging a person to talk by waiting for the answers.
Accepting	Indicates that the person has been understood. The statement does not necessarily indicate agreement but is nonjudgmental. However, nurses do not imply that they understand when they do not understand.	"Yes." "Uh-huh." "I follow what you say."
Giving recognition	Indicates awareness of change and personal efforts. Does not imply good or bad, or right or wrong.	"Good morning, Mr. James." "You've combed your hair today." "I notice that you shaved today."
Offering self	Offers presence, interest, and a desire to understand. Is not offered to get the person to talk or behave in a specific way.	"I would like to spend time with you." "I'll stay here and sit with you awhile."
Offering general leads	Allows the other person to take direction in the discussion. Indicates that the nurse is interested in what comes next.	"Go on." "And then?" "Tell me about it."
Giving broad openings	Clarifies that the lead is to be taken by the patient. However, the nurse discourages pleasantries and small talk.	"Where would you like to begin?" "What are you thinking about?" "What would you like to discuss?"
Placing the events in time or sequence	Puts events and actions in better perspective. Notes cause-and-effect relationships and identifies patterns of interpersonal difficulties.	"What happened before?" "When did this happen?"
Making observations	Calls attention to the person's behavior (e.g., trembling, nail biting, restless mannerisms). Encourages the person to notice the behavior to describe thoughts and feelings for mutual understanding. Helpful with mute and withdrawn people.	"You appear tense." "I notice you're biting your lips." "You appear nervous whenever John enters the room."
Encouraging description of perception	Increases the nurse's understanding of the patient's perceptions. Talking about feelings and difficulties can lessen the need to act them out inappropriately.	"What do these voices seem to be saying?" "What is happening now?" "Tell me when you feel anxious."
Encouraging comparison	Brings out recurring themes in experiences or interpersonal relationships. Helps the person clarify similarities and differences.	"Has this ever happened before?" "Is this how you felt when . . .?" "Was it something like . . .?"
Restating	Repeats the main idea expressed. Gives the patient an idea of what has been communicated. If the message has been misunderstood, the patient can clarify it.	*Patient:* "I can't sleep. I stay awake all night." *Nurse:* "You have difficulty sleeping?" *Patient:* "I don't know . . . he always has some excuse for not coming over or keeping our appointments." *Nurse:* "You think he no longer wants to see you?"
Reflecting	Directs questions, feelings, and ideas back to the patient. Encourages the patient to accept his or her own ideas and feelings. Acknowledges the patient's right to have opinions and make decisions and encourages the patient to think of self as a capable person.	*Patient:* "What should I do about my husband's affair?" *Nurse:* "What do you think you should do?" *Patient:* "My brother spends all of my money and then has the nerve to ask for more." *Nurse:* "You feel angry when this happens?"
Focusing	Concentrates attention on a single point. It is especially useful when the patient jumps from topic to topic. If a person is experiencing a severe or panic level of anxiety, the nurse should not persist until the anxiety lessens.	"This point you are making about leaving school seems worth looking at more closely." "You've mentioned many things. Let's go back to your thinking of 'ending it all.'"

Continued

TABLE 6-2	Techniques That Enhance Communication—cont'd	
Technique	**Discussion**	**Examples**
Exploring	Examines certain ideas, experiences, or relationships more fully. If the patient chooses not to elaborate by answering no, the nurse does not probe or pry. In such a case, the nurse respects the patient's wishes.	"Tell me more about that." "Would you describe it more fully?" "Could you talk about how it was that you learned your mom was dying of cancer?"
Giving information	Makes available facts the person needs. Supplies knowledge from which decisions can be made or conclusions drawn. For example, the patient needs to know the role of the nurse; the purpose of the nurse-patient relationship; and the time, place, and duration of the meetings.	"My purpose for being here is . . ." "This medication is for . . ." "The test will determine . . ."
Seeking clarification	Helps patients clarify their own thoughts and maximize mutual understanding between nurse and patient.	"I am not sure I follow you." "What would you say is the main point of what you just said?" "Give an example of a time you thought everyone hated you."
Presenting reality	Indicates what is real. The nurse does not argue or try to convince the patient, just describes personal perceptions or facts in the situation.	"That was Dr. Todd, not a man from the Mafia." "That was the sound of a car backfiring." "Your mother is not here; I am a nurse."
Voicing doubt	Undermines the patient's beliefs by not reinforcing the exaggerated or false perceptions.	"Isn't that unusual?" "Really?" "That's hard to believe."
Seeking consensual validation	Clarifies that both the nurse and patient share mutual understanding of communications. Helps the patient become clearer about what he or she is thinking.	"Tell me whether my understanding agrees with yours."
Verbalizing the implied	Puts into concrete terms what the patient implies, making the patient's communication more explicit.	*Patient:* "I can't talk to you or anyone else. It's a waste of time." *Nurse:* "Do you feel that no one understands?"
Encouraging evaluation	Aids the patient in considering people and events from the perspective of the patient's own set of values.	"How do you feel about . . .?" "What did it mean to you when he said he couldn't stay?"
Attempting to translate into feelings	Responds to the feelings expressed, not just the content. Often termed *decoding*.	*Patient:* "I am dead inside." *Nurse:* "Are you saying that you feel lifeless? Does life seem meaningless to you?"
Suggesting collaboration	Emphasizes working with the patient, not doing things for the patient. Encourages the view that change is possible through collaboration.	"Perhaps you and I can discover what produces your anxiety." "Perhaps by working together we can come up with some ideas that might improve your communications with your spouse."
Summarizing	Brings together important points of discussion to enhance understanding. Also allows the opportunity to clarify communications so that both nurse and patient leave the interview with the same ideas in mind.	"Have I got this straight?" "You said that . . ." "During the past hour, you and I have discussed . . ."
Encouraging formulation of a plan of action	Allows the patient to identify alternative actions for interpersonal situations the patient finds disturbing (e.g., when anger or anxiety is provoked).	"What could you do to let anger out harmlessly?" "The next time this comes up, what might you do to handle it?" "What are some other ways you can approach your boss?"

Adapted from Hays, J.S., & Larson, K. (1963). *Interacting with patients.* New York: Macmillan. Copyright © 1963 Macmillan Publishing Company.

TABLE 6-3   Nontherapeutic Communication

Nontherapeutic Technique	Examples	Discussion	More Helpful Response
Giving premature advice	"Get out of this situation immediately."	Assumes the nurse knows best and the patient can't think for self. Inhibits problem solving and fosters dependency.	*Encouraging problem solving:* "What are the pros and cons of your situation?" "What were some of the actions you thought you might take?" "What are some of the ways you have thought of to meet your goals?"
Minimizing feelings	***Patient:*** "I wish I were dead." ***Nurse:*** "Everyone gets down in the dumps." "I know what you mean." "You should feel happy you're getting better." "Things get worse before they get better."	Indicates that the nurse is unable to understand or empathize with the patient. Here the patient's feelings or experiences are being belittled, which can cause the patient to feel small or insignificant.	*Empathizing and exploring:* "You must be feeling very upset. Are you thinking of hurting yourself?"
Falsely reassuring	"I wouldn't worry about that." "Everything will be all right." "You will do just fine, you'll see."	Underrates a person's feelings and belittles a person's concerns. May cause the patient to stop sharing feelings if the patient thinks he or she will be ridiculed or not taken seriously.	*Clarifying the patient's message:* "What specifically are you worried about?" "What do you think could go wrong?" "What are you concerned might happen?"
Making value judgments	"How come you still smoke when your wife has lung cancer?"	Prevents problem solving. Can make the patient feel guilty, angry, misunderstood, not supported, or anxious to leave.	*Making observations:* "I notice you are still smoking even though your wife has lung cancer. Is this a problem?"
Asking "why" questions	"Why did you stop taking your medication?"	Implies criticism; often has the effect of making the patient feel defensive.	*Asking open-ended questions; giving a broad opening:* "Tell me some of the reasons that led up to your not taking your medications."
Asking excessive questions	***Nurse:*** "How's your appetite? Are you losing weight? Are you eating enough?" ***Patient:*** "No."	Results in the patient's not knowing which question to answer and possibly being confused about what is being asked.	*Clarifying:* "Tell me about your eating habits since you've been depressed."
Giving approval; agreeing	"I'm proud of you for applying for that job." "I agree with your decision."	Implies that the patient is doing the *right* thing—and that not doing it is wrong. May lead the patient to focus on pleasing the nurse or clinician; denies the patient the opportunity to change his or her mind or decision.	*Making observations:* "I noticed that you applied for that job. What factors will lead up to your changing your mind?" *Asking open-ended questions; giving a broad opening:* "What led to that decision?"

Continued

TABLE 6-3	Nontherapeutic Communication—cont'd		
Nontherapeutic Technique	**Examples**	**Discussion**	**More Helpful Response**
Disapproving; disagreeing	"You really should have shown up for the medication group." "I disagree with that."	Can make a person defensive.	*Exploring:* "What was going through your mind when you decided not to come to your medication group?" "That's one point of view. How did you arrive at that conclusion?"
Changing the subject	*Patient:* "I'd like to die." *Nurse:* "Did you go to Alcoholics Anonymous like we discussed?"	May invalidate the patient's feelings and needs. Can leave the patient feeling alienated and isolated and increase feelings of hopelessness.	*Validating and exploring:* *Patient:* "I'd like to die." *Nurse:* "This sounds serious. Have you thought of harming yourself?"

Adapted from Hays, J.S., & Larson, K. (1963). *Interacting with patients.* New York: Macmillan. Copyright © 1963, Macmillan Publishing Company.

Disapproving is moralizing and implies that the nurse has the right to judge the patient's thoughts or feelings. Again, an observation should be made instead.

Disapproving: "You really should not cheat, even if you think everyone else is doing it."

More therapeutic approach: "Can you give me two examples of how cheating could negatively affect your goal of graduating?"

Advising

Although we ask for and give advice all the time in daily life, **giving advice** to a patient is rarely helpful. Often when we ask for advice, our real motive is to discover if we are thinking along the same lines as someone else or if they would agree with us. When the nurse gives advice to a patient who is having trouble assessing and problem solving in conflicted areas of the patient's life, the nurse is interfering with the patient's ability to make personal decisions. When the nurse offers the patient solutions, the patient eventually begins to think that the nurse does not view the patient as capable of making effective decisions.

People often feel inadequate when they are given no choices over decisions in their lives. Giving advice to patients can foster dependency ("I'll have to ask the nurse what to do about . . .") and can undermine their sense of competence and adequacy. However, people do need information to make informed decisions. Often the nurse can help the patient define a problem and identify what information might be needed to come to an informed decision. A more useful approach would be, "What do you see as some possible actions you can take?" It is much more constructive to encourage problem solving by the patient. At times the nurse can suggest several alternatives that a patient might consider (e.g., "Have you ever thought of telling your friend about the incident?"). The patient is then free to say yes or no and make a decision from among the suggestions.

Asking "Why" Questions

"Why did you come late?" "Why didn't you go to the funeral?" "Why didn't you study for the exam?" Very often **"why" questions** imply criticism. We may ask our friends or family such questions and, in the context of a solid relationship, the "Why?" may be understood more as "What happened?" With people we do not know—especially an anxious person who may be feeling overwhelmed—a "why" question from a person in authority (nurse, physician, teacher) can be experienced as intrusive and judgmental, which serves only to make the person defensive.

It is much more useful to ask *what* is happening rather than *why* it is happening. Questions that focus on who, what, where, and when often elicit important information that can facilitate problem solving and further the communication process.

COMMUNICATION AND CULTURE: NEGOTIATING BARRIERS

Ethnically diverse populations are a rapidly growing segment of the American population. Health care professionals are gradually becoming aware of the need to become more familiar with the verbal and nonverbal communication characteristics of the diverse multicultural populations now using the health care system. The nurse's awareness of the cultural meaning of certain verbal and nonverbal communications in initial face-to-face encounters with a patient can lead to the formation of positive therapeutic alliances with members of culturally diverse populations (Kavanaugh, 2003).

Unrecognized differences between aspects of the cultural identities of patient and nurse can result in assessment and interventions that are not optimally respectful of the patient and can be inadvertently biased or prejudiced (Lu et al., 1995). Lu and colleagues further emphasized that health care workers need to have not only knowledge of various patients' cultures but also awareness of their own cultural identities. Especially important are nurses' attitudes and beliefs toward those from ethnically diverse populations, because these will affect their relationships with patients (Kavanaugh, 2003). Four areas that may prove problematic for the nurse interpreting specific verbal and nonverbal messages of the patient include the following:

1. Communication styles
2. Use of eye contact
3. Perception of touch
4. Cultural filters

Communication Styles

People from some ethnic backgrounds may communicate in an intense and highly emotional manner. For example, from the perspective of a non-Hispanic person, Hispanic Americans may appear to use dramatic body language when describing their emotional problems. Such behavior may be perceived as out of control and thus viewed as having a degree of pathology that is not actually present. Within the Hispanic culture, however, intensely emotional styles of communication often are culturally appropriate and are to be expected (Kavanaugh, 2003). French and Italian Americans also show animated facial expressions and expressive hand gestures during communication that can be mistakenly interpreted by others.

Conversely, in other cultures, a calm facade may mask severe distress. For example, in Asian cultures, expression of either positive or negative emotions is a private affair, and open expression of emotions is considered to be in bad taste and possibly to be a weakness. A quiet smile by an Asian American may express joy, an apology, stoicism in the face of difficulty, or even anger (USDHHS, 2001). German and British Americans also value highly the concept of self-control and may show little facial emotion in the presence of great distress or emotional turmoil.

It is important to understand an ethnic minority in light of the historical context in which it evolved and its relationship to the dominant culture. For example, African Americans, whose historical background in the United States is one of slavery and oppression, are likely to be aware of a basic need for survival. As a result of their experiences, many African Americans have become highly selective and guarded in their communication with those outside their cultural group. Therefore, a tendency toward guarded and selective communication among African American patients may represent a healthy cultural adaptation (Smedley et al., 2002; USDHHS, 2001).

Eye Contact

Culture also dictates a person's comfort or lack of comfort with direct eye contact. Some cultures consider direct eye contact disrespectful and improper. For example, Hispanic individuals have traditionally been taught to avoid eye contact with authority figures such as nurses, physicians, and other health care professionals. Avoidance of direct eye contact is seen as a sign of respect to those in authority. To nurses or other health care workers from non-Hispanic backgrounds, however, this lack of eye contact may be wrongly interpreted as disinterest in the interview or even as a lack of respect. Conversely, the nurse is expected to look directly at the patient when conducting the interview (Kavanaugh, 2003).

Similarly, in Asian cultures, respect is shown by avoiding eye contact. For example, in Japan, direct eye contact is considered to show lack of respect and to be a personal affront; preference is for shifting or downcast eyes. With many Chinese, gazing around and looking to one side when listening to another is considered polite. However, when speaking to an older adult, direct eye contact is used (Kavanaugh, 2003). Philippine Americans may try to avoid eye contact; however, once it is established, it is important to return and maintain eye contact.

Many Native Americans also believe it is disrespectful or even a sign of aggression to engage in direct eye contact, especially if the speaker is younger. Direct eye contact by members of the dominant culture in the health care system can and does cause discomfort for some patients (Kavanaugh, 2003).

Among German Americans, direct and sustained eye contact indicates that the person listens, trusts, is somewhat aggressive, or in some situations is sexually interested. Russians also find direct, sustained eye contact the norm for social interactions (Giger & Davidhizar, 2004). In Haiti, it is customary to hold eye contact with everyone but the poor (Kavanaugh, 2003; USDHHS, 2001). French, British, and many African Americans maintain eye contact during conversation; avoidance of eye contact by another person may be interpreted as being disinterested, not telling the truth, or avoiding the sharing of important information. In some Arab cultures, for a woman to make direct eye contact with a man may imply a sexual interest or even promiscuity. In Greece, staring in public is acceptable (Kavanaugh, 2003).

Touch

The therapeutic use of touch is a basic aspect of the nurse-patient relationship, and touch is normally perceived as a gesture of warmth and friendship. However, touch can be perceived as an invasion of privacy or an invitation to intimacy by some patients (Dee, 1991). The response to touch is often culturally defined. For example, many Hispanic Americans are accustomed to frequent physical contact. Holding the patient's hand in response to a distressing situation or giving the patient a reassuring pat on the shoulder may be experienced as supportive and thus help facilitate openness early in the therapeutic relationship (Kavanaugh, 2003).

When the nurse is working with parents of a Mexican American, the nurse should touch the child since, in the minds of some Mexican Americans, this action can both prevent and treat illness (Giger & Davidhizar, 2004). However, the degree of comfort conveyed by touch in the nurse-patient relationship depends on the country of origin. People of Italian and French backgrounds may also be accustomed to frequent touching during conversation (USDHHS, 2001). In the Russian culture, touch is also an important part of nonverbal communication used freely with intimate and close friends (Giger & Davidhizar, 2004).

In other cultures personal touch within the context of an interview might be experienced as patronizing, intrusive, aggressive, or sexually inviting. For example, among German, Swedish, and British Americans, touch practices are infrequent, although a handshake may be common at the beginning and end of an interaction. In India, men may shake hands with other men but not with women; an Asian Indian man may greet a woman by nodding and holding the palms of his hands together but not touching the woman. In Japan, handshakes are acceptable; however, a pat on the back is not. Chinese Americans may not like to be touched by strangers. Some Native Americans extend

their hand and lightly touch the hand of the person they are greeting rather than shake hands (Kavanaugh, 2003).

Even among people of the same culture, the use of touch has different interpretations and rules when the touch is between individuals of different genders and classes. Students are urged to check the policy manual of their facility because some facilities have a "no touch" policy, particularly with adolescents and children who may have experienced inappropriate touch and would not know how to interpret the touch of the health care worker.

Cultural Filters

It is important to recognize that it is impossible to listen to people in an unbiased way. In the process of socialization we develop **cultural filters** through which we listen to ourselves, others, and the world around us (Egan, 2001). Cultural filters are a form of cultural bias or cultural prejudice that determines what we pay attention to and what we ignore.

Egan (1994) stated that we need these cultural filters to provide structure for ourselves and to help us interpret and interact with the world. However, unavoidably, these cultural filters also introduce various forms of bias into our listening because they are bound to influence our personal, professional, familial, and sociological values and interpretations.

We all need a frame of reference to help us function in our world. The trick is to understand that other people use many other frames of reference to help them function in their worlds. Acknowledging that others view the world quite differently and trying to understand other people's ways of experiencing and living in the world can go a long way toward minimizing our personal distortions in listening. Building acceptance and understanding of those culturally different from ourselves is a skill, too.

EVALUATION OF CLINICAL SKILLS

After you have had some introductory clinical experience, you may find the facilitative skills checklist in Figure 6-2 useful for evaluating your progress in developing interviewing skills. Note that some of the items might not be relevant for some of your patients (e.g., numbers 11 through 13 may not be possible to do when a patient is highly psychotic). Self-evaluation of clinical skills is a way to focus on therapeutic improvement. Role playing can be a useful tool for preparation for the clinical experience as well as a practice in acquiring more effective and professional communication skills.

FACILITATIVE SKILLS CHECKLIST

Instructions: Periodically during your clinical experience, use this checklist to identify areas where growth is needed and progress has been made. Think of your clinical client experiences. Indicate the extent of your agreement with each of the following statements by marking the scale: *SA*, strongly agree; *A*, agree; *NS*, not sure; *D*, disagree; *SD*, strongly disagree.

	SA	A	NS	D	SD
1. I maintain good eye contact.	SA	A	NS	D	SD
2. Most of my verbal comments follow the lead of the other person.	SA	A	NS	D	SD
3. I encourage others to talk about feelings.	SA	A	NS	D	SD
4. I am able to ask open-ended questions.	SA	A	NS	D	SD
5. I can restate and clarify a person's ideas.	SA	A	NS	D	SD
6. I can summarize in a few words the basic ideas of a long statement made by a person.	SA	A	NS	D	SD
7. I can make statements that reflect the person's feelings.	SA	A	NS	D	SD
8. I can share my feelings relevant to the discussion when appropriate to do so.	SA	A	NS	D	SD
9. I am able to give feedback.	SA	A	NS	D	SD
10. At least 75% or more of my responses help enhance and facilitate communication.	SA	A	NS	D	SD
11. I can assist the person to list some alternatives available.	SA	A	NS	D	SD
12. I can assist the person to identify some goals that are specific and observable.	SA	A	NS	D	SD
13. I can assist the person to specify at least one next step that might be taken toward the goal.	SA	A	NS	D	SD

Figure 6-2 ■ Facilitative skills checklist. (Adapted from Myrick, D., & Erney, T. [2000]. *Caring and sharing* [2nd cd., p. 168]. Copyright © 2000 by Educational Media Corporation, Minncapolis, Minnesota.)

KEY POINTS TO REMEMBER

- Knowledge of communication and interviewing techniques is the foundation for development of any nurse-patient relationship. Goal-directed professional communication is referred to as therapeutic communication.
- Communication is a complex process. Berlo's communication model has five parts: stimulus, sender, message, medium, and receiver. Feedback is a vital component of the communication process for validating the accuracy of the sender's message.
- A number of factors can minimize or enhance the communication process. For example, differences in culture, language, and knowledge levels; noise; lack of privacy; the presence of others; and expectations all can influence communication.
- There are verbal and nonverbal elements in communication; the nonverbal elements often play the larger role in conveying a person's message. Verbal communication consists of all words a person speaks. Nonverbal communication consists of the behaviors displayed by an individual, in addition to the actual content of speech.
- Communication has two levels: the content level (verbal) and the process level (nonverbal behavior). When content is con-gruent with process, the communication is said to be healthy. When the verbal message is not reinforced by the communicator's actions, the message is ambiguous; we call this a double (or mixed) message.
- Cultural background (as well as individual differences) has a great deal to do with what nonverbal behavior means to different individuals. The degree of eye contact and the use of touch are two nonverbal aspects that can be misunderstood by individuals of different cultures.
- There are a number of communication techniques that nurses can use to enhance their nursing practices. Many widely used communication enhancers are cited in Table 6-2.
- There are also a number of nontherapeutic techniques that nurses can learn to avoid to enhance their effectiveness with people. Some are cited in Table 6-3 along with suggestions for more helpful responses.
- Most nurses are most effective when they use nonthreatening and open-ended communication techniques.
- Effective communication is a skill that develops over time and is integral to the establishment and maintenance of a therapeutic alliance.

CRITICAL THINKING

1. Keep a log for 30 minutes a day of your communication pattern (a tape recorder is ideal). Pick out four effective techniques that you notice you use frequently. Identify two techniques that are obstructive. In your log, rewrite these nontherapeutic communications and replace them with statements that would better facilitate discussion of thoughts and feelings. Share your log and discuss the changes you are working on with one classmate.

2. Role play with a classmate at least five nonverbal communications and have your partner identify the message he or she was receiving.

3. Using touch and use of eye contact, act out how the nurse would use the nonverbal messages in three different cultural groups.

CHAPTER REVIEW

Choose the most appropriate answer.

1. Paraphrasing, restating, reflecting, and exploring are techniques used for the purpose of:
   1. clarifying.
   2. summarizing.
   3. encouraging comparison.
   4. placing events in time and sequence.

2. Which communication technique would yield positive results within the context of a therapeutic relationship?
   1. Advising
   2. Giving approval
   3. Listening actively
   4. Asking "why" questions

3. When the patient makes the statement, "I get all balled up when I try to talk to him," and the nurse responds, "Give me an example of getting all balled up," the nurse is using the technique called:
   1. exploring.
   2. reflecting.
   3. interpreting.
   4. paraphrasing.

4. Which statement by the nurse to a patient would be considered nontherapeutic?
   1. "I know exactly how you feel."
   2. "I'm not sure I understand what you mean."
   3. "Tell me more about what happened when you resigned."
   4. "I see that you are wringing your hands as we talk about the job interview."

REFERENCES

Alderman, C. (2000). The art of listening. *Nursing Standards, 14*(20), 18-19.

Arnold, E.C., & Boggs, K.U. (2007). *Interpersonal relationships: Professional communication skills for nurses* (5th ed.). St. Louis: Saunders.

Bateson, G., Jackson, D., & Haley, J. (1956). Toward a theory of schizophrenia. *Behavioral Sciences, 1*(4), 251-264.

Berlo, D.K. (1960). *The process of communication.* San Francisco: Reinhart Press.

Collins, M. (1983). *Communication in health care: The human connection in the life cycle* (2nd ed.). St. Louis: Mosby.

Dee, V. (1991). How can we become more aware of culturally specific body language and use this awareness therapeutically? *Journal of Psychosocial Nursing, 29*(11), 39-40.

Egan, G. (1994). *The skilled helper: A problem management approach* (5th ed.). Pacific Grove, CA: Brooks/Cole.

Egan, G. (2001). *The skilled helper: A systematic approach to effective helping* (7th ed.). Pacific Grove, CA: Wadsworth.

Ellis, R.B., Gates, B., & Kenworthy, N. (2003). *Interpersonal communicating in nursing* (2nd ed.). London: Churchill Livingstone.

Giger, J.N., & Davidhizar, R.E. (2004). *Transcultural nursing: Assessment and intervention* (4th ed.). St. Louis: Mosby.

Haber, J. (2000). Hildegard E. Peplau: The psychiatric nursing legacy of a legend. *Journal of the American Psychiatric Nursing Association, 6*(2), 56-62.

Kavanaugh, K.H. (2003). Transcultural perspectives in mental health nursing. In M. Andrews & J. Boyle (Eds.), *Transcultural concepts in nursing care.* Philadelphia: Lippincott Williams & Wilkins.

Lu, F.G., & Mezzich, J.E. (1995). Issues in the assessment and diagnosis of culturally diverse individuals. In J.M. Oldhan & M.B. Riba (Eds.), *Review of psychiatry* (vol. 14, pp. 477-510). Washington, DC: American Psychiatric Press.

Mohl, P.C. (2003). Listening to the patient. In A. Tasman, J. Kay, & J.A. Lieberman (Eds.), *Psychiatry* (2nd ed.). West Sussex, England: Wiley.

Peplau, H.E. (1952). *Interpersonal relations in nursing: A conceptual frame of reference for psychodynamic nursing.* New York: Putnam.

Rankin, J.A. (2001). *Body language in negotiations and sales* (2nd ed.) Springfield, VA: Rankin File.

Shea, S.C. (1998). *Psychiatric interviewing: The art of understanding* (2nd ed.). Philadelphia: Saunders.

Smedley, B., Stith, A., & Nelson, A. (2002). *Unequal treatment: Confronting racial and ethnic disparities in healthcare* (Institute of Medicine Report). Washington, DC: National Academies Press.

Sommers-Flanagan, J., & Sommers-Flanagan, R. (2003). *Clinical interviewing* (3rd ed.). Hoboken, NJ: Wiley.

U.S. Department of Health and Human Services (USDHHS). (2001). *Mental health: Culture, race, and ethnicity: Supplement to mental health: A report of the surgeon general.* Rockville, MD: U.S. Department of Health and Human Services, Substance Abuse and Mental Health Services Administration, Center for Mental Health Services.

CHAPTER 7

Therapeutic Relationships and the Clinical Interview

Elizabeth M. Varcarolis

Key Terms and Concepts

Objectives

1. Compare and contrast the three phases of the nurse-patient relationship.
2. Compare and contrast a social relationship and a therapeutic relationship regarding purpose, focus, communications style, and goals.
3. Identify at least four patient behaviors a nurse may encounter in the clinical setting.
4. Explore aspects that foster a therapeutic nurse-patient relationship and those that are inherent in a nontherapeutic nursing interactive process.
5. Define and discuss the role of empathy, genuineness, and positive regard on the part of the nurse in a nurse-patient relationship.
6. Identify two attitudes and four actions that may reflect the nurse's positive regard for a patient.
7. Analyze what is meant by boundaries and the influence of transference and countertransference on boundary blurring.
8. Understand the use of attending behaviors (eye contact, body language, vocal qualities, and verbal tracking).
9. Discuss the influences of disparate values and cultural beliefs on the therapeutic relationship.

evolve

For additional resources related to the content of this chapter, visit the Evolve website at http://evolve.elsevier.com/Varcarolis/essentials.

- Chapter Outline
- Chapter Review Answers

- Nurse, Patient, and Family Resources
- Concept Map Creator

Psychiatric mental health nursing is based on principles of *science*. A background in anatomy, physiology, and chemistry is the basis for the safe and effective provision of biological treatments. For example, it is assumed the nurse has knowledge of how medications work, indications for use, and adverse effects based on best-evidenced studies and trials. However, it is the caring relationship and the development of the skills needed to enhance and maintain these relationships that make up the *art* of psychiatric nursing. Quinlan (1996) states that "the development of that very human relationship allows a place for caring and healing to occur. This use of the essential humanness of the nurse as a person is the most critical part of the way nurses make themselves available to both patients and colleagues" (p. 7). Quinlan goes on to say that how this is achieved remains within the domain of the individual nurse.

NURSE-PATIENT RELATIONSHIPS

The therapeutic nurse-patient relationship is the basis of all psychiatric nursing treatment approaches regardless of the specific aim. The very first connections between nurse and patient are to establish an understanding that the nurse is safe, confidential, reliable, consistent, and that the relationship is conducted within appropriate and clear boundaries (LaRowe, 2004).

It is true that many disorders, such as schizophrenia and major affective disorders have strong biochemical and genetic components. However, many accompanying emotional problems such as poor self-image, low self-esteem, and difficulties with adherence to treatment regimen can be significantly improved through a therapeutic nurse-patient alliance or relationship (LaRowe, 2004). All too commonly, those entering treatment have taxed or exhausted their familial and social resources and have found themselves in a position of isolation from people who will listen for more than a few minutes.

The nurse-patient relationship is a creative process and unique to each nurse. Each person brings his or her own uniqueness to the nurse-patient relationship. Each of us has unique gifts that we can learn to use creatively to form positive bonds with others. Historically this has been referred to as the "therapeutic use of self." Therapeutic use of self is an example of the practice of the "art of nursing." *Important to remember,* the efficacy of this therapeutic use of self has been scientifically substantiated as an evidence-based intervention. Randomized clinical trials have repeatedly found that development of a positive alliance (therapeutic relationship) is one of the best predictors of outcomes in therapy (Kopta et al., 1999).

Korn (2001) states that therapeutic success is a result of the personal characteristics of the clinician and the patient, not necessarily on the particular process employed. Furthermore, there is evidence that psychotherapy (talk therapy) and a therapeutic alliance actually change brain chemistry in much the same way as medication, thus the adage that the best treatment for most psychiatric problems (less so with psychotic disorders) is a combination of medication and psychotherapy. Cognitive-behavioral therapy, in particular, has met with great success in the treatment of depression, phobias, obsessive-compulsive disorders, and others.

Establishing a therapeutic alliance or relationship with a patient takes time. Skills in this area gradually improve with guidance from those with more skill and experience. When patients do not engage in a therapeutic alliance, chances are that no matter what plans of care or planned interventions are made, nothing much will happen except mutual frustration and mutual withdrawal.

Therapeutic Versus Other Types of Relationships

The nurse-patient relationship is often loosely defined, but a therapeutic relationship incorporating principles of mental health nursing is more clearly defined and differs from other relationships. A therapeutic nurse-patient relationship has specific goals and functions. Goals in a therapeutic relationship include the following:

- **Facilitating** communication of distressing thoughts and feelings
- **Assisting** patients with problem solving to help facilitate activities of daily living
- **Helping** patients examine self-defeating behaviors and test alternatives
- **Promoting** self-care and independence

A relationship is an interpersonal process that involves two or more people. Throughout life we meet people in a variety of settings and share a variety of experiences. With some individuals we develop long-term relationships; with others the relationship lasts only a short time. Naturally the kinds of relationships we enter vary from person to person and from situation to situation. Generally, relationships can be defined as (1) social or (2) therapeutic.

Social Relationships

A **social relationship** can be defined as a relationship that is primarily initiated for the purpose of friendship, socialization, enjoyment, or accomplishment of a task. Mutual needs are met during social interaction (e.g., participants share ideas, feelings, and experiences). Communication skills used in social relationships may include giving advice and (sometimes) meeting basic dependency needs, such as lending money and helping with jobs. Often the content of the communication remains superficial. During social interactions, roles may shift. Within a social relationship there is little emphasis on the evaluation of the interaction:

Patient: "Oh, gosh, I just hate to be alone. It is getting me down and sometimes it hurts so much."

Nurse: "I know just how you feel. I don't like it either. What I do is get a friend and go to a movie or something. Do you have someone to hang with?" (In this response the nurse is minimizing the patient's feelings and giving advice prematurely.)

Patient: "No, not really, but often I don't even feel like going out. I just sit at home feeling scared and lonely."

Nurse: "Most of us feel like that at one time or another. Maybe if you took a class or joined a group you could meet more people. I know of some great groups you could join. It's not good to be stuck in by yourself all of the time." (Again, the nurse is not "hearing" the patient's distress, and in so doing, is minimizing again her pain and isolation. The nurse goes on to give the patient banal advice thus closing off the patient's feelings and experience.)

Therapeutic Relationships

The **therapeutic relationship** between nurse and patient differs from both a social and an intimate relationship in that the nurse maximizes his or her communication skills, understanding of human behaviors, and personal strengths to enhance the patient's growth. The focus of the relationship is on the patient's ideas, experiences, and feelings. Inherent in a therapeutic relationship is the nurse's focus on significant personal issues introduced by the patient during the clinical interview. The nurse and the patient identify areas that need exploration and periodically evaluate the degree of change in the patient.

Although the nurse may assume a variety of roles (e.g., teacher, counselor, socializing agent, liaison), **the relationship is consistently focused on the patient's problem and needs.** Nurses must get their needs met outside the relationship. When nurses begin to want the patient to "like them," "do as they suggest," "be nice to them," or "give them recognition," the needs of the patient cannot be adequately met, and the interaction could be detrimental (nontherapeutic) to the patient.

Working under supervision is an excellent way to keep the focus and boundaries clear. Communication skills and knowledge of the stages of and phenomena occurring in a therapeutic relationship are crucial tools in the formation and maintenance of that relationship. Within the context of a helping relationship, the following occur:

• The needs of the patient are identified and explored.
• Alternate problem-solving approaches are taken.
• New coping skills may develop.
• Behavioral change is encouraged.

Staff nurses as well as students may struggle with the boundaries between social and therapeutic relationships. There is a fine line. In fact, students often feel more comfortable "being a friend" because it is a more familiar role, especially with people close to their own age. However, when this occurs, the nurse or student needs to make it clear (to themselves and the patient) that the relationship is a therapeutic one. This does *not* mean that the nurse is not friendly toward the patient, and it does *not* mean that talking about less than heavy topics (television, weather, children's pictures) is forbidden. It does mean, however, that the nurse follows the prior stated guidelines regarding a therapeutic relationship; essentially, the focus is on the patient, and the relationship is not designed to meet the nurse's needs. The patient's problems and concerns are explored, potential solutions are discussed by both patient and nurse, and solutions are implemented by the patient:

Patient: "Oh, gosh, I just hate to be alone. It is getting me down and sometimes it hurts so much."

Nurse: "Loneliness can be painful. What is going on now that you are feeling so alone?"

Patient: "Well, my mom died 2 years ago, and last month, my—oh, I am so scared." (*Patient takes a deep breath, looks down, and looks like she might cry.*)

Nurse: (*Sits in silence while the patient recovers.*) "Go on . . ."

Patient: "My boyfriend left for Iraq. I haven't heard from him, and they say he is missing. He was my best friend and we were going to get married, and if he dies I don't want to live."

Nurse: "Have you thought of harming yourself?"

Patient: "Well, if he dies I will. I can't live without him."

Nurse: "Have you ever felt like this before?"

Patient: Yes, when my mom died. I was depressed for about a year until I met my boyfriend."

Nurse: "It sounds like you are going through a very painful and scary time. Perhaps you and I can talk some more and come up with some ways for you to feel less anxious, scared, and overwhelmed. Would you be willing to work on this together?"

The ability of the nurse to engage in interpersonal interactions in a goal-directed manner for the purpose of assisting patients with their emotional or physical health needs is the foundation of the nurse-patient relationship. The nurse-patient relationship is synonymous with a professional helping relationship. Behaviors that have relevance to health care workers, including nurses, are as follows:

- **Accountability.** Nurses assume responsibility for their conduct and the consequences of their actions.
- **Focus on patient needs.** The interest of the patient rather than the nurse, other health care workers, or the institution is given first consideration. The nurse's role is that of patient advocate.
- **Clinical competence.** The criteria on which the nurse bases his or her conduct are principles of knowledge and those that are appropriate to the specific situation. This involves awareness and incorporation of the latest knowledge made available from research (evidence-based practice).
- **Delaying judgment.** Ideally, nurses refrain from judging patients and avoid putting their own values and beliefs on others.
- **Supervision** by a more experienced clinician or team is essential to developing one's competence in this area.

Nurses interact with patients in a variety of settings, such as emergency departments, medical-surgical units, obstetric and pediatric units, clinics, community settings, schools, and patients' homes. Nurses who are sensitive to patients' needs and have effective assessment and communication skills can significantly help patients confront current problems and anticipate future choices.

Sometimes the type of relationship that occurs may be informal and not extensive, such as when the nurse and patient meet for only a few sessions. However, even though it is brief, the relationship may be substantial, useful, and important for the patient. This limited relationship is often referred to as a **therapeutic encounter.** When the nurse really is concerned with another's circumstances (has positive regard, empathy), even a short encounter with the individual can have a powerful effect on that individual's life.

At other times, the encounters may be longer and more formal, such as in inpatient settings, mental health units, crisis centers, and mental health facilities. This longer time span allows the development of a therapeutic nurse-patient relationship.

Establishing Relationship Boundaries

A well-defined therapeutic relationship allows the establishment of clear patient boundaries that provide a safe space through which the patient can explore feelings and treatment issues (Peternelj-Taylor, 2002). The nurse's role in the therapeutic relationship is theoretically rather well defined. The patient's needs are separated from the nurse's needs, and the patient's role is different from that of the nurse. Therefore the boundaries of the relationship seem to be well stated. In reality, boundaries are at risk of blurring, and a shift in the nurse-patient relationship may lead to nontherapeutic dynamics. Pilette and associates (1995) described the following two common circumstances that can produce blurring of boundaries:

- When the relationship slips into a social context
- When the nurse's needs are met at the expense of the patient's needs

There are warning signals that indicate a nurse may be blurring boundaries. According to Pilette and colleagues (1995), they are:

- **Overhelping:** doing for patients what they are able to do themselves or going beyond the wishes or needs of patients
- **Controlling:** asserting authority and assuming control of patients "for their own good"
- **Narcissism:** having to find weakness, helplessness, and/or disease in patients to feel helpful, at the expense of recognizing and supporting patients' healthier, stronger, and more competent features

When situations such as these arise, the relationship has ceased to be a helpful one and the phenomenon of control becomes an issue. Role blurring is often a result of unrecognized transference or countertransference.

Transference

Transference is a phenomenon originally identified by Sigmund Freud when he used psychoanalysis to treat patients. **Transference** is the process whereby a person unconsciously and inappropriately displaces (transfers) onto individuals in his or her current life those patterns of behavior and emotional reactions that originated in relation to significant figures in childhood. The patient may even say, "You remind me of my _____ (mother, sister, father, brother, etc.). See the following example:

Patient: "Oh, you are so high and mighty. Did anyone ever tell you that you are a cold, unfeeling machine, just like others I know?"

Nurse: "Tell me about one person who is cold and unfeeling toward you." *(In this example, the patient is experiencing the nurse in the same way she did with significant other(s) during her formative years. In this case, the patient's mother was very aloof, leaving her with feelings of isolation, worthlessness, and anger.)*

Although the transference phenomenon occurs in all relationships, transference seems to be intensified in relationships of authority. Because the process of transference is accelerated toward a person in authority, physicians, nurses, and social workers all are potential objects of transference. It is important to realize that the patient may experience thoughts, feelings, and reactions toward a health care worker that are realistic and appropriate; these are *not* transference phenomena.

Common forms of transference include the desire for affection or respect and the gratification of dependency needs. Other transferential feelings the patient might experience are hostility, jealousy, competitiveness, and love. Requests for special favors (e.g., cigarettes, water, extra time in the session) are concrete examples of transference phenomena.

Countertransference

Countertransference refers to the tendency of the nurse to displace onto the patient feelings related to people in his or her past. Frequently, the patient's transference to the nurse evokes countertransference feelings in the nurse. For example, it is normal to feel angry when attacked persistently, annoyed when frustrated unreasonably, or flattered when idealized. A nurse might feel extremely important when depended on exclusively by a patient. If the nurse does not recognize his or her own omnipotent feelings as countertransference, encouragement of independent growth in the patient might be minimized at best. Recognizing our countertransference reactions maximizes our ability to *empower* our patients. When we fail to recognize our countertransferences toward our patients, the therapeutic relationship stalls, and essentially we *disempower* our patients by experiencing them not as individuals but rather as inner projections. See the following examples:

> *Patient:* "Yeah, well I decided not to go to that dumb group. 'Hi, I'm so and so, and I'm an alcoholic.' Who cares?" *(Patient sits slumped in a chair chewing gum, nonchalantly looking around.)*
>
> *Nurse: (In a very impassioned tone)* "You always sabotage your chances. You need AA to get in control of your life. Last week you were going to go and now you have disappointed everyone." *(Here the nurse is reminded of her mother who was an alcoholic. The nurse had tried everything to get her mother into treatment and took it as a personal failure and deep disappointment that her mother never sought recovery. After the nurse sorts out her thoughts and feelings and realizes the frustration and feelings of disappointment and failure belonged with her mother and not the patient, the nurse starts out the next session with the following approach.)*
>
> *Nurse:* "Look, I was thinking about last week and I realize the decision to go to AA or find other help is solely up to you. It is true that I would like you to live a fuller and more satisfying life, but it is your

decision. I am wondering, however, what happened to change your mind to not go to AA."

If the nurse feels either a strongly positive or a strongly negative reaction to a patient, the feeling most often signals countertransference in the nurse. One common sign of countertransference in the nurse is overidentification with the patient. In this situation the nurse may have difficulty recognizing or understanding problems the patient has that are similar to the nurse's own. For example, a nurse who is struggling with an alcoholic family member may feel disinterested, cold, or disgusted toward an alcoholic patient. Other indications of countertransference occur when the nurse gets involved in power struggles, competition, or arguments with the patient.

Identifying and working through various transference and countertransference issues is crucial if the nurse is to achieve professional and clinical growth and allow for positive change in the patient. These issues are best dealt with through the use of supervision by either the peer group or therapeutic team. Regularly scheduled supervision sessions provide the nurse with the opportunity to increase self-awareness, clinical skills, and growth, as well as allow for continued growth of the patient.

Self-Check on Boundary Issues

It is helpful for all of us to take time out to be reflective and to try to be aware of our thoughts and actions with patients, as well as with colleagues, friends, and family. Figure 7-1 is a helpful self-test you can use throughout your career, no matter what area of nursing you choose.

Phases of the Nurse-Patient Relationship

Hildegard Peplau introduced the concept of the nurse-patient relationship in 1952 in her ground-breaking book *Interpersonal Relations in Nursing.* This model of the nurse-patient relationship is well accepted in the United States and Canada and has become an important tool for all nursing practice. Peplau (1952) proposed that the nurse-patient relationship "facilitates forward movement" for both the nurse and the patient (p. 12). Peplau's interactive nurse-patient process is designed to facilitate the patient's boundary management, independent problem solving, and decision making that promotes autonomy (Haber, 2000).

It is most likely that in the brief period you have for your psychiatric nursing rotation, all the phases of the nurse-patient relationship will not have time to develop. However, it is important for you to be aware of these phases because you must be able to recognize and use them later. It is also important to remember that any contact that is

NURSING BOUNDARY INDEX SELF-CHECK

Please rate yourself according to the frequency with which the following statements reflect your behavior, thoughts, or feelings within the past 2 years while providing patient care.*

1. Have you ever received any feedback about your behavior being overly intrusive with patients and their families?	Never _____	Rarely _____	Sometimes _____	Often _____
2. Do you ever have difficulty setting limits with patients?	Never _____	Rarely _____	Sometimes _____	Often _____
3. Do you ever arrive early or stay late to be with your patient for a longer period?	Never _____	Rarely _____	Sometimes _____	Often _____
4. Do you ever find yourself relating to patients or peers as you might to a family member?	Never _____	Rarely _____	Sometimes _____	Often _____
5. Have you ever acted on sexual feelings you have for a patient?	Never _____	Rarely _____	Sometimes _____	Often _____
6. Do you feel that you are the only one who understands the patient?	Never _____	Rarely _____	Sometimes _____	Often _____
7. Have you ever received feedback that you get "too involved" with patients or families?	Never _____	Rarely _____	Sometimes _____	Often _____
8. Do you derive conscious satisfaction from patients' praise, appreciation, or affection?	Never _____	Rarely _____	Sometimes _____	Often _____
9. Do you ever feel that other staff members are too critical of "your" patient?	Never _____	Rarely _____	Sometimes _____	Often _____
10. Do you ever feel that other staff members are jealous of your relationship with your patient?	Never _____	Rarely _____	Sometimes _____	Often _____
11. Have you ever tried to "match-make" a patient with one of your friends?	Never _____	Rarely _____	Sometimes _____	Often _____
12. Do you find it difficult to handle patients' unreasonable requests for assistance, verbal abuse, or sexual language?	Never _____	Rarely _____	Sometimes _____	Often _____

* Any item that is responded to with "Sometimes" or "Often" should alert the nurse to a possible area of vulnerability. If the item is responded to with "Rarely," the nurse should determine whether it is an isolated event or a possible pattern of behavior.

Figure 7-1 ■ Nursing boundary index self-check. (From Pilette, P., Berck, C., & Achber, L. [1995]. Therapeutic management. *Journal of Psychosocial Nursing, 33*[1], 45.)

caring, respectful, and demonstrates concern for the situation of another person can have an enormous positive impact on that person.

Peplau (1952, 1999) described the nurse-patient relationship as evolving through interlocking, overlapping phases. The distinctive phases of the nurse-patient relationship are generally recognized as the:

- Orientation phase
- Working phase
- Termination phase

Although various phenomena and goals are identified for each phase, they often overlap. Even before the first meeting, the nurse may have many thoughts and feelings related to the first clinical session. This is sometimes referred to as the *preorientation phase.*

Preorientation Phase

Beginning health care professionals usually have many concerns and experience a mild to moderate degree of anxiety on their first clinical day. Commonly, nursing instructors will encourage students to identify concerns about working with psychiatric patients in preconference on the first clinical day. These concerns focus on being afraid of people with psychiatric problems, saying "the wrong thing," and what to do in response to certain patient behaviors. There really are no magic words. Talking with the instructor and supervised peer group discussion will add confidence, feedback, and suggestions. Chapter 6 discusses the use of communication strategies in clinical practice.

Often, students new to the mental health setting are concerned about being in situations that they may not know how to handle. These concerns are universal and often arise in the clinical setting. Table 7-1 identifies common patient behaviors (e.g., crying, asking the nurse to keep a secret, threatening to commit suicide, giving a gift) and gives examples of an appropriate response, the rationale for the response, and a possible verbal statement. The exact words depend on the situation, but understanding the

TABLE 7-1   Common Patient Behaviors and Nurse Responses

Possible Reactions by Nurse	Useful Responses by Nurse
What to Do If the Patient Says He or She Wants to Kill Himself or Herself	
The nurse may feel overwhelmed or responsible for "talking the patient out of it." The nurse may pick up some of the patient's feelings of hopelessness.	The nurse assesses whether the patient has a plan and the lethality of the plan. The nurse tells the patient that this is serious, that the nurse does not want harm to come to the patient, and that this information needs to be shared with other staff. "This is very serious, Mr. Lamb. I do not want any harm to come to you. I will have to share this with the other staff." The nurse can then discuss with the patient the feelings and circumstances that led up to this decision. (Refer to Chapter 20 for strategies in suicide intervention.)
What to Do If the Patient Asks the Nurse to Keep a Secret	
The nurse may feel conflict because the nurse wants the patient to share important information but is unsure about making such a promise.	The nurse *cannot* make such a promise. The information may be important to the health or safety of the patient or others. "I cannot make that promise. It might be important for me to share it with other staff." The patient then decides whether to share the information.
What to Do If the Patient Asks the Nurse a Personal Question	
The nurse may think that it is rude not to answer the patient's question. A new nurse might feel relieved to put off having to start the interview. The nurse may feel put on the spot and want to leave the situation. New nurses are often manipulated by a patient into changing roles. This keeps the focus off the patient and prevents the building of a relationship.	The nurse may or may not answer the patient's query. If the nurse decides to answer a natural question, he or she answers in a word or two, then refocuses back on the patient. *Patient:* Are you married? *Nurse:* Yes. Do you have a spouse? *Patient:* Do you have any children? *Nurse:* This time is for you—tell me about yourself. *Patient:* You can just tell me if you have any children. *Nurse:* This is your time to focus on your concerns. Tell me something about your family.
What to Do If the Patient Makes Sexual Advances	
The nurse feels uncomfortable but may feel conflicted about "rejecting" the patient or making him or her feel "unattractive" or "not good enough."	The nurse needs to set clear limits on expected behavior. "I am not comfortable having you touch (kiss) me. This time is for you to focus on your problems and concerns." Frequently restating the nurse's role throughout the relationship can help maintain boundaries. If the patient doesn't stop the nurse might say, "If you can't stop this behavior, I'll have to leave. I'll be back at [time] to spend time with you then." Leaving gives the patient time to gain control. The nurse returns at the stated time.
What to Do If the Patient Cries	
The nurse may feel uncomfortable and experience increased anxiety or feel somehow responsible for making the person cry.	The nurse should stay with the patient and reinforce that it is all right to cry. Often it is at that time that feelings are closest to the surface and can be best identified. "You seem ready to cry." "You are still upset about your brother's death." "What are you thinking right now?" The nurse offers tissues when appropriate.

TABLE 7-1	Common Patient Behaviors and Nurse Responses—cont'd

Possible Reactions by Nurse	Useful Responses by Nurse
What to Do If the Patient Leaves Before the Session Is Over	
The nurse may feel rejected, thinking it was something that he or she did. The nurse may experience increased anxiety or feel abandoned by the patient.	Some patients are not able to relate for long periods without experiencing an increase in anxiety. On the other hand, the patient may be testing the nurse. "I will wait for you here for 15 minutes, until our time is up." During this time, the nurse does not engage in conversation with any other patient or even with the staff. When the time is up, the nurse approaches the patient, says the time is up, and restates the day and time the nurse will see the patient again.
What to Do If the Patient Says He or She Does Not Want to Talk	
The nurse new to this situation may feel rejected or ineffectual.	At first, the nurse might say something to this effect: "It's all right. I would like to spend time with you. We don't have to talk." The nurse might spend short, frequent periods (e.g., 5 minutes) with the patient throughout the day. "Our 5 minutes is up. I'll be back at 10 AM and stay with you 5 more minutes." This gives the patient the opportunity to understand that the nurse means what he or she says and is back on time consistently. It also gives the patient time between visits to assess how he or she feels and what he or she thinks about the nurse, and perhaps to feel less threatened.
What to Do If the Patient Gives the Nurse a Present	
The nurse may feel uncomfortable when offered a gift. The meaning needs to be examined. Is the gift (1) a way of getting better care, (2) a way to maintain self-esteem, (3) a way of making the nurse feel guilty, (4) a sincere expression of thanks, or (5) a cultural expectation?	Possible guidelines: If the gift is expensive, the only policy is to graciously refuse. If it is inexpensive, then (1) if it is given at the end of hospitalization when a relationship has developed, graciously accept; (2) if it is given at the beginning of the relationship, graciously refuse and explore the meaning behind the present. "Thank you, but it is our job to care for our patients. Are you concerned that some aspect of your care will be overlooked?" If the gift is money, it is always graciously refused.
What to Do If Another Patient Interrupts During Time with Your Selected Patient	
The nurse may feel a conflict. The nurse does not want to appear rude. Sometimes the nurse tries to engage both patients in conversation.	The time the nurse had contracted with a selected patient is that patient's time. By keeping his or her part of the contract, the nurse demonstrates that the nurse means what he or she says and views the sessions as important. "I am with Mr. Rob for the next 20 minutes. At 10 AM, after our time is up, I can talk to you for 5 minutes."

rationale will aid you in applying the information later on.

Most experienced psychiatric nursing faculty and staff monitor the unit atmosphere and have a sixth sense as it pertains to behaviors that indicate escalating tension. They are trained in crisis interventions, and formal security is often available onsite to give the staff support. Your instructor will set the ground rules for safety during the first clinical day. For example, don't go into a patient's room alone, know if there are any patients not to engage, stay where other people are around in an open area, know the signs and symptoms of escalating anxiety. There are certain rules of thumb regarding actions a nurse can take if a patient's anger begins to escalate (see Chapter 21). You should always trust your own instincts. If you feel uncomfortable for any reason, excuse yourself for a moment and discuss your feelings with your instructor or staff member. In addition to getting reassurance and support, students can often provide valuable information about the patient's condition by sharing these perceptions.

Orientation Phase

The **orientation phase** can last for a few meetings or can extend over a longer period. It is the first time the nurse and the patient meet, and they are strangers to each other. When strangers meet, they interact according to their own backgrounds, standards, values, and experiences. This fact—that each person has a unique frame of reference—underlies the need for self-awareness on the part of the nurse. The initial interview includes the following:

* An atmosphere is established in which rapport can grow.
* The nurse's role is clarified, and the responsibilities of both the patient and the nurse are defined.
* The contract containing the time, place, date, and duration of the meetings is discussed.
* Confidentiality is discussed and assumed.
* The terms of termination are introduced (these are also discussed throughout the orientation phase and beyond).
* The nurse becomes aware of transference and countertransference issues
* Patient problems are articulated, and mutually agreed goals are established.

Establishing Rapport

A major emphasis during the first few encounters with the patient is on providing an atmosphere in which trust and understanding, or **rapport**, can grow. As in any relationship, rapport can be nurtured by demonstrating genuineness and empathy, developing positive regard, showing consistency, and offering assistance in problem solving and in providing support.

Parameters of the Relationship

The patient needs to know about the nurse (who the nurse is and the nurse's background) and the purpose of the meetings. For example, a student might furnish the following information:

> *Student:* "Hello, Mrs. Rodriquez, I am Jim Thompson from Scottsdale Community College. I am in my psychiatric rotation and will be coming here for the next six Thursdays. I would like to spend time with you each Thursday if you are still here. I'm here to

be a support person for you as you work on your treatment goals."

Formal or Informal Contract

A contract emphasizes the patient's participation and responsibility because it shows that the nurse does something *with* the patient rather than *for* the patient. The **contract**, either stated or written, contains the place, time, date, and duration of the meetings. During the orientation phase, the patient may begin to express thoughts and feelings, identify problems, and discuss realistic goals. Therefore the mutual agreement on goals is also part of the contract.

> *Student:* "Mrs. Rodriquez, we will meet at 10 AM each Thursday in the consultation room at the clinic for 45 minutes from September 15 to October 27. We can use that time for further discussion of your feelings of loneliness and anger and explore some things you could do to make the situation better for yourself."

Confidentiality

The patient has a right to know who else will be given the information shared with the nurse and that the information may be shared with specific people, such as a clinical supervisor, the physician, the staff, or other students in conference. The patient also needs to know that the information will *not* be shared with relatives, friends, or others outside the treatment team, except in extreme situations. Safeguarding the privacy and confidentiality of individuals is not only the nurse's ethical obligation, but a legal responsibility as well (Erickson & Miller, 2005).

Extreme situations include (1) child or elder abuse, (2) threats of self-harm or harm to others, or (3) intention not to follow through with the treatment plan. If information must be given to others, this is usually done by the physician, according to legal guidelines (see Chapter 26). The nurse must be aware of the patient's right to **confidentiality** and must not violate that right.

> *Student:* "Mrs. Rodriquez, I will be sharing some of what we discuss with my nursing instructor, and at times I may discuss certain concerns with my peers in conference or with the staff. However, I will *not* be sharing this information with your husband or any other members of your family or anyone outside the hospital without your permission."

Termination

Termination begins in the orientation phase. It also may be mentioned when appropriate during the working phase if the nature of the relationship is time limited (e.g., six or nine sessions). The date of the termination phase should be clear from the beginning. In some situations the nurse-patient contract may be renegotiated when the termination date has been reached. In other situations, when the therapeutic nurse-patient relationship is an open-ended one, the termination date is not known.

> *Student:* "Mrs. Rodriquez, as I mentioned earlier, our last meeting will be on October 27. We will have three more meetings after today."

Working Phase

The development of a strong working relationship can allow the patient to experience increased levels of anxiety and demonstrate dysfunctional behaviors in a safe setting while trying out new and more adaptive coping behaviors. Moore and Hartman (1988) identified specific tasks of the **working phase** of the nurse-patient relationship that remain relevant in current practice:

- Maintain the relationship.
- Gather further data.
- Promote the patient's problem-solving skills, self-esteem, and use of language.
- Facilitate behavioral change.
- Overcome resistance behaviors.
- Evaluate problems and goals, and redefine them as necessary.
- Promote practice and expression of alternative adaptive behaviors.

During the working phase, the nurse and patient together identify and explore areas in the patient's life that are causing problems. Often, the patient's present ways of handling situations stem from earlier means of coping devised to survive in a chaotic and dysfunctional family environment. Although certain coping methods may have worked for the patient at an earlier age, they now interfere with the patient's interpersonal relationships and prevent him or her from attaining current goals. The patient's dysfunctional behaviors and basic assumptions about the world are often defensive, and the patient is usually unable to change the dysfunctional behavior at will. Therefore, most of the problem behaviors or thoughts continue because of unconscious motivations and needs that are beyond the patient's awareness.

The nurse can work with the patient to identify these unconscious motivations and assumptions that keep the patient from finding satisfaction and reaching potential. Describing, and often reexperiencing, old conflicts generally awakens high levels of anxiety in the patient. Patients may use various defenses against anxiety and displace their feelings onto the nurse. Therefore during the working phase, intense emotions such as anxiety, anger, self-hate, hopelessness, and helplessness may surface. Defense mechanisms, such as acting out anger inappropriately, withdraw-

ing, intellectualizing, manipulating, and denying are to be expected.

During the working phase, the patient may unconsciously transfer strong feelings into the present and onto the nurse that belong to significant others from the past (transference). The emotional responses and behaviors in the patient may also awaken strong countertransference feelings in the nurse. **The nurse's awareness of personal feelings and reactions to the patient are vital for effective interaction with the patient.**

Termination Phase

The **termination phase** is the final, integral phase of the nurse-patient relationship. Termination is discussed during the first interview, and again during the working stage at appropriate times. Termination may occur when the patient is discharged or when the student's clinical rotation ends. Basically, the tasks of termination are as follows:

- Summarizing the goals and objectives achieved in the relationship is part of the termination process
- Discussing ways for the patient to incorporate into daily life any new coping strategies learned during the time spent with the nurse
- Reviewing situations that occurred during the time spent together
- Exchanging memories, which can help validate the experience for both nurse and patient and facilitate closure of that relationship

Termination often awakens strong feelings in both nurse and patient. Termination of the relationship signifies a loss for both, although the intensity and meaning of termination may be different for each. If a patient has unresolved feelings of abandonment, loneliness, not being wanted, or rejection, these feelings may be reawakened during the termination process. This process can be an opportunity for the patient to express these feelings, perhaps for the first time.

Important reasons for the student or nurse to address the termination phase are as follows:

- Feelings are aroused in both the patient and the nurse with regard to the experience they have had; when these feelings are recognized and shared, patients learn that it is acceptable to feel sadness and loss when someone they care about leaves.
- Termination can be a learning experience; patients can learn that they are important to at least one person.
- By sharing the termination experience with the patient, the nurse demonstrates caring for the patient.
- This may be the first successful termination experience for the patient.

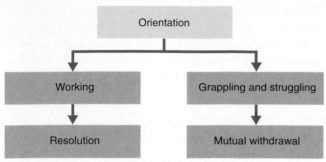

Figure 7-2 ■ Phases of therapeutic and nontherapeutic relationships. (From Forchuk, C., Westwell, J., Martin, M., et al. [2000]. The developing nurse-client relationship: Nurses' perspectives. *Journal of the American Psychiatric Nurses Association,* 6[1], 3-10.)

If a nurse has been working with a patient for a while, it is important for her to bring into awareness any feelings and reactions the patient may be experiencing related to separations. If a patient denies that the termination is having an effect (assuming the nurse-patient relationship was strong), the nurse may say something like, "Goodbyes are difficult for people. Often they remind us of other goodbyes. Tell me about another separation in the past." If the patient appears to be displacing anger, either by withdrawing or by being overtly angry at the nurse, the nurse may use generalized statements such as, "People may experience anger when saying goodbye. Sometimes they are angry with the person who is leaving. Tell me how you feel about my leaving." New practitioners as well as students in the psychiatric setting need to give thought to their last clinical experience with their patient and work with their supervisor or instructor to facilitate communication during this time.

A common response of beginning practitioners, especially students, is feeling guilty about terminating the relationship. These feelings may, in rare cases, be manifested by the student's giving the patient his or her telephone number, making plans to get together for coffee after the patient is discharged, continuing to see the patient afterward, or exchanging letters. Maintaining contact after discharge is not acceptable and is in opposition to the goals of a therapeutic relationship. Often this is in response to the student's need to (1) feel less guilty for "using the patient for learning needs," (2) maintain a feelings of being "important" to the patient, or (3) sustain the illusion that the student is the only one that "understands" the patient, among other student-centered rationales.

Indeed, part of the termination process may be to explore, after discussion with the patient's case manager, the patient's plans for the future: where the patient can go for help, which agencies to contact, and which people may best help the patient find appropriate and helpful resources.

What Hinders and What Helps

Not all nurse-patient relationships follow the classic phases as outlined by Peplau. Some nurse-patient relationships start in the orientation phase but move to a mutually frustrating phase and finally to mutual withdrawal (Figure 7-2).

Forchuk and associates (2000) conducted a qualitative study of the nurse-patient relationship. They examined the phases of both the therapeutic and the nontherapeutic relationship. From this study they identified certain behaviors that were beneficial to the progression of the nurse-patient relationship as well as those that hampered the development of this relationship. The study emphasized the importance of consistent, regular, and private interactions with patients as essential to the development of a therapeutic alliance. Nurses in this study stressed the importance of listening, pacing, and consistency.

Specifically, Forchuk and associates (2000) found evidence that the following factors enhanced the nurse-patient relationship, allowing it to progress in a mutually satisfying manner:

- **Consistency** includes ensuring that a nurse is always assigned to the same patient and that the patient has a regular routine for activities. Interactions are facilitated when they are frequent and regular in duration, format, and location. Consistency also refers to the nurse's being honest and consistent (congruent) in what is said to the patient.
- **Pacing** includes letting the patient set the pace and letting the pace be adjusted to fit the patient's moods. A slow approach helps reduce pressure, and at times it is necessary to step back and realize that developing a strong relationship may take a long time.
- **Listening** includes letting the patient talk when needed. The nurse becomes a sounding board for the patient's concerns and issues. Listening is perhaps the most important skill for nurses to master. Truly listening to another person, attending to what is behind the words, is a learned skill.
- **Initial impressions,** especially positive initial attitudes and preconceptions, are significant considerations in how the relationship will progress. Preconceived negative impressions and feelings toward the patient usually bode poorly for the positive growth of the relationship. In contrast, the nurse's feeling that

the patient is "interesting" or "a challenge" and a positive attitude about the relationship are usually favorable signs for the developing therapeutic alliance.

- **Comfort and control,** that is, promoting patient comfort and balancing control, usually reflect caring behaviors. Control refers to keeping a balance in the relationship: not too strict and not too lenient.
- **Patient factors** that seem to enhance the relationship include trust on the part of the patient and the patient's active participation in the nurse-patient relationship.

In relationships that did not progress to therapeutic levels, there seemed to be evidence that two major factors hampered the development of positive relationships: **inconsistency** and **unavailability** (e.g., lack of contact, infrequent meetings, meetings in the hallway) on the part of the nurse, patient, or both. When nurse and patient are reluctant to spend time together and meeting times become sporadic and or superficial, the term **mutual avoidance** is used. This is clearly a lose-lose situation.

The nurse's feelings and lack of self-awareness are major elements that contribute to the lack of progression of positive relationships. Negative preconceived ideas about the patient and negative feelings (e.g., discomfort, dislike, fear, and avoidance) seem to be a constant in relationships that end in frustration and mutual withdrawal. Sometimes these feelings are known, and sometimes the nurse is only vaguely aware of them.

Factors That Enhance Growth

Rogers and Truax (1967) identified three personal characteristics that help promote change and growth in patients, which are still valued today as vital components for establishing a therapeutic alliance or relationship: (1) genuineness, (2) empathy, and (3) positive regard. These are some of the intangibles that are at the heart of the art of nursing.

Genuineness
Genuineness, or self-awareness of one's feelings as they arise within the relationship and the ability to communicate them when appropriate, is a key ingredient in building trust. When a person is genuine, one gets the sense that what is displayed on the outside of the person is congruent with the internal processes. It is conveyed by listening to and communicating with others without distorting their messages, and being clear and concrete in communications with patients. Being genuine in a therapeutic relationship implies the ability to use therapeutic communication tools in an appropriately spontaneous manner, rather than rigidly or in a parrot-like fashion.

Empathy
Empathy is a complex multidimensional concept that has moral, cognitive, emotional, and behavioral components (Mercer & Reynolds, 2002). Perhaps Carl Rogers (1980) explained empathy most clearly:

> "It means entering the private perceptual world of the other and becoming thoroughly at home with it. It involves being sensitive, moment by moment, to the changing felt meanings which flow in this other person, to the fear or rage or tenderness or confusion or whatever that he or she is experiencing. It means temporarily living in the other's life, moving about in it delicately without making judgments" (p. 142).

Therefore, empathy signifies a central focus and feeling with and in the patient's world. According to Mercer and Reynolds (2002) it involves the following:

- Accurately perceiving the patient's situation, perspective, and feelings
- Communicating one's understanding to the patient and checking with the patient for accuracy
- Acting on this understanding in a helpful (therapeutic) way toward the patient

Empathy Versus Sympathy
There is much confusion regarding empathy versus sympathy. A simple way to distinguish them is that in empathy we *understand* the feelings of others. In sympathy we *feel* the feelings of others. When a helping person is feeling sympathy for another, objectivity is lost, and the ability to assist the patient in solving a personal problem ceases. Furthermore, sympathy is associated with feelings of pity and commiseration. Although these are considered nurturing human traits, they may not be particularly useful in a therapeutic relationship. When people express sympathy, they express agreement with another, which in some situations may discourage further exploration of a person's thoughts and feelings.

The following examples are given to clarify the distinction between empathy and sympathy. A friend tells you that her mother was just diagnosed with inoperable cancer. Your friend then begins to cry and pounds the table with her fist.

> *Sympathetic response:* "I know exactly how you feel. My mother was hospitalized last year and it was awful. I was so depressed. I still get upset just thinking about it." You go on to tell your friend about the incident.

Sometimes when nurses try to be sympathetic, they are apt to project their own feelings onto the patient's, which thus limits the patient's range of responses. A more useful response might be as follows:

> *Empathic response:* "How upsetting this must be for you. Something similar happened to my mother last year and I had so many mixed emotions. What thoughts and feelings are you having?" You continue to stay with your friend and listen to his or her thoughts and feelings.

In the practice of psychotherapy or counseling, empathy is an essential ingredient in a therapeutic relationship both for the better-functioning patient and for the patient who functions at a more primitive level.

Positive Regard

Positive regard implies respect. It is the ability to view another person as being worthy of caring about and as someone who has strengths and achievement potential. Positive regard is usually communicated indirectly by actions rather than directly by words.

Attitudes

One attitude through which a nurse might convey respect is willingness to work with the patient. That is, the nurse takes the patient and the relationship seriously. The experience is viewed not as "a job," "part of a course," or "time spent talking" but as an opportunity to work with patients to help them develop personal resources and actualize more of their potential in living.

Actions

Some actions that manifest an attitude of respect are attending, suspending value judgments, and helping patients develop their own resources.

Attending. Attending behavior is the foundation of interviewing (Ivey & Ivey, 1999). To succeed, nurses must pay attention to their patients in culturally and individually appropriate ways (Sommers-Flanagan & Sommers-Flanagan, 2003). *Attending* is a special kind of listening that refers to an intensity of presence, or being with the patient. At times, simply being with another person during a painful time can make a difference.

Body posture, eye contact, and body language are non-verbal behaviors that reflect the degree of attending and are highly culturally influenced. The cultural component of body posture, eye contact, and body language are covered in more depth in the Clinical Interview section of this chapter.

Suspending Value Judgments. Although we will always have personal opinions, nurses are more effective when they guard against using their own value systems to judge patients' thoughts, feelings, or behaviors. For example, if a patient is taking drugs or is involved in sexually risky behavior, you might recognize that these behaviors are hindering the patient from living a more satisfying life, posing a potential health threat, or preventing the patient from developing satisfying relationships. However, labeling these activities as bad or good is not useful. Rather, focus on exploring the behavior of the patient and work toward identifying the thoughts and feelings that influence this behavior. Judgmental behavior on the part of the nurse will most likely interfere with further exploration.

The first steps in eliminating judgmental thinking and behaviors are to (1) recognize their presence, (2) identify how or where you learned these responses to the patient's behavior, and (3) construct alternative ways to view the patient's thinking and behavior. Denying judgmental thinking will only compound the problem.

> *Patient:* "I am really sexually promiscuous and I love to gamble when I have money. I have sex whenever I can find a partner and spend most of my time in the casino. This has been going on for at least 3 years."

A judgmental response would be the following:

> *Nurse A:* "So your promiscuous sexual and compulsive gambling behaviors really haven't brought you much happiness, have they? You are running away from your problems and could end up with AIDS and broke."

A more helpful response would be the following:

> *Nurse B:* "So, your sexual and gambling activities are part of the picture also. You sound as if these activities are not making you happy."

In this example, Nurse B focuses on the patient's behaviors and the possible meaning they might have to the patient. Nurse B does not introduce personal value statements or prejudices regarding promiscuous behavior, as does Nurse A. Empathy and positive regard are essential qualities in a successful nurse-patient relationship.

Helping Patients Develop Resources. The nurse becomes aware of patients' strengths and encourages patients to work at their optimal level of functioning. The nurse does not act for patients unless absolutely necessary, and then only as a step toward helping them act on their own. It is important that patients remain as independent as possible to develop new resources for problem solving.

> *Patient:* "This medication makes my mouth so dry. Could you get me something to drink?"
>
> *Nurse:* "There is juice in the refrigerator. I'll wait here for you until you get back."
>
> or
>
> *Nurse:* "I'll walk with you while you get some juice from the refrigerator."

or

Patient: "Could you ask the doctor to let me have a pass for the weekend?"

Nurse: "Your doctor will be on the unit this afternoon. I'll let her know that you want to speak with her."

Consistently encouraging patients to use their own resources helps minimize the patients' feelings of helplessness and dependency and validates their potential for change.

THE CLINICAL INTERVIEW

The content and direction of the clinical interview are decided by the patient. The patient leads. The nurse employs communication skills and active listening to better understand the patient's situation. During the clinical interview, the nurse provides the opportunity for the patient to reach specific goals, including the following:

- To feel understood and comfortable
- To identify and explore problems relating to others
- To discuss healthy ways of meeting emotional needs
- To experience a satisfying interpersonal relationship

Preparing for the Interview

Helping a person with an emotional or medical problem is rarely a straightforward task. The goal of assisting a patient to regain psychological or physiological stability can be difficult to achieve. Extremely important to any kind of counseling is permitting the patient to set the pace of the interview, no matter how slow the progress may be (Arnold & Boggs, 2007).

Setting

Effective communication can take place almost anywhere. However, because the quality of the interaction—whether in a clinic, a clinical unit, an office, or the patient's home—depends on the degree to which the nurse and patient feel safe; establishing a setting that enhances feelings of security can be important to the helping relationship. A health care setting, a conference room, or a quiet part of the unit that has relative privacy but is within view of others is ideal. When the interview takes place in the home, it offers the nurse a valuable opportunity to assess the person in the context of everyday life.

Seating

In all settings, chairs need to be arranged so that conversation can take place in normal tones of voice and eye contact can be comfortably maintained or avoided. For example, a nonthreatening physical environment for nurse and patient would involve the following:

- Assuming the same height, either both sitting or both standing.
- Avoiding a face-to-face stance when possible; a 90- to 120-degree angle or side-by-side position may be less intense, and patient and nurse can look away from each other without discomfort.
- Providing safety and psychological comfort in terms of exiting the room. The patient should not be positioned between the nurse and the door, nor should the nurse be positioned in such a way that the patient feels trapped in the room.
- Avoiding a desk barrier between the nurse and the patient.

Introductions

In the orientation phase, students tell the patient who they are, what the purpose of the meeting is, and how long and at what time they will be meeting with the patient. The issue of confidentiality is brought up during the initial interview. Please remember that all health care professionals must respect the private, personal, and confidential nature of the patient's communication except in specific situations as outlined earlier (e.g., harm to self or others, child abuse, elder abuse). What is discussed with staff and your clinical group in conference should not be discussed outside with others, no matter who they are (e.g., patient's relatives, news media, friends, etc.). The patient needs to know that whatever is discussed will stay confidential unless permission is given for it to be disclosed.

The nurse can then ask the patient how he or she would like to be addressed. This question accomplishes a number of tasks (Arnold & Boggs, 2007). For example:

- It conveys respect.
- It gives the patient direct control over an important ego issue. (Some patients like to be called by their last names; others prefer being on a first-name basis with the nurse.)

Initiating the Interview

Once introductions have been made, the nurse can turn the interview over to the patient by using one of a number of open-ended statements such as the following:

- "Where should we start?"
- "Tell me a little about what has been going on with you."
- "What are some of the stresses you have been coping with recently?"

- "Tell me a little about what has been happening in the past couple of weeks."
- "Perhaps you can begin by letting me know what some of your concerns have been recently."
- "Tell me about your difficulties."

Communication can be facilitated by appropriately **offering leads** (e.g., "Go on"), making **statements of acceptance** (e.g., "Uh-huh"), or otherwise conveying interest.

Tactics to Avoid

The nurse needs to avoid certain behaviors (Moscato, 1988). For example:

Do Not:	Try To:
Argue with, minimize, or challenge the patient.	Keep focus on facts and the patient's perceptions.
Give false reassurance.	Make observations of the patient's behavior. "Change is always possible."
Interpret to the patient or speculate on the dynamics	Listen attentively, use silence, and try to clarify the patient's problem.
Question or probe patients about sensitive areas that they do not wish to discuss.	Pay attention to nonverbal communication. Strive to keep the patient's anxiety decreased.
Try to sell the patient on accepting treatment.	Encourage the patient to look at pros and cons.
Join in attacks patients launch on their mates, parents, friends, or associates.	Focus on facts and the patient's perceptions; be aware of nonverbal communication.
Participate in criticism of another nurse or any other staff member.	Focus on facts and the patient's perceptions.
	Check out serious accusations with the other nurse or staff member.
	Have the patient meet with the nurse or staff member in question and senior staff or clinician and clarify perceptions.

Helpful Guidelines

Some guidelines for conducting the initial interviews are offered by Meier and Davis (2001), including the following:

- Speak briefly.
- When you don't know what to say, say nothing.
- When in doubt, focus on feelings.
- Avoid advice.
- Avoid relying on questions.
- Pay attention to nonverbal cues.
- Keep the focus on the patient.

Attending Behaviors: The Foundation of Interviewing

Engaging in attending behaviors and listening well are two key principles of counseling on which just about everyone agree (Sommers-Flanagan & Sommers-Flanagan, 2003). Attending behaviors were addressed earlier but are covered more thoroughly here as they relate to the clinical interview. Ivey and Ivey (1999) define attending behaviors as "culturally and individually appropriate . . . eye contact, body language, vocal qualities, and verbal tracking" (p. 15). Sommers-Flanagan and Sommers-Flanagan (2003) state that positive attending behaviors can open up communication and encourage free expression. However, negative attending behaviors are more likely to inhibit expression. These behaviors need to be evaluated in terms of cultural patterns and past experiences of both the interviewer and the interviewee. There are no universals; however, there are guidelines that students can follow.

Eye Contact

Even among people from similar cultural backgrounds there may be variation in what an individual is personally comfortable with in terms of eye contact. For some patients and interviewers, sustained eye contact is normal and comfortable, whereas for other patients and interviewers it may be more comfortable and natural to make brief eye contact but look away or down much of the time. Sommers-Flanagan and Sommers-Flanagan (2003) state that it is appropriate for most nurse clinicians to maintain more eye contact when the patient speaks and less constant eye contact when the nurse speaks. However, in general, white patients are more comfortable with more sustained eye contact much of the time, whereas Native Americans, African Americans, and Asian patients often prefer less eye contact.

Body Language

Body language involves two elements: kinesics and proxemics. *Kinesics* is associated with physical characteristics such as body movements and postures. The way someone holds the head, legs, and shoulders, facial expressions, eye contact or lack thereof, and so on convey a multitude of messages. For example, a person who slumps in a chair, rolls the eyes, and sits with arms crossed in front of the chest can be perceived as resistant and unreceptive to what another wants to communicate.

On the other hand, positive body language may include leaning in slightly toward the speaker, maintaining a relaxed and attentive posture, making direct eye contact, making hand gestures that are unobtrusive and smooth while minimizing the number of other movements, and matching one's facial expressions to one's feelings or to the patient's feelings.

Proxemics refers to personal space and what distance between oneself and others is comfortable for an individual. Proxemics takes into account that these distances may be different for different cultural groups. **Intimate distance** in the United States is 0 to 18 inches and is reserved for those we trust most and with whom we feel most safe. **Personal distance** (18 to 40 inches) is for personal communications such as those with friends or colleagues. **Social distance** (4 to 12 feet) is applied to strangers or acquaintances, often in public places or formal social gatherings. **Public distance** (12 feet or more) relates to public space (e.g., public speaking). In public space one may hail another, and the parties may move about while communicating with one another.

Vocal Qualities

Vocal quality, or **paralinguistics,** encompasses voice loudness, pitch, rate, and fluency. Sommers-Flanagan and Sommers-Flanagan (2003) state that "effective interviewers use vocal qualities to enhance rapport, communicate interest and empathy and to emphasize special issues or conflicts" (p. 56). This supports the old adage, "It's not *what* you say, but *how* you say it." Speaking in soft and gentle tones is apt to encourage a person to share thoughts and feelings, whereas speaking in a rapid, high-pitched tone may convey anxiety and create it in the patient. Consider, for example, how tonal quality can affect communication in a simple sentence like "I will see you tonight."

1. "*I* will see you tonight." (I will be the one who sees you tonight.)
2. "I *will* see you tonight." (No matter what happens; or whether you like it or not, I will see you tonight.)
3. "I will see *you* tonight." (Even though others are present, it is you I want to see.)
4. "I will see you *tonight*." (It is definite, tonight is the night we will meet.)

Verbal Tracking

Verbal tracking is just that: tracking what the patient is saying. Individuals cannot know if you are hearing or understanding what they are saying unless you provide them with cues. Verbal tracking is giving neutral feedback in the form of restating or summarizing what the patient has already said. It does not include personal or professional opinions of what the patient has said (Sommers-Flanagan & Sommers-Flanagan, 2003). For example:

Patient: "I don't know what the fuss is about. I smoke marijuana to relax and everyone makes a fuss."

Nurse: "Do you see this as a problem for you?"

Patient: "No, I don't. It doesn't affect my work . . . well, most of the time, anyway. I mean, of course, if I have to think things out and make important decisions, then obviously it can get in the way. But most of the time I'm cool."

Nurse: "So when important decisions have to be made, then it interferes; otherwise, you don't see it affecting your functioning."

Patient: "Yeah, well, most of the time I'm cool."

Meier and Davis (2001) state that verbal tracking involves pacing the interview with the patient by sticking closely with the patient's speech content (as well as speech volume and tone as discussed earlier). It can be difficult to know which leads to follow if the patient introduces many topics at once.

Clinical Supervision and Process Recordings

Communication and interviewing techniques are acquired skills. Nurses learn to increase their ability to use communication and interviewing skills through practice and clinical supervision. In **clinical supervision**, the focus is on the nurse's behavior in the nurse-patient relationship. The nurse and the supervisor examine and analyze the nurse's feelings and reactions to the patient and the way they affect the relationship.

Farkas-Cameron (1995) stated that "the nurse who does not engage in the clinical supervisory process stagnates both theoretically and clinically, while depriving him- or herself of the opportunity to advance professionally" (p. 44). She observed that clinical supervision can be a therapeutic process for the nurse. During the process, feelings and concerns are ventilated as they relate to the developing nurse-patient relationship. The opportunity to examine interactions, obtain insights, and devise alternative strategies for dealing with various clinical issues enhances clinical growth and minimizes frustration and burnout. Clinical supervision is a necessary professional activity that fosters professional growth and helps minimize the development of nontherapeutic nurse-patient relationships.

The best way to increase communication and interviewing skills is to review clinical interactions exactly as they occur. This process offers students the opportunity to identify themes and patterns in their own, as well as their patients', communications. Students also learn to deal with the variety of situations that arise in the clinical interview.

The use of process recordings is a popular way to identify patterns in the student's and the patient's communication. **Process recordings** are written records of a segment of the nurse-patient session that reflect as closely as possible the verbal and nonverbal behaviors of both patient and nurse. Process recordings have some disadvantages because they rely on memory and are subject to distortions. However, they can be a useful tool for identifying communication patterns. It is usually best if the student can write notes verbatim (word for word) in a private area immediately after the interaction has taken place. Sometimes a clinician takes notes during the interview. This practice also has disadvantages, for example, it may be distracting for both interviewer and patient, or some patients (especially those with a paranoid disorder) may resent or misunderstand the nurse's intent.

VALUES, CULTURAL INFLUENCES, AND THE THERAPEUTIC RELATIONSHIP

Relationships are complex. We bring into our relationships a multitude of thoughts, feelings, beliefs, and attitudes—some rational and some irrational. We form these from families or culture, our spiritual beliefs and experiences, and our "heroes." It is helpful, even crucial, that we have an understanding of our own values and attitudes so that we may become aware of the beliefs or attitudes we hold that may interfere with the establishment of positive relationships with those under our care.

Increasingly we are working with, living with, and caring for people from diverse cultures and subcultures whose life experiences and life values may be quite different from our own. **Values** are abstract standards and represent an ideal, either positive or negative. For example, in the United States, to create a social order in which people can live peaceably together and feel secure in their person and property, society has adopted the two values of respecting one another's liberty and working cooperatively for a common goal. Not all the nation's people live up to these ideals all the time.

You may have noticed that there may be a dichotomy between theory and practice in the lives of some. For example, some people may pay lip service to the values of authority, but their behavior contradicts these values. They may stress honesty and respect for the law, yet cheat on their taxes and in their business practices. They may love their neighbors on Sunday and preach the love of God but demean or downgrade others around them for the rest of the week. They may declare themselves patriots, but label others traitors or even deny freedom of speech to any dissenters whose concept of patriotism differs from theirs.

A person's value system greatly influences both everyday and long-range choices. Values and beliefs provide a framework for what life goals people develop and for what they want their life to include. Our values are usually culturally oriented and influenced in a variety of ways through our parents, teachers, religious institutions, workplaces, peers, and political leaders as well as through Hollywood and the media. All these influences attempt to instill their values and to form and influence ours (Simon et al., 1995).

We also form our values through the example of others. **Modeling** is perhaps one of the most potent means of value education because it presents a vivid example of values in action (Simon et al., 1995). We all need role models to guide us in negotiating life's many choices. Young people in particular are hungry for role models and will find them among peers as well as adults. As nurses, parents, bosses, co-workers, friends, lovers, teachers, spouses, and singles, we are constantly (in either a positive or negative manner) providing a role model to others.

Our culture, and more precisely our subculture, defines the guidelines that provide structure to our lives. It is through this that our beliefs, thoughts, behaviors, and feelings are interpreted (Korn, 2001). Culture provides meaning to our lives and our environment in the form of an operating system or interpretive system. How we view the world and how we are supposed to behave, think, believe, and live are influenced by this interpretive system. Problems arise when the interpretive system of the clinician and that of the individual seeking guidance are glaringly different. When the nurse is working with an individual from a culturally distinct environment, the interpretive system between them might be so distinct at times that it is difficult for the patient and clinician to connect in a clinically meaningful way (Korn, 2001).

There are many ways this can be problematic. Although we emphasize that the patient and the nurse identify outcomes together, what happens when the nurse's beliefs, values, and interpretive system are very different from those of a patient? For example, the patient wants an abortion, which is against the nurse's values (or vice versa). The patient engages in irresponsible sex with multiple partners, and that is against the nurse's values. The patient puts material gain and objects far ahead of loyalty to friends and family, in direct contrast with the nurse's values (or vice versa). The patient's lifestyle includes taking illicit drugs, and substance abuse is against the nurse's values. The patient is deeply religious, and the nurse is a nonbeliever who shuns organized religion. Can nurses develop a working relationship and help patients solve a problem when the values, goals, and interpretive systems of the patients are so different from their own?

As nurses, it is useful for us to understand that our values and beliefs are not necessarily right and certainly not right for everyone. It is helpful to realize that our values and beliefs (1) reflect our own culture, (2) are derived from a whole range of choices, and (3) are those we have *chosen* for ourselves from a variety of influences and role models. These chosen values guide us in making decisions and taking the actions we hope will make our lives meaningful, rewarding, and full.

Personal values may change over time; indeed, they may change many times over the course of a lifetime. The values you held as a child are different from those you held as an adolescent and so forth. Self-awareness requires that we understand what we value and those beliefs that guide our behavior. It is critical that as nurses we not only understand and accept our own values and beliefs but also are sensitive to and accepting of the unique and different values and beliefs of others.

KEY POINTS TO REMEMBER

- The nurse-patient relationship is well defined, and the roles of the nurse and the patient must be clearly stated.
- It is important that the nurse be aware of the differences between a therapeutic relationship and a social or intimate relationship. In a therapeutic nurse-patient relationship, the focus is on the patient's needs, thoughts, feelings, and goals. The nurse is expected to meet personal needs outside this relationship in other professional, social, or intimate arenas.
- Genuineness, positive regard, and empathy are personal strengths in the helping person that foster growth and change in others.
- Although the boundaries of the nurse-patient relationship generally are clearly defined, they can become blurred; this blurring can be insidious and may occur on an unconscious level. Usually, transference and countertransference phenomena are operating when boundaries are blurred.
- It is important to have a grasp of common countertransferential feelings and behaviors and of the nursing actions to counteract these phenomena.
- Supervision aids in promoting the professional growth of the nurse as well as in the nurse-patient relationship, allowing the patient's goals to be worked on and met.

- The phases of the nurse-patient relationship include the orientation, working, and termination phases.
- The clinical interview is a key component of psychiatric mental health nursing. Presented are considerations needed for establishing a safe setting and planning for appropriate seating, introduction, and initiation of the interview.
- Attending behaviors (e.g., eye contact, body language, vocal qualities, and verbal tracking) are a key element in effective communication.
- Cultural background (as well as individual differences) has a great deal to do with what nonverbal behavior means to different individuals. The degree of eye contact and the use of touch are two nonverbal aspects that can be misunderstood by individuals of different cultures.
- A meaningful therapeutic relationship is facilitated when values and cultural influences are considered. It is the nurse's responsibility to seek to understand the patient's perceptions.

CRITICAL THINKING

1. On your first clinical day you spend time with an older woman, Mrs. Schneider, who is very depressed. Your first impression is "Oh, my, she looks like my mean Aunt Helen. She even sits like her." Mrs. Schneider asks you, "Who are you and how can you help me?" She tells you that "a student" could never understand what she is going through. She then says, "If you really wanted to help me you could get me a good job after I leave here."
    A. Identify transference and countertransference issues in this situation. What is your most important course of action? What in the study of Forchuk and associates (2000) indicates that this is a time for you to exercise self-awareness and self-insight to establish the potential for a therapeutic encounter or relationship?
    B. How could you best respond to Mrs. Schneider's question about who you are? What other information will

you give her during this first clinical encounter? Be specific.
    C. What are some useful responses you could give her regarding her legitimate questions about ways you could be of help to her?
    D. Analyze Mrs. Schneider's request that you find her a job. How does this request relate to boundary issues, and how can this be an opportunity for you to help Mrs. Schneider develop resources? Keeping in mind the aim of Peplau's interactive nurse-patient process, describe some useful ways you could respond to this request.
2. You are attempting to conduct a clinical interview with a very withdrawn patient. You have tried silence and open-ended statements, but all you get is one-word answers. What other actions could you take at this time?

CHAPTER REVIEW

Choose the most appropriate answer.

1. Which of the following is an accurate statement about transference?
   1. Transference occurs when the patient attributes thoughts and feelings toward the therapist that pertain to a person in the patient's past.
   2. Transference occurs when the therapist attributes thoughts and feelings toward the patient that pertain to a person in the patient's past.
   3. Transference occurs when the therapist understands and builds a value system consistent with the patient's value system.
   4. Transference occurs when the therapist recalls circumstances in his or her life similar to those the patient is experiencing and shares this with the patient.
2. A basic tool the nurse uses when establishing a relationship with a patient with a psychiatric disorder is:
   1. narcissism.
   2. role blurring.
   3. consistency.
   4. formation of value judgments.
3. Which nurse behavior jeopardizes the boundaries of the nurse-patient relationship?
   1. Focusing on patient needs
   2. Suspending value judgments
   3. Recognizing the value of supervision
   4. Allowing the relationship to become social
4. Which nurse behavior would not be considered a boundary violation?
   1. Narcissism
   2. Controlling
   3. Genuineness
   4. Keeping secrets about the relationship
5. Which statement describes an event that would occur during the working phase of the nurse-patient relationship?
   1. The nurse summarizes the objectives achieved in the relationship.
   2. The nurse assesses the patient's level of psychological functioning, and mutual identification of problems and goals occurs.
   3. Some regression and mourning occur about the nurse-patient relationship, although the patient demonstrates satisfaction and competence.
   4. The patient strives for congruence among actions, thoughts, and feelings and engages in problem solving and testing of alternative behaviors.

REFERENCES

Arnold, E.C., & Boggs, K.U. (2007). *Interpersonal relationships: Professional communication skills for nurses* (5th ed.). St. Louis: Saunders.

Erickson, J.I., & Miller, S. (2005). Caring for patients while respecting their privacy: Renewing our commitment. *Online Journal of Issues in Nursing, 10*(2).

Farkas-Cameron, M.M. (1995). Clinical supervision in psychiatric nursing. *Journal of Psychosocial Nursing and Mental Health Services, 33*(2), 40-47.

Forchuk, C., Westwell, J., Martin, M., et al. (2000). The developing nurse-client relationship: Nurse's perspectives. *Journal of the American Psychiatric Nurses Association, 6*(1), 3-10.

Haber, J. (2000). Hildegard E. Peplau: The psychiatric nursing legacy of a legend. *Journal of the American Psychiatric Nurses Association, 6*(2), 56-62.

Ivey, A.E., & Ivey, M. (1999). *Intentional interviewing and counseling* (4th ed.). Pacific Grove, CA: Brooks/Cole.

Kopta, S.M., Saunders, S.M., Lueger, R.L., & Howard, K.I. (1999). Individual psychotherapy outcome and process research: Challenge leading to great turmoil or positive transition? *Annual Review of Psychology, 50*, 441-469.

Korn, M.L. (2001). *Cultural aspects of the psychotherapeutic process.* Retrieved June 20, 2006, from http://doctor.medscape.com/viewarticle/418608.

LaRowe, K. (2004). *The therapeutic relationship.* Retrieved February 3, 2005, from http://compassion-fatigue.com/Index.asp?PG=89.

Meier, S.T., & Davis, S.R. (2001). *The elements of counseling* (4th ed.). Pacific Grove, CA: Brooks/Cole.

Mercer, S. W., & Reynolds, W. (2002). Empathy and quality of care. *British Journal of General Practice, 52*(Suppl.), S9-S12.

Moore, J.C., & Hartman, C.R. (1988). Developing a therapeutic relationship. In C.K. Beck, R.P. Rawlins, & S.R. Williams (Eds.), *Mental health–psychiatric nursing.* St. Louis: Mosby.

Moscato, B. (1988). The one-to-one relationship. In H.S. Wilson & C. S. Kneisel (Eds.), *Psychiatric nursing* (3rd ed.). Menlo Park, CA: Addison-Wesley.

Peplau, H.E. (1952). *Interpersonal relations in nursing: A conceptual frame of reference for psychodynamic nursing.* New York: Putnam.

Peplau, H.E. (1999). *Interpersonal relations in nursing: A conceptual frame of reference for psychodynamic nursing.* New York: Springer.

Peternelj-Taylor, C. (2002). Professional boundaries. A matter of therapeutic integrity. *Journal of Psychosocial Nursing and Mental Health Services, 40*(4), 22-29.

Pilette, P.C., Berck, C.B., & Achber, L.C.(1995). Therapeutic management of helping boundaries. *Journal of Psychosocial Nursing and Mental Health Services, 33*(1), 40-47.

Quinlan, J.C.F. (1996). *Co-creating personal and professional knowledge through peer support and peer approval in nursing.* Submitted for degree of PhD of the University of Bath, England, 1996. Retrieved July 17, 2006, from www.bath.ac.uk/carpp/jquinlan/titlepage.htm.

Rogers, C.R. (1980). *A Way of Being*. Boston: Houghton Mifflin.

Rogers, C.R., & Truax, C.B. (1967). The therapeutic conditions antecedent to change: A theoretical view. In C.R. Rogers (Ed.), *The therapeutic relationship and its impact*. Madison: University of Wisconsin Press.

Simon, S.B., Howe, L.W., & Kirschenbaum, H. (1995). *Values clarification*. New York: Warner Books.

Sommers-Flanagan, J., & Sommers-Flanagan, R. (2003). *Clinical interviewing* (3rd ed.). Hoboken: Wiley.

Caring for Patients with Psychobiological Disorders

CHAPTER 8

Anxiety and Anxiety Disorders

Elizabeth M. Varcarolis

Key Terms and Concepts

Objectives

1. Differentiate among normal anxiety, acute anxiety, and chronic anxiety.
2. Contrast and compare the four levels of anxiety in relation to perceptual field, ability to learn, and physical and other defining behavioral characteristics.
3. Summarize five properties of the defense mechanisms.
4. Give a definition for at least six defense mechanisms.
5. Rank the defense mechanisms from harmless to highly detrimental.
6. Identify genetic, biological, psychological, and cultural factors associated with anxiety disorders.
7. Describe clinical manifestations of each anxiety disorder.

continued

Edited by Nancy Christine Shoemaker in the fifth edition of *Foundations of Psychiatric Mental Health Nursing*.

Objectives—cont'd

8. Formulate four NANDA International nursing diagnoses that might be appropriate in the care of an individual with an anxiety disorder.
9. Name three defense mechanisms commonly used in excess by patients with anxiety disorders.
10. Propose realistic outcome criteria for patients with (a) generalized anxiety disorder, (b) panic disorder, and (c) posttraumatic stress disorder.
11. Discuss three classes of medications appropriate for patients or patients experiencing anxiety disorders.

evolve

For additional resources related to the content of this chapter, visit the Evolve website at http://evolve.elsevier.com/Varcarolis/essentials.

- Chapter Outline
- Chapter Review Answers
- Case Studies and Nursing Care Plans

- Nurse, Patient, and Family Resources
- Concept Map Creator

An understanding of anxiety and anxiety defense mechanisms is basic to the practice of psychiatric nursing. One of the greatest legacies of Hildegard Peplau (1909-1999) in nursing is her operational definition of the four levels of anxiety and suggestions for interventions appropriate to the level of anxiety the person is experiencing. **Anxiety** is a universal human experience to which no one is a stranger. It is the most basic of emotions. Dysfunctional behavior is often a defense against anxiety. When behavior is recognized as dysfunctional, interventions to reduce anxiety can be initiated by the nurse. As anxiety decreases, dysfunctional behavior will frequently decrease, and vice versa.

ANXIETY

Anxiety can be defined as a feeling of apprehension, uneasiness, uncertainty, or dread resulting from a real or perceived threat whose actual source is unknown or unrecognized. **Fear** is a reaction to a specific danger, whereas anxiety is a vague sense of dread relating to an unspecified danger. However, the body reacts in similar ways physiologically to both anxiety and fear.

An important distinction between anxiety and fear is that anxiety affects us at a deeper level than does fear. Anxiety invades the central core of the personality. It erodes the individual feelings of self-esteem and personal worth that contribute to a sense of being fully human.

Normal anxiety is a healthy life force that is necessary for survival. It provides the energy needed to carry out the tasks involved in living and striving toward goals. Anxiety motivates people to make and survive change. It prompts constructive behaviors, such as studying for an examination, being on time for job interviews, preparing for a presentation, and working toward a promotion.

Acute anxiety is also referred to as state anxiety. **Acute (state) anxiety** is precipitated by an imminent loss or change that threatens an individual's sense of security. It may be seen in performers before a concert. For example, many entertainers experience acute anxiety before live concerts or theater performances. Students may experience acute anxiety before an examination. Patients preparing for surgery often experience acute anxiety. The death of a loved one can stimulate acute anxiety when there is great disruption in the life of the bereaved person. In general, crisis involves the experience of acute anxiety.

Trait anxiety is another name for chronic anxiety. **Chronic (trait) anxiety** is anxiety that a person has lived with for a time. Ego psychologists suggest that in a nurturing environment the developing personality incorporates the primary caregivers' positive attributes, which allows the child to tolerate anxiety. When conditions for personality growth are less than adequate, positive values may not be incorporated, and the child may become anxiety ridden, a state that often covers up overwhelming, angry, and hostile impulses (Sullivan, 1953).

An understanding of the types, levels, and defensive patterns used in response to anxiety is basic to psychiatric nursing care. This understanding is essential for effectively assessing and planning interventions to help patients lower their levels of anxiety, as well as one's own. With practice, one becomes more skilled at identifying levels of anxiety as well as the defenses used to alleviate it, and at evaluating the possible stressors contributing to increases in a person's level of anxiety.

EXAMINING THE EVIDENCE   Gender Influences on Stress Responses

Fight or flight seems to ignore other possibilities for coping with stressful situations. What about other less drastic strategies such as negotiating or compromising?

Yes, fight or flight evokes images of western shoot-outs, wilderness confrontations with savage animals, battle scenes, cops and villains crouched behind cars, and other masculine struggles. In fact, the fight-or-flight response may be more descriptive of men than women for a very simple reason. Most of the groundwork for Canon's theory was based on research with human males' and even nonhuman males' physiological responses to stress. However, new research indicates that women may have unique physiological and social responses to stress (Motzer & Hertig, 2004).

Physically, women have lower hypothalamic-pituitary-adrenal axes and autonomic responses to stress at all ages, especially during pregnancy (Kajantie & Phillips, 2006). Researchers hypothesize that estrogen exposure reduces stress responses for women. Men and women also have different neural responses to stress: whereas men experience altered prefrontal blood flow and increased salivary cortisol, women respond with increased limbic activity and less significantly altered salivary cortisol (Wang, et al., 2007).

The tend-and-befriend model has been posed as an alternate response to non–life-threatening stress. This model asserts that women have historically banded together to provide mutual support during times of adversity (Taylor et al., 2000). This response may have a physiological basis. Whereas the fight response in men is promoted by testosterone, women's aggressive responses seem to be mediated by the relaxing effects of oxytocin, which promotes tending of and caring for others. In terms of the flight responses, the authors contend that fleeing is not a good strategy to promote survival of offspring. Instead, women are likely to seek out the support of others, particularly other women, to deal with stressful situations.

How does this model relate to nursing? According to Taylor (2002), "Social ties are the cheapest medicine we have" (p. 199). Stressful situations, including struggling with the direct effects of mental illness and its life-altering complications, can be reduced by the presence of skilled, caring, and competent nurses. Furthermore, the model suggests that promoting family support and involvement would improve outcomes.

You are probably asking yourself, "Ok, this kind of caring focus might be good for female patients, but how about the guys?" Well, once men get past fighting or fleeing (which may well affect men's decreased tendency to seek help for mental health issues), it is logical to conclude that men, too, benefit from tending and befriending. Multiple studies indicate that social support is essential to improved psychological functioning regardless of gender (Skarsater & Willem, 2006; Vanderhorst & McLaren, 2005). There is evidence to suggest that an interpersonal connection and cooperation between men and the health care team is facilitated by empowering, "You are the expert in your care," conveying strength; "It took courage to come here for treatment"; and recognizing progress and change, "Let's look at how you felt when you first got here and where you are now" (Smith & Robertonson, 2006).

Motzer, S.A., & Hertig, V. (2004). Stress, stress response, and health. *Nursing Clinics of North America, 39*(1), 1-17.

Skarsater, I., & Willman, A. (2006). The recovery process in major depression: An analysis employing Meleis' transition framework for deeper understanding as a foundation for nursing interventions. *Advances in Nursing Science, 29,* 245-259.

Smith, J.M., & Robertson, S. (2006). Nurses' tending instinct as a conduit for men's access to mental health counseling. *Issues in Mental Health Nursing, 27,* 559-574.

Taylor, S. (2002). *The tending instinct.* New York: Holt.

Taylor, S.E., Klein, L.C., Lewis, B.P., et al. (2000). Biobehavioral responses to stress in females: Tend-and-befriend, not fight-or-flight. *Psychological Review, 107,* 411-429.

Vanderhorst, R.K., & McLaren, S. (2005). Social relationship as predictors of depression and suicidal ideation in older adults. *Aging and Mental Health, 9,* 517-525.

Wang, J., Korczykowski, M., Rao, H., et al. (2007). Gender difference in neural response to psychological stress. *Social cognitive and affective neuroscience advance access* [online]. Oxford.

LEVELS OF ANXIETY

Levels of anxiety range from mild to moderate to severe to panic. Peplau's classic delineation of these four levels of anxiety (1968) is based on the work of Harry Stack Sullivan (American psychiatrist and theorist, 1892-1949). Assessment of a patient's level of anxiety is basic to therapeutic intervention in any setting—psychiatric, hospital, or community. Identification of a specific level of anxiety can be used as a guideline in selecting interventions. Although four levels of anxiety from mild to panic have been defined, the boundaries between these levels are not distinct, and the behaviors and characteristics shown by individuals experiencing anxiety can and often do overlap these categories. Use Table 8-1 as a guide for making observations.

Mild Anxiety

Mild anxiety occurs in the normal experience of everyday living. A person's ability to perceive reality is brought into

TABLE 8-1	Anxiety Levels and Their Characteristics		
Mild	**Moderate**	**Severe**	**Panic**
Perceptual Field			
May have heightened perceptual field	Has narrow perceptual field; grasps less of what is going on	Has greatly reduced perceptual field	Unable to focus on the environment
Is alert and can see, hear, and grasp what is happening in the environment	Can attend to more *if pointed out by another* (selective inattention)	Focuses on details or one specific detail	Experiences the utmost state of terror and emotional paralysis; feels he or she "ceases to exist"
Can identify things that are disturbing and are producing anxiety		Attention scattered	In panic, may have hallucinations or delusions that take the place of reality
		Completely absorbed with self	
		May not be able to attend to events in environment *even when pointed out by others*	
		In severe to panic levels of anxiety, the environment is blocked out. It is as if these events are not occurring.	
Ability to Learn			
Able to work effectively toward a goal and examine alternatives	Able to solve problems but not at optimal ability	Unable to see connections between events or details	May be mute or have extreme psychomotor agitation leading to exhaustion
	Benefits from guidance of others	Has distorted perceptions	Shows disorganized or irrational reasoning
Mild and moderate levels of anxiety can alert the person that something is wrong and can stimulate appropriate action.		*Severe and panic levels prevent problem solving and discovery of effective solutions. Unproductive relief behaviors are called into play, thus perpetuating a vicious cycle.*	
Physical or Other Characteristics			
Slight discomfort	Voice tremors	Feelings of dread	Experience of terror
Attention-seeking behaviors	Change in voice pitch	Ineffective functioning	Immobility or severe hyperactivity or flight
Restlessness	Difficulty concentrating	Confusion	Dilated pupils
Irritability or impatience	Shakiness	Purposeless activity	Unintelligible communication or inability to speak
Mild tension-relieving behavior: foot or finger tapping, lip chewing, fidgeting	Repetitive questioning	Sense of impending doom	Severe shakiness
	Somatic complaints, (e.g., urinary frequency and urgency, headache, backache, insomnia)	More intense somatic complaints (e.g., dizziness, nausea, headache, sleeplessness)	Sleeplessness
	Increased respiration rate	Hyperventilation	Severe withdrawal
	Increased pulse rate	Tachycardia	Hallucinations or delusions; likely out of touch with reality
	Increased muscle tension	Withdrawal	
	More extreme tension-relieving behavior; pacing, banging hands on table	Loud and rapid speech	
		Threats and demands	

sharp focus. A person sees, hears, and grasps more information, and problem solving becomes more effective. A person may display physical symptoms such as slight discomfort, restlessness, irritability, or mild tension-relieving behaviors (e.g., nail biting, foot or finger tapping, fidgeting).

Moderate Anxiety

As anxiety escalates, the patient's perceptual field narrows and some details are excluded from observation. An indi-

vidual experiencing **moderate anxiety** sees, hears, and grasps less information than someone who is not in that state. Individuals may demonstrate **selective inattention,** in which only certain things in the environment are seen or heard. The ability to think clearly is hampered, but learning and problem solving can still take place, although not at an optimal level. At the moderate level of anxiety, the person's ability to solve problems is enhanced greatly by the supportive presence of another. Physical symptoms include tension, pounding heart, increased pulse and respiration rate, perspiration, and mild somatic symptoms (gastric discomfort, headache, urinary urgency). Voice tremors and shaking may be noticed. Mild or moderate anxiety levels can be constructive, because anxiety can be viewed as a signal that something in the person's life needs attention.

evolve

> For a comprehensive case study of a patient experiencing moderate anxiety, visit the Evolve website at http://evolve.elsevier.com/Varcarolis/ essentials/.

Severe Anxiety

The perceptual field of a person experiencing severe anxiety is greatly reduced. A person with **severe anxiety** may focus on one particular detail or many scattered details. The person will have difficulty noticing what is going on in the environment, even when it is pointed out by another. Learning and problem solving are not possible at this level, and the person may be dazed and confused. Behavior is automatic and aimed at reducing or relieving anxiety. Often the individual complains of increased severity of somatic symptoms (headache, nausea, dizziness, insomnia), trembling, and pounding heart. The most classic experiences are hyperventilation and a sense of impending doom or dread.

evolve

> For a comprehensive case study of a patient experiencing severe anxiety, visit the Evolve website at http://evolve.elsevier.com/Varcarolis/ essentials.

Panic Level of Anxiety

The **panic level of anxiety** is the most extreme form and results in markedly disturbed behavior. An individual is not able to process what is going on in the environment and may lose touch with reality. The resulting behavior may be confusion, shouting, screaming, or withdrawal. Hallucinations, or false sensory perceptions such as seeing people or objects that are not there, may be experienced by people at panic levels of anxiety. Physical behavior may be erratic, uncoordinated, and impulsive. Automatic behaviors are used to reduce and relieve anxiety, although such efforts may be ineffective. Acute panic may lead to exhaustion. Review Table 8-1 to identify the levels of anxiety through their effects on (1) perceptual field, (2) ability to learn, and (3) physical and other defining characteristics.

INTERVENTIONS
Mild to Moderate Levels of Anxiety

A patient experiencing a mild to moderate level of anxiety is still able to solve problems; however, the ability to concentrate decreases as anxiety increases. The nurse can help the patient focus and solve problems with the use of specific communication techniques, such as employing open-ended questions, giving broad openings, and exploring and seeking clarification. These techniques can be useful to a patient experiencing mild to moderate anxiety. Closing off topics of communication and bringing up irrelevant topics can increase a person's anxiety and are tactics that usually make the *nurse,* not the patient, feel better.

Reducing the patient's level of anxiety and preventing escalation of anxiety can be accomplished by being calm, recognizing the anxious patient's distress, and being willing to listen. Evaluation of effective past coping mechanisms is useful. Often the nurse can help the patient consider alternatives to problem situations and offer activities that may temporarily relieve feelings of inner tension. Table 8-2 identifies counseling interventions useful in assisting people experiencing mild to moderate levels of anxiety.

Severe to Panic Levels of Anxiety

A patient experiencing a severe to panic level of anxiety is unable to solve problems and may have a poor grasp of what is happening in the environment. Unproductive relief behaviors may take over and the person may not be in control of his or her actions. Extreme regression and running about aimlessly are behavioral manifestations of a person's intense psychic pain. The nurse must be concerned with the patient's safety and, at times, with the safety of others. Physical needs (e.g., for fluids and rest) must be met to prevent exhaustion.

Anxiety reduction measures may take the form of removing the person to a quiet environment in which there is minimal stimulation and providing gross motor activities to drain some of the tension. The use of medications may have to be considered, but medications and restraints should be used only after other more personal and less restrictive interventions have failed to decrease anxiety to safer levels. Although communication may be scattered and disjointed, themes can often be heard that the nurse must address. The feeling that one is understood can decrease the sense of isolation and reduce anxiety.

Because individuals experiencing severe to panic levels of anxiety are unable to solve problems, techniques suggested for communicating with people with mild to moderate levels of anxiety are not always effective. Patients experiencing severe to panic anxiety levels are out of control,

TABLE 8-2	Interventions for Mild to Moderate Levels of Anxiety

NURSING DIAGNOSIS: *Anxiety* (moderate) related to situational event or psychological stress, as evidenced by increase in vital signs, moderate discomfort, narrowing of perceptual field, and selective inattention

Intervention	Rationale
1. Help the patient identify anxiety. "Are you comfortable right now?"	1. It is important to validate observations with the patient, name the anxiety, and start to work with the patient to lower anxiety.
2. Anticipate anxiety-provoking situations.	2. Escalation of anxiety to a more disorganizing level is prevented.
3. Use nonverbal language to demonstrate interest (e.g., lean forward, maintain eye contact, nod your head).	3. Verbal and nonverbal messages should be consistent. The presence of an interested person provides a stabilizing focus.
4. Encourage the patient to talk about his or her feelings and concerns.	4. When concerns are stated aloud, problems can be discussed and feelings of isolation decreased.
5. Avoid closing off avenues of communication that are important for the patient. Focus on the patient's concerns.	5. When staff anxiety increases, changing the topic or offering advice is common but leaves the person isolated.
6. Ask questions to clarify what is being said. "I'm not sure what you mean. Give me an example."	6. Increased anxiety results in scattering of thoughts. Clarifying helps the patient identify thoughts and feelings.
7. Help the patient identify thoughts or feelings before the onset of anxiety. "What were you thinking right before you started to feel anxious?"	7. The patient is assisted in identifying thoughts and feelings, and problem solving is facilitated.
8. Encourage problem solving with the patient.*	8. Encouraging patients to explore alternatives increases sense of control and decreases anxiety.
9. Assist in developing alternative solutions to a problem through role play or modeling behaviors.	9. The patient is encouraged to try out alternative behaviors and solutions.
10. Explore behaviors that have worked to relieve anxiety in the past.	10. The patient is encouraged to mobilize successful coping mechanisms and strengths.
11. Provide outlets for working off excess energy (e.g., walking, playing Ping-Pong, dancing, exercising).	11. Physical activity can provide relief of built-up tension, increase muscle tone, and increase endorphin levels.

*Patients experiencing mild to moderate anxiety levels can problem solve.

so they need to know that they are safe from their own impulses. **Firm, short, and simple statements are useful.**

Reinforcing commonalities in the environment and pointing out reality when there are distortions can also be useful interventions for severely anxious persons. Table 8-3 suggests some basic nursing interventions for patients with severe to panic levels of anxiety.

DEFENSE MECHANISMS

Responses to stress and anxiety are affected by factors such as age, sex, culture, life experiences, and lifestyle. Vaillant and Vaillant (2004) identify three classes of coping mechanisms that people use to overcome stressful and anxiety-provoking situations. It is important to note that social

support is one mediating factor that has been heavily researched and has significant implications for nurses and other health care professionals. The fact that strong social support from significant others can enhance mental and physical health and act as a significant buffer against distress has been well documented in the literature. Numerous studies have found a strong correlation between lower mortality rates and intact support systems (Koenig et al., 2001).

Defense mechanisms protect people from painful awareness of feelings and memories that can provoke overwhelming anxiety (Sonnenberg et al., 2003). Adaptive use of defense mechanisms helps people lower anxiety to achieve goals in acceptable ways.

Defense mechanisms operate all the time. However, when an individual is faced with a situation that triggers

TABLE 8-3	Interventions for Severe to Panic Levels of Anxiety

NURSING DIAGNOSIS: *Anxiety* (severe, panic) related to severe threat (biochemical, environmental, psychosocial), as evidenced by verbal or physical acting out, extreme immobility, sense of impending doom, inability to differentiate reality (possible hallucinations or delusions), and inability to problem solve

Intervention	Rationale
1. Maintain a calm manner.	1. Anxiety is communicated interpersonally. The quiet calm of the nurse can serve to calm the patient. The presence of anxiety can escalate anxiety in the patient.
2. Always remain with the person experiencing an acute severe to panic level of anxiety.	2. Alone with immense anxiety, a person feels abandoned. A caring face may be the patient's only contact with reality when confusion becomes overwhelming.
3. Minimize environmental stimuli. Move to a quieter setting and stay with the patient.	3. Helps minimize further escalation of patient's anxiety.
4. Use clear and simple statements and repetition.	4. A person experiencing a severe to panic level of anxiety has difficulty concentrating and processing information.
5. Use a low-pitched voice; speak slowly.	5. A high-pitched voice can convey anxiety. Low pitch can decrease anxiety.
6. Reinforce reality if distortions occur (e.g., seeing objects that are not there or hearing voices when no one is present).	6. Anxiety can be reduced by focusing on and validating what is going on in the environment.
7. Listen for themes in communication.	7. In severe to panic levels of anxiety, verbal communication themes may be the only indication of the patient's thoughts or feelings.
8. Attend to physical and safety needs when necessary (e.g., need for warmth, fluids, elimination, pain relief, family contact).	8. High levels of anxiety may obscure the patient's awareness of physical needs.
9. Because safety is an overall goal, physical limits may need to be set. Speak in a firm, authoritative voice: "You may not hit anyone here. If you can't control yourself, we will help you."	9. A person who is out of control is often terrorized. Staff must offer the patient and others protection from destructive and self-destructive impulses.
10. Provide opportunities for exercise (e.g., walk with nurse, punching bag, Ping-Pong game).	10. Physical activity helps channel and dissipate tension and may temporarily lower anxiety.
11. When a person is constantly moving or pacing, offer high-calorie fluids.	11. Dehydration and exhaustion must be prevented.
12. Assess need for medication or seclusion after other interventions have been tried and not been successful.	12. Exhaustion and physical harm to self and others must be prevented.

high anxiety, that person may become more rigid in the use of defense mechanisms and may revert to using less mature defenses (Sonnenberg et al., 2003). The degree of distortion of reality and disruption in interpersonal relationships determines if the use of a defense mechanism is adaptive (healthy) or maladaptive (unhealthy) (Vaillant, 1994).

Sigmund Freud and his daughter Anna Freud outlined most of the defense mechanisms that we recognize today. Vaillant (1994) summarized five of the most important properties of defense mechanisms:

1. Defenses are a major means of managing conflict and affect.
2. Defenses are relatively unconscious.
3. Defenses are discrete from one another.
4. Although defenses are often the hallmarks of major psychiatric syndromes, they are reversible.
5. Defenses are adaptive as well as pathological.

All defense mechanisms except sublimation and altruism can be used in both healthy and not-so-healthy ways. (Sublimation and altruism are commonly very healthy coping mechanisms.) Most people use a variety of defense mechanisms but not always at the same level. Keep in mind that whether the use of defense mechanisms is adaptive or maladaptive is determined for the most part by their *frequency*, *intensity*, and *duration* of use.

The defense mechanisms are discussed in the following sections starting with the most mature and healthy, followed by those that are less healthy, and then by those that result in a greater degree of reality distortion and disruption in relationships and personal functioning.

Healthy Defenses

Altruism. In **altruism**, emotional conflicts and stressors are dealt with by meeting the needs of others. Unlike in self-sacrificing behavior, in altruism the person receives gratification either vicariously or from the response of others (APA, 2000).

VIGNETTE

Six months after losing her husband in a car accident, Jeanette began to spend one day a week doing grief counseling with families who had lost a loved one. She found that she was effective in helping others in their grief, and she obtained a great deal of satisfaction and pleasure from helping others work through their pain.

Sublimation. **Sublimation** is an unconscious process of substituting constructive and socially acceptable activity for strong impulses that are not acceptable in their original form. Often these impulses are sexual or aggressive. A man with strong hostile feelings may choose to become a butcher, or he may be involved in rough contact sports. A person who is unable to experience sexual activity may channel this energy into something creative, such as painting or gardening.

Humor. Humor makes life easier. An individual may deal with emotional conflicts or stressors by emphasizing the amusing or ironic aspects of the conflict or stressor through **humor** (APA, 2000).

VIGNETTE

A man goes to an interview that means a great deal to him. He is being interviewed by the top executives of the company. He has recently had foot surgery and, on entering the interview room, he stumbles and loses his balance. There is a stunned silence, and then the man states calmly, "I was hoping I could put my best foot forward." With everyone laughing, the interview continues in a relaxed manner.

Suppression. **Suppression** is the conscious denial of a disturbing situation or feeling. For example, a student who has been studying for the state board examinations says, "I can't worry about paying my rent until after my exam tomorrow."

Intermediate Defenses

Repression. **Repression** is the exclusion of unpleasant or unwanted experiences, emotions, or ideas from conscious awareness. Forgetting the name of a former boyfriend or girlfriend, or forgetting an appointment to discuss poor grades are examples. Repression is considered the cornerstone of the defense mechanisms, and it is the first line of psychological defense against anxiety.

Displacement. Transfer of emotions associated with a particular person, object, or situation to another person, object, or situation that is nonthreatening is called **displacement**. The frequently cited example in which the boss yells at the man, the man yells at his wife, the wife yells at the child, and the child kicks the cat demonstrates the successive use of displaced hostility. The use of displacement is common but not always adaptive. Spousal, child, and elder abuse are often cases of displaced hostility.

Reaction Formation. In **reaction formation** (also termed **overcompensation**), unacceptable feelings or behaviors are kept out of awareness by developing the opposite behavior or emotion. For example, a person who harbors hostility toward children becomes a Boy Scout leader.

Somatization. Transforming anxiety on an unconscious level into a physical symptom that has no organic cause is a form of **somatization**. Often the symptom functions as an attention getter or as an excuse.

VIGNETTE

A professor develops laryngitis on the day he is scheduled to defend a research proposal to a group of peers.

A woman who does not want to go out with her boss's brother calls to say "her back went out," and she cannot make the date (and, in fact, her back is sore).

Undoing. **Undoing** makes up for an act or communication (e.g., giving a gift to undo an argument). A common behavioral example of undoing is compulsive handwashing. This can be viewed as cleansing oneself of an act or thought perceived as unacceptable.

Rationalization. **Rationalization** consists of justifying illogical or unreasonable ideas, actions, or feelings by developing acceptable explanations that satisfy the teller as well as the listener. Common examples are, "If I had Lynn's brains, I'd get good grades, too," or "Everybody cheats, so why shouldn't I?" Rationalization is a form of self-deception.

Immature Defenses

Passive Aggression. A passive-aggressive individual deals with emotional conflict or stressors by indirectly and unassertively expressing aggression toward others. On the surface, there is an appearance of compliance that masks covert resistance, resentment, and hostility (APA, 2000). In **passive aggression**, aggression toward others is expressed through procrastination, failure, inefficiency, passivity, and illnesses that affect others more than oneself. Such passive-aggressive behaviors occur especially in response to assigned tasks or demands for independent action, responsibilities, or obligations (Widiger & Mullins, 2003).

VIGNETTE

Sam promises his boss that he is working on the presentation for important patients, even though he constantly "forgets" to bring in samples of the presentation. The day of the presentation, Sam calls in sick with the flu.

Acting-Out Behaviors. In acting out, an individual deals with emotional conflicts or stressors by actions rather than reflections or feelings (APA, 2000). For example, a person may lash out in anger verbally or physically to distract the self from threatening thoughts or feelings. The verbal or physical expression of anger can make a person feel temporarily less helpless or vulnerable. By lashing out at others, an individual can transfer the focus from personal doubts and insecurities to some other person or object. **Acting-out behaviors** are a destructive coping style.

VIGNETTE

When Harry was turned down a third time for a promotion, he went to his office and tore apart every patient file in his file cabinet. His initial feelings of worthlessness and lowered self-esteem related to the situation were interpreted by Harry to mean "I am no good." This thinking resulted in Harry's quickly transforming these painful feelings into actions of anger and destruction. Temporarily, Harry felt more powerful and less vulnerable.

Dissociation. A disruption in the usually integrated functions of consciousness, memory, identity, or perception of the environment is known as **dissociation**.

VIGNETTE

A young mother who saw her son run over by a car was taken to a neighbor's house while the police dealt with the accident. Later she told the policeman, "I really don't remember what happened. The last thing I remember is going out the door to check on Johnny." At that moment, to protect herself from an unbearable situation, she split off the threatening event from awareness until she could begin to deal with her feelings of devastation.

Devaluation. **Devaluation** occurs when emotional conflicts or stressors are dealt with by attributing negative qualities to self or others (APA, 2000). When devaluing another, the individual then appears good by contrast.

VIGNETTE

A woman who is very jealous of a co-worker says, "Oh, yes, she won the award. Those awards don't mean anything anyway, and I wonder what she had to do to be chosen." In this way she minimizes the other's accomplishments and keeps her own fragile self-esteem intact.

Idealization. In **idealization**, emotional conflicts or stressors are dealt with by attributing exaggerated positive qualities to others (APA, 2000). Idealization is an important aspect of the development of the self. Children who grow up with parents they can respect and idealize develop healthy standards of conduct and morality (Merikangas & Kupfer, 1995).

When people idealize and overvalue a person in a new relationship, they are sure to be disappointed when the object of the idealization turns out to be human. This leads to a great deal of disappointment and painful lowering of self-esteem. Such individuals may then end up devaluing and rejecting the object of their affection to protect their own self-esteem. This pattern can be repeated over and over on a job, in friendships, in intimate relationships, and in marriage.

VIGNETTE

Mary met the most "wonderful and perfect" man. No one could tell Mary that Jim was nice but had some quirks, like everyone else. Mary wouldn't listen. When Jim failed to live up to Mary's expectations of giving her constant attention, adoration, and gifts, Mary was devastated. Shortly thereafter, she started saying that Jim was, like all men, a brute, and that she wanted no more to do with such an insensitive person.

Splitting. **Splitting** is the inability to integrate the positive and negative qualities of oneself or others into a cohesive image. Aspects of the self and of others tend to alternate between opposite poles; for example, either good, loving, worthy, and nurturing, or bad, hateful, destructive, rejecting, and worthless (APA, 2000). Use of this defense mechanism is prevalent in personality disorders, especially the borderline ones, and will be discussed at greater length in Chapter 10.

VIGNETTE

Alice viewed her therapist as the most wonderful, loving, and insightful therapist she had ever had. When her therapist refused to write her a prescription for Valium, Alice shouted at her that she was the "stupidest, most uncaring, and thickheaded person," and she demanded another therapist "right away."

Projection. A person unconsciously rejects emotionally unacceptable personal features and attributes them to other people, objects, or situations through **projection**. This is the hallmark of blaming or scapegoating, which is the root of prejudice. People who always feel that others are out to deceive or cheat them may be projecting onto others those characteristics in themselves that they find distasteful and cannot consciously accept.

Projection of anxiety can often be seen in systems (family, hospital, school, business). In a family in which there are problems, the child is often scapegoated, and the pain and anxiety within the family are projected onto the child: "The problem is Tommy." In a larger system in which anxiety and conflict are present, the weakest members are scapegoated: "The problem is the nurses' aides . . . the students . . . the new salesman." When pain and anxiety exist within a system, projection can be an automatic relief behavior. Once the cause of the anxiety is identified, changes in relief behavior can ensue, and the system can become more functional and productive.

Denial. **Denial** involves escaping unpleasant realities by ignoring their existence. For example, a man believes that physical limitations reflect negatively on one's manhood. Thus he may deny chest pains, even though heart attacks run in his family, because of a threat to his self-image as a man. A woman whose health has deteriorated because of alcohol abuse denies she has a problem with alcohol by saying she can stop drinking whenever she wants. Table 8-4 gives examples of adaptive and maladaptive uses of some common defense mechanisms.

ANXIETY DISORDERS

Anxiety is a normal response to threatening situations, and everyone experiences occasional distress. Anxiety becomes a problem when it interferes with adaptive behavior, causes physical symptoms, or exceeds a tolerable level. With people who have anxiety disorders, the experience is often one of considerable functional impairment and distress.

Individuals with anxiety disorders use rigid, repetitive, and ineffective behaviors to try to control anxiety. The common element in anxiety disorders is that individuals experience a degree of anxiety that is so high that it interferes with personal, occupational, or social functioning. Anxiety disorders are common, chronic, and tend to be persistent and often disabling.

PREVALENCE AND COMORBIDITY

Anxiety disorders are the most prevalent lifetime psychiatric disorders in the United States and estimated at 28.8% (Kessler et al 2005), that means that approximately one in four individuals in the United States will experience an anxiety disorder in his or her lifetime (Charney, 2005). People with anxiety disorders frequently seek health care services for relief of physical symptoms. Women are reported to be more frequently affected than men.

Anxiety disorders are frequently **comorbid** with other psychiatric problems. Several studies suggest that up to 90% of people with an anxiety disorder develop another psychiatric disorder during their lifetime (Overbeek et al., 2002). Major depression often co-occurs in 50% of people with anxiety disorders and produces a greater impairment with poorer response to treatment (Satcher et al., 2005; Simon & Rosenbaum, 2003). Substance abuse is encountered frequently and has a similar negative effect on treatment (Myrick & Brady, 2003). Other comorbid conditions include other anxiety disorders, eating disorders, and medical illness (e.g., cancer, heart disease, high blood pressure, irritable bowel syndrome, etc.) (Satcher et al., 2005).

THEORY

There is no longer any doubt that biological correlates predispose some individuals to pathological anxiety states (e.g., phobias, panic attacks). By the same token, traumatic life events, psychosocial factors, and sociocultural factors also are etiologically significant.

A **genetic** component is substantiated by numerous studies that find anxiety disorders tend to cluster in families. Twin studies indicate the existence of a genetic component

TABLE 8-4	Defense Mechanisms	
Defense Mechanism	**Adaptive**	**Maladaptive**
Repression	Man forgets his wife's birthday after a marital fight.	Woman is unable to enjoy sex after having pushed out of awareness a traumatic sexual incident from childhood.
Sublimation	Woman who is angry with her boss writes a short story about a heroic woman. By definition, use of sublimation is always constructive.	None
Regression	Four-year-old boy with a new baby brother starts sucking his thumb and wanting a bottle.	Man who loses a promotion starts complaining to others, hands in sloppy work, misses appointments, and comes in late for meetings.
Displacement	Patient criticizes a nurse after his family fails to visit.	Child who is unable to acknowledge fear of his father becomes fearful of animals.
Projection	Man who is unconsciously attracted to other women teases his wife about flirting.	Woman who has repressed an attraction toward other women refuses to socialize. She fears another woman will make homosexual advances toward her.
Compensation	Short man becomes assertively verbal and excels in business.	Individual drinks alcohol when self-esteem is low to diffuse discomfort temporarily.
Reaction formation	Recovering alcoholic constantly preaches about the evils of drink.	Mother who has an unconscious hostility toward her daughter is overprotective and hovers over her to protect her from harm, interfering with her normal growth and development.
Denial	Man reacts to news of the death of a loved one by saying, "No, I don't believe you. The doctor said he was fine."	Woman whose husband died 3 years earlier still keeps his clothes in the closet and talks about him in the present tense.
Conversion	Student is unable to take a final examination because of a terrible headache.	Man becomes blind after seeing his wife flirt with other men.
Undoing	After flirting with her male secretary, a woman brings her husband tickets to a show.	Man with rigid and moralistic beliefs and repressed sexuality is driven to wash his hands to gain composure when around attractive women.
Rationalization	Employee says, "I didn't get the raise because the boss doesn't like me."	Father who thinks his son was fathered by another man excuses his malicious treatment of the boy by saying, "He is lazy and disobedient," when that is not the case.
Identification	Five-year-old girl dresses in her mother's shoes and dress and meets her father at the door.	Young boy thinks a neighborhood pimp with money and drugs is someone to look up to.
Introjection	After his wife's death, husband has transient complaints of chest pains and difficulty breathing—the symptoms his wife had before she died.	Young child whose parents were overcritical and belittling grows up thinking that she is not any good. She has taken on her parent's evaluation of her as part of her self-image.
Suppression	Businessman who is preparing to make an important speech later in the day is told by his wife that morning that she wants a divorce. Although visibly upset, he puts the incident aside until after his speech, when he can give the matter his total concentration.	A woman who feels a lump in her breast shortly before leaving for a 3-week vacation puts the information in the back of her mind until after returning from her vacation.

to both panic disorder and obsessive-compulsive disorder (OCD) (APA, 2000; Hemmings & Stein, 2006). First-degree biological relatives of people with panic disorder are up to eight times more likely to experience panic attacks (Brown, 2003). Even for posttraumatic stress disorder (PTSD) and generalized anxiety disorder (GAD), there is evidence of inherited components (APA, 2000).

There are various **biological** theories regarding the causes of anxiety disorders. One is the GABA benzodiazepine theory. Recently discovered benzodiazepine receptors are linked to a receptor that inhibits the activity of the neurotransmitter GABA. The release of GABA slows neural transmission, which has a calming effect. Binding of the benzodiazepine medications to the benzodiazepine receptors facilitates the action of GABA (Brown, 2003). This theory proposes that abnormalities of these benzodiazepine receptors may lead to unregulated anxiety levels.

Studies of patients with PTSD suggest that the stress response of the hypothalamus-pituitary-adrenal system is abnormal in these individuals. Repeated trauma or stress not only alters the release of neurotransmitters but also changes the anatomy of the brain—neuroimaging shows that the size of the hippocampus is actually reduced (Gorman, 2000).

Learning theories provide another view. Behavioral psychologists conceptualize anxiety as a learned response that can be unlearned. Some individuals may learn to be anxious from the modeling provided by parents or peers. For example, a mother who is fearful of thunder and lightning and who hides in closets during storms may transmit her anxiety to her children, who continue to adopt her behavior even into adult life. Such individuals can unlearn this behavior by observing others who react normally to a storm.

Cognitive theorists take the position that anxiety disorders are caused by distortions in an individual's thinking and perceiving. Because individuals with such distortions believe that any mistake they make will have catastrophic results, they experience acute anxiety. Brain scans taken before and after cognitive therapy treatment support the hypothesis that learning to reframe one's thinking can literally change the chemistry and function of the brain. Cognitive-behavioral therapy seems to have the best evidence not only for effective psychotherapeutic treatment of anxiety disorders but also for more lasting results in many incidences.

CULTURAL CONSIDERATIONS

Reliable data on the incidence of anxiety disorders among cultures are sparse, but sociocultural variation in symptoms of anxiety disorders has been noted. In some cultures, individuals express anxiety through somatic symptoms, whereas in other cultures, cognitive symptoms predominate. Panic attacks in Latin Americans and Northern Europeans often involve sensations of choking, smothering, numbness, or tingling, as well as fear of dying. In other cultural groups, panic attacks involve fear of magic or witchcraft. Social phobias in Japanese and Korean cultures may relate to a belief that the individual's blushing, eye contact, or body odor is offensive to others (APA, 2000).

One of the barriers for some cultural groups seeking health care for anxiety disorders is the stigma that various cultures associate with mental disorders. For example, African Americans are much less likely to seek mental health services than the majority of the population, and Asian Americans even more so (Satcher et al., 2005).

CLINICAL PICTURE

The term *anxiety disorders* refers to a number of disorders, including panic disorders, phobias, obsessions, compulsions, and posttraumatic stress disorder, among others. Figure 8-1 presents the *DSM-IV-TR* criteria for various anxiety disorders.

Panic Disorders

The panic attack is the key feature of **panic disorders**. A **panic attack** is the sudden onset of extreme apprehension or fear, usually associated with feelings of impending doom. The feelings of terror present during a panic attack are so severe that normal function is suspended, the perceptual field is severely limited, and misinterpretation of reality may occur. Severe personality disorganization is evident. People experiencing panic attacks may believe that they are losing their minds or are having a heart attack. The attacks are often accompanied by highly uncomfortable physical symptoms, such as palpitations, chest pain, breathing difficulties, nausea, feelings of choking, chills, and hot flashes. Typically, panic attacks occur suddenly (not necessarily in response to stress), are extremely intense, last a matter of minutes, and then subside.

Panic Disorder with Agoraphobia

Panic disorder with agoraphobia is a combination of the above symptoms and agoraphobia. **Agoraphobia**, a phobic disorder, is intense, excessive anxiety or fear about being in places or situations from which escape might be difficult or embarrassing, or in which help might not be available if a panic attack occurred (APA, 2000). The feared places are avoided by the individual in an effort to control anxiety. Examples of situations that are commonly avoided by

DSM-IV-TR CRITERIA FOR ANXIETY DISORDERS

ANXIETY DISORDERS

Panic Disorder

1. Both A and B
   A. Recurrent episodes of panic attacks
   B. At least one of the attacks has been followed by 1 month (or more) of the following:
   1. Persistent concern about having additional attacks
   2. Worry about consequences ("going crazy," having a heart attack, losing control)
   3. Significant change in behavior

2. A. Absence of agoraphobia = **Panic disorder without agoraphobia**
   B. Presence of agoraphobia = **Panic disorder with agoraphobia**

Phobias

1. Irrational fear of an object or situation that persists although the person may recognize it as unreasonable

2. Types include:
   - **Agoraphobia**: Fear of being alone in open or public places where escape might be difficult; may not leave home
   - **Social phobia**: Fear of situations where one might be seen and embarrassed or criticized (e.g., speaking to authority figures, public speaking, or performing)
   - **Specific phobia**: Fear of a single object, activity, or situation (e.g., snakes, closed spaces, flying)

3. Anxiety is severe if the object, situation, or activity cannot be avoided.

Obsessive-Compulsive Disorder (OCD)

1. Either obsessions or compulsions
   A. Preoccupation with persistent intrusive thoughts, impulses, or images (obsession) **or**
   B. Repetitive behaviors or mental acts that the person feels driven to perform in order to reduce distress or prevent a dreaded event or situation (compulsion)

2. Person knows the obsessions/compulsions are excessive and unreasonable.

3. The obsession/compulsion can cause increased distress and is time-consuming.

Generalized Anxiety Disorder (GAD)

1. A. Excessive anxiety or worry more days than not over 6 months
   B. Inability to control the worrying

2. Anxiety and worry associated with three or more of the following symptoms:
   A. Restless, keyed-up
   B. Easily fatigued
   C. Difficulty concentrating, mind goes blank
   D. Irritability
   E. Muscle tension
   F. Sleep disturbance

3. Anxiety or worry or physical symptoms cause significant impairment in social, occupational, or other areas of important functioning.

Figure 8-1 ■ Diagnostic criteria for anxiety disorders. (Adapted from American Psychiatric Association. [2000]. *Diagnostic and statistical manual of mental disorders* [4th ed., text rev.]. Washington, DC: Author.)

patients with agoraphobia are being alone outside; being alone at home; traveling in a car, bus, or airplane; being on a bridge; and riding in an elevator. Avoidance behaviors can be debilitating and life constricting. Consider the effect on a father whose avoidance renders him unable to leave home and who thus cannot see his child's high school graduation, or the businesswoman whose avoidance of flying prevents her from attending distant business conferences. See Figure 8-1 for the *DSM-IV-TR* criteria for panic disorders.

Phobias

A **phobia** is a persistent, irrational fear of a specific object, activity, or situation that leads to a desire for avoidance, or

actual avoidance, of the object, activity, or situation (APA, 2000).

Specific phobias are characterized by the experience of high levels of anxiety or fear in response to specific objects or situations, such as dogs, spiders, heights, storms, water, blood, closed spaces, tunnels, and bridges (APA, 2000). Specific phobias are common and usually do not cause much difficulty because people can contrive to avoid the feared object. Clinical names for common phobias are given in Table 8-5.

Social phobia, or **social anxiety disorder,** is characterized by severe anxiety or fear provoked by exposure to a social situation or a performance situation (e.g., fear of saying something that sounds foolish in public, not being

TABLE 8-5	Clinical Names for Common Phobias
Clinical Name	**Feared Object or Situation**
Acrophobia	Heights
Agoraphobia	Open spaces
Astraphobia	Electrical storms
Claustrophobia	Closed spaces
Glossophobia	Talking
Hematophobia	Blood
Hydrophobia	Water
Monophobia	Being alone
Mysophobia	Germs or dirt
Nyctophobia	Darkness
Pyrophobia	Fire
Xenophobia	Strangers
Zoophobia	Animals

able to answer questions in a classroom, eating in public, and performing on stage). Fear of public speaking is the most common social phobia.

Agoraphobia, described above, can be the most limiting and debilitating of all of the phobias. In its most extreme form, patients may simply refuse to leave their house, putting great strain on family and friends and result in problems within the marriage. Characteristically, phobic individuals experience overwhelming and crippling anxiety when they are faced with the object or situation provoking the phobia. Phobic people go to great lengths to avoid the feared object or situation. A phobic person may not be able to think about or visualize the object or situation without becoming severely anxious. The life of a phobic person becomes more restricted as activities are given up so that the phobic object can be avoided. All too frequently, complications ensue when people try to decrease anxiety through self-medication with alcohol or drugs. See Figure 8-1 for the *DSM-IV-TR* criteria for phobias.

Obsessive-Compulsive Disorder (OCD)

Obsessions are defined as thoughts, impulses, or images that persist and recur so that they cannot be dismissed from the mind. Obsessions often seem senseless (ego-dystonic) to the individual who experiences them, although they still cause the individual to experience severe anxiety. **Ego-dystonic** refers to those symptoms that an individual experiences that are unacceptable, objectionable, and "alien" to themselves.

Compulsions are ritualistic behaviors that an individual feels driven to perform in an attempt to reduce anxiety. Performing the compulsive act temporarily reduces high levels of anxiety. Primary gain is achieved by compulsive rituals, but because the relief is only temporary, the compulsive act must be repeated again and again.

Although obsessions and compulsions can exist independently of each other, they most often occur together as in **obsessive-compulsive disorder (OCD)**. OCD behavior exists along a continuum. "Normal" individuals may experience mildly obsessive-compulsive behavior. Nearly everyone has had the experience of having a tune run persistently through the mind, despite attempts to push it away. Many people have had nagging doubts as to whether a door is locked or the stove is turned off. These doubts require the person to go back to check the door or stove. Minor compulsions, such as touching a lucky charm, knocking on wood, and making the sign of the cross upon hearing disturbing news, are not harmful to the individual. Mild compulsions (timeliness, orderliness, and reliability) are valued traits in selective contexts in the U.S. society.

At the pathological end of the continuum are obsessive-compulsive symptoms that typically involve issues of sexuality, violence, contamination, illness, or death. These obsessions or compulsions cause marked distress to the individual. People often feel humiliation and shame regarding these behaviors. The rituals are time consuming and interfere with normal routine, social activities, and relationships with others. Severe OCD consumes so much of the individual's mental processes that the performance of cognitive tasks may be impaired. See Figure 8-1 for the *DSM-IV-TR* criteria for OCD.

evolve

For a comprehensive case study and associated care plans for a patient with OCD, visit the Evolve website at http://evolve.elsevier.com/Varcarolis/essentials.

Generalized Anxiety Disorder

Generalized anxiety disorder (GAD) is characterized by excessive anxiety or worry about numerous things that lasts for 6 months or longer (APA, 2000). The individual with GAD also displays many of the following symptoms: restlessness, fatigue, poor concentration, irritability, tension, and sleep disturbance.

The individual's worry is out of proportion with the true effect of the event or situation about which the individual is worried. Examples of worries typical in GAD are inadequacy in interpersonal relationships, job responsibilities, finances, health of family members, household chores, and lateness for appointments. Sleep disturbance is common because the individual worries about the day's events and real or imagined mistakes, reviews past problems, and anticipates future difficulties. Decision making is difficult because of poor concentration and dread of making a mistake. See Figure 8-1 for the *DSM-IV-TR* criteria for GAD.

Posttraumatic Stress Disorder

Posttraumatic stress disorder (PTSD) is characterized by repeated re-experiencing of a highly traumatic event that involved actual or threatened death or serious injury to self or others, to which the individual responded with intense fear, helplessness, or horror (APA, 2000). PTSD may occur after any traumatic event that is outside the range of usual experience. Examples are military combat; detention as a prisoner of war; natural disasters such as floods, tornados, earthquakes, tsunamis; human disasters such as plane and train accidents; crime-related events such as bombing, assault, mugging, rape, incest, and being taken hostage; or diagnosis of a life-threatening illness.

PTSD symptoms often begin within 3 months after the trauma, but a delay of months or years is not uncommon. After 2 or 3 months, survivors benefit from receiving treatments for chronic PSTD. After a year, if severe symptoms are not treated, they become chronic and natural recovery is unlikely (Foa, 2005). The major features of PTSD are the following:

- Persistent re-experiencing of the trauma through recurrent intrusive recollections of the event, dreams, and flashbacks (**flashbacks** are dissociative experiences during which the event is relived and the person behaves as though he or she is experiencing the event at that time)
- Persistent avoidance of stimuli associated with the trauma, which results in the individual's avoiding talking about the event or avoiding activities, people, or places that arouse memories of the trauma
- After the trauma, experience of persistent numbing of general responsiveness, as evidenced by the individual's feeling detached or estranged from others, feeling empty inside, or feeling turned off to others
- After the trauma, experiencing of persistent symptoms of increased arousal, as evidenced by irritability, difficulty sleeping, difficulty concentrating, hypervigilance, or exaggerated startle response

Difficulty with interpersonal, social, or occupational relationships nearly always accompanies PTSD, and trust is a common issue of concern. Child and spousal abuse

may be associated with hypervigilance and irritability. Chemical abuse (alcohol or other mind-altering substances) may begin as an attempt to self-medicate to relieve anxiety.

It is important for health care workers to realize that exposure to stimuli reminiscent of those associated with the original trauma may cause an exacerbation of the trauma. For example, one nurse therapist observed that the attack on the World Trade Center on September 11, 2001, caused an exacerbation of PTSD symptoms in veterans of World War II (Kaiman, 2003). The incidence of PTSD in Afghanistan and Iraq war veterans is as high or higher than 20% (Ritchie & Cavazos, 2005).

evolve

For a comprehensive case study of a patient experiencing posttraumatic stress disorder, visit the Evolve website at http://evolve.elsevier.com/Varcarolis/essentials.

Acute Stress Disorder

Acute stress disorder occurs within 1 month after exposure to a highly traumatic event, such as those listed in the section on PTSD. To be diagnosed with acute stress disorder, the individual must display at least three dissociative symptoms either during or after the traumatic event: a subjective sense of numbing, detachment, or absence of emotional responsiveness; a reduction in awareness of surroundings; derealization (a sense of unreality related to the environment); depersonalization (experience of a sense of unreality or self-estrangement); or dissociative amnesia (loss of memory) (APA, 2000). By definition, acute stress disorder resolves within 4 weeks. Critical incident stress debriefing is often valuable in ameliorating symptoms and helping the individual in the resolution process.

Anxiety Caused by Medical Conditions

In anxiety due to medical conditions, the individual's symptoms of anxiety are a direct physiological result of a medical condition, such as hyperthyroidism, pulmonary embolism, or cardiac dysrhythmias (APA, 2000). To determine whether the anxiety symptoms are caused by a medical condition, a careful and comprehensive assessment of multiple factors is necessary. Once again, evidence must be present in the history, physical examination, or laboratory findings to diagnose the medical condition.

TABLE 8-6	Defenses Used in Anxiety Disorders

Phenomenon	Defense	Purpose	Example
Phobia	Displacement	In phobias, anxiety is reduced when strong feelings about the original object are directed at a less-threatening object and that object is avoided.	Patient has abnormal fear of cats. In therapy, it is discovered that the patient unconsciously links cats to a feared and cruel mother.
Compulsion	Undoing	Performing a symbolic act cancels out an unacceptable act or idea.	Patient performs symbolic rituals (e.g., handwashing, cleaning, and checking). Handwashing removes guilt. Cleaning removes dirty thoughts. Checking protects against hostile thoughts.
Obsession	Reaction formation	Anxiety-producing unacceptable thoughts or feelings are kept out of awareness by the opposite feeling or idea.	Patient with strong aggressive feelings toward husband repeatedly thinks the opposite ("I love him with all my heart") to keep hostile feelings out of awareness.
	Intellectualization	Excessive use of reasoning, logic, or words prevents the person from experiencing associated feelings.	Person talks in detail about parents' funeral but is unable to feel the associated pain of loss.
Posttraumatic stress	Isolation disorder	Facts associated with anxiety-laden events remain conscious, but associated painful feelings are separated from the experience.	Patient describes feeling "numb and empty inside."
	Repression		Patient is unable to trust authority figures at work after taking orders from commanding officer to kill civilians while in combat.

Application of the Nursing Process

ASSESSMENT
Symptoms of Anxiety

People with anxiety disorders rarely need hospitalization unless they are suicidal or have compulsions causing injury (cutting self, banging a body part). Therefore, most patients prone to anxiety are encountered in a variety of community settings. A common example of an acute anxiety episode occurs when an individual who is taken to an emergency department to rule out a heart attack is found to be experiencing a panic attack. Therefore one of the first things that may need to be determined is whether the anxiety is from a secondary source (medical condition or substances) or a primary source, as in an anxiety disorder.

Defenses Used in Anxiety Disorders

People use a variety of ego defenses and behaviors to lessen the uncomfortable levels of anxiety. Psychodynamic theo-

rists believe that people who suffer from anxiety disorders employ specific defenses (Table 8-6). A comprehensive and sophisticated assessment is the Hamilton Rating Scale for Anxiety. *A word of caution:* The Hamilton scale highlights important areas in the assessment of anxiety. Because many answers are subjective, experienced clinicians use this tool as a guide when planning care and draw on their knowledge of their patients.

Assessment Guidelines

Anxiety Disorders

1. Ensure that a sound physical and neurological examination is performed to help determine whether the anxiety is primary or secondary to another psychiatric disorder, a medical condition, or substance use.
2. Assess for potential for self-harm and suicide because it is known that people suffering from high levels of intractable anxiety may become desperate and attempt suicide.
3. Perform a psychosocial assessment. Always ask the person, "What has happened recently that might be increasing your anxiety?" The patient may identify a

problem that should be addressed through counseling or therapy (stressful marriage, recent loss, stressful job or school situation).

4. Assess cultural beliefs and background. Differences in culture can affect how anxiety is manifested.

DIAGNOSIS

NANDA International (NANDA-I, 2007) provides many nursing diagnoses that can be considered for patients experiencing anxiety and anxiety disorders. The "related-to" component will vary with the individual patient. Table 8-7 identifies potential nursing diagnoses for the anxious patient. Included are the signs and symptoms that might be found on assessment that support the diagnoses.

OUTCOMES IDENTIFICATION

The Nursing Outcomes Classification (NOC) identifies a number of desired outcomes for patients with anxiety or anxiety-related disorders (Moorhead et al., 2008). *Psychiatric–Mental Health Nursing: Scope and Standards of Practice* (ANA, 2007) emphasizes that outcomes should, among other considerations:

- Reflect patient values and ethical and environmental situations
- Are culturally appropriate
- Be documented as measurable goals
- Include a time estimate of expected outcomes.

Table 8-8 identifies short- and long-term outcomes using the criteria from *Psychiatric–Mental Health Nursing: Scope and Standards of Practice* (ANA, 2007).

PLANNING

Anxiety disorders are encountered in numerous settings. Nurses care for people with concurrent anxiety disorders in medical-surgical units and in outpatient settings, such as homes, day programs, and clinics. Usually patients with anxiety disorders do not require admission to inpatient

TABLE 8-7	Potential Nursing Diagnoses for the Anxious Patient
Signs and Symptoms	**Nursing Diagnoses**
• Concern that a panic attack will occur • Exposure to phobic object or situation • Presence of obsessive thoughts • Recurrent memories of traumatic event • Fear of panic attacks	*Anxiety (moderate, severe, panic)* *Fear*
• High levels of anxiety that interfere with the ability to work, disrupt relationships, and change ability to interact with others • Avoidance behaviors (phobia, agoraphobia) • Hypervigilance after a traumatic event • Inordinate time taken for obsession and compulsions	*Ineffective coping* *Deficient diversional activity* *Social isolation* *Ineffective role performance*
• Difficulty with concentration • Preoccupation with obsessive thoughts • Disorganization associated with exposure to phobic object • Intrusive thoughts and memories of traumatic event • Excessive use of reason and logic associated with overcautiousness and fear of making a mistake	*Disturbed thought processes* *Post-trauma syndrome*
• Inability to go to sleep related to intrusive thoughts, worrying, replaying of a traumatic event, hypervigilance, fear	*Sleep deprivation* *Fatigue*
• Feelings of hopelessness, inability to control one's life, low self-esteem related to inability to have some control in one's life	*Hopelessness* *Chronic low self-esteem* *Spiritual distress*
• Inability to perform self-care related to rituals	*Self-care deficit*
• Skin excoriation related to rituals of excessive washing or excessive picking at the skin	*Impaired skin integrity*
• Inability to eat because of constant ritual performance • Feeling of anxiety or excessive worrying that overrides appetite and need to eat	*Imbalanced nutrition: less than body requirements*
• Excessive overeating to appease intense worrying or high anxiety levels	*Imbalanced nutrition: more than body requirements*

TABLE 8-8	Short- and Long-Term Outcomes for Specific Anxiety Disorders
Anxiety Disorder	**Short- or Long-Term Outcomes**
Phobia	Patients will: • Develop skills at reframing anxiety-provoking situation (date) • Work with nurse to desensitize self to feared object or situation (date) • Demonstrate one new relaxation skill that works well for them (date)
Generalized anxiety disorder	Patients will: • State increased ability to make decisions and problem solve • Demonstrate ability to perform usual tasks even though still moderately anxious by (date) • Demonstrate one cognitive or behavioral coping skill that helps reduce anxious feelings by (date)
Obsessive-compulsive disorder	Patients will: • Demonstrate techniques that can distract and distance self from thoughts that are anxiety producing by (date) • Decrease time spent in ritualistic behaviors • Demonstrate increased amount of time spent with family, friends, and on pleasurable activities • State they have more control over intrusive thoughts and rituals by (date)
Posttraumatic stress disorder	Patients will: • Attend support group at least once a week by (date) • Increase social support by one each month with aid of nurse/counselor • Report increase in restful sleep periods • Report decrease in nightmares or flashbacks • Demonstrate at least one new anxiety-reduction technique (cognitive or behavioral) that work well for them

psychiatric units. Therefore, planning for care usually involves selecting interventions that can be implemented in a community setting.

Whenever possible, the patient should be encouraged to participate actively in planning. By sharing decision making with the patient, the nurse increases the likelihood of positive outcomes. Shared planning is especially appropriate for a patient with mild or moderate anxiety. When the patient is experiencing severe levels of anxiety, he or she may be unable to participate in planning, which requires the nurse to take a more directive role.

IMPLEMENTATION

The nurse follows the *Psychiatric–Mental Health Nursing: Scope and Standards of Practice* (ANA, 2007) when intervening with patients. Whenever possible, interventions should be based on the best evidence available. Overall guidelines for basic nursing interventions are as follows:

1. Identify community resources that can offer specialized treatment that is proven to be highly effective for people with a variety of anxiety disorders.
2. Identify community support groups for people with specific anxiety disorders and their families.

3. Use therapeutic communications, milieu therapy, promotion of self-care activities, and psychobiological and health teaching and health promotion as appropriate.

Communication Guidelines

Psychiatric mental health nurses use therapeutic communication skills to assist patients with anxiety disorders to reduce anxiety, enhance coping and communication skills, and intervene in crises. When patients request or prefer to use integrative therapies, the nurse performs assessment and teaching as appropriate.

Refer to the "Applying the Art" on p 144 for an example of a nurse using therapeutic communication with a patient experiencing obsessive-compulsive disorder.

Health Teaching and Health Promotion

Health teaching is a significant nursing intervention for patients with anxiety disorders. Patients may conceal symptoms for years before seeking treatment and often come to the attention of the nurse due to a co-occurring problem. For example, one study found that only 60% of people who

APPLYING THE ART   A Person with Obsessive-Compulsive Disorder

SCENARIO: Eight-year-old Tommy came to see the school nurse I worked with during my community nursing leadership rotation. His productive cough and a temperature of 101.2° F prompted a call to his mother. While we waited, Tommy looked worried. "Germs make people sick," he said. I nodded. "But how did I get sick when [holding out his red dry hands] I wash my hands lots of times just like Mommy does?" Tommy took a tissue for a cough. "Maybe I got sick because I forgot to use a tissue to hold the doorknob like Mommy does." When Mrs. Jansen arrived, I introduced myself and we talked privately while Tommy's make-up assignments were being gathered.

THERAPEUTIC GOAL: By the end of this interaction, Tommy will acknowledge needing help to manage her anxiety and ritualistic washing.

Student-Patient Interaction	Thoughts, Communication Techniques, and Mental Health Nursing Concepts
Mrs. Jansen: "I'm going to get Tommy to his pediatrician this afternoon. He didn't carry a fever this morning, though he did act a little grouchy." *Student's feelings: Poor little guy—I wonder about that.*	Tommy looked relieved to see his mother. I don't observe any signs of abuse or neglect. *He's already a worrier at 8 years old. Sounds like he's afraid that getting sick is his fault.*
Student: "You're concerned about him." *She nods.* "Mrs. Jansen, Tommy worried that he got sick from germs, despite, as he said, 'washing my hands lots of times like Mommy.' " *Student's feelings: I just met this person yet here I am jumping in, which means I might make a mistake. I guess I'd rather make a mistake by trying to help than by saying nothing. Guess I'm anxious.*	I *give information* about Tommy. From looking at Tommy's hands and from what he is saying, this could be a problem. I am concerned that his mother has some obsessive-compulsive traits.
Mrs. Jansen: *Looking stricken.* "My poor baby! I didn't want my problem to affect him."	
Student: "Your problem?"	I use *restatement.* Because Mrs. Jansen is able to identify a problem, she may be showing some *insight.*
Mrs. Jansen: "Until now I've been convincing myself that I just wanted my house clean." *Student's feelings: How could she not see that her behavior represents more than just keeping her house clean?*	She uses *denial* and *rationalization.*
Student: "How do you explain all the handwashing and using tissues to not touch doorknobs?" *Student's feelings: I didn't mean to sound like I'm blaming her. This isn't about a logical decision. It's about a disorder.*	Although I asked an *open* question, this came out like I was being critical of her, like I'm *challenging* or even accusing her.
Mrs. Jansen: *Looks down. Silent.*	
Student: "I'm sorry I pushed you for an explanation. This must be so difficult."	I work on restoring trust by attempt to *translate into feelings.* *I hope I did the right thing by saying I'm sorry.*

APPLYING THE ART   A Person with Obsessive-Compulsive Disorder—cont'd

Student-Patient Interaction	Thoughts, Communication Techniques, and Mental Health Nursing Concepts
Mrs. Jansen: *Nods, then makes brief eye contact.* "Since Tommy's dad went to Iraq, I worry all the time. I know I sound crazy, but when I try to stop washing my house, my hands, the doorknobs, I see Tom, Sr. getting blown up by a suicide bomber." ***Student's feelings:*** *I would worry too with my loved one in Iraq. She worries about "sounding crazy." The stigma of mental illness interferes with people feeling okay about seeking treatment. I feel concern toward her.*	Worrying "all the time" sounds like *generalized anxiety disorder*. The obsessive worry that gets relieved by the washing rituals sounds like *OCD*. Both disorders cause such distress. Her *self-esteem* sounds low, especially about her *mothering role*.
Student. "You feel kind of scared so often and so alone." ***Student's feelings:*** *I want to always show nonjudgmental acceptance. I show empathy when I reflect underlying feelings. I feel sad at all she has to carry. She obviously cares about her son.*	I attempt to *translate* into feelings.
Mrs. Jansen: *Tears in her eyes.* "While I wash things, my mind rests a minute. Then I look at my bloody raw hands! Now, I've worried Tommy. Poor kid deserves better than me."	
Student: "Mrs. Jansen, sounds like you're feeling really down on yourself."	I assess about her *self-esteem*. Low self-esteem, *depressed mood*, and *suicide* ideation go hand-in-hand. I *validate* to see if I've understood her meaning.
Mrs. Jansen: "Sometimes I feel panicky . . . like giving up."	
Student: "Like giving up . . . as in suicide?" ***Student's feelings:*** *I feel awkward asking about suicide, but I would rather feel funny asking, than overlook a suicide cue.*	*Asking* about suicide does not plant the idea of suicide.
Mrs. Jansen: "No, never. I wouldn't do that to Tommy, Jr. The only time I can resist cleaning for a while is when Tommy needs me to help him with something at home or when I watch him play soccer." ***Student's feelings:*** *I'm so relieved that she answered "no" immediately even if the reason is Tommy rather than self.*	She focuses so many of her responses in terms of her son. Mrs. Jansen recognizes that resisting the compulsion is healthy behavior. I *validate* the meaning.
Student. "So sometimes you are able to delay the compulsive washing behavior. How do you feel, then?" ***Student's feelings:*** *I called the behavior "compulsive." I hope that naming the behavior with the word "compulsive" does not threaten her.*	I *give support* by saying, "you are able to. . . ." I then ask an *open question*.
Mrs. Jansen: "Proud of myself, but also scared for Tom, Sr. You said 'compulsive.' I've heard of that on Dr. Phil."	Mrs. Jansen identified hearing about *OCD* on television. Maybe that helped her readiness to talk about her ritualistic behaviors.
Student: *Nods.* "Obsessive-compulsive disorder responds to medication and therapy. You don't have to do this all by yourself." ***Student's feelings:*** *I feel hopeful that Mrs. Jansen really will seek treatment.*	I *validate* the meaning and *assess* her feelings. I do a little teaching as I give information that OCD responds to treatment.
Mrs. Jansen: *Looking down at her red raw hands.* "I'm ready for Tommy's sake." *I watch and wait.* "And for myself." *As Tommy rejoins us, Mrs. Jansen asks the school nurse for the community mental health number.*	

experience panic attacks seek medical treatment (Katerndahl, 2002, p. 464). Teaching about the specific disorder and available effective treatments is a major step to improving the quality of life of these patients.

In the community or hospital setting, the nurse teaches the patient about signs and symptoms of the disorder; theory regarding causes or risk factors; risk of co-occurrence with other disorders, especially substance abuse; medication use; use of relaxation exercises; and availability of specialized treatment such as cognitive-behavioral therapy.

Patients with anxiety disorders are usually able to meet their own basic physical needs. Sleep, however, can be a real problem. Patients with GAD, PTSD, and acute stress disorder often experience sleep disturbance and nightmares. Teaching patients ways to promote sleep (e.g., warm bath, warm milk, relaxing music) and monitoring sleep through a journal are useful interventions.

Milieu Therapy

As mentioned, most patients with anxiety disorders can be treated successfully as outpatients. Hospital admission is necessary only if severe anxiety or symptoms that interfere with the individual's health are present, or if the individual is suicidal. If or when hospitalization is necessary, the following features of the therapeutic milieu can be especially helpful to the patient:

- Structuring the daily routine to offer physical safety and predictability, thus reducing anxiety over the unknown
- Providing daily activities to promote sharing and cooperation
- Providing therapeutic interactions, including one-on-one nursing care and behavior contracts
- Including the patient in decisions about his or her own care

Psychotherapy

Among the most useful therapies are the cognitive-behavioral therapies (CBT), which provide education, address cognitive distortions, and provide behavioral approaches in an attempt to reduce symptoms and increase involvement with others and the environment. Therapists teach people to restructure their thinking and examine their assumptions, problems or concerns so that problems or concerns seem more amenable to change, and hold less negative emotional impact. Teaching people to successfully redefine their fears and look at themselves in a new and more positive way can make chemical changes in the brain similar to those of medications.

CBT essentially challenges core beliefs that are causing a person distress. Examples of such beliefs include (Sadock & Sadock, 2007):

- Panic attacks: Catastrophic misinterpretations of bodily and mental disturbances.
- Phobias: Danger in specific avoidable situations.
- Obsessive compulsive disorders: Repeated warnings or doubting about safety and repetitive acts to ward off threats.
- Anxiety disorders: Fear of physical or psychological threats.

Pharmacological, Biological, and Integrative Therapies

Anxiety disorders are chronic and incurable conditions, but many helpful treatments are available. Several classes of medications have been found to be effective in the treatment of anxiety disorders. Best evidence research points to the fact that when the serotonergic system is modulated (SSRIs, CBT) by itself, or with the noradrenergic system (SNRIs), anxiety symptoms are alleviated (Masand, 2005), much more than with traditional antidepressants. The following medications have been shown to be helpful (Satcher et al., 2005):

1. Benzodiazepines: *short-term treatment only*; not for use if the patient has substance dependence problems
2. Buspirone: management of anxiety disorders or short-term relief of anxiety symptoms
3. SSRIs: first-line treatment for all anxiety disorders
4. SNRIs: venlafaxine, milnacipran, and duloxetine. Only venlafaxine is currently approved for panic disorder (PD), generalized anxiety disorder (GAD), and seasonal affective disorder (SAD).
5. Tricyclic antidepressants: second- or third-line use in people with PD, GAD, and SAD. Clomipramine is effective in obsessive-compulsive disorder (OCD).

Refer to Table 8-9 for names and dosages of common medications and Table 8-10 for medications used to treat specific anxiety disorders.

Antidepressants

As stated, selective serotonin reuptake inhibitors (SSRIs) are the first-line treatment for anxiety disorders. They are preferable to the tricyclic antidepressants (TCAs) because they have more rapid onset of action, fewer problematic side effects, and are more effective. Monoamine oxidase inhibitors (MAOIs) are reserved for treatment-resistant conditions because of the risk of life-threatening hypertensive crisis if the patient does not follow dietary restrictions. (Patients cannot eat foods containing tyramine and must be given specific dietary instructions.) Venlafaxine (Effexor) and duloxetine (Cymbalta) are serotonin-norepinephrine

TABLE 8-9   Medications Commonly Used in the Treatment of Anxiety Disorders

Generic Name	Trade Name	Usual Daily Dose (mg/Day)	Comments
Benzodiazepines			
Alprazolam*	Xanax	0.5-6	Anxiolytic effects result from depressing
	Xanax XR	3-6	neurotransmission in the limbic system and cortical
Diazepam	Valium	4-40	areas. Useful for short-term treatment of anxiety;
Lorazepam*	Ativan	2-6	dependence and tolerance develop. These drugs are
Oxazepam	Serax	30-120	NOT indicated as a primary treatment for OCD
Chlordiazepoxide	Librium	15-100	or PTSD
Clorazepate	Tranxene	15-60	
Buspirone			
Buspirone hydrochloride†	BuSpar	30-60	Alleviates anxiety, but works best before benzodiazepines have been tried. Less sedating than benzodiazepines. Does not appear to produce physical or psychological dependence. Requires 3 or more weeks to be effective.
Selective Serotonin Reuptake Inhibitors (SSRIs)			
First Line			
Citalopram	Celexa	20-60	
Escitalopram	Lexapro	10-20	Escitalopram not useful with SAD or PD.
Fluoxetine	Prozac	20-80	
Fluvoxamine	Luvox	100-300	
Paroxetine	Paxil	20-50	
Sertraline	Zoloft	50-200	
Dual-Action Reuptake Inhibitors (Serotonin & Norepinephrine) (SNRIs)			
First Line			
Duloxetine	Cymbalta	40-60	Acts within 1 to 2 weeks.
Venlafaxine	Effexor	75-225	
Tricyclic Antidepressants (TCAs)			
Second or Third Line			
Amitriptyline	Elavil	100-200	Clomipramine effective with OCD, PD, GAD,
Clomipramine	Anafranil	100-200	SAD; may also respond to Surmontil
Desipramine	Norpramin	100-200	
Doxepin	Sinequan	75-150	
Imipramine	Tofranil	75-150	
Maprotiline	Ludiomil	100-150	
Nortriptyline	Pamelor	75-150	
Trimipramine	Surmontil	50-150	
Amoxapine	Asendin	200-300	
β-Blockers			
Propranolol	Inderal	20-160	Used to relieve physical symptoms of anxiety, as in
Atenolol	Tenormin	25-100	performance anxiety (stage fright). Act by attaching to sensors that direct arousal messages.

GAD, Generalized anxiety disorder; *OCD*, obsessive-compulsive disorder; *PTSD*, posttraumatic stress disorder; *PD*, panic disorder; *SAD*, seasonal affective disorder.

*Most commonly used benzodiazepines for treating chronic or unpredictable anxiety syndromes.

†Useful as a first-line treatment in GAD.

Adapted from Varcarolis, E.M. (2006). *Manual of psychiatric mental health nursing care plans* (3rd ed.). St. Louis: Saunders, p. 151.

Benzodiazepines dosage updated from Lehne, R.A. (2007). *Pharmacology for nursing care* (6th ed.). St. Louis, MO: Saunders.

TABLE 8-10	Medications and Psychotherapy for Specific Anxiety Disorders	
Disorder	**Pharmacotherapy**	**Psychotherapy**
Generalized anxiety disorder	Selective serotonin reuptake inhibitors (SSRIs) Buspirone (BuSpar) Serotonin-norepinephrine reuptake inhibitor (SNRI): venlafaxine XR Valproic acid (Depakene) Tricyclic antidepressants (TCAs)	Cognitive-behavioral therapy
Obsessive-compulsive disorder	SSRIs, especially fluvoxamine (Luvox) TCAs, especially clomipramine (Anafranil)	Behavioral therapy
Panic disorder	SSRI: venlafaxine TCAs Monoamine oxidase inhibitors (MAOIs) β-Blockers Valproic acid (Depakote)	Cognitive-behavioral therapy
Posttraumatic stress disorder	SSRIs TCAs Benzodiazepines SNRIs MAOIs β-Blockers Carbamazepine (Tegretol)	Cognitive-behavioral therapy Family therapy Group therapy with survivors
Social phobia or social anxiety disorder	SSRIs Benzodiazepines Buspirone β-Blockers Gabapentin (Neurontin)	Cognitive-behavioral therapy

reuptake inhibitors (SNRIs) used to treat anxiety disorders.

Antidepressants have the secondary benefit of treating comorbid depressive disorders in patients. Because anxiety and depression frequently occur together, these agents may bring welcome benefits to patients. However, there are three notes of caution. First, when treatment is started, low doses of SSRIs must be used because of the activating effect, which temporarily increases anxiety symptoms. Second, in patients with co-occurring bipolar disorder, use of an antidepressant may cause a manic episode, which requires the addition of mood stabilizers or even antipsychotic agents. Third, use of MAOIs is contraindicated in patients with comorbid substance abuse because of the risk of hypertensive crisis with use of stimulant drugs.

Anxiolytics

Anxiolytic drugs (also called *antianxiety drugs*) are often used to treat the somatic and psychological symptoms of anxiety disorders. When moderate or severe anxiety is reduced, patients are better able to participate in treatment directed at their underlying problems. Benzodiazepines are most commonly used because they have a quick onset of action. Because of the potential for dependence, however, these medications should ideally be used for *short periods only* until other medications or treatments reduce symptoms. It is important for the nurse to monitor for side effects of the benzodiazepines, including sedation, ataxia, and decreased cognitive function. Benzodiazepines are not recommended for patients with a known substance use problem and should not be given to women during pregnancy or breast feeding. Box 8-1 lists important information on patient and family medication teaching.

Buspirone (BuSpar) is an alternative anxiolytic medication that does not cause dependence, but 2 to 4 weeks are required for it to reach full effects. Its usefulness in the anxiety disorders is probably limited to the treatment of GAD (Stein, 2005).

Other Classes of Medication

Other classes of medication sometimes used to treat anxiety disorders include β-blockers, antihistamines, and anticon-

BOX 8-1

Patient and Family Medication Teaching: Anxiolytic Drugs

1. Caution the patient
   - Not to increase dose or frequency of ingestion without prior approval of therapist.
   - That these medications reduce the ability to handle mechanical equipment (e.g., cars, saws, and other machinery).
   - Not to drink alcoholic beverages or take other antianxiety drugs because depressant effects of both would be potentiated.
   - To avoid drinking beverages containing caffeine because they decrease the desired effects of the drug.
2. Recommend that the patient taking benzodiazepines avoid becoming pregnant because these drugs increase the risk of congenital anomalies.
3. Advise the patient not to breast-feed because these drugs are excreted in the milk and would have adverse effects on the infant.
4. Teach a patient who is taking monoamine oxidase inhibitors about the details of a tyramine-restricted diet.
5. Teach the patient that:
   - Cessation of benzodiazepine use after 3 to 4 months of daily use may cause withdrawal symptoms such as insomnia, irritability, nervousness, dry mouth, tremors, convulsions, and confusion
   - Medications should be taken with, or shortly after, meals or snacks to reduce gastrointestinal discomfort
   - Drug interactions can occur: antacids may delay absorption; cimetidine interferes with metabolism of benzodiazepines, causing increased sedation; central nervous system depressants, such as alcohol and barbiturates, cause increased sedation; serum phenytoin concentration may build up because of decreased metabolism

vulsants. These agents are often added if the first course of treatment is ineffective. The β-blockers have been used to treat panic disorder and SAD. Anticonvulsants have shown some benefit in management of GAD, SAD, and comorbid depression with SAD or panic disorder. See Box 8-1 for information on patient and family medication teaching.

Complementary Interventions

Among the "natural" substances purported to relieve anxiety are kava kava, valerian root, gotu kola, and St. John's wort. Although randomized control studies are under way, available scientific evidence for any of these treating anxiety disorders is sparse (Stein, 2005).

Herbs and dietary supplements are not subject to the same rigorous testing as prescription medications. Also, herbs and dietary supplements are not required to be uniform, and there is no guarantee of bioequivalence of the active compound across preparations (McEnany, 2000). Problems that can occur with the use of psychotropic herbs include toxic side effects and herb-drug interactions.

EVALUATION

Identified outcomes serve as the basis for evaluation. In general, evaluation of outcomes for patients with anxiety disorders deals with questions such as the following:

- Is the patient experiencing a reduced level of anxiety? Describe level of anxiety supported by the patient's present symptoms.
- Does the patient recognize symptoms as anxiety related? What symptoms does he or she experience when anxiety levels are rising?
- Does the patient continue to display obsessions, compulsions, phobias, worrying, or other symptoms of anxiety disorders? If so, ask the patient to identify the number in increase or decrease during the day/night/situation. How does the patient describe change in the level of intensity?
- What newly learned behaviors does the patient use to help manage anxiety?
- Can the patient adequately perform self-care activities? Describe changes in ability to manage health care abilities.
- Can the patient maintain satisfying interpersonal relations? How does the patient describe close relationships now as compared with initially?
- Can the patient assume usual roles? Describe the ways certain role performances have improved, and identify roles performance that still require interventions.
- Is the patient compliant with medication?

KEY POINTS TO REMEMBER

- The basic emotion of anxiety is differentiated from fear in that anxiety has an unknown or unrecognized source, whereas fear is a reaction to a specific threat.
- Anxiety can be normal, acute, or chronic, as well as adaptive or maladaptive.
- Peplau operationally defined four levels of anxiety. The patient's perceptual field, ability to learn, and physical and other characteristics are different at each level (see Table 8-1).
- Effective psychosocial interventions are different for people experiencing mild to moderate levels of anxiety and individuals experiencing severe to panic levels of anxiety. Effective psychosocial nursing approaches are suggested in Tables 8-2 and 8-3.
- Defenses against anxiety can be adaptive or maladaptive. Defenses are presented in a hierarchy from healthy to intermediate to immature. Table 8-4 provides examples of adaptive and maladaptive uses of many of the more common defense mechanisms.

- Anxiety disorders are the most common psychiatric disorders in the United States and frequently co-occur with depression or substance abuse.
- Research has identified genetic and biological factors in the etiology of anxiety disorders.
- Psychological theories and cultural influences also are pertinent to the understanding of anxiety disorders.
- Patients with anxiety disorders suffer from panic attacks, irrational fears, excessive worrying, uncontrollable rituals, or severe reactions to stress.
- People with anxiety disorders are often too embarrassed or ashamed to seek psychiatric help. Instead, they go to primary care providers with multiple somatic complaints.
- Psychiatric treatment is effective for anxiety disorders, especially cognitive-behavioral therapy (CBT).
- Interventions include counseling, milieu therapy, promotion of self-care activities, psychobiological intervention, and health teaching.

CRITICAL THINKING

1. Ms. Smith, a patient with OCD, washes her hands until they are cracked and bleeding. Your nursing goal is to promote healing of her hands. What interventions will you plan?
2. This is Mr. Olivetti's third emergency department visit in a week. He is experiencing severe anxiety accompanied by many physical symptoms. He clings to you, desperately crying, "Help me! Help me! Don't let me die!" Diagnostic tests have ruled out a physical disorder. The patient outcome has been identified as "Patient anxiety level will be reduced

to moderate/mild within 1 hour." What interventions should you use?
3. Mrs. Zeamans is a patient with GAD. She has a history of substance abuse and is a recovering alcoholic. During a clinic visit, she tells you she plans to ask the psychiatrist to prescribe diazepam (Valium) to use when she feels anxious. She asks whether you think this is a good idea. How would you respond? What action could you take?

CHAPTER REVIEW

Choose the most appropriate answer.

1. Shortly after being told that he has 90% blockage of three major coronary arteries and needs emergency coronary artery bypass surgery, Paul is noted by the nurse to appear dazed. His thoughts are scattered, as evidenced by the fact that his conversation jumps from topic to topic. He frequently states, "I'm overwhelmed. I don't know what to do." He is unable to give direction to his wife when she asks him whom he wants her to notify. His pulse rate rises 15 points. The nurse can assess the type of anxiety Paul is experiencing as:
    1. normal anxiety at a mild level.
    2. sublimated anxiety at a panic level.
    3. acute (state) anxiety at a severe level.
    4. chronic (trait) anxiety at a moderate level.
2. Which characteristic is true of mature ego defenses but not true of ego defenses that are immature?

1. Mature defenses arise from experiencing panic-level anxiety.
2. Mature defenses do not distort reality to a significant degree.
3. Mature defenses disguise reality to make it less threatening.
4. Mature defenses are exclusively maladaptive.
3. One possible reason for panic disorder may be:
    1. faulty learning.
    2. dopamine deficiency.
    3. inhibition of GABA.
    4. clomipramine (Anafranil) excess.
4. Mrs. T. is preoccupied with persistent thoughts and impulses that intrude on her daily functioning. She performs ritualistic acts repetitively, such as cleaning the kitchen counter over and over again. She expresses distress that her attention is so

CHAPTER REVIEW—cont'd

consumed that she cannot accomplish her usual activities. These symptoms are most consistent with the *DSM-IV-TR* diagnosis of:
1. panic disorder.
2. social phobia.
3. GAD.
4. OCD.

5. In addition to prescribing an SSRI to treat Mr. G.'s panic disorder, the nurse psychotherapist is likely to recommend:
1. family therapy.
2. psychoanalysis.
3. vocational rehabilitation.
4. cognitive-behavioral therapy.

REFERENCES

American Nurses Association, American Psychiatric Nurses Association, & International Society of Psychiatric-Mental Health Nurses. (2007). *Psychiatric-mental health nursing: Scope and standards of practice.* Silver Springs, MD: Nursesbooks.org.

American Psychiatric Association. (2000). *Diagnostic and statistical manual of mental disorders (DSM-IV-TR)* (4th ed., text rev.). Washington, DC: Author.

Brown, A.B. (2003). Panic disorder: Highly disabling, yet treatable. *NARSAD Research Newsletter, 15*(3), 24-28.

Charney, D. (2005). Anxiety disorders: Introduction and overview. In B.J. Sadock & V.A. Sadock (Eds.), *Kaplan and Sadock's comprehensive textbook of psychiatry* (8th ed., vol. 1). Philadelphia: Lippincott Williams & Wilkins.

Foa, E.B. (2005). The psychological aftermath of hurricane Katrina: An expert interview with Edna B. Foa. *Medscape Psychiatry & Mental Health, 10*(2).

Gorman, J.M. (2000). Anxiety disorders: Introduction and overview. In B.J. Sadock & V.A. Sadock (Eds.), *Comprehensive textbook of psychiatry* (7th ed., vol. 1, pp. 1441-1444). Philadelphia: Lippincott Williams & Wilkins.

Hemmings, S.M.J., & Stein, D.J. (2006). The current status of association studies in obsessive-compulsive disorder. In D.J. Stein (Ed.), Obsessive compulsive spectrum disorders; *Psychiatric Clinics of North America,* June 2006, *29*(2), 441-444.

Kaiman, C. (2003). PTSD in the World War II combat veteran. *American Journal of Nursing, 103*(11), 32-40.

Katerndahl, D.A. (2002). Factors influencing care seeking for a self-defined worst panic attack. *Psychiatric Services, 53*(4), 464-470.

Kessler, R.C, Berglulnd, P., Demler,O., et al.(2005). Lifetime prevalence and age-of-onset distributions of DSM-IV disorders in the national comorbidity survery replication. *Arch Gen Psychiatry, 62,* 593-602.

Koenig, H.G., McCullough, M.E., & Larson, D.B. (2001). *Handbook of religion and health.* New York: Oxford University Press.

McEnany, G. (2000). Herbal psychotropics: III. Focus on kava, valerian, and melatonin. *Journal of the American Psychiatric Nurses Association, 6*(4), 126-132.

Merikangas, K.R., & Kupfer, D.J. (1995). Mood disorders: Genetic aspects. In H.I. Kaplan & B.J. Sadock (Eds.), *Comprehensive textbook of psychiatry/VI* (6th ed., vol. 1, pp. 1102-1115). Baltimore: Williams & Wilkins.

Moorhead, S., Johnson, M., Maas, M.L, & Swanson, E. (2008). *Nursing outcomes classification (NOC)* (4th ed.). St. Louis: Mosby.

Myrick, H., & Brady, K. (2003). Editorial review: Current review of the comorbidity of affective, anxiety, and substance use disorders. *Current Opinions in Psychiatry, 16*(3), 261-270.

North American Nursing Diagnosis Association International (NANDA-I). (2007). *NANDA nursing diagnoses: Definitions and classification 2007-2008.* Philadelphia: Author.

Overbeek, T., Sachruers, K., Vermetten, E., et al. (2002). Comorbidity of obsessive-compulsive disorder and depression: Prevalence, symptom severity, and treatment effect. *Journal of Clinical Psychiatry, 63*(12), 1106-1112.

Peplau, H.E. (1968). A working definition of anxiety. In S.F.Burd & M.A. Marshall (Eds.), *Some clinical approaches to psychiatric nursing.* New York: Macmillan.

Ritchie, E.C., & Cavazos (2005). *Meeting the mental health needs of veterans of wars in Iraq and Afghanistan: An expert interview with Colonel Elspeth Cameron Ritchie, MD, MPH. Medscape Psychiatry & Mental Health, 10*(2).

Sadock, B.J., & Sadock, V.A.. (2007). *Kaplan and Sadock's Synopsis of psychiatry* (10th Ed.). Philadelphia: Wolters/Lippincott Williams & Wilkins.

Satcher, D., Delgado, & Masand, P.S. (2005). A surgeon general's perspective on the unmet needs of patients with anxiety disorders. Medscape Psychiatry & Mental Health, 10(2).

Simon, N.M., & Rosenbaum, J.F. (2003). *Anxiety and depression comorbidity: Implications and intervention. Medscape Psychiatry & Mental Health, 8*(1).

Sonnenberg, S.M., Ursano, A.M., & Ursano, R.J. (2003). Physician-patient relationship. In A. Tasman, J. Kay, & J.A. Lieberman (Eds.), *Psychiatry* (2nd ed.). West Sussex, England: Wiley.

Stein, M.B. (2005). Anxiety disorders: Somatic treatment. In B.J. Sadock & V.A. Sadock (Eds.), *Kaplan and Sadock's comprehensive textbook of psychiatry* (8th ed., vol. 1). Philadelphia: Lippincott Williams & Wilkins.

Sullivan, H.S. (1953). *The interpersonal theory of psychiatry.* New York: Norton.

Vaillant, G.E. (1994). Ego mechanisms of defense and personality psychopathology. *Journal of Abnormal Psychology, 103*(1), 44-50.

Vaillant, G.E., & Vaillant, C.O. (2004). Normality and mental health. In B.J. Sadock & V.A. Sadock (Eds.), *Kaplan and Sadock's comprehensive textbook of psychiatry* (8th ed., vol. 1, pp. 583-597). Philadelphia: Lippincott Williams & Wilkins.

Widiger, T.A., & Mullins, S. (2003). Personality disorders. In A. Tasman, J. Kay, & J.A. Lieberman (Eds.). *Psychiatry* (2nd ed.). West Sussex, England: Wiley.

CHAPTER 9

Somatoform and Dissociative Disorders

Elizabeth M. Varcarolis and Helene (Kay) Charron

Key Terms and Concepts

alternate personality (alter), or subpersonality, p. 165

body dysmorphic disorder, p. 157

conversion disorder, p. 157

depersonalization disorder, p. 164

dissociative amnesia, p. 164

dissociative disorders, p. 153

dissociative fugue, p. 165

dissociative identity disorder (DID), p. 165

factitious disorder, p. 153

hypochondriasis, p. 157

la belle indifférence, p. 158

malingering, p. 153

pain disorder, p. 157

psychosomatic illness, p. 153

secondary gains, p. 158

somatization, p. 153

somatization disorder, p. 157

somatoform disorders, p. 153

Objectives

1. Compare and contrast essential characteristics of somatoform and dissociative disorders.
2. Differentiate among symptoms of somatoform disorders and those of malingering and factitious disorder.
3. Describe five psychosocial interventions that would be appropriate for a patient with somatic complaints.
4. Explain the key symptoms of the four dissociative disorders.
5. Compare and contrast dissociative amnesia and dissociative fugue.
6. Identify three specialized elements in the assessment of a patient with a dissociative disorder.

evolve

For additional resources related to the content of this chapter, visit the Evolve site at http://evolve.elsevier.com/Varcarolis/essentials.

- Chapter Outline
- Chapter Review Answers
- Case Study and Nursing Care Plans

- Nurse, Patient, and Family Resources
- Concept Map Creator

Edited by Nancy Christine Shoemaker in the fifth edition of *Foundations of Psychiatric Mental Health Nursing.*

Somatoform disorders are a group of disorders characterized by the presence of physical symptoms in the absence of pathology or known pathophysiology. Somatization is the tendency to experience and to report bodily symptoms that have no physical explanation. Somatization is associated with increased health care use, functional impairment, provider dissatisfaction, and psychiatric comorbidity. For some people, somatization progresses to a form of chronic illness behavior. In the most extreme cases of somatization, the sick role becomes the person's predominant mode of relating to the world (e.g., hypochondriasis).

The *DSM-IV-TR* defines **dissociative disorders** as disturbances in the normally well-integrated continuum of consciousness, memory, identity, and perception. Dissociation is an unconscious defense mechanism to protect the individual against overwhelming anxiety. Patients with dissociative disorders have intact reality testing; that is, they are not delusional or hallucinating. When the ability to integrate memories is impaired, the individual has *dissociative amnesia*. When the ability to maintain one's identity is affected, the individual may develop a *dissociative fugue* or *dissociative identity disorder (DID)*, sometimes referred to as *multiple personality disorder*. When there is a persistent or recurrent disruption in perception, the individual has *depersonalization disorder*, with a feeling of detachment from the mind or body.

SOMATOFORM DISORDERS

The somatoform disorders currently recognized by the *DSM-IV-TR* include the following: somatization disorder, undifferentiated somatoform disorder, conversion disorder, pain disorder, hypochondriasis, body dysmorphic disorder, and somatoform disorder not otherwise specified. This chapter addresses the five main *DSM-IV-TR* diagnoses presented in Figure 9-1.

Soma is the Greek word for body, and **somatization** is defined as the expression of psychological stress through physical symptoms. It is important to know that these disorders are grouped together merely because of their similarities in presentation and not because of any sound underlying theory or laboratory findings (Guggenheim, 2000). Somatoform disorders demonstrate complex mind-body interactions, and they cause real distress to the patient with significant impairment in social and occupational functioning. Often the patient has another psychiatric disorder as well.

In somatoform disorders, symptoms are not intentional or under the conscious control of the patient, unlike in malingering or factitious disorders. **Malingering** involves a conscious process of intentionally producing symptoms for an obvious benefit; for example, an employee complains of nonexistent back pain to get disability income. **Factitious disorder** refers to deliberate fabrication of symptoms or self-inflicted injury for the purpose of assuming the sick role and receiving nurturance, comfort, and attention. For example, people with factitious disorder may inject a caustic substance into the skin to form an abscess.

Munchausen syndrome is the most severe and chronic form of factitious disorder, and results in self-harm severe enough for hospitalization, doctor shopping, and seeking invasive diagnostic tests. *Munchausen syndrome by proxy* is manifested in a caregiver (usually a mother with a health care background) injuring a child to get attention or sympathy.

The somatoform disorders are also differentiated from **psychosomatic illness**, in which there is evidence of a general medical condition that may be affected by stress or psychological factors (e.g., ulcerative colitis or essential hypertension).

PREVALENCE AND COMORBIDITY

Prevalence rates for these disorders in the general population are unknown; however, it is estimated that 38% of primary care patients present with symptoms that have no serious medical basis. Almost half (46%) of new complaints or new symptoms contain some element of somatization, and at least 10% of these represent pure somatization (Calabrese & Stern, 2004).

Differentiating somatoform disorders from physical disorders and identifying **comorbid conditions** are significant issues for the primary care provider. Research shows that half of all frequent users of medical care have psychological problems. Psychiatric disorders are frequently present in people who have medically unexplained complaints. A **depressive disorder** can be diagnosed 50% to 60% of the time, and an **anxiety disorder** can be diagnosed 40% to 50% of the time in patients who present with physical complaints that are unexplained medically (Kroenke & Rosmalen, 2006). Excessive co-occurrence of **substance use and personality disorders** also has been found.

Therefore, a comprehensive physical examination with appropriate diagnostic studies is necessary to rule out medical conditions, which can be confused with somatoform disorders. Along with a comprehensive medical examination, a thorough psychosocial history is required to clarify a somatoform diagnosis as well as any co-occurring psychiatric disorders.

DSM-IV-TR CRITERIA FOR SOMATOFORM DISORDERS

SOMATOFORM DISORDERS

Somatization Disorder

1. History of many physical complaints beginning before 30 years of age, occurring over a period of years and resulting in impairment in social, occupational, or other important areas of functioning.

2. Complaints must include all of the following:
   - History of pain in at least **four** different sites or functions
   - History of at least **two** gastrointestinal symptoms other than pain
   - History of at least **one** sexual or reproduction symptom
   - History of at least **one** symptom defined as or suggesting a neurological disorder

Conversion Disorder

1. Development of one or more symptoms or deficits suggesting a neurological disorder (blindness, deafness, loss of touch) or general medical condition.

2. Psychological factors are associated with the symptom or deficit because the symptom is initiated or exacerbated by psychological stressors.

3. Not due to malingering or factitious disorder and not culturally sanctioned.

4. Cannot be explained by general medical condition or effects of a substance.

5. Causes impairment in social or occupational functioning, causes marked distress, or requires medical attention.

Hypochondriasis

For at least 6 months:

1. Preoccupation with fears of having, or the idea that one has, a serious disease.

2. Preoccupation persists despite appropriate medical tests and reassurances.

3. Other disorders are ruled out (e.g., somatic delusional disorders).

4. Preoccupation causes significant impairment in social or occupational functioning or causes marked distress.

Pain Disorder

1. Pain in one or more anatomical sites is a major part of the clinical picture.

2. Causes significant impairment in occupational or social functioning or causes marked distress.

3. Psychological factors thought to cause onset, severity, or exacerbation. **Pain associated with psychological factors.**

4. Symptoms not intentionally produced or feigned. If medical condition present, it plays minor role in accounting for pain.

5. **Pain may be associated with a psychological and/or medical condition.** Both factors are judged to be important in onset, severity, exacerbation, and maintenance of pain.

Body Dysmorphic Disorder (BDD)

1. Preoccupation with some imagined defect in appearance. If the defect is present, concern is excessive.

2. Preoccupation causes significant impairment in social or occupational functioning or causes marked distress.

3. Preoccupation not better accounted for by another mental disorder.

Figure 9-1 ▪ Diagnostic criteria for somatoform disorders. (Adapted from American Psychiatric Association. [2000]. *Diagnostic and statistical manual of mental disorders* [4th ed., text rev.]. Washington, DC: Author.)

THEORY

Genetic and Familial Factors

There is no direct evidence of a genetic etiology for any *specific* somatoform disorder (Hollifield, 2005). Some physiological data support a genetic theory that somatization disorder tends to run in families, occurring in 10% to 20% of first-degree female relatives of women with somatization disorder. Twin studies show an increased risk of conversion disorder in monozygotic twin pairs. First-degree biological relatives of people with chronic pain disorder are more likely to have chronic pain, depressive disorder, and alcohol dependence.

Cely-Serrano and Floet (2006) state that genetic and familial factors play a significant role in the predisposition to somatoform disorders. These disorders are associated with:

* Low pain threshold
* Impaired verbal communication
* Patterns of information processing characterized by distractibility, impulsiveness, and failure to habituate to repetitive stimuli

Genetic and Environmental Origins

A study by Taylor and associates (2006) supports previous twin studies that report somatoform disorders are moderately heritable. The study included monozygotic (MZ) as well as dizygotic twin groups. They evaluated for "health anxiety," which ranges from mild to severe, with severe meeting the criteria for hypochondriasis. There are several facets of "health anxiety" that include health-related fears, disease conviction, excessive health-related behaviors (e.g., doctor shopping), and impairment in occupational functioning. They found that less than 40% of health anxiety is genetically correlated. The majority 60% to 90% of health anxiety correlated with environmental factors. These findings left the authors to conclude that since excessive health anxiety (hypochondriacal symptoms) involves genetic as well as environmental factors; optimum treatment would involve a combination of pharmacological and psychosocial interventions.

Learning and Sociocultural Factors

Research supports the idea that early experiences and learning are the primary factors of somatic sensitivity and bodily preoccupations. An adult with somatoform symptoms will present with symptoms that were given attention to by parents during the adult's childhood (Hollifield, 2005). Constant attention to a specific body part enhances the ability of a person to direct sensations to that body part. Therefore symptoms are reinforced by constant parental attention, and the child learns the benefits of the sick role.

Psychodynamic Theory

These are complex theories. According to Hollifield (2005) there is some empirical evidence to support one of the psychodynamic theories. This theory, simply put, is that the development of narcissism is turned into bodily preoccupation during the separation and individuation phase of development. If the parents are not available, are harsh, or are inconsistent and fail to acknowledge the needs of the child during this transition, a process of self-focus ensues. The child, and later adult, learns to focus on the body as a defense against stress and mental pain because the emotional and nurturing needs as a child were not met from the outside world.

Interpersonal Model

There is growing evidence that childhood adversity is linked to adult hypochondriasis. A study by Noyes and colleagues (2002) found that patients diagnosed with hypochondriasis more frequently report traumatic events and substance abuse in their families compared with controls. According to Cely-Serrano and Floet (2006), recent studies point to an association between childhood physical or sexual abuse and conversion, somatization, and dissociative disorders. Table 9-1 provides clinical examples of each of the somatoform disorders and their associated defense mechanisms.

CULTURAL CONSIDERATIONS

Cultural factors can influence an individual's tendency to somatize, as well as the types of symptoms that unconsciously might be used. In some cultures, somatic symptoms may be the first symptoms that indicate a patient may have an underlying anxiety or depressive disorder (Cely-Serrano & Floet, 2006).

The *DSM-IV-TR* provides information about the role of culture in somatoform disorders and states that the type and the frequency of somatic symptoms vary across cultures. Burning hands and feet or the sensation of worms in the head or ants under the skin is more common in Africa and southern Asia than in North America. Alteration of consciousness with falling is a symptom commonly associated with culture-specific religious and healing rituals. Somatization disorder, which is rarely seen in men in the United States is often reported in Greek and Puerto Rican men, which suggests that cultural mores may permit these men to use somatization as an acceptable approach to dealing with life stress.

TABLE 9-1	Examples of Somatoform Disorders and Associated Defense Mechanisms	
Disorder	**Defense Mechanism**	**Example**
Conversion disorder	Conversion	Jan, a 28-year-old former secretary, awakens one morning to find that she has a tingling in both hands and cannot move her fingers. Two days earlier, her husband had told her that he wanted a separation and that she would have to go back to work to support herself. The conversion of anxiety relates the separation and increase in dependency needs to "paralysis of her fingers" so that she is unable to work.
Pain disorder	Displacement	Henry, 47, a laborer, "pulled a muscle" in his back a year ago. Two weeks before this, his wife, a waitress, told him that she wanted to go back to school to get her bachelor's degree. He suffers severe, constant pain, despite negative results from myelography, computed tomography, magnetic resonance imaging, and neurological examinations. He watches television all day and collects disability. His wife, unable now to go back to school, waits on him and has assumed his home responsibilities. Henry displaces his anxiety over the threat to his own self-esteem by his wife's potential change of status onto "pain in his back." The focus of his anxiety is now on his back and not on his threatened self-esteem.
Body dysmorphic disorder	Symbolism and projection	Michele, a young, attractive woman, is preoccupied with her nose, which she considers too long and ugly. She is constantly concerned by and distressed over her perception. Two plastic surgeons she consulted are hesitant to reshape her nose, but this has not altered her thinking that her nose makes her ugly.
Somatization disorder	Somatization	Deanna, 27, presents at the physician's office with excessively heavy menstruation. She tells the nurse that recently she experienced pain "first in my back and then going to every part of my body." She states that she is often bothered by constipation and vomiting when she "eats the wrong food." She says that she was "unwell" and had suffered from seizures and still has them occasionally. The nurse becomes confused, not knowing what symptoms Deanna wants the physician to evaluate. Deanna tells the nurse that she lives at home with her parents because her poor health makes it hard for her to hold a job.
Hypochondriasis	Denial and somatization	Julio, 52, lost his wife to colon cancer 5 months earlier, which he "took very well." Recently he saw a sixth physician with the same complaint. He believes that he has liver cancer, despite repeated and extensive diagnostic tests, results of which are all negative. He has ceased seeing his friends, has dropped his hobbies, and spends much of his time checking his sclera and "resting his liver." His son finally demands that he see a doctor.

In some cultures, certain physical symptoms are believed to result from the casting of spells on the individual. Spellbound individuals often seek the help of traditional healers in addition to modern medical staff. The medical provider may diagnose a non–life-threatening somatoform disorder, whereas the traditional healer may offer an entirely different explanation and prognosis. The individual may not show improvement until the traditional healer removes the spell.

CLINICAL PICTURE

Refer to Figure 9-1 for the *DSM-IV-TR* criteria for various somatoform disorders.

Somatization Disorder

The diagnosis of **somatization disorder** requires the presence of a certain number of symptoms accompanied by significant functional impairment. The most frequent symptoms are pain (head, chest, back, joints, pelvis), dysphagia, nausea, bloating, constipation, palpitations, dizziness, and shortness of breath. Patients report significant distress and seek out multiple providers for medical care. Anxiety and depression are common comorbid conditions.

Somatoform disorders are relatively more common in those who are unmarried, nonwhite, poorly educated, and from a rural area (Hollifield, 2005). The course of the illness is chronic and relapsing, and it rarely remits completely.

Hypochondriasis

Hypochondriasis is a widespread phenomenon: it is estimated that 1 out of 20 people who seek outpatient medical attention suffer from this disorder (APA, 2002). Patients with this disorder misinterpret innocent physical sensations as evidence of a serious illness. They cannot be reassured by negative diagnostic test findings, and they seek extensive medical care with frustrating results. Most patients refuse referral to a psychiatrist. Approximately two thirds of the patients with hypochondriasis have a comorbid psychiatric disorder of depression or anxiety disorder (APA, 2002). People with this disorder experience severe distress, and their ability to function in personal, social, and occupational roles often is impaired.

No specific socioeconomic factors are associated with this disorder (Barsky, 2001). However, many patients have a history of sexual or physical trauma, parental upheaval, or absence from school during childhood for health reasons. The course of the illness is chronic and relapsing, with symptoms exacerbated during times of stress (Guggenheim, 2000). Yet improvement is noted in up to 50% of patients who receive treatment.

Pain Disorder

Pain is one of the most frequent reasons people seek medical attention. When testing rules out any organic cause for the pain, and the discomfort leads to significant impairment, **pain disorder** is diagnosed. Although most pain can be reduced, chronic pain results in significant disability and high costs for health care. In 2000, it was estimated that 7 million Americans suffered from low back pain. Suicide is a serious risk in patients with chronic pain: the suicide rate is nine times higher in such patients than in the general population (Guggenheim, 2000).

Pain is difficult to measure objectively, and individuals react differently to the same injury. Typical sites of pain include the head, face, lower back, and pelvis (Guggenheim, 2000). Frequent comorbid conditions include depression, substance dependence, and personality disorders. These patients are at risk for excessive use of narcotic or sedative medications (Guggenheim, 2000). Some research suggests that a background of sexual abuse or trauma is common in women with pain disorder.

The course of pain disorder varies according to the acuity of the symptoms. Acute pain disorders have a favorable prognosis, but chronic pain is more difficult to treat. Antidepressants tend to decrease pain intensity (Hollifield, 2005).

Body Dysmorphic Disorder

Body dysmorphic disorder (BDD) is a highly distressing and impairing disorder. Patients with body dysmorphic disorder usually have a normal appearance, although a small number do show minor defects (Hollifield, 2005). Preoccupation with an imagined "defective body part" results in obsessional thinking and compulsive behavior, such as mirror checking and camouflaging. Individuals with BDD may feel great shame and hide or withdraw from others. Many will alter their appearance through plastic surgeries wrongly perceiving themselves to be ugly or having "hideous physical flaws" (PsychCentral, 2007). Unfortunately even when cosmetic surgery is sought, there is no relief of symptoms (Guggenheim, 2000).

Normal social activities related to academic or occupational functioning are impaired (Carroll et al., 2002). Patients are frequently concerned with the face, skin, genitalia, thighs, hips, and hair. In one study, women were found to be more focused on weight and hips, whereas men were found to be concerned about body build and genitalia (Carroll et al., 2002).

Common comorbid diagnoses include major depression, obsessive-compulsive disorder, and social phobia (Guggenheim, 2000). A study by Rief and associates (2006) found that individuals with BDD reported higher rates of suicidal ideation (19% versus 3%) and suicide attempts due to appearance concerns (7% versus 1%) than individuals who did not meet criteria for BDD. The disorder is often kept secret for many years, and the patient does not respond to reassurance. The disorder is chronic and the response to treatment is limited.

Conversion Disorder

Conversion disorder is marked by symptoms or deficits that affect voluntary motor or sensory functions, which suggest another medical condition (Hollifield, 2005). The dysfunction does not correspond to current scientific understanding of the nervous system and they are judged because of psychological factors. Many patients show a lack of emotional concern about the symptoms (**la belle indifférence**), although others are quite distressed. Common symptoms are involuntary movements, seizures, paralysis, abnormal gait, anesthesia, blindness, and deafness.

Conversion disorder is among the most common of the somatoform disorders. Socioeconomic factors that seem to be related are lower education and income levels, residence in a rural area, and military service, especially in combat zones (Guggenheim, 2000). Some studies have found an association between childhood physical or sexual abuse and conversion disorder (Roelofs et al., 2002). Common comorbid psychiatric conditions include depression, anxiety, other somatoform disorders, and personality disorders. There are also cases in which a comorbid medical or neurological condition exists and the conversion symptom is an exaggeration of the original problem.

The course of the disorder is related to its acuity: in cases with acute onset during stressful events, the remission rate is approximately 95%. If symptoms have been present for 6 months or more, there is only about a 50% chance that symptoms will remit (Hollifield, 2005).

evolve

For a comprehensive case study and associated care plans for a patient with conversion disorder, visit the Evolve website at http://evolve.elsevier.com/Varcarolis/essentials.

Assessment of patients with somatoform disorders is a complex process that requires careful and complete documentation. The following sections outline several areas that are not normally included in a nursing assessment but are of considerable importance in the assessment of a patient with suspected somatoform disorder.

Application of the Nursing Process
ASSESSMENT
Symptoms and Unmet Needs

Assessment should begin with collection of data about the nature, location, onset, character, and duration of the symptom or symptoms. Often, patients with conversion disorder report having a sudden loss in function of a body part. "I woke up this morning and couldn't move my arm." Patients with somatization disorder, hypochondriasis, or

somatoform pain disorder usually discuss their symptoms in dramatic terms. They may use colorful metaphors and exaggerations: "The pain was searing, like a hot sword drawn across my forehead" or "My symptoms are so rare that I've stumped hundreds of doctors." Individuals with body dysmorphic disorder are concerned about only one part of the body, display disgust with the offending part, and often seek cosmetic surgery.

Information should be sought about patients' ability to meet their own basic needs. Tachypnea and tachycardia may be brought on by anxiety. Nutrition, fluid balance, and elimination needs should be evaluated because patients with somatization disorders often complain of gastrointestinal distress, diarrhea, constipation, and anorexia. The physiological need for sex may be altered by patient experiences of painful intercourse, pain in another part of the body, or lack of interest in sex.

Rest, comfort, activity, and hygiene needs may be altered as a result of patient problems such as fatigue, weakness, insomnia, muscle tension, pain, and avoidance of diversional activity. Safety and security needs may be threatened by patient experiences of blindness, deafness, loss of balance and falling, and anesthesia of various parts of the body.

Voluntary Control of Symptoms

During assessment it is important to determine if the symptoms are under the patient's voluntary control. True somatoform symptoms are *not* under the individual's voluntary control. The patient cannot see the relationship between symptoms and interpersonal conflicts that may be obvious to others, and often suffer extreme physical discomfort and mental anguish.

Secondary Gains

The nurse tries to identify secondary gains the patient may be receiving from the symptoms. Secondary gains are those benefits derived from the symptoms alone; for example, in the sick role, the patient is not able to perform the usual family, work, and social functions, and receives extra attention from loved ones. If a patient derives personal benefit from the symptoms, giving up the symptoms is more difficult. The clinician works with the patient to achieve the same benefits through healthier avenues (e.g., assertiveness training). One approach to identifying the presence of secondary gains is to ask the patient questions such as the following:

- What can't you do now that you used to be able to do?
- How has this problem affected your life?

Cognitive Style

In general, patients with these disorders misinterpret physical stimuli and distort reality regarding their symptoms. For example, sensations a normal individual might interpret as a headache might suggest a brain tumor to a patient with hypochondriasis. Exploring the patient's cognitive style is helpful in distinguishing between hypochondriasis and somatization disorder. The patient with hypochondriasis exhibits more anxiety and an obsessive attention to detail, along with a preoccupation with the fear of serious illness. The patient with somatization disorder is often rambling and vague about the details of his or her many symptoms and gives a disorganized history.

Ability to Communicate Feelings and Emotional Needs

Patients with somatoform disorders have difficulty communicating their emotional needs. As children, many of these patients had difficulty with expressing emotions in their families and would somatize as an unconscious expression of anxiety, depression, or fear. As adults, patients are able to describe their physical symptoms, but are unable to verbalize feelings, especially those related to anger, guilt, and dependence. As a consequence, the somatic symptom may be the patient's chief means of communicating emotional needs. Psychogenic blindness or hearing loss may represent the symbolic statement, "I can't face this knowledge." For example, after a wife overheard friends discussing her husband's sexual infidelity, she developed total deafness.

Dependence on Medication

Individuals experiencing many somatic complaints often become dependent on medication to relieve pain or anxiety or to induce sleep. Physicians prescribe anxiolytic agents for patients who seem highly anxious and concerned about their symptoms. Patients often return to the physician for prescription renewal or seek treatment from numerous physicians. It is important that the nurse assess the type and the amount of medications being used.

Assessment Guidelines

It is always important to ensure that an underlying medical condition has been ruled out. Some important differential diagnostic considerations for hypochondriasis are multiple sclerosis, myasthenia gravis, thyroid or parathyroid disease, and other autoimmune disorders (e.g., systemic lupus and others). However, the presence of a general medical condition does not exclude the possibility of a coexisting hypochondriasis.

Somatoform Disorders

1. Assess for nature, location, onset, characteristics, and duration of the symptom(s).
2. Assess the patient's ability to meet basic needs.
3. Assess risks to safety and security needs of the patient as a result of the symptom(s).
4. Determine whether the symptoms are under the patient's voluntary control.
5. Identify any secondary gains that the patient is experiencing from symptom(s).
6. Explore the patient's cognitive style and ability to communicate feelings and needs.
7. Assess type and amount of medication the patient is using.

DIAGNOSIS

Patients with somatoform disorders present various nursing problems. *Ineffective coping* is frequently diagnosed. Causal statements might include the following:

- Distorted perceptions of body functions and symptoms
- Chronic pain of psychological origin
- Dependence on pain relievers or anxiolytics

Table 9-2 identifies potential nursing diagnoses for patients with somatoform disorders.

OUTCOMES IDENTIFICATION

The overall goal in treating somatoform disorders is that people with these disorders will eventually be able to live as normal a life as possible. They may never be pain free or free of other symptoms, but it is hoped the quality of their lives can be improved.

The following are examples of potential outcome criteria:

- Patient will articulate feelings such as anger, shame, guilt, and remorse.
- Patient will resume performance of work role behaviors.
- Patient will identify ineffective coping patterns.
- Patient will make realistic appraisal of strengths and weaknesses.
- Patient will allow family to be involved in decision making.

PLANNING

Because patients with somatoform disorders are seldom admitted to psychiatric units specifically because of these

TABLE 9-2	Potential Nursing Diagnoses for Somatoform Disorders
Signs and Symptoms	**Nursing Diagnoses**
• Inability to meet occupational, family, or social responsibilities because of symptoms	*Ineffective coping*
	Ineffective role performance
• Inability to participate in usual community activities or friendships because of psychogenic symptoms	*Impaired social interaction*
• Dependence on pain relievers	*Powerlessness*
• Distortion of body functions and symptoms	*Disturbed body image*
• Presence of secondary gains by adoption of sick role	*Pain (Acute or Chronic)*
• Inability to meet family role function and need for family to assume role function of the somatic individual	*Interrupted family processes*
	Ineffective sexuality pattern
• Assumption of some of the roles of the somatic parent by the children	*Impaired parenting*
• Shifting of the sexual partner's role to that of caregiver or parent and of the patient's role to that of recipient of care	*Risk for caregiver role strain*
• Feeling of inability to control symptoms or understand why he or she cannot find help	*Chronic low self-esteem*
	Spiritual distress
• Development of negative self-evaluation related to losing body function, feeling useless, or not feeling valued by significant others	
• Inability to take care of basic self-care needs related to conversion symptom (paralysis, seizures, pain, fatigue)	*Those that focus on Self-care deficit, e.g. bathing/hygiene, dressing/grooming, feeding, toileting*
• Inability to sleep related to psychogenic pain	*Disturbed sleep pattern*

disorders, long-term interventions usually take place on an outpatient basis or in the home. Short-term planning may be initiated if the patient is admitted to a medical-surgical unit. Such a stay is usually short, and discharge will occur as soon as diagnostic tests are completed and negative results are received.

Nursing interventions should focus initially on establishing a helping relationship with the patient. The therapeutic relationship is vital to the success of the care plan, given the patient's resistance to the concept that no physical cause for the symptom exists and the patient's tendency to go from caregiver to caregiver.

To be successful, therapeutic interventions must address ways to help the patient get needs met without resorting to somatization. The secondary gains the patient has derived from illness behaviors become less important to the patient when underlying needs can be met directly. Collaboration with family or significant others is essential for success.

IMPLEMENTATION
Communication Guidelines

Generally, for patients with somatoform disorders, nursing interventions take place in the home or clinic setting. The nurse attempts to help the patient improve overall functioning through the development of effective coping and com-

munication strategies. Remember, when patients complain of physical symptoms, take the symptoms seriously, because even if a medical explanation is not found, the symptoms are real and troublesome to the patient. Table 9-3 lists several possible interventions for patients with somatoform disorders.

Working with people who have somatoform disorders can be frustrating, and you may find yourself avoiding interaction with them. However, it is important to note that when people feel cared for, the intensity of symptoms tends to diminish. As the symptoms diminish, it becomes easier to address emotional issues.

Health Teaching and Health Promotion

When somatization is present, the patient's ability to perform self-care activities may be impaired, and nursing intervention is necessary. In general, interventions involve the use of a matter-of-fact approach to support the highest level of self-care of which the patient is capable. For patients manifesting paralysis, blindness, or severe fatigue, an effective nursing approach is to support patients while expecting them to feed, bathe, or groom themselves. For example, the patient who demonstrates arm paralysis can be expected to eat using the other arm. The patient who is experiencing blindness can be told at what numbers on an imaginary

TABLE 9-3	Interventions for Somatoform Disorders

Intervention	Rationale
1. Offer explanations and support during diagnostic testing.	1. Reduces anxiety while ruling out organic illness
2. After physical complaints have been investigated, avoid further reinforcement (e.g., do not take vital signs each time patient complains of palpitations).	2. Directs focus away from physical symptoms
3. Spend time with patient at times other than when summoned by patient to voice physical complaint.	3. Rewards non–illness-related behaviors and encourages repetition of desired behavior
4. Observe and record frequency and intensity of somatic symptoms. (Patient or family can give information.)	4. Establishes a baseline and later enables evaluation of effectiveness of interventions
5. Do not imply that symptoms are not real.	5. Acknowledges that psychogenic symptoms are real to the patient
6. Shift focus from somatic complaints to feelings or to neutral topics.	6. Conveys interest in patient as a person rather than in patient's symptoms; reduces need to gain attention via symptoms
7. Assess secondary gains that "physical illness" provides for patient (e.g., attention, increased dependency, and distraction from another problem).	7. Allows these needs to be met in healthier ways and thus minimizes secondary gains
8. Use matter-of-fact approach to patient exhibiting resistance or covert anger.	8. Avoids power struggles; demonstrates acceptance of anger and permits discussion of angry feelings
9. Have patient direct all requests to case manager.	9. Reduces manipulation
10. Show concern for patient, but avoid fostering dependency needs.	10. Shows respect for patient's feelings while minimizing secondary gains from "illness"
11. Reinforce patient's strengths and problem-solving abilities.	11. Contributes to positive self-esteem; helps patient realize that needs can be met without resorting to somatic symptoms
12. Teach assertive communication.	12. Provides patient with a positive means of getting needs met; reduces feelings of helplessness and need for manipulation
13. Teach patient stress reduction techniques, such as meditation, relaxation, and mild physical exercise.	13. Provides alternate coping strategies; reduces need for medication

clock the food is located on the plate and encouraged to feed him- or herself. These strategies are effective in reducing secondary gain.

Assertiveness training is often appropriate to teach patients with somatoform disorders. Use of assertiveness techniques gives patients a direct means of getting needs met and thereby decreases the need for somatic symptoms. Teaching an exercise regimen, such as doing range-of-motion exercises for 15 to 20 minutes daily, can help the patient feel in control, increases endorphin levels, and may help decrease anxiety.

Case Management

"Doctor shopping" is common among patients with somatoform disorders. The patient goes from physician to physician, clinic to clinic, or hospital to hospital, hoping to establish a physical basis for distress. Repeated computed

CT/MRI

tomography scans, magnetic resonance images, and other diagnostic tests are often documented in the medical record. Case management can help limit health care costs associated with such visits. The case manager can recommend to the physician that the patient be scheduled for brief appointments every 4 to 6 weeks at set times rather than on demand and that laboratory tests be avoided unless they are absolutely necessary. The patient who establishes a relationship with the case manager often feels less anxiety because the patient has someone to contact and knows that someone is "in charge."

Psychotherapy

Cognitive and behavioral approaches can be effective and may prove to be the therapy of choice for patients with somatoform disorders (Cely-Serrano & Floet, 2006). Behavior modification can provide incentives, motivation, and rewards to help patients control their symptoms. Family

TABLE 9-4	Somatoform Disorders		
Disorder	**Characteristics**	**Comorbidity**	**Therapeutic Approach**
Conversion disorder	One or two neurological complaints	Major depression; dissociative disorder; personality disorder	Behavioral therapy; family therapy; hypnosis; anxiolytics
Somatization disorder	Many physical complaints affecting many organs	Major depression; panic disorder; personality disorder; substance dependence	Consultation with primary care provider to arrange regular patient visits, limited tests; group therapy; cognitive-behavioral therapy
Hypochondriasis	Characterized less by a focus on symptoms than by the patients' beliefs that they have a specific disease	Depressive disorder; anxiety disorder; other somatoform disorders	Cognitive-behavioral therapy; antidepressants; cognitive group therapy; stress management
Pain disorder	Symptoms of pain that are either solely related to or significantly exacerbated by psychosocial factors	Anxiety disorder; depressive disorder; substance dependence	Group therapy; family; cognitive-behavioral therapy; antidepressants; hypnosis
Body dysmorphic disorder	A false belief or exaggerated perception that a body part is defective	Major depression; obsessive-compulsive disorder; social phobia	Cognitive-behavioral therapy; antidepressants

and group therapy can increase awareness of communication and interaction patterns, help patients improve interpersonal communication, and learn strategies to improve social skills (Cely-Serrano & Floet, 2006). Nurses may be involved with teaching patients alternative coping skills (relaxation techniques, cognitive restructuring, and refocusing) to aid in controlling anxiety and reappraising thinking in an effort to better mediate their symptoms. Refer to Table 9-4 for a summary of the characteristics of somatoform disorders, their comorbidities, and specific therapeutic approaches that have the potential to improve the lives of these patients.

Pharmacological, Biological, and Integrative Therapies

Presently antidepressants, specifically the selective serotonin reuptake inhibitors, show the greatest promise for helping patients with somatoform disorders (Phillips et al., 2002; Stahl, 2003). Patients may also benefit from short-term use of antianxiety medication, which must be monitored carefully because of the risk of dependence. The nurse may administer these medications in certain settings, but teaching about the medication to patients and families is helpful in all settings.

EVALUATION

Evaluation of patients with somatoform disorders is a simple process when measurable behavioral outcomes have been written clearly and realistically. For these patients, nurses often find that goals and outcomes are only partially met. This should be considered a positive finding, because these patients often exhibit remarkable resistance to change. Patients are likely to report the continuing presence of somatic symptoms, but they often say that they are less concerned about the symptoms. Families are likely to report relatively high satisfaction with outcomes, even without total eradication of the patient's symptoms.

DISSOCIATIVE DISORDERS

Patients who have dissociative disorders routinely experience significant emotional pain and struggle with overall functioning and safety (Turkus & Kahler, 2006). Dissociative disorders are characterized by altered mind-body connections and are believed to be related to stress or anxiety. For dissociative patients, consciousness itself is altered in a dramatic way, whereas thinking, feeling, and perceptions are less impaired. These disorders can be quite severe.

We all dissociate. Fantasy, daydreaming, absorption in activities, and night dreaming are considered by dissociative theorists to be the four most common examples of non-pathological dissociation (Butler, 2006). For example, we say we are on "automatic pilot" when we drive home from work but cannot recall the last 15 minutes before reaching home. However, research shows that these common experiences are distinctly different from the processes of pathological dissociation (Simeon et al., 2001).

PREVALENCE AND COMORBIDITY

The actual **prevalence of dissociative disorders** in the general population is hard to know. However, Sar and associates (2007) report the results of a recent study in which the prevalence of dissociate disorders in general psychiatric settings can range from 5% to 20%, and between 12% and 29% among outpatients.

Dissociative processes and/or dissociative disorders often exist with patients who present at a psychiatric emergency department with self-harming behaviors (suicide or self-mutilation), addictions, eating disorders, "rapid cycling," mood changes, pseudoseizures, trauma-related flashbacks, and many other conditions. Often identification of the dissociative process goes undiagnosed by mental health clinicians who are not trained in dissociation or dissociative disorders (Chefetz, 2006). **Dissociative disorders can co-occur** with a wide range of other psychiatric disorders. Besides the disorders mentioned, potential dissociative processes may occur in posttraumatic stress disorder, profound body dysmorphic syndrome, borderline personality disorders, childhood sexual abuse, attention deficit problems, and others.

THEORY

The actual cause of dissociative disorders is unknown. However, childhood physical, sexual, or emotional abuse and other traumatic life events are associated with adult dissociative symptoms. Several factors related to etiology are reviewed in the following sections.

Biological Factors

Current research suggests that the limbic system is involved in the development of dissociative disorders. Traumatic memories are processed in the limbic system, and the hippocampus stores this information. Animal studies show that early prolonged detachment from the caretaker negatively affects the development of the limbic system. For humans, early trauma or detachment from the caregiver could impair memory processing, leading to dissociation (Kreidler et al., 2000). Significant early trauma and lack of attachment have also been demonstrated to have effects on neurotransmitters, specifically on serotonin.

Research indicates that people with dissociative identity disorder may have hippocampuses that are about 19% smaller and amygdalas that are about 32% smaller as compared with control subjects (Vermetten et al., 2006). The hippocampus is the part of the brain essential for memory and learning, and the amygdala regulates emotion.

Depersonalization disorder and dissociative fugue have a possible neurological link. Altered perceptions of self and fugue states occur with neurological diseases such as brain tumors and epilepsy, especially complex partial seizure disorder (Coons, 2000). Depersonalization is also experienced by individuals under the influence of certain drugs, such as alcohol, barbiturates, and hallucinogens (Steinberg, 2000a).

Genetic Factors

Several studies suggest that DID is more common among first-degree biological relatives of individuals with the disorder than in the population at large.

Psychosocial Factors

Learning theory suggests that dissociative disorders can be explained as learned methods for avoiding stress and anxiety. The pattern of avoidance occurs when an individual deals with an unpleasant event by consciously deciding not to think about it. The more anxiety-provoking the event, the greater the need not to think about it. The more this technique is used, the more likely it is to become automatically invoked as dissociation. When stress is intolerable—for example, in an abused child—the individual develops dissociation to defend against pain and the memory of it.

CULTURAL CONSIDERATIONS

Certain culturally bound disorders exist in which there is a high level of activity, a trancelike state, and running or fleeing, followed by exhaustion, sleep, and amnesia regarding the episode. These syndromes include *piblokto* seen in native people of the Arctic, Navajo *frenzy* witchcraft, and *amok* among western Pacific natives. These syndromes, if observed in individuals native to the corresponding geographical areas, must be differentiated from dissociative disorders.

CLINICAL PICTURE

At present, there is major debate and disagreement with the current *DSM-IV-TR* criteria as related to the status of dissociative disorders. *DSM-IV-TR* lists four major dissociative disorders: (1) depersonalization disorder, (2) dissociative amnesia, (3) dissociative fugue, and (4) DID, which are presented in this chapter. Refer to Figure 9-2 for the *DSM-IV-TR* diagnostic criteria for each disorder.

Depersonalization Disorder

The *DSM-IV-TR* describes **depersonalization disorder** as a persistent or recurrent alteration in the perception of the self while reality testing remains intact. The person experiencing depersonalization may feel mechanical, dreamy, or detached from the body. These experiences of feeling a sense of deadness of the body, of seeing oneself from a distance, or of perceiving the limbs to be larger or smaller than normal are described by patients as being very disturbing. In some cases, depersonalization may be preceded by severe stress; in other cases, there may be an association with childhood emotional abuse (Lowenstein & Putnam, 2005).

> **VIGNETTE**
>
> Margaret describes becoming very distressed at perceiving changes in her appearance when she looks in a mirror. She thinks that her image looks wavy and indistinct. Soon after, she describes feeling as though she is floating in a fog with her feet not actually touching the ground. Questioning reveals that Margaret's son has recently confided to her that he tested positive for HIV.

Dissociative Amnesia

Dissociative amnesia is marked by the inability to recall important personal information, often of a traumatic or stressful nature, that is too pervasive to be explained by ordinary forgetfulness. A patient with generalized amnesia is unable to recall information about his or her entire lifetime. The amnesia may also be localized (the patient is unable to remember all events in a certain period) or selective (the patient is able to recall some but not all events in a certain period).

DSM-IV-TR CRITERIA FOR DISSOCIATIVE DISORDERS

DISSOCIATIVE DISORDERS

Dissociative Amnesia*

1. One or more episodes of inability to recall important information — usually of a traumatic or stressful nature.

2. Causes significant distress or impairment in social, occupational, or other important areas of functioning.

*Not due to substance, medical, neurological, or other psychiatric disorder.

Dissociative Fugue*

1. Sudden, unexpected travel away from home or one's place of work with inability to remember past.

2. Confusion about personal identity or assumption of new identity.

3. Symptoms cause significant distress or impairment in social, occupational, or other important areas of functioning.

*Not due to substance, medical, neurological, or other psychiatric disorder.

Dissociative Identity Disorder* (DID)

1. Existence of two or more distinct subpersonalities, each with its own patterns of relating, perceiving, and thinking.

2. At least two of these subpersonalities take control of the person's behavior.

3. Inability to recall important information too extensive to be explained by ordinary forgetfulness.

*Not due to substance, medical, neurological, or other psychiatric disorder.

Depersonalization Disorder*

1. Persistent or recurrent experience of feeling detached from and outside of one's mental processes or body.

2. Reality testing remains intact.

3. The experience causes significant impairment in social or occupational functioning or causes marked distress.

*Not due to substance, medical, neurological, or other psychiatric disorder.

Figure 9-2 ■ Diagnostic criteria for dissociative disorders. (Adapted from American Psychiatric Association. [2000]. *Diagnostic and statistical manual of mental disorders* [4th ed., text rev.]. Washington, DC: Author.)

VIGNETTE

A young woman found wandering in a Florida park is partly dressed and poorly nourished. She has no knowledge of who she is. Her parents identify her 2 weeks later when she appears in an interview on a national television show. She had just broken up with her boyfriend of 3 years.

Dissociative Fugue

Dissociative fugue is characterized by sudden, unexpected travel away from the customary locale and inability to recall one's identity and information about some or all of the past. In rare cases, an individual with dissociative fugue assumes a whole new identity. During a fugue state, individuals tend to lead rather simple lives, rarely calling attention to themselves. After a few weeks to a few months, they may remember their former identities and become amnesic of the time spent in the fugue state. Usually a dissociative fugue is precipitated by a traumatic event.

VIGNETTE

A middle-aged woman awakens one morning and notices snow outside the window swirling around unfamiliar buildings and streets. The radio tells her it is December. She is perplexed to find herself in a residential hotel in Chicago with no idea of how she got there. She feels confused and shaken. As she leaves the hotel, she is surprised to find that strangers recognize her and say, "Good morning, Sally." The name Sally does not seem right, but she cannot remember her true identity. She finds her way to a hospital, where she is evaluated and referred to the psychiatric nurse in the emergency department. A day later, "Sally" is able to remember her true identity, Mary Hunt. She tells the nurse tearfully that she can now recall that her husband came home one day and "out of the blue" told her he wanted a divorce to marry a younger woman. Mary calls her sister in New York, who comes to Chicago to take her home.

Dissociative Identity Disorder

The essential feature of **dissociative identity disorder (DID)**, formerly known as multiple personality disorder, is the presence of two or more distinct personality states that recurrently take control of behavior. Each **alternate personality (alter), or subpersonality,** has its own pattern of perceiving, relating to, and thinking about the self and the environment. It is believed that severe sexual, physical, or psychological trauma in childhood predisposes an individual to the development of DID. One way to operationally define the steps in development of a dissociated identity was theorized by McAllister (2000):

1. The child being harmed by a trusted caregiver splits off the awareness and memory of the traumatic event to survive in the relationship.
2. The memories and feelings go into the subconscious and are experienced later as a separate personality.
3. This process happens repeatedly at different times so that different personalities develop, containing different memories and performing different functions that are helpful or destructive.
4. Dissociation becomes a coping mechanism for the individual when faced with further stressful situations.

Each alternate personality, or subpersonality, is a complex unit with its own memories, behavior patterns, and social relationships that dictate how the person acts when that personality is dominant. Often the original or primary personality is religious and moralistic, and the subpersonalities are pleasure seeking and nonconforming. The alters may behave as individuals of a different sex, race, or religion. The dominant hand and the voice may be different; intelligence and electroencephalographic findings also may be altered. Subpersonalities often exhibit signs of emotional disturbance: common ones are a fearful child and a persecutor who inflicts pain and may try to kill the individual.

Typical **cognitive distortions** include the insistence that alternate personalities inhabit separate bodies and are unaffected by the actions of one another. The primary personality or host is usually not aware of the subpersonalities and is perplexed by lost time and unexplained events. Experiences such as finding unfamiliar clothing in the closet, being called a different name by a stranger, or not having childhood memories are characteristic of DID. Subpersonalities are often aware of the existence of each other to some degree. Transition from one personality to another occurs during times of stress and may range from a dramatic to a barely noticeable event. Some patients experience the transition when awakening. Shifts may last from minutes to months, although shorter periods are more common.

VIGNETTE

Andrea, a conservative 28-year-old electrical engineer, is the primary personality. Three alternate personalities coexist and vie for supremacy:

- Michele is a 5-year-old who is sometimes playful and sometimes angry. She speaks with a slight lisp and with the facial expressions, voice inflections, and vocabulary of a precocious child. She likes to play on swings, draw with a crayon, and eat ice cream. She likes to cuddle a teddy

continued

bear and occasionally sucks her thumb. Her favorite outfit is jeans and a Mickey Mouse sweatshirt.

- Ann is an accomplished ballet dancer. She is shy but firm about needing time to practice. When she is dominant, she likes to wear white and fixes her hair in a severe, pulled-back style. She does little but dance when she is in control.
- Bridget is near Andrea's age, although she says a lady never tells her age. She dresses seductively in bright colors, wears her hair tousled, and likes to frequent bars and stay out late. She often drinks to excess and has several male admirers. Bridget has many moods. She states that she would like to get rid of Ann and Andrea because they're such "goody-goodies."

Andrea does not drink, hates ice cream, and sees herself as somewhat awkward. She does not dance. She is a paid soloist in a church choir. Andrea takes public transportation,

but Ann and Bridget have driver's licenses. Andrea goes to bed and arises early, but Bridget and Michele like to stay up late.

Andrea seeks treatment when she finds herself behind the wheel of a moving car and realizes that she does not know how to drive. She has been concerned for some time because she has found strange clothes in her closet. She has also received phone calls from men who insist that she has flirted with them in bars. She sometimes misses appointments and cannot account for periods of time. Although she goes to bed early, she is often unaccountably tired in the morning.

The student is encouraged to see the classic film *Sybil* (1976), which is an actual case study of a person with DID, or *The Three Faces of Eve* (1957).

EXAMINING THE EVIDENCE   Proving Multiple Personality Disorder

How do we know that people actually have multiple personalities?

There is, in fact, a significant controversy over the diagnosis of dissociative identity disorder (DID), which was first included as multiple personality disorder in the second edition of the *Diagnostic and Statistical Manual (DSM-II)* in 1968. *Sybil* was a hugely popular book and film in the 1970s about a woman who suffered unspeakable and horrendous psychological and physical abuse at the hands of her mother. She survived this abuse by dissociating into 16 alter personalities and spent years in therapy to reintegrate into her core personality. This story paved the way for an explosion of multiple personality disorder diagnoses in the 1980s. Since that time, there have been allegations that Sybil's symptoms were a result of suggestions made by her therapist.

Scientific interest in DID appears to be waning. A systematic review of the literature for the years 1984-2003 by Pope, Berry, Bodkin, and Hudson (2006) revealed that scholarly publications involving DID peaked in the mid-1990s and fell off sharply thereafter to only 25% of the peak years. The authors concluded that these disorders are not widely accepted in the scientific community. The reasons for this lack of acceptance include difficulty in diagnosing, scant support that childhood

trauma actually causes DID, the rarity of childhood cases of DID, and charges of iatrogenesis (i.e., conditions brought forth or suggested by the healer).

Less than 40% of psychiatrists in the United States support DID's inclusion in the *DSM*, and nearly 70% question it as a valid diagnosis (Escobar, 2004). Yet some scholars and mental health professionals continue to affirm the existence of DID. Bolstering this belief are reports that there is measurable evidence of pathology in people with DID. Vermetten and colleagues (2006) describe observable differences in brain structure, specifically in reduced amygdalar and hippocamapal volume, in individuals with DID. Alters have been found to have unique cardiovascular responses and cerebral blood flow patterns (Reinders et al., 2006).

Understanding this complex constellation of symptoms is imperative as we provide care and treatment for people who are subjected to significant childhood trauma. Empirical research and expert opinion will provide support for both sides of the DID controversy. As our diagnostic procedures and understanding of neurochemistry, brain structure, and brain function becomes increasingly sophisticated, perhaps we'll know if Sybil was one talented actress or the unwilling host to 16 unique personalities and biological responses.

Escobar, J.I. (2004). Transcultural aspects of dissociative and somatoform disorders. *Psychiatric Times, 21*(5).

Pope, H.G., Barry, S., Bodkin, A., & Hudson, J.I. (2006). Tracking scientific interest in the dissociative disorders: A study of scientific publication output 1984-2003. *Psychotherapy and Psychosomatics, 75,* 19-24.

Reinders, A.A.T.S., Nijenhuis, E.R.S., Ouak, J., et al. (2006). Psychobiological characteristics of dissociative identity disorder: A symptom provocation study. *Biological Psychiatry, 60*(7), 730-740.

Vermetten, E., Schmahl, C., Lindner, S., et al. (2006). Hippocampal and amygdalar volumes in dissociative identity disorder. *American Journal of Psychiatry, 163,* 630-636.

Application of the Nursing Process

ASSESSMENT

Medical Workup

In order for one of the dissociative disorders to be diagnosed, medical and neurological illnesses, substance use, and other coexisting psychiatric disorders must be ruled out or identified as coexisting with a dissociative disorder. Medical personnel collect objective data from physical examination, electroencephalography, imaging studies, projective tests, structured personality tests, and specific questionnaires designed to identify dissociative symptoms, such as the *Structured Clinical Interview for DSM-IV Dissociative Disorders—Revised (SCID-D-R)* (Brand et al., 2006).

Identity and Memory

Assessing patients' ability to identify themselves requires more than asking patients to state their names. Changes in patient behavior, voice, and dress might signal the presence of an alternate personality. Referring to self by another name or in the third person and using the word *we* instead of *I* are indications that the patient may have assumed a new identity. The nurse should consider the following when assessing memory:

- Can the patient remember recent and past events?
- Is the patient's memory clear and complete or partial and fuzzy?
- Is the patient aware of gaps in memory, such as lack of memory for events such as a graduation or a wedding?
- Do the patient's memories place the self with a family, in school, in an occupation?

Patients with amnesia and fugue may be disoriented with regard to time and place as well as person. Relevant assessment questions include the following:

- Do you ever lose time or have blackouts?
- Do you find yourself in places with no idea how you got there?

Patient History

The nurse must gather information about events in the person's life. Has the patient sustained a recent injury, such as a concussion? Does the patient have a history of epilepsy, especially temporal lobe epilepsy? Does the patient have a history of early trauma, such as physical, mental, or sexual abuse? If DID is suspected, pertinent questions include the following:

- Have you ever found yourself wearing clothes that you can't remember buying?

- Have you ever had strange people greet and talk to you as though they were old friends?
- Does your ability to engage in things such as athletics, artistic activities, or mechanical tasks seem to change?
- Do you have differing sets of memories about childhood?

Mood

Is the individual depressed, anxious, or unconcerned? Many patients with DID seek help when the primary personality is depressed. The nurse also observes for mood shifts. When subpersonalities of DID take control, their predominant moods may be different from that of the principal personality. If the subpersonalities shift frequently, marked mood swings may be noted.

Use of Alcohol and Other Drugs

Specific questions should be asked to identify drug or alcohol use. Dissociative episodes may be associated with recent use of alcohol or other substances—cocaine, opioids, sedatives, or stimulants (Steinberg, 2000b).

Effect on Patient and Family

Has the patient's ability to function been impaired? Have disruptions in family functioning occurred? Is secondary gain evident? In fugue states, individuals often function adequately in their new identities by choosing simple, undemanding occupations and having few intimate social interactions. The families of patients in fugue states report being highly distressed over the patient's disappearance. Patients with amnesia may be more dysfunctional. Their perplexity often renders them unable to work, and their memory loss impairs normal family relationships.

Families often direct considerable attention toward the patient but may exhibit concern over having to assume roles that were once assigned to the patient. Patients with DID often have both family and work problems. Families find it difficult to accept the seemingly erratic behaviors of the patient. Employers dislike the lost time that may occur when subpersonalities are in control. Patients with depersonalization disorder are often fearful that others may perceive their appearance as distorted and may avoid being seen in public. If they exhibit high anxiety, the family is likely to find it difficult to keep relationships stable.

Suicide Risk

Whenever a patient's life has been substantially disrupted, he or she may have thoughts of suicide. The nurse gathering data should be alert for expressions of hopelessness, help-lessness, or worthlessness and for verbalization or other behavior of a subpersonality that indicates the intent to engage in self-destructive or self-mutilating behaviors.

Assessment Guidelines

Dissociative Disorders

1. Assess for a history of a similar episode in the past with benign outcomes.
2. Establish whether the person suffered abuse, trauma, or loss as a child.
3. Identify relevant psychosocial distress issues by performing a basic psychosocial assessment. (See Chapter 5 for information on the basic psychosocial assessment.)

DIAGNOSIS

Nursing diagnoses for patients with dissociative disorders are suggested in Table 9-5.

OUTCOMES IDENTIFICATION

Outcomes must be established for each nursing diagnosis. General goals are to develop trust, correct faulty perceptions, and encourage the patient to live in the present instead of dissociating (Kreidler et al., 2000). NOC outcomes potentially appropriate for patients with dissociative disorders include *Identity, Role Performance, Coping, Anxiety Self-Control, Self-Mutilation Restraint,* and *Aggression Self-Control* (Moorhead, 2008). Specific examples of indicators that the outcomes are being achieved include the following:

- Patient will verbalize clear sense of personal identity.
- Patient will report decrease in stress (using a scale of 1-10).
- Patient will report comfort with role expectations.
- Patient will plan coping strategies for stressful situations.
- Patient will refrain from injuring self.

PLANNING

The planning of nursing care for the patient with a dissociative disorder is influenced by the setting and presenting problem. Nurses may encounter such a patient in times of crisis either in the emergency department or when the patient is admitted to the hospital for suicidal or homicidal behavior. The care plan will focus on safety and crisis intervention. The patient also may seek treatment of a comorbid depression or anxiety disorder in the community setting. Planning will address the major complaint with appropriate referrals for treatment of the dissociative disorder.

IMPLEMENTATION

Most of the time the DID patient is treated in the community. However, a patient with DID is admitted to a psychiatric unit when suicidal or in need of crisis stabilization. At that time, the nurse gathers specific information

---

TABLE 9-5   Potential Nursing Diagnoses for Dissociative Disorders

Signs and Symptoms	Nursing Diagnoses
• Amnesia or fugue related to a traumatic event	*Disturbed personal identity*
• Symptoms of depersonalization; feelings of unreality or body image distortions	*Disturbed body image*
• Alterations in consciousness, memory, or identity	*Ineffective coping*
• Abuse of substances related to dissociation	*Ineffective role performance*
• Disorganization or dysfunction in usual patterns of behavior (absence from work, withdrawal from relationships, changes in role function)	
• Disturbances in memory and identity	*Interrupted family processes*
• Interrupted family processes related to amnesia or erratic and changing behavior	*Impaired parenting*
• Feeling of being out of control of memory, behaviors, and awareness	*Anxiety*
• Inability to explain actions or behaviors when in altered state	*Spiritual distress*
	Risk for other-directed violence
	Risk for self-directed violence
• Obsessive fear of contracting or having a serious or terminal illness	*Death anxiety*

TABLE 9-6	Interventions for Dissociative Disorders

Intervention	Rationale
1. Ensure patient safety by providing safe, protected environment and frequent observation.	1. Sense of bewilderment may lead to inattention to safety needs; some subpersonalities may be thrill seeking, violent, or careless
2. Provide nondemanding, simple routine.	2. Reduces anxiety
3. Confirm identity of patient and orientation to time and place.	3. Supports reality and promotes ego integrity
4. Encourage patient to do things for self and make decisions about routine tasks.	4. Enhances self-esteem by reducing sense of powerlessness and reduces secondary gain associated with dependence
5. Assist with other decision making until memory returns.	5. Lowers stress and prevents patient from having to live with the consequences of unwise decisions
6. Support patient during exploration of feelings surrounding the stressful event.	6. Helps lower the defense of dissociation used by patient to block awareness of the stressful event
7. Do not flood patient with data regarding past events.	7. Memory loss serves the purpose of preventing severe to panic levels of anxiety from overtaking and disorganizing the individual
8. Allow patient to progress at own pace as memory is recovered.	8. Prevents undue anxiety and resistance
9. Provide support during disclosure of painful experiences.	9. Can be healing while minimizing feelings of isolation
10. Accept patient's expression of negative feelings.	10. Conveys permission to have negative or unacceptable feelings
11. Teach stress reduction methods.	11. Provides alternatives for anxiety relief

about identity, memory, consciousness, life events, mood, suicide risk, and the effect of the disorder on the patient and the family.

Communication Guidelines

Nurses can offer emotional presence during the recall of painful experiences, provide a sense of safety, and encourage an optimal level of functioning. Table 9-6 offers examples of interventions for patients with dissociative disorders.

Health Teaching and Health Promotion

Patients with dissociative disorders need teaching about the illness and instruction in coping skills and stress management. They may need to develop a plan to interrupt a dissociative episode, such as singing or doing a specific activity. Staff and significant others are made aware of the plan in order to foster their cooperation. Patients need to keep a daily journal to increase their awareness of feelings and to identify triggers to dissociation. If a patient has never written a journal, the nurse should suggest beginning with a 5- to 10-minute daily writing exercise.

Milieu Therapy

When the patient is in a crisis that requires hospitalization, providing a safe environment is fundamental. Other desirable characteristics include that the environment be quiet, simple, structured, and supportive. Confusion and noise increase anxiety and the potential for depersonalization, delayed memory return, or shifts among subpersonalities. Task-oriented therapy or occupational and art therapy can be useful for these patients if used in isolation from one another.

Psychotherapy

Psychotherapy has been proven to be the primary and most effective treatment modality in dissociative identify disorder patients (Lowenstein & Putnam, 2005). Therapists who treat this population need special training in dissociation. Turkus and Kahler (2006) state that therapy needs to be very flexible. From their years of experience they found applying specific techniques within an overall psychodynamic framework effective. Such techniques include psychoeducation, "talking through," traumatic reenactment, safety planning, journaling, and artwork.

APPLYING THE ART   A Person with Dissociative Disorder

SCENARIO: Last week I noticed 25-year-old Sammy restlessly reading a magazine while she waited for her teenage brother to finish his outpatient psychotherapy with the advanced practice nurse. Today she again made eye contact with me, and she looked like she'd been crying. I offered her a tissue as I sat near her in the waiting area, empty except for the receptionist at the far end.

THERAPEUTIC GOAL: By the end of this interaction, Sammy will express at least one indication that she is ready to access help for feelings related to trauma.

Student-Patient Interaction	Thoughts, Communication Techniques, and Mental Health Nursing Concepts
Student: "Hi. We've smiled at each other before. I'm _____ a nursing student from _____. May I sit with you while you wait?" **Student's feelings:** *I remember her. Who would think that smiling and making eye contact could open a nurse-patient interaction a week later.*	Even though this relationship hasn't been planned, the *contract* sets boundaries. I'll need to let her know about confidentiality as soon as possible.
Sammy: *Nods and takes the tissue.* "I'm Samantha, 'Sammy,' here with my 14-year-old brother. Sometimes I wonder if I'm not the one who should be seeing someone. But I need to be the strong one."	
Student: "I've found that sometimes a person still qualifies as 'the strong one' yet lets it be okay to get a little help along the way." **Student's feelings:** *It's frustrating that mental illness still carries so many stigmas.*	I chose *restatement* because her words "the strong one" are significant to her self-esteem.
Sammy glances at me, holding eye contact 1 or 2 seconds.	
Student's feelings: *I hope I didn't push that too much. I keep thinking about my friend who almost waited too long to get help. Good timing that my clinical teacher made rounds just now.*	I need to think HIPAA (patient confidentiality, Heath Insurance Portability and Accountability Act) at all times.
Sammy: "I've sort of been a mother to my brother his whole life. When he was born I was just starting middle school."	
Student: "You really care about your brother. I want to listen, but let's move to that side room so the receptionist can still see you to tell us when your brother's done." *We move and the receptionist lets my instructor know where I am.*	I use *reflection* and *offer self*. The patient can't feel safe if I don't, so I stay in visual range and let my instructor know where I am.
Sammy: *Doodles on scrap paper as she talks.* "I don't know what I'd do if anything ever happened to my brother. He's only 14, you know." **Student's feelings:** *I feel that way about my family, too.*	
Student: "That's the second time you've told me he's only 14. His age seems important to you."	I use *validation*. Is her brother's age a *theme*?
Sammy: *Eyes widen.* "Fourteen is how old I was when my dad left for good."	

APPLYING THE ART   A Person with Dissociative Disorder—cont'd

Student-Patient Interaction	Thoughts, Communication Techniques, and Mental Health Nursing Concepts
Student: "You still remember how rough that time was." ***Student's feelings:*** *Sad. So young to lose her dad.*	Using *reflection* shows *empathy*.
Sammy: "Yeah. My 'nice' mom turned into a mean and bitter mom. I tried to help her all I could, especially after we lost the house and had to move."	
Student: "That must've been scary to lose your dad, your home, and your 'nice' mom all at once." ***Student's feelings****: I feel overwhelmed just thinking about all she lost when just a young teen.*	I use *reflection* and *restatement*. "Loss" is definitely a *theme*. I wonder to what extent she's been able to work through the *grief process*.
Sammy: "First, I lost my 'nice' mom, then last year she really dies and Billy moved into my apartment." *Eyes tearing.* "He just couldn't handle everything and started messing up and getting in fights at school." ***Student's feelings:*** *No wonder Billy had trouble.*	I remember that *depression* may manifest as irritability in teens.
Student: "You say your mother really died. Sounds like you believe part of her died long before last year." ***Student's feelings:*** *My mother loves me, and I know this even when we argue. I need to keep tuning into Sammy.*	I use *restatement*.
Sammy avoids eye contact. Suddenly her doodles become purposeful as she now draws with dark lines.	
Student: "What are you drawing?"	I use an *open question* as Sammy's attention turns to the drawing.
Sammy: *Silently draws a simple house. She gives only one of the windows a shade, which she darkens with forceful scribbles.*	
Student: "Sammy, you seem upset. I am concerned about what you are going through. Talk a little about what is going on with you." ***Student's feelings:*** *Whatever is going on, I feel Sammy's intensity. I hope I can handle this.*	Her *anxiety level* starts to escalate. I *reflect* then assess with an *open question*.
Sammy: "It was in that room." *She points to the picture of the closed window shade.* "I'm just . . ." *Sobs, wrings her hands, and breathes rapidly.* ***Student's feelings:*** *Should I stop and go get my teacher? I don't want to interrupt the process. I'm scared of what's happening but others are nearby. I can get help. I'm not alone.*	Is she having an *abreaction*?
Student: "I'm _____. I'm right here with you, Sammy."	I *offer self*.
Sammy: *Suddenly rapidly looks around over each shoulder.* "Don't make me do that! Please, Mommy! Make him stop touching there." *She holds her cheek like she's just been slapped, then whimpers.*	She is hyperventilating, *hypervigilent*, and appears not aware of her present environment. She seems to be escalating into *severe levels of anxiety*. I think she's reliving something awful that she had *dissociated*. Is this a *flashback*?

Continued

APPLYING THE ART   A Person with Dissociative Disorder—cont'd

Student-Patient Interaction	Thoughts, Communication Techniques, and Mental Health Nursing Concepts
Student: "Sammy, you are a grownup now. You are safe here at the clinic. No one can hurt you like that now." *I wait quietly while leaning toward her.* **Student's feelings:** *I don't know if I'm saying the right things but I have to try.*	I use *attending behavior.*
Sammy: *Sobs loudly, then cries, then looks up and breathes more slowly.* "I feel like I want to vomit. I'm scared. I don't want to think about that ever again! What's happening to me?" *Wringing hands.* **Student's feelings:** *Something sexual happened. I feel like I could vomit, too. Was she forced to have oral sex?*	Could she have *posttraumatic stress disorder?*
Student: "I don't know for sure, but it seems like you recovered a memory from a time when you were younger. Something terribly hurtful happened." **Student's feelings:** *I really feel for Sammy.*	I *give information* and use *reflection.*
Sammy: *Nods, cries softly.* "I've always felt so dirty. My mom had lots of boyfriends. One of them . . . maybe more than one of them . . . it's just too awful." *Shudders.* **Student's feelings:** *I feel furious at Sammy's mother!*	How would a nurse be able to intervene therapeutically if Sammy's mother were the patient? What about if the perpetrator were the patient? Would I be able to care about either of them? Could I be therapeutic?
Student: "You are safe now. You're in charge of you. You decide how much, if, and when you feel ready to visit those memories."	I remember that working through *repressed dissociated trauma* takes a long, painful time.
Sammy: "I've always felt different from other women, like I'm not good enough. I should've been strong enough to stop it." **Student's feelings:** *I grieve for her. She was raped. Probably repeatedly. Imagine how terrified and powerless a young girl would feel.*	I remember that sometimes women who are raped blame themselves so they at least feel some sense of control. In other words, the trauma won't happen again if only I do this or don't do that.
Student: "Whatever happened when you were a child was not your fault. You did the best you could. These feelings are left over from your childhood when you felt powerless." **Student's feelings:** *I so want to make this all better and I can't! I believe all I've said but I must not overdo or I'm reassuring rather than supporting her. This is not about me; I cannot protect her. I can support her to empower herself.*	*Support* is therapeutic while *reassurance* is nontherapeutic like I'm trying to talk her into something. She'll feel like it's not okay to say and feel whatever she needs to feel. I think interspersing rather than saying all that at once would be better.
Sammy: "I can't handle all this."	
Student: "You don't have to handle it alone. Let me get my instructor. She works here part-time." **Student's feelings:** *We got through the deeply emotional part. I'm relieved, but ready for my instructor's help.*	I think it is okay for me to briefly leave Sammy. My teacher knows all the resources here at the clinic.
Sammy nods. I ask the receptionist to page my instructor.	

APPLYING THE ART   A Person with Dissociative Disorder—cont'd

Student-Patient Interaction	Thoughts, Communication Techniques, and Mental Health Nursing Concepts
Student: "That took courage to let some of your feelings out."	
Sammy: *Shudders.* "I have a lot more stuff where that came from." *She manages a small smile at me.* "I guess I was assaulted or something." *Looks to me as though checking my reaction.*	Her anxiety level is returning to *mild.*
Student: "I'm so sorry for all this pain in your life." *I wait.* **Student's feelings:** *She needs my nonjudgmental acceptance.*	I show *empathy.*
Sammy nods, stifles a sob.	
Student: "I see strength in you. You are here helping your brother and somehow coping with all this in your life despite such trauma." **Student's feelings:** *I really feel she's pretty amazing. I don't know if I'd do so well, though I know this is only the beginning of all she has to go through as she heals.*	*Offering support* and *making an observation.*
Sammy: *Surprised.* "I guess I am. Thanks. It really helps to talk." *She breathes deeply and stops crying.*	
My instructor comes, and after a while Sammy agrees to see an advanced practice nurse-psychotherapist and maybe later a group for adult survivors of child sexual abuse.	A *group for survivors* could really help Sammy find meaning and support from others with similar trauma.
Sammy: "I feel worn out."	
Student: "No wonder! Sammy, you took some giant steps today. It's exhausting to feel so much, so intensely." **Student's feelings:** *I probably shouldn't have said "no wonder." But really—no wonder!*	I give *support* and use *reflection* again. I think these are becoming my favorites.
Sammy: "Yes. Thanks."	
Student: "Thank you." **Student's feelings:** *I'd like to work with her again, but the work she has to do requires an advanced practice nurse. Still, I helped her connect with help, and that feels good!*	

Pharmacological, Biological, and Integrative Therapies

There are no specific medications for dissociative disorders, but appropriate antidepressants or anxiolytic medications are given for comorbid conditions. Substance use disorders and suicidal risk, which are common, must be assessed carefully if medication is to be used. In the acute setting, the nurse may witness dramatic memory retrieval in patients with dissociative amnesia or fugue after treatment with intravenous benzodiazepines (Ballew et al., 2003).

EVALUATION

Treatment is considered successful when outcomes are met. In the final analysis, the evaluation is positive when:

- Patient safety has been maintained
- Anxiety has been reduced and the patient has returned to a functional state
- Conflicts have been explored

- New coping strategies have permitted the patient to function at a better level
- Stress is handled adaptively, without the use of dissociation

KEY POINTS TO REMEMBER

- Somatoform disorders are characterized by the presence of multiple, real physical symptoms for which there is no evidence of medical illness.
- Dissociative disorders involve a disruption in consciousness with a significant impairment in memory, identity, or perceptions of self.
- The emergence of somatoform and dissociative symptoms are believed to be responses to psychological stress, although the patient shows no insight into the potential stressors.
- Patients with somatoform and dissociative disorders often have a number of comorbid psychiatric illnesses, primarily depression, anxiety, and substance abuse, as well as many others.

- The course of these disorders may be brief, with acute onset and spontaneous remission, or chronic, with a gradual onset and prolonged impairment.
- Because these patients may not seek psychiatric treatment, the nurse does not usually see them in the acute psychiatric setting, except during a period of crisis such as suicidal risk.
- The nursing assessment is especially important to clarify the history and course of past symptoms, as well as to obtain a complete picture of the current physical and mental status.
- Although these patients do respond to crisis intervention, they usually require referral for psychotherapy to attain sustained improvement in level of functioning.

CRITICAL THINKING

1. A patient with suspected somatization disorder has been admitted to the medical-surgical unit after an episode of chest pain with possible electrocardiographic changes. While on the unit, she frequently complains of palpitations, asks the nurse to check her vital signs, and begs staff to stay with her. Some nurses take her pulse and blood pressure when she asks. Others evade her requests. Most staff try to avoid spending time with her. Consider why staff wish to avoid her. Design interventions to cope with the patient's behaviors. Give rationales for your interventions.
2. A patient with body dysmorphic disorder talks incessantly about how big her nose is, how those around her are offended

by her appearance, and how her appearance has negatively affected her employment and her social life. What interventions could you make to reduce her anxiety?
3. A patient with DID has been admitted to the crisis unit for a short-term stay after a suicide threat. On the unit, the patient has repeated the statement that she will kill herself to get rid of "all the others," meaning her subpersonalities. The patient refuses to sign a "no harm" contract. Design a care plan to meet her safety and security needs.

CHAPTER REVIEW

Choose the most appropriate answer(s).
1. Nurses working with patients with somatization and dissociative disorders can expect that these patients will fit on the continuum of psychobiological disorders at the:
    1. mild level.
    2. moderate to severe level.
    3. severe to psychotic level.
    4. They do not belong on the continuum, because anxiety has been reduced by ego defense mechanisms.
2. Mr. R. presents with a history of having assumed a new identity in a distant locale. He has no recollection of his former identity. Which *DSM-IV-TR* diagnosis can the nurse expect the psychiatrist to make?

1. Hypochondriasis
2. Conversion disorder
3. Dissociative fugue
4. Depersonalization disorder

3. When considering a diagnosis of a somatoform disorder, which information, among the four types below, is *least* likely to require detailed assessment by the nurse?
    1. Patient's level of ability to voluntarily control symptoms
    2. Results of patient's diagnostic laboratory tests
    3. Patient's limitations in carrying out activities of daily living
    4. Patient's potential for violent behavior

CHAPTER REVIEW—cont'd

4. Nurse S. is developing outcome criteria with her patient, who has a nursing diagnosis of *Ineffective coping*. The diagnosis is related to the patient's dependence on pain relievers to treat chronic pain of psychological origin. Which of the following are appropriate outcome criteria?
   1. Patient will resume performance of work role behaviors.
   2. Patient will identify ineffective coping patterns.
   3. Patient will make realistic appraisal of strengths and weaknesses.

4. Patient will make realistic appraisal of family's capacity to be involved in decision making.
5. Which sign or symptom would be *least* likely to occur for a patient with hypochondriasis?
   1. Impairment in occupational functioning
   2. Repetitive, time-consuming rituals
   3. Misinterpretation of physical sensations
   4. Loss of interest in formerly pleasurable activities

REFERENCES

American Psychiatric Association. (2000). *Diagnostic and statistical manual of mental disorders (DSM-IV-TR)* (4th ed., text rev.). Washington, DC: Author.

American Psychiatric Association. (2002). Consumer and family information: Hypochondriasis. *Psychiatric Services, 53*(4), 383.

Ballew, L, Morgan, Y., & Lippmann, S. (2003). Intravenous diazepam for dissociative disorder: Memory lost and found. *Psychosomatics, 44,* 346-347.

Barsky, A.J. (2001). The patient with hypochondriasis. *New England Journal of Medicine, 345*(19), 1395-1399.

Brand, B.L., Armstrong, J.G., & Lowenstein, R.J. (2006). Psychological assessment of patients with dissociative identity disorders. *Psychiatric Clinics of North America, 29*(1), 145-168.

Butler, L.D. (2005). Normative dissociation. *Psychiatric Clinics of North America, 29*(1), 45-62.

Calabrese, L., & Stern, T.A. (2004) The patient with multiple physical complaints. In T.A. Stern, J.B. Herman, & P.L. Slavin (Eds.), *Massachusetts General Hospital Guide to Primary Care Psychiatry* (2nd ed.) New York: McGraw-Hill.

Carroll, D.H., Scahill, L., & Phillips, K.A. (2002). Current concepts in body dysmorphic disorder. *Archives of Psychiatric Nursing, 16*(2), 72-79.

Cely-Serrano, M.S., & Floet, A.M.W. (2006). *Somatoform disorder: Hypochondriasis.* Retrieved July 5, 2007, from www.emedicine.com/ped/topic2911.htm.

Chefetz, R.A. (2006). Why should you read these articles on dissociative processes?. *Psychiatric Clinics of North America, 29*(1), xv-xxiii.

Coons, P.M. (2000). Dissociative fugue. In B.J. Sadock & V.A. Sadock (Eds.), *Comprehensive textbook of psychiatry* (7th ed., vol. 1, pp. 1549-1552). Philadelphia: Lippincott Williams & Wilkins.

Guggenheim, F.G. (2000). Somatoform disorders. In B.J. Sadock & V.A. Sadock (Eds.), *Comprehensive textbook of psychiatry* (7th ed., vol. 1, pp. 1504-1532). Philadelphia: Lippincott Williams & Wilkins.

Hollifield, M.A. (2005). Somatoform disorders. In B.J. Sadock & V.A. Sadock (Eds.), *Comprehensive textbook of psychiatry* (8th ed., vol. 1, pp. 1800-1828). Philadelphia: Lippincott Williams & Wilkins.

Kreidler, M.C., Zupancic, M.K., & Bell, C. (2000). Trauma and dissociation: Treatment perspectives. *Perspectives in Psychiatric Care, 36*(3), 77-85.

Kroenke, K., & Rosmalen, J.G.M. (2006). Symptoms, syndromes, and the value of psychiatric diagnostics, in patients who have functional somatic disorders. *Medical Clinics of North America, 90,* 603-626.

Lowenstein, R.J., & Putnam, R.W. (2005). Dissociative disorders. Dissociative identity disorder. In B.J. Sadock & V.A. Sadock (Eds.), *Comprehensive textbook of psychiatry* (8th ed., vol. 1, pp. 1844-1901). Philadelphia: Lippincott Williams & Wilkins.

McAllister, M.M. (2000). Dissociative identity disorder: A literature review. *Journal of Psychiatric and Mental Health Nursing, 7,* 25-33.

Moorhead, S., Johnson, M., Maas, M.L., & Swanson, E. (2008). *Nursing outcomes classification (NOC)* (4th ed.). St. Louis: Mosby.

Noyes, R., Stuart, S., Langbehn, D.R., et al. (2002). Childhood antecedents of hypochondriasis. *Psychosomatics, 43*(4), 282-289.

PsychCentral. (2007). New hope for body image disorder. Retrieved June 30, 2007, from http://psychcentral.com/news/2007/06/29/new-hope-for-body-image-disorder.

Phillips, K.A., Albertini, R.S., & Rasmussen, S.A. (2002). A randomized placebo-controlled trial of fluoxetine in body dysmorphic disorder. *Archives of General Psychiatry, 59,* 381-388.

Rief, W., Buhlmann, U., Wilhelm, S., et al. (2006). The prevalence of body dysmorphic disorder: A population-based survey. *Psychological Medicine, 36,* 877-885.

Roelofs, K., Keijsers, G.P., Houduin, K.S., et al. (2002). Childhood abuse in patients with conversion disorder. *American Journal of Psychiatry, 159*(11), 1908-1913.

Sar, V., Lpuimca. A., Ozturk, E., et al. (2007). Dissociative disorders in the psychiatric emergency ward. *General Hospital Psychiatry, 29,* 45-50.

Simeon, D., Guralnik,O., Schmeidler, J., et al. (2001). The role of childhood interpersonal trauma in depersonalization disorder. *American Journal of Psychiatry, 158*(7), 1027-1033.

Stahl, S.M. (2003). Antidepressants and somatic symptoms: Therapeutic actions are expanding beyond affective spectrum disorders to functional somatic syndromes. *Journal of Clinical Psychiatry, 64*(7), 745-746.

Steinberg, M. (2000a). Depersonalization disorder. In B. J. Sadock & V. A. Sadock (Eds.), *Comprehensive textbook of psychiatry* (7th ed., Vol. 1, pp. 1564-1570). Philadelphia: Lippincott Williams & Wilkins.

Steinberg, M. (2000). Dissociative amnesia. In B.J. Sadock & V.A. Sadock (Eds.), *Comprehensive textbook of psychiatry* (7th ed., vol. 1, 1544-1549). Philadelphia: Lippincott Williams & Wilkins.

Taylor, S., Thordarson, D., Jang, K.L., & Asmundson, G.J.G. (2006). Genetic and environmental origins of health anxiety: A twin study. *World Psychiatry, 5*(1), 47-50.

Turkus, J.A., & Kahler, J.A. (2006). Therapeutic interventions in the treatment of dissociative disorders. *Psychiatric Clinics of North America, 29,* 245-262.

Vermetten, E., Schmahl, C., Lindner, S., et al. (2006). Hippocampal and amygdalar volumes in dissociative identity disorder. *American Journal of Psychiatry, 163,* 630-636.

CHAPTER 10

Personality Disorders

Elizabeth M. Varcarolis

Key Terms and Concepts

Objectives

1. Identify four characteristics that people with personality disorders share.
2. Describe comorbid conditions that are often present in people with a personality disorder.
3. Give some examples of primitive or immature defenses.
4. Compare and contrast the behaviors seen in borderline personality disorder and narcissistic personality disorder.
5. Understand some of the feelings that are experienced by health care professionals when working with a person with a personality disorder.
6. Identify four communication guidelines when working with a manipulative patient.
7. Identify four communication guidelines when working with a patient who has impulsive behaviors.

evolve

For additional resources related to the content of this chapter, visit the Evolve website at http://evolve.elsevier.com/Varcarolis/essentials.

- Chapter Outline
- Chapter Review Answers
- Case Studies and Nursing Care Plans

- Nurse, Patient, and Family Resources
- Concept Map Creator

Edited by Nancy Christine Shoemaker in the fifth edition of
Foundations of Psychiatric Mental Health Nursing.

Personality is essentially the "style" of how a person deals with the world. Personality traits then are stylistic peculiarities that all people bring to social relationships, including traits such as shyness, seductiveness, rigidity, or suspiciousness (Groves, 2004). In people with a **personality disorder (PD)**, these traits are exaggerated to the point that they cause dysfunction in their relationships (Groves, 2004).

People with PDs present the most complex, difficult behavioral challenges for themselves and people around them. In the health care community a "difficult patient" is almost always an individual with a PD, which is also among the most frequently treated disorders by psychiatrists (Zimmerman et al., 2005), although the initial focus of treatment is usually a co-occurring symptom or disorder. Personality disorders range from mild to severe.

The *DSM-IV-TR* classifies personality disorders as Axis II diagnoses (along with mental retardation). It also defines a PD as:

An enduring pattern of inner experience and behavior that deviates markedly form the expectations of he individual's culture, is pervasive and inflexible, has an onset in adolescent or early adulthood, is stable over time and leads to distress or impairment.

All people with PDs share common characteristics:
- *Inflexible and maladaptive responses to stress.* Individuals have difficulty responding flexibly and adaptively to the environment and to the changing demands of life. They often are unable to cope with stress and react by using maladaptive behaviors, which exposes the disorder.
- *Disability in working and loving, which is generally more serious and pervasive than the similar disability found in other disorders.* Individuals with PDs assume that everyone thinks and functions as they do; therefore, within relationships, they do not see their behavior as a problem, nor do they see a need to make changes or accommodate others. They believe that they are normal and that others have a problem. This thinking leads to problems with self-concept, relationships, and ability to function in society. Although some individuals with PDs may desire closer relationships with others, some of the reasons personal and work relationships often fail are:
  - Avoidance and fear of rejection
  - Blurring of boundaries between the self and others so that closeness seems to lead to fusion, which may terrify both parties
  - Insensitivity to the needs of others
  - Demanding and fault finding
  - Inability to trust

- Lack of individual accountability
- *The tendency to evoke intense interpersonal conflict.* Because people with PDs fail to see themselves objectively, and they lack the desire to alter aspects of their behavior to enrich or maintain important relationships. Relationships are often marked by intense emotional upheavals and hostility that lead to serious interpersonal conflict, and in some cases violence (self-violence or violence toward others).
- *Capacity to "get under the skin" of others.* People with PDs often have an uncanny ability to merge personal boundaries with others, which has an intense and undesirable effect on others.

People with PDs do suffer. Their relationships with others are problematic, and they rarely reach their potential. They are often socially isolated because of their rigidity, maladaptive coping skills, and control issues that complicate their interactions with society. These patients can act bizarre, anxious, withdrawn, manipulative, or violent, and their behaviors tend to alienate them from the population. Because they are unaware that their personalities cause problems, they often blame others for their difficulties or even deny they have a problem.

PREVALENCE AND COMORBIDITY

According to results of the 2001-2003 National Epidemiological Survey on Alcohol and Related Conditions, an estimated 14.8% met the standard diagnostic criteria for at least one PD as defined by the *Diagnostic and Statistical Manual of Mental Disorders* (fourth edition, text revision; *DSM-IV-TR*) (Bender, 2004). Excluded from the study were borderline, schizotypal, and narcissistic PDs, which are to be included in another phase of the study. Surprisingly, obsessive-compulsive disorder was the most common of the seven disorders surveyed, with an occurrence of 7.9%; then came paranoid PD at 4.4%; third was antisocial PD at 3.6%. Others were schizoid (3.1%), avoidant (2.4%), histrionic (1.8%), and dependent (0.5%). Data from the APA (2000) put the prevalence of borderline PD in clinical setting from 10% to 20%. There do not seem to be data for the prevalence of schizoid or schizotypal personality disorder (APA, 2000).

A number of PDs are associated with significant emotional disability as well as problems with social functioning and occupational impairment, in particular avoidant, dependent, paranoid, schizoid, and antisocial. Interestingly, many people with obsessive-compulsive disorder seem to be high functioning, with no correlation to high disability.

Co-occurring Disorders

Personality disorders often co-occur with other PDs, other Axis I disorders (e.g., substance abuse, somatization, eating disorders, posttraumatic stress disorder [PTSD], depression, anxiety disorders), or with general medical conditions. Because most people with PDs do not believe there is anything wrong with them and that problems with their lives are caused by outside people or events, they rarely come into treatment for their disorder alone. Most often the disorder is not the initial focus of treatment. Zimmerman and colleagues (2005) state that PDs should be evaluated in all psychiatric patients because their presence can influence the course and treatment of an Axis I disorder or a medical disorder for which the patient sought help initially.

THEORY

It is unlikely that there is any single cause for a discrete PD. Personality traits and their exaggerations are probably largely caused by a combination of hereditary temperamental traits and environmental and developmental events. The contribution of genetic, biological, and environmental factors will vary with each specific disorder. The personality traits are thought to be present from infancy but in most cases, it is not until adolescence that the disorder emerges.

Genetic Factors

PDs have historically been considered to be environmentally mediated. However, research is beginning to support a more dominant role of genetics. In a study of 128 pairs of twins who were raised apart, identical twins were found to have more similar personality traits than fraternal twins (Markon et al., 2002).

Genetics seem to play a significant role in the development of schizotypal personality disorder, schizoid personality disorder, and paranoid personality disorder, which are more common in families with a history of schizophrenia. Obsessive-compulsive personality disorder seems to have a genetic link as well. A family history of antisocial PD increases the risk of a person developing this condition.

Neurobiological Factors

More recent work with brain imaging studies suggest abnormalities in prefrontal, coricostriatal, and limbic networks that may be related to lowered serotonin neurotransmission and behavioral disinhibition in people with borderline personality disorder (BPD) (Oldham, 2005).

Psychological Influences

Childhood abuse and trauma seem to be influential in the development of all PDs; neglect seems to be particularly damaging. Childhood trauma may be a risk factor for antisocial personality disorder; those with the disorder often have histories of excessively harsh or erratic discipline, alcoholic parent(s), or an abusive or chaotic home life.

People who have borderline personality disorder frequently were raised in families in which they were subject to constant belittling, devaluation, and invalidation (Linehan, 1995). There is consistent evidence that sexual abuse is a common risk factor for borderline PD, which also may entail significant parental conflict or loss. If the history of sexual abuse was before the age of 13, PTSD also may be part of the picture.

Cultural Considerations

It appears that certain subgroups of the population are at a greater risk than others for certain PDs (Bender, 2004). For example, Native Americans are 1.6 times as likely to have avoidant PDs as whites. African Americans, Native Americans, and Hispanics are at greater risk for paranoid PD than are whites. In general, other risk factors include being Native American or African American, being a young adult, having low socioeconomic status, and being divorced, separated, widowed, or never married.

CLINICAL PICTURE

Figure 10-1 presents the *DSM-IV-TR* grouping of **personality disorder clusters**.

DSM-IV-TR Cluster A Disorders— Odd or Eccentric Behavior

Cluster A disorders, often referred to as "odd" or "eccentric," comprise those PDs that have been established to have some relationship to schizophrenia. Of the Cluster A disorders, schizotypal is the most strongly related to schizophrenia. Individuals with Cluster A disorders avoid interpersonal relationships, have unusual beliefs, and may be indifferent to the reactions of others in their lives. People with these disorders come into the health care system either because of a comorbid disorder, or for a brief psychotic episode. They refuse responsibility of their own feelings and assign responsibility to others. Prominent features for the following disorders are listed and illustrated by the vignettes.

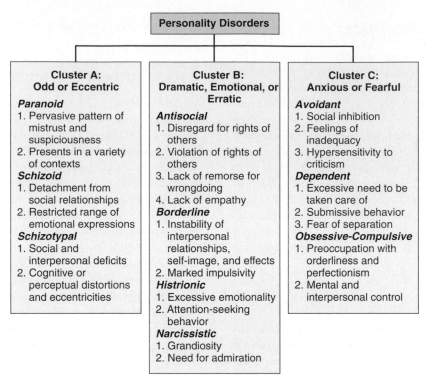

Figure 10-1 ■ Clusters of personality disorders. (Adapted from American Psychiatric Association. [2000]. Personality disorders. In *Diagnostic and statistical manual of mental disorders* [4th ed., text rev., pp. 685-729]. Washington, DC: Author.)

Paranoid Personality Disorder

People with **paranoid personality disorder** traits are not strangers to the health care system. Nurses encounter people who are hostile, irritable, angry, injustice collectors, pathologically jealous of partner, and litigious cranks. Often these people are the ones with paranoid PD (Sadock & Sadock, 2004). They lack warmth, pay close attention to power and rank, and express disdain to those who are weak, sickly, and impaired. Although they may appear business-like and efficient, they often generate fear and conflict in others (Sadock & Sadock, 2004). They are constantly suspicious of the intentions of others, and often project their own fears and intentions onto others. They usually make others uncomfortable, and are keenly aware of the weaknesses of others and exploit these weaknesses in order to keep interpersonal distance. Grace Sills used to say these people "lack the milk of human kindness."

The following are characteristics of paranoid PD:

- Belief that others are lying, cheating, exploiting, or trying to harm them
- Perception of hidden malicious meaning in benign comments
- Inability to work collaboratively with others
- Emotionally detached
- Hostility toward others

VIGNETTE

Mr. Cole, a 58-year-old, comes into the emergency department (ED) with chest pains. He refuses to give background information "because the information could be used against me," and is haughty and demeaning to the nurse saying, "Get someone in here who knows something." When the nurse turned her back to Mr. Cole to speak to the doctor, Mr. Cole shouted, "What lies is she telling you about me? What kind of hole is this?"

Schizoid Personality Disorder

People with a **schizoid personality disorder** are seen by others as eccentric, isolated, or lonely. They may exist on the periphery of society, avoiding relationships of even the most superficial nature. Although they invest no interest or energy into human relationships of any kind, they may invest enormous energy into nonhuman interests such as mathematics and astronomy, and be much attached to animals. Although aloof, some may conceive, develop, and give the world genuinely original, creative ideas.

The following are characteristics of schizoid PD:

- Neither desires nor enjoys human relationships
- Fixated on personal thoughts; fantasizes
- Shows emotional coldness, detachment, flattened affect

- Appears indifferent to praise or criticism
- Most always chooses solitary activities.

Mr. Sed is a 38-year-old unmarried bookkeeper. He was mugged on his way home from work. A bystander called 911 and he was taken to the ED unconscious. Once awake, he answers in mono-syllables never making eye contact. When spoken to he often looks away and does not respond. He was compliant, and remained a passive recipient of his treatment once he got to the ED. He rejects all nursing interventions aimed at increasing socialization.

Schizotypal Personality Disorder

People with **schizotypal personality disorder** exhibit markedly strange behavior. They most closely resemble people with schizophrenia. These patients may have magical thinking and rituals, or hold beliefs that they can control the actions of others. Their speech is peculiar in phrasing and syntax and may have meaning only to them. Reactions of confusion to their apparent illogical speech by others may cause them to become suspicious of others. Their eccentric and unkempt behaviors and inattention to social conventions make it impossible for them to have give-and-take conversations. People with this disorder are unhappy about their lack of relationships, and their social anxiety and unhappiness just increase over time. Under stress these individuals may have brief psychotic symptoms.

The following are characteristics of schizotypal PD:

- Behavior or appearance that is odd, eccentric, or peculiar
- Odd elaborate style of dressing, speaking, and inter-acting with others
- "Magical thinking," odd beliefs and ideas of reference
- Unusual perceptual experiences
- Lack of close friends and confidants
- Excessive and unrelieved social anxiety frequently associated with paranoid fears

Ms. Sands is 36 years old, lives alone, and is a "writer" on social security benefits. She goes out every night, only at night, to a nearby grocery store (because "their magic does not work at night"). She dresses in several layers of multicolored and mis-matched clothes even in warmer weather. She wears a turban on her head to "keep them from seeing my thoughts." Each night she tells the grocer in a flat and formal manner that she is going to be a famous director and star. She knows this because "it hasn't snowed yet, and that means the coast is clear."

DSM-IV-TR Cluster B Disorders— Dramatic, Emotional, or Erratic

The four disorders in this cluster appear to share dramatic, erratic, or flamboyant behaviors as part of their presenting symptoms. There is a great deal of overlapping among these disorders as well as comorbidity with Axis I disorders (e.g., substance abuse, depression, eating disorders). People with these PDs are more apt to be seen in the health care system It may be through attempted suicide and affective distress (borderline individuals) or though the courts (antisocial individuals). **Manipulation** is a common defensive mecha-nism among these disorders, and it is always challenging no matter what part of the health care system is caring for their needs.

Antisocial Personality Disorder

Antisocial personality disorder is characterized by deceit, manipulation, revenge, and harm to others with an absence of guilt or anxiety. People with antisocial PD have a sense of **entitlement**, which means they believe they have the right to hurt others, take what they want, treat others unfairly, destroy the property of others, and so on. They do not adhere to traditional values or standards of morality as boundaries for their actions. Therefore, there is no restraint on their behavior with any assumption of guilt, remorse, or responsibility for their actions. However, they do count on others to conform to the social norms. Verbally these patients may be charming, engaging, and uncanny in their ability to find just the right angle to lure a person into their intrigue with the intent to exploit them for money, favors, or more sadistic purposes. Promiscuity, partner abuse, child abuse, and drunk driving are common events in their lives.

The following are characteristics of antisocial PD:

- Chronic irresponsibility and unreliability
- Lack of regard for the law and the rights of others
- Persistent lying and stealing
- Deceitfulness, use of alias, conning others for personal profit or pleasure
- Lack of remorse for hurting others
- Reckless disregard for safety of self or others

Mr. Jones has been extorting money from lonely widows by charming them, "helping them with their finances," promising to marry them, and then taking off with their money. When in court, he laughed when he was asked if he felt guilty for taking their life savings. "Hey, I gave them what they wanted." Fingerprints revealed that his name was really Oliver Torres, and he had a history of assaults, burglary, and abandoning his wife and child 4 years previous.

Borderline Personality Disorder

Central to people with **borderline personality disorder** is their characteristic instability of affect, lack of a sense of identity, and instability in relationships. Feelings of anxiety, dysphonia, and irritability can be intense though short lived. Chronic depression is common. Linehan (1995) refers to the pattern of high emotional sensitivity, acute responsiveness, and slow return to normal as "emotional dysregulation." This cycle may lead to feelings of deadness, panic, and fury. *Self-mutilation* and *suicide-prone behaviors* are responses to threats of separation or rejection; unfortunately, suicide is a significant risk in these patients.

Other self-destructive behaviors include such things as impulsive gambling, substance abuse, engaging in unsafe sex, driving recklessly, and binge eating. Psychosis-like symptoms are possible under periods of stress. These patients experience overwhelming needs, both internal and external, that they seek to have met in relationships, but their excessive demands, unstable anger, and impulsive behavior result in driving people away. A major defense mechanism is **splitting**. This idealizing then devaluing the same person results in unstable and difficult interpersonal relationships. People with this disorder have little tolerance of being alone and intense fear of abandonment.

The following are characteristics of borderline PD:
- Difficulty controlling emotions
- Stormy relationships involving intense anger and possibly physical fights
- Identity disturbance, markedly and persistently unstable self-image
- Frantic efforts to avoid real or perceived abandonment
- Frequent dramatic changes in mood, opinions, and plans
- Chronic feelings of emptiness
- Impulsive self-damaging behaviors
- Recurrent suicide attempts or self-mutilation

VIGNETTE

Mrs. Kit is twice divorced and has been hospitalized several times for suicidal ideation and self-injury. She comes in for therapy session. Her nurse therapist is leaving for a 2-week vacation and has been preparing Mrs. Kit for the separation for weeks. Mrs. Kit comes in with fresh razor marks on her arms and tells the nurse that she is quitting therapy because the nurse really doesn't like her anyway, and she might as well kill herself. "Go, have a good time; I might not be here when you get back." She then storms out of the office, and refuses to answer the phone all day long.

Histrionic Personality Disorder

Patients with **histrionic personality disorder** are dramatic, charming, flamboyant, and excessively emotional in order to seek the constant attention, love, and admiration that they require. They may act out with displays of temper, tears, and accusations when they are not getting the attention or praise they believe they deserve. Interactions are often characterized by a seductiveness or provocation in order to draw others into a relationship or work project, but then their attention is usually short lived. Their relationships tend to be superficial and shallow. Histrionic people lack insight as to their roles in why their relationships do not last. They may seek treatment for depression or another comorbid condition.

The following are characteristics of histrionic PD:
- Attention grabbing through self-dramatization and exaggerated expressions of emotion
- Use of sexually provocative clothing and behavior
- Excessive concern with physical appearance
- Extremely sensitive to others' approval
- False sense of intimacy with others
- Constant sudden emotional shifts
- Speech may be impressionistic and lack detail

VIGNETTE

Ms. Todd, a 45-year-old, meets her therapist, Dr. Jim, for the fist time dressed in a tight top and short skirt and wearing a lot of makeup. She becomes flirtatious with him and tells Dr. Jim that she wants extra time today because her story is so long and she is most likely more interesting than his other patients. When he reiterates the terms of the contract and reminds her that they have 20 minutes remaining in today's session to discuss her issues, she becomes angry and insulting and tells him he better admit her to the hospital right now because she is going to commit suicide if he doesn't.

EXAMINING THE EVIDENCE   Are Personality Disorders Treatable?

I heard one of the nurses refer to a patient as borderline. When she did so, she sort of rolled her eyes. What's the deal?

People with personality disorders (PDs) lead lives that are filled with uncertainty and overanalysis; simple interactions can create tremendous emotional turmoil. These Axis II diagnosed individuals meet with even more stigma and prejudice than do Axis I diagnosed individuals (e.g., major depression, anxiety, schizophrenia). This is likely because of a perception that these problems are within personal control, even more so than are Axis I problems (Halter, 2004). Health care providers get frustrated by what seems to be nothing more than "bad behavior." Practitioners may be reluctant to take them on as patients because of their marked inability to get along with others, an inability that not surprisingly extends to therapists (Dingfelder, 2004). Further, therapists often consider such work as futile. Insurance companies have been reluctant to reimburse care for PDs, citing a lack of empirical evidence that shows it is helpful (Kersting, 2004).

This is beginning to change as researchers demonstrate that PDs can improve, either on their own as a function of maturation (Lenzenweger et al., 2004), and discover effective pharma-

cological and psychological treatment (Dingfelder, 2004). Investigations using molecular genetics are particularly promising in our understanding of PDs (Howland, 2007). Genetic variation has been implicated in stress responsiveness, that is, how strongly a person responds to a difficult life event. Researchers also have identified links between Axis I and Axis II disorders (e.g., psychotic disorders and Cluster A personality disorders) that may suggest medication strategies.

The most researched treatment is dialectical behavior therapy (DBT) for the most commonly treated personality disorder, borderline personality disorder (BPD) (Dingfelder, 2004). It involves replacing extremes of emotion and behavior with more moderate responses. DBT is particularly useful for nurses to help improve adaptive coping strategies in people with BPD (Osborne & McComish, 2006). Linehan (1993), the originator of DBT, has developed a manual with handouts and assignments to address self-awareness, interpersonal skills, emotional regulation, and learning to tolerate distress. Patients are encouraged to record their progress on diary cards, and nurses can help by reviewing the cards. Students are encouraged to access the 2006 Osborne and McComish article listed in the references if they are working with patients with BPD.

Dingfelder, S.F. (2004). Treatment for the "untreatable." *APA Online: Monitor on Psychology.* Available at www.apa.org/monitor/mar04/treatment.html.

Halter, M.J. (2004). The influence of stigma on help seeking for depression. *Archives of Psychiatric Nursing, 18*(5), 178-184.

Howland, R.H. (2007). Pharmacotherapy in personality disorders. *Journal of Psychosocial Nursing, 45*(6), 15-19.

Kersting, K. (2004). Axis II gets short shrift. *APA Online: Monitor on Psychology.* Available at www.apa.org/monitor/mar04/axis.html.

Lenzenweger, M.F., Johnson, M.D., & Willett, J.B. (2004). Individual growth curve analysis illuminates stability and change in personality disorder features: The longitudinal study of personality disorders. *Archives of General Psychiatry, 61,* 1015-1024.

Linehan, M. (1993). *Skills training manual for treating borderline personality disorder.* New York: Guilford.

Osborne, L.L., & McComnish, J.F. (2006). Working with borderline personality disorder: Nursing interventions using dialectical behavioral therapy. *Journal of Psychosocial Nursing and Mental Health Services, 44*(6), 40-49.

Narcissistic Personality Disorder

Narcissistic personality disorder is a maladaptive social response characterized by a person's grandiose sense of personal achievements. People with this disorder consider themselves special and expect special treatment. Their demeanor is arrogant and haughty and their sense of entitlement is striking. They lack empathy for the needs or feelings of others and in fact exploit others to meet their own needs. At times, people who have narcissistic PD are admired and envied by others for what appears to be a rich and talented life. However, they require this admiration in greater and greater quantities. On the other hand, they often envy others their successes or possession, believing that it is they that deserve the admiration and privileges more. Because of their fragile self-esteem, they are prone to depression, interpersonal difficulties, occupational problems, and rejection

(Sadock & Sadock, 2004). Common characteristics of narcissistic people are manipulation (splitting), tantrums, and arrogance with sadistic and often paranoid tendencies.

The following are characteristics of narcissistic PD:

- Inflated sense of importance, achievements, and talents
- Constant attention-grabbing and admiration-seeking behaviors
- Manipulation of others for personal gain
- No regard for the feelings or situations of others
- Behaving in an arrogant and haughty manner toward others
- Unreasonable expectation for special treatment or compliance with wishes
- Often envious of others and believes others are envious of him or her

DSM-IV-TR Cluster C Disorders— Anxious or Fearful Behaviors

The common feature of the Cluster C disorders is the experience of high levels of anxiety and outward signs of fear. These personalities also show social inhibitions mostly in the sexual sphere (e.g., shy and awkward with potential sexual partners, impotence, or frigidity). They are often fearful and reluctant to express irritation and anger with others even when it is justified. People with these disorders (avoidant, dependent, and obsessive-compulsive) are inhibited and tend to internalize blame for the frustration in their lives, even when they are not to blame. This is directly opposed to paranoid, antisocial, borderline, and narcissistic personalities who tend to blame others.

Avoidant Personality Disorder

People with **avoidant personality disorder** are very sensitive to rejection and avoid situations that require socialization. They have a strong desire for affection and acceptance but are fearful of disappointment and criticism. Unlike schizoid PD, they are openly distressed by their isolation and their difficulty relating to others, and unlike borderline PD, they do not respond with anger to rejection, but rather withdraw. Virtually all people with avoidant PDs have social phobias.

The following are characteristics of avoidant PDs:

- Hypersensitive to criticism or rejection
- Self-imposed social isolation
- Preoccupation with being criticized or rejected in social situations
- Strongly desires close relationships, but shies away for fear of being shamed or ridiculed
- Avoids occupational activities that involve significant interpersonal contact
- View themselves as socially inept, personally unappealing, or inferior to others

Obsessive-Compulsive Personality Disorder

People with **obsessive-compulsive personality disorder** are preoccupied with orderliness, perfectionism, control, neatness, and the achievement of perfection. They are cautious and weigh everything in a methodical and inflexible manner. They are obsessed with rules and details and follow them rigidly. They are often unable to make decisions and may have trouble completing tasks. They are high achievers and do well in the sciences and intellectually demanding fields that require attention to detail.

They often have a very formal demeanor, lack a sense of humor, and have limited interpersonal skills. Although they are excessive in verbosity, these patients are miserly with material goods and emotions. They are uncomfortable with their feelings, relationships, and situations they cannot control or in which events are unpredictable. Even though they may have deep and genuine affection for others, their intimacy in relationships is superficial and rigidly controlled. Unlike people with the Axis I anxiety disorder or obsessive-compulsive disorder (OCD), people with this disorder do not display unwanted obsessions and ritualistic behavior.

The following are characteristics of obsessive-compulsive PD:

- Preoccupation with details, rules, lists, order, or organization to the point that the purpose of the activity may be lost
- Perfectionism often so pronounced that tasks cannot be completed
- Inability to share responsibility with others
- Devotion to work may exclude pleasurable activities and friendships
- Financial stinginess
- Inability to throw out even broken, worthless objects
- Discomfort with emotions and aspect of personal relationships that the person cannot control

Mike is a 45-year-old middle manager for a microchip company. He works late, and sometimes on the weekends, avoiding social and recreational activities. He has a need to get everything done to perfection, which has pushed back the deadline on many projects. He has had some heartburn now for a month, and his wife has been insisting he see a doctor. He tells her when this project is finished he will go but hates to "waste" his money on doctors. In the doctor's office he says he does not have time to take a treadmill test. When the doctor tells him that he cannot tell him what is wrong with him until he gets all the test results, Mike gets very anxious.

Dependent Personality Disorder

People with a **dependent personality disorder** believe that they are incapable of survival if left alone. They solicit caretaking by clinging and being perversely and excessively submissive. By early adulthood, these people perceive themselves as being unable to separate from others, work independently, or function at all on their own. If others do not initiate or take responsibility for them, their needs remain neglected. Their intense fear of being alone is so great that they tolerate poor, even abusive treatment in order to stay in a relationship, and once a relationship ends, there is an urgent need to get into another.

They may obsessively ruminate and fantasize about abandonment even when it is not threatened.

The patient with a dependent PD is at greater risk for anxiety and mood disorders, and this disorder can occur with borderline, avoidant, and histrionic PDs. This condition commonly occurs in individuals who have a general medical condition or disability that requires them to be dependent on others.

The following are characteristics of a dependent PD:

- Difficulty making everyday decisions without excessive advice and reassurance
- Others assume responsibility for most major areas of a PD person's life

Mr. Collins, 48 years old, has lived with his mother since high school. His mother cooks, cleans, and shops for him. He works as a shipping dock clerk and has had the job for 30 years. He even has to ask his mother's advice on what to wear each day for work. He has become extremely anxious and fearful because his mother has to have an operation and will be away for 5 days. He is terrified that he cannot cope without her there to care for him.

- Fear of disagreeing with others for fear of loss of support or approval
- Preoccupied with fear of being left alone; exaggerated fears of not able to care for self

Application of the Nursing Process
ASSESSMENT
Primitive Defenses

People with personality disorders often tend to behave in outrageous and troublesome behaviors because they are unable to use the higher-level defense mechanisms most of us use to modulate painful feelings and channel needs or aggression into creative outlets; ambivalence is poorly tolerated and impulse control is dismal (Groves, 2004). "Normal people," or at least those who live full and satisfying lives amid the inevitable personal crises and environmental negative surprises that seem to dot life, have at their disposal a variety of higher-level defense mechanisms that they use to help them through such events and eventually move on with their lives. The "ego weakness" of people with PDs relies on more immature or primitive defenses (e.g., splitting, dissociation, psychotic denial). (See Chapter 8 for definitions of immature or primitive defenses.)

These intense and outrageous behaviors are thought to arise from intense affect, distorted cognitions, and inadequate or primitive defenses (Groves, 2004). Figure 10-2 identifies the unmodulated affects (rage, envy, shame), some of the challenging behaviors, and the cognitive processes that contribute to the behaviors. To add to the difficulties, personal boundaries are often blurred in many people with PDs. Closeness can seem like fusion and the boundaries where one person begins and where one leaves off are blurred. Needs are experienced as rage, and sexuality and dependency are confused with aggression (Groves, 2004).

The intense and inappropriate behaviors that characterize the lives of people with PDs tend to uproot their relationships in all settings, and are no less disruptive in the health care setting. These primitive defenses are an attempt to control their inner chaos.

For nurses, clinicians, and other health care workers, much of the challenge is dealing with many of the PD defenses and **behaviors.** This is especially true with those of the borderline and antisocial PD because nurses deal with them most often in all medical settings.

The *DSM-IV-TR* presented the first overreaching definition of personality disorders; however, after data from studies and clinical experience have become available, it is

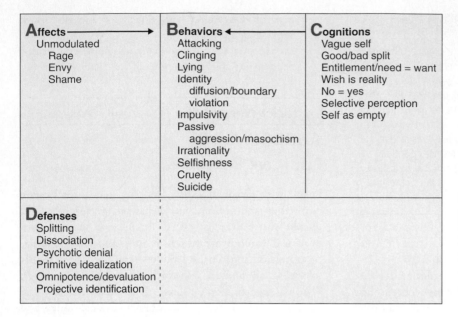

Figure 10-2 ■ ABCs of difficult patients' problem behaviors: how troublesome behaviors arise. (From Groves, J.E. [2004]. Personality disorders I: Approaches to difficult patients. In T.A. Stern, J.B. Herman, & P.E. Slavin [Eds.], *Massachusetts General Hospital guide to primary care psychiatry* [2nd ed.]. New York: McGraw-Hill.)

felt by many that the definitions are poorly validated. Even borderline and antisocial PDs, which are the most valid categories, contain controversies. Personality disorders are difficult to diagnose; people with these disorders present complicated problems, and their response to psychotherapy and medication is unpredictable (Paris, 2006). Paris also states that some of the personality disorders—specifically schizotypal and avoidant personality disorders—might belong on Axis I (Mental Disorders) and not Axis II (Personality Disorders).

Another more recent finding is that many of the problematic symptoms and behaviors may decline over time (McGlashan et al., 2005). However, Paris (2006) states that even when people stop meeting the *DSM* criteria, their functional scores do not change. They continue to have serious problems. In their study, McGlashan and colleagues (2005) concluded that PDs appear to be a combination of stable traits (personality traits), and less stable symptomatic behaviors that vary over time. Therefore it is concluded that sets of criteria are key to defining PDs, one set highlighting personality and the other set highlighting the disorder. Most likely there will be a five-factor dimensional model of personality added to the *DSM-V,* scheduled to publish in 2011.

Assessment Tools

Several structured interview tools are used to diagnose PDs. These tools are not used in all clinical settings because of the need for lengthy interviews (2 hours or longer) and evaluation.

Assessment of History

Taking a full medical history can help determine if the problem is psychiatric, medical, or both. Medical illness should never be ruled out as the cause for problem behavior until the data support this conclusion. Important issues in assessment for PDs include the following: a history of suicidal or aggressive ideation or actions, current use of medicines and illegal substances, ability to handle money, and legal history.

Important areas about which further details must be obtained include current or past physical, sexual, or emotional abuse and level of current risk of harm from self or others. At times, immediate interventions may be needed to ensure the safety of the patient or others. Information regarding prior use of any medication, including psychopharmacological agents, is important. This information gives evidence of other contacts the patient has made for help and indicates how the health care provider found the patient at that time.

Self-Assessment

Finding an approach for helping patients with PDs who have overwhelming needs can be overwhelming for caregivers. The intense feelings evoked in the nurse often mirror the feelings being experienced by the patient. Caregivers may feel confused, helpless, angry, and frustrated. These patients tell the nurse that they are inadequate, incompetent, and abusive of authority and are often successful in using splitting behaviors with the staff by praising or disparaging the nurse to peers in such a way that the peers begin to react negatively. Usually this is the peer's attempt to defend against his or her own feelings of frustration and powerlessness, but the result is that substantial conflict can ensue in the treatment team.

Nurses and other health care workers should practice self-health management. This includes acknowledging and accepting their own emotional responses, and attempting to ensure personal well-being (Haas et al., 2005).

Assessment Guidelines

Personality Disorders

1. Assess for suicidal or homicidal thoughts. If these are present, the patient will need immediate attention.
2. Determine whether the patient has a medical disorder or another psychiatric disorder that may be responsible for the symptoms (especially a substance use disorder).
3. View the assessment about personality functioning from within the person's ethnic, cultural, and social background.
4. Ascertain whether the patient experienced a recent important loss. PDs are often exacerbated after the loss

of significant supporting people or in a disruptive social situation.
5. Evaluate for a change in personality in middle adulthood or later, which signals the need for a thorough medical workup or assessment for unrecognized substance use disorder.
6. Be aware of the strong negative emotions these patients may evoke in you.

DIAGNOSIS

People with PDs are usually admitted to psychiatric institutions because of symptoms of comorbid disorders, dangerous behavior, or a court order for treatment. Borderline as well as antisocial PDs present a challenge for health care providers. Because the behaviors central to these disorders often cause disruption in psychiatric and medical-surgical settings, nursing care is emphasized. Emotions such as anxiety, rage, and depression and behaviors such as withdrawal, paranoia, and manipulation are among the most frequent that health care workers need to address. See Table 10-1 for common potential nursing diagnoses.

TABLE 10-1 Potential Nursing Diagnoses for Personality Disorders	
Signs and Symptoms	**Nursing Diagnoses**
Crisis, high levels of anxiety	*Ineffective coping*
Anger and aggression; child, elder, or spouse abuse	*Risk for other-directed violence*
	Ineffective coping
	Impaired parenting
	Disabled family coping
Withdrawal	*Social isolation*
Paranoia	*Fear*
	Disturbed sensory perception
	Disturbed thought processes
	Defensive coping
Depression	*Hopelessness*
	Risk for suicide
	Self-mutilation
	Chronic low self-esteem
	Spiritual distress
Difficulty in relationships, manipulation	*Ineffective coping*
	Impaired social interaction
	Defensive coping
	Interrupted family processes
	Risk for loneliness
Failure to keep medical appointments, late arrival for appointments, failure to follow prescribed medical procedure or medication regimen	*Ineffective therapeutic regimen management*
	Noncompliance

OUTCOMES IDENTIFICATION

Realistic goal setting comes from the perspective that personality change happens one behavioral solution and one learned skill at a time. This can be expected to take much time and repetition. No matter how intelligent they may appear or how insightful they can be about themselves and others, these patients find that change is slow and occurs via trial and error with the support of affect management and much interpersonal reinforcement—no shortcuts occur. In permanent change the learning can be integrated at the cellular level, which means that by the time they come for help, these patients may have already seen several caregivers and are likely to take whatever the nurse or counselor can give and then move on to the next caregiver. Theirs is a long and circuitous road, and the nurse is their most recent attempt to find healing.

Because larger steps are not realistic, outcomes need to be very modest and obtainable. For some individuals, overall outcome criteria might include:

- Minimizing self-destructive or aggressive behaviors
- Reducing the effect of manipulating behaviors
- Linking consequences to functional as well as dysfunctional behaviors
- Practicing the substitution of functional alternatives during a crisis
- Initiating functional alternatives to prevent a crisis
- Practicing ongoing management of anger, anxiety, shame, and happiness
- Creating a lifestyle that prevents regressing

PLANNING

Basically, patients with PDs do not voluntarily seek treatment. People with antisocial and borderline PDs are, however, frequently seen in health care settings for other reasons, and manifestations of both these disorders can cause a disruption for the nurse, staff, or system in which they are seen.

IMPLEMENTATION

It is often difficult to create a therapeutic relationship with patients with PD. Because most have experienced a series of interrupted therapeutic alliances, their suspiciousness, aloofness, and hostility can be a setup for failure. The guarded and secretive style of these patients tends to produce an atmosphere of combativeness. When patients blame and attack others, the nurse needs to understand the context of their complaints; these attacks spring from feeling threatened, and the more intense the complaints, the greater the fear of potential harm or loss.

Lacking the ability to trust, patients require a sense of control over what is happening to them. Giving them choices—whether to come to a clinic appointment in the morning or afternoon, for example—may enhance compliance with treatment. Because these individuals are hypersensitive to criticism yet have no strong sense of autonomy, the most effective teaching of new behaviors builds on their own existing skills.

When people with PDs exhibit fantasies that attribute malevolent intentions to the nurse or others, it is important to orient them to reality. They need to know that even though they have insulted or threatened their caregiver, they will still be helped and protected from being hurt. When they are hurt by others, as naturally happens in everyday life, the nurse takes time to dissect the situation with them, asking when, where, and how it happened, and honestly maps out for them how people, systems, families, and relationships work. It is important to be honest about their limitations and assets. The patient may already be aware of them, but acknowledging them demonstrates trustworthiness.

Communication Guidelines

People with PDs may be excessively dependent, demanding, manipulative, or stubborn, or they may self-destructively refuse treatment (Haas et al., 2005). Nurses greatly enhance their ability to be therapeutic when they combine limit-setting, trustworthiness, dealing with manipulations, and authenticity with their own natural style. People with borderline PD are impulsive (e.g., suicidal, self-mutilating), aggressive, manipulative, and even psychotic under periods of stress. People with antisocial PD most often are seen in the health care systems through court order. They are also manipulative, aggressive, and impulsive.

Refer to Table 10-2 for interventions for manipulation and Table 10-3 for interventions for impulsive behaviors.

Milieu Therapy

Individuals with PDs may at times be treated within a therapeutic milieu: inpatient, partial hospital, or day treatment settings. The primary therapeutic goal of milieu therapy is affect management in a group context. Community meetings, problem-solving groups, coping skills groups, and socializing groups are all areas in which patients can interact with peers, discuss relationship problems, delegate and take responsibility for certain tasks, discuss goals, collectively deal with problems that arise in the milieu, and learn problem-solving skills.

Through desensitization via social group experience, overwhelming and painful internal states can be felt and

TABLE 10-2   Interventions for Manipulation

Intervention	Rationale
1. Assess your own reactions toward patient. If you feel angry, discuss with peers ways to reframe your thinking to defray feelings of anger.	1. Anger is a natural response to being manipulated. It is also a block to effective nurse-patient interaction.
2. Assess patient's interactions for a short period before labeling as manipulative.	2. A patient might respond to one particular, high-stress situation with maladaptive behaviors, bur use appropriate behaviors in other situations.
3. Set limits on any manipulative behaviors: Arguing or begging Flattery or seductiveness Instilling guilt, clinging Constantly seeking attention Pitting one person, staff, group against another Frequently disregarding the rules Constant engagement in power struggles Angry, demanding behaviors	3. From the beginning, limits need to be clear. It will be necessary to refer to these limits frequently because it is to be expected that the patient will test these limits repeatedly.
4. Intervene in manipulative behavior. All limits should be adhered to by all staff involved. Objective physical signs in managing clinical problems should be carefully documented. Behaviors should be documented objectively (give time, dates, circumstances). Provide clear boundaries and consequences. Enforce the consequences.	4. Patients will test limits, and, once they understand the limits are solid, this understanding can motivate them to work on other ways to get their needs met. It is hoped that this will be done with the nurse clinician through problem-solving alternative behaviors and learning new effective communication skills.
5. Be vigilant; avoid: Discussing yourself or other staff members with patient. Promising to keep a secret for the patient Accepting gifts from the patient Doing special favors for the patient	5. Patients can use this kind of information to manipulate you and/or split staff. Decline all invitations in a firm, but matter-of-fact manner; for example: "I am here to focus on you." "I cannot keep secrets from other staff. If you tell me something I may have to share it." "I cannot accept gifts, but I am wondering what this means to you." "You are to return to the unit by 4 PM on Sunday, period."

TABLE 10-3   Interventions for Impulsive Behaviors

Intervention	Rationale
1. Identify the needs and feelings preceding the impulsive acts.	1. Identify triggers to impulsive actions.
2. Discuss current and previous impulsive acts.	2. Helps link pattern of thoughts or events that trigger impulsive action.
3. Explore effects of such acts on self and others.	3. Helps patients evaluate the results of their behaviors on self and others—may motivate change.
4. Recognize cues of impulsive behaviors that may injure others.	4. Once cues are recognized, planning alternatives to impulsive actions is possible.
5. Identify situations that trigger impulsivity, and discuss alternative behaviors.	5. Once aware of cause and effect, patient can make choices.
6. Teach or refer patient to appropriate place to learn needed coping skills (anger management, assertive skills).	6. Special skills training can potentiate positive change in behaviors.

APPLYING THE ART   A Person with Borderline Personality Disorder

SCENARIO: Eighteen-year-old Maria had already met with me three times on the young adult unit. She always wore long sleeves even though the unit was warm. The last time we'd met, Maria shared her poetry, which expressed themes of loneliness amid the beauty of nature. Each time she seemed glad to see me while simultaneously disparaging the evening shift staff.

THERAPEUTIC GOAL: By the end of this interaction, Maria will choose to express her feelings using a nondestructive form of communication rather than through self-mutilating behavior.

Student-Patient Interaction	Thoughts, Communication Techniques, and Mental Health Nursing Concepts
Maria: "I wondered if you'd actually come back."	According to her chart, she's had lots of reasons to mistrust, starting with her dad, who sexually abused her. She started self-mutilating in middle school when her parents divorced.
Student: "Hi, Maria. I came back as I said I would, but next Tuesday is my last day here." **Student's feelings:** *Sometimes I feel guilty to enter my patients' lives only to leave again. I don't want to be one more person to let her down.*	I *give information* reminding Maria of our *original nurse-patient contract.* Maria reacts with surprise, but avoids any discussion about *termination* of the *nurse-patient relationship.*
Maria: Avoids eye contact. "Read this." Hands me her poem. **Student's feelings:** *I feel okay about her bossiness. I recognize that I'm in charge of my own boundaries. Actually I'm relieved that Maria and I get along. She gets in so much trouble with the staff. I've seen the staff get frustrated with Maria.*	Maria says, "Read this" almost as a command. The abuse in her childhood left her feeling powerless. She needs to feel in charge of something.
Student: "Your poem describes the mother as 'daisy.' 'Daisy deigning to decorate my life.' Maria nods. "The 'my life' person might feel lonely with such a powerful mother who drops by to decorate only." We make eye contact. "Is this about you, Maria?"	I reflect the feeling "lonely" and seek to clarify that the poem actually refers to Maria and her mother.
Maria: "She loves me, she loves me not." **Student's feelings:** *I'm beginning to feel a little lost in the poetry. I need to pay better attention in my English classes!*	Through the poem, Maria uses *symbolism* to safely express her thoughts and sad feelings.
Student: "At first I didn't catch the meaning of 'daisy' in your poems. 'She loves me, she loves me not.' You're sharing about your mother." **Student's feelings:** *I feel so sad that she's so young yet still must battle this mental torment that so disrupts her life and her happiness. She shows so much talent in her writings.*	
Maria: "She says I can't come back to live with her! She's such a ____!"	Maria shows anger in her swearing. Fear and loss fuel her anger. Her mood changes so fast! *Labile,* that's the term.
Student: "You feel abandoned. Maybe thrown away like the daisy petals." **Student's feelings:** *I know from her history the chaos evident in her family. I also recognize that Maria pulls people close then pushes them away. Still, I can't image not being able to turn to my family. I feel lonely at the thought.*	I use *reflection* remembering that patients with *borderline personality disorder* vacillate between feeling *engulfed* by the person they move close to and needing to push that person away to *individuate* self again. Unfortunately they often *devalue* the other person, get rejected, then experience *abandonment depression* until once again, they move too close.

APPLYING THE ART A Person with Borderline Personality Disorder—cont'd

Student-Patient Interaction	Thoughts, Communication Techniques, and Mental Health Nursing Concepts
Maria: "I don't feel anything. Just numb. I have to go to the bathroom."	Maria says she's numb, not *depressed*. The numbness *isolates* her feelings from awareness.
Student: "Okay." *When Maria leaves, I tell my instructor and the nurse what just happened. The nurse immediately goes to find Maria.* **Student's feelings:** *I feel upset with myself for not immediately understanding that after this exchange Maria might cut herself!*	I probably should have gone with her or asked if she felt like cutting when she said she felt numb. Self-mutilating breaks through the numbness that has its roots in Maria's past. As a child Maria had to *dissociate* to survive the sexual abuse.
Maria: *Standing in front of me.* "You told on me!" *Raises voice but sits down two chairs away.* **Student's feelings:** *I feel uncomfortable being yelled at, and my anxiety level begins to elevate some.*	I understand her behavior; it will just take me a while to not take a patient's behavior so personally and look beyond the behavior to the patient's reason for the behavior.
Student: "Maria, I talked to the nurse that you felt upset about your mom and maybe about my leaving. I was concerned that you would be okay." **Student's feelings:** *I feel anxious, but I know that in reporting, I did the right thing. I want Maria to know I am concerned for her safety.*	When Maria confronts me, I *give truthful information*. When we *contracted* I said I would need to share important information with the *treatment team*.
Maria: "I don't want to talk to you anymore." **Student's feelings:** *I feel sad as Maria rejects me. I know this isn't really about me, but still I feel sad.*	
Student: *Quietly.* "You're really upset at me and at your mother, yet you were still able to stop from cutting yourself." **Student's feelings:** *I feel good that so far I'm able to contain my feelings in light of her angry and rejecting behavior toward me. I do know she needs me to stay calm and not be pushed away no matter how hard she tries.*	I *reflect* feelings and make an observation and give *support* by identifying her nondestructive choice and that she has some control over not cutting herself.
Maria: "I'm so _____ at you. A fine nurse you'll be!" *Storms away.*	With the sarcasm, Maria *devalues* me. I remember devaluing as the other pole to *idealizing* others, also part of the disorder. Nevertheless, using words to express her anger shows some progress. She uses *withdrawal* in leaving me. The closeness threatens her safety by encroaching on her *ego boundaries*. Maria's deeper loss, which pertains to her mother, gets *displaced* into the anger at me.
I stay seated about 5 minutes. I notice Maria glancing over at me a few times before she leaves for lunch. **Student's feelings:** *Maria acts so very angry at me. I feel my heart rate pick up (guess it makes me anxious). Okay, I'll take some mindful breaths. It's hard to wait here but I want Maria to know she's worth waiting for.*	Because I promised Maria that the 45 minutes we contracted for was for her, I will make myself available to her for the contracted period of time.
I leave to debrief with my clinical group. **Student's feelings:** *I hope Maria will let me talk to her later today or at least on the last day I come.*	Maria's self-esteem and even her sense of identify are fragile. She restores some kind of control or power by leaving me before I terminate with her.

endured, even while the task of the group is accomplished. Viewing and acting out as unconscious communication that needs to be made conscious and verbal, so that it is possible to understand the need that it communicates, enables the group and the individual to decide how to meet that need.

Psychotherapy

Paris (2006) states that several psychotherapies have been shown to be effective in treating personality disorders, although they are lengthy and expensive.

Psychodynamic Psychotherapy

This approach may help patients recognize their responsibility in the existence of turmoil in their lives and learn healthier ways of reacting to other people and problems. Individual, family, and group therapy all can be helpful.

Cognitive-Behavioral Therapy

This form of therapy helps people recognize how they draw faulty conclusions by becoming aware of their thought processes. The focus is then on reframing one's faulty thinking into a rational and realistic way of thinking about the world. Behavioral techniques include social skills training and assertiveness training, and helping patients learn more effective ways to deal with their feelings, frustrations, and interpersonal issues.

Dialectical Behavior Therapy

Dialectical behavior therapy (DBT) was developed by Marsha Linehan (1993) for the treatment of borderline PD. Its theory and philosophy borrow from biological, social, cognitive-behavioral, and spiritual orientations. It is a four-stage treatment. In stage one the primary focus is on stabilizing the patient and achieving behavioral control. According to Blennerhassett and O'Raghallaigh (2005), the target behaviors are:

- Decreasing life-threatening suicidal behaviors
- Decreasing therapy-interfering behaviors
- Decreasing quality-of-life–interfering behaviors
- Increasing behavioral skills

Dialectical behavior therapy has been extremely effective in helping borderline individuals gain hope and quality of life.

Pharmacological, Biological, and Integrative Therapies

There are no medications for the treatment of these disorders, but at times treating the symptoms is helpful. By and large, benzodiazepines for anxiety are not appropriate because the potential is great for abuse, and many of these patients present with comorbid substance abuse problems. Most people do not seek treatment, but those with borderline and antisocial PDs are seen most often in the health care system.

Because of their propensity for suicidal gestures and self-harm, medications with low toxicity are appropriate for patients with borderline PD. Because borderline patients may become psychotic under stress, the atypical antipsychotic can be helpful. Depression is often comorbid in these patients, so the selective serotonin reuptake inhibitors (SSRIs) trazodone and venlafaxine are good choices because they are the least toxic in overdose. The SSRIs can also help borderline patients who have comorbid panic attacks. Carbamazepine (anticonvulsant) to help target impulsivity, dyscontrol, and self-harm has been useful. Some people with antisocial PD have problems with anger and acting out. Lithium, anticonvulsants, or SSRIs may be helpful to minimize aggression. Anticonvulsants may be used with other PDs as well to help curb impulsive and aggressive behaviors.

People with schizotypal PD, although they rarely voluntarily seek treatment, may be helped with low-dose antipsychotic mediations that help ameliorate anxiety and psychosis-like features associated with this disorder. People with paranoid PD are distrustful of medications, but may benefit from antipsychotics to treat overtly psychotic decompensations that these patients might experience under stress. Obsessive-compulsive PD is often helped with clomipramine (a tricyclic) and SSRIs for both their obsessional thinking and comorbid depression.

EVALUATION

Evaluating treatment effectiveness in this patient population is difficult. Health care providers may never know the real results of their interventions, particularly in acute care settings. Even in long-term outpatient treatment, many patients find the relationship too intimate an experience to remain long enough for successful treatment. However, some motivated patients may be able to learn to change their behavior, especially if positive experiences are repeated. Each therapeutic episode offers an opportunity for patients to observe themselves interacting with caregivers who consistently try to teach positive coping skills. Perhaps effectiveness can be measured by how successfully the nurse is able to be genuine with the patient, maintain a helpful posture, offer substantial instruction, and still care for him- or herself. Specific short-term outcomes may be accomplished, and overall, the patient can be given the message of hope that quality of life can always be improved.

KEY POINTS TO REMEMBER

- People with personality disorders (PDs) present with the most complex, difficult behavioral challenges for themselves and the people around them.
- All people with a PD have (1) inflexible and maladaptive responses to stress, (2) disability in working and loving, (3) ability to evoke strong, intense personal conflict, and (4) capacity to get "under the skin" of others.
- PDs often co-occur with other Axis I disorders (e.g., depression, substance abuse, somatization, eating disorders, PTSD, anxiety disorders), other personality disorders, and general medical conditions.
- People with PDs do not believe there is anything wrong with them, but rather that their problems occur because of other people or events.
- It is unlikely there is any single cause for discrete PDs—most seem to have genetic and environmental risk factors.
- People with these disorders respond to stress (frustration, anger, loneliness, etc.) with more primitive defenses resulting in outrageous behaviors unmodified by "normal" defenses.
- Needs are experienced as rage, and sexuality and dependency are confused with aggression.
- Cluster A, B, and C PDs are defined here using *DSM-IV-TR* criteria, and a clinical example of each disorder is given.
- Self-assessment is an important part of the assessment with a person with a PD because if personal feelings are not recognized or dealt with, substantial interpersonal conflict may ensue.
- Determining if there is a history of suicide/homicide/self-mutilation, and if there are co-occurring disorders as well, is a vital part of the initial assessment interview.
- Nursing diagnoses are given and reflect the problematic behaviors of the PD at the time.
- Communication guidelines for manipulative and impulsive behaviors are outlined.
- Careful evaluation for antidepressants, anticonvulsants (for aggression and impulsive behaviors), and antipsychotics (for stress induced psychotic thinking) may offer the patient relief.
- Therapy has been used with patients with PDs; however, there is little evidence-based research except for how each therapy works for different disorders except for dialectical behavior therapy (DBT), which has been extremely effective in people with borderline PD.
- Much needs to be done to better understand PDs:
  - More and better biological research
  - Prospective community studies of psychosocial risk factors such as trauma
  - Developing medications specifically for borderline PD
  - Creating a common approach to psychotherapy

CRITICAL THINKING

1. Mr. Rogers is undergoing surgery for a broken leg. He is very suspicious of the staff and believes that everyone is trying to harm him and to "do him in." He scans his environment constantly for danger (hypervigilance) and speaks very little to the nurses or the other patients. He has paranoid PD.
   1. Explain why being friendly and outgoing may be threatening to Mr. Rogers.
   2. Explain how being matter of fact and neutral and sticking to the facts would be the most useful to Mr. Rogers.
   3. What could be done to give Mr. Rogers some control over his situation in a hospital setting?
   4. How would you best handle his sarcasm and hostility so that both you and he would feel most comfortable?
2. Ms. Pemrose is brought to the ED after slashing her wrist with a razor. She has previously been in the ED for drug overdose and has a history of addictions. Ms. Pemrose can be sarcastic, belittling, and aggressive to those who try to care for her. She has a history of difficulty with interpersonal relationships at her job. When the psychiatric triage nurse comes in to see her, Ms. Pemrose is at first adoring and compliant, telling him, "You are the best nurse I've ever seen, and I truly want to change." But when he refuses to support her request for diazepam (Valium) and meperidine (Demerol) for "pain," she yells at him, "You are a stupid excuse for a nurse. I want a doctor immediately." Ms. Pemrose has borderline PD.
   1. What defense mechanism is Ms. Pemrose using?
   2. How could the nurse best handle this situation in keeping with setting limits and offering concern and useful interventions?

CHAPTER REVIEW

Choose the most appropriate answer(s).

1. Which of the following best describes people with PDs?
   1. They readily assume the roles of compromiser and harmonizer.
   2. They often seek help to change maladaptive behaviors.
   3. They have the ability to tolerate high levels of anxiety.
   4. They have difficulty working and loving.

2. After experiencing a social rejection, which patient is most likely to need a nursing plan to monitor self-destructive behavior?
   1. Mr. A., who has been diagnosed with obsessive-compulsive PD
   2. Ms. B., who has been diagnosed with borderline PD
   3. Mr. C., who has been diagnosed with paranoid PD
   4. Ms. D., who has been diagnosed with schizoid PD

3. For the nurse working with patients with PDs, which nursing intervention must be an ongoing priority?
   1. Offering professional advice
   2. Probing for etiological factors
   3. Encouraging diversional activity
   4. Setting appropriate limits

4. Which statement provides a foundation for understanding patients with PDs?
   1. The background of a patient with a PD is usually trouble free.
   2. The tendency to develop a PD may have genetic determinants.
   3. A patient with a PD functions with a highly developed sense of autonomy.
   4. A PD is more amenable to treatment than an anxiety disorder.

5. When nurses are caring for a patient with a PD, which of the emotional states listed below are they likely to experience themselves?
   1. Anger
   2. Confusion
   3. Frustration
   4. Helplessness

REFERENCES

American Psychiatric Association. (2000). Personality disorders. In *Diagnostic and statistical manual of mental disorders* (4th ed., text rev., pp. 685-729). Washington, DC: Author.

Bender, E. (2004). Personality disorder prevalence surprises research. *Psychiatric News, 39*(17), 12.

Blennerhassett, R.C., & O'Raghallaigh, J.W. (2005). Dialectical behavior therapy in the treatment of borderline personality disorder. *The British Journal of Psychiatry, 186,* 278-280.

Groves, J.E. (2004). Personality disorders I: Approaches to difficult patients. In T.A. Stern, J.B. Herman, & P.E. Slavin (Eds.), *Massachusetts General Hospital guide to primary care psychiatry* (2nd ed.). New York: McGraw-Hill.

Haas, L.J., Leiser, J.P., Macgill, M.K., & Sanyer, O.N. (2005). Management of the difficult patient. *American Family Physician, 72*(10), 2063-2068.

Linehan, M.M. (1993). *Understanding borderline personality disorder: A dialectical approach.* New York: Guilford.

Markon, K.E., Krueger, R.F., Bouchard, T.J., & Gottesman, I.I. (2002). Normal and abnormal personality traits: Evidence for genetic and environmental relationships in the Minnesota study of twins reared apart. *Journal of Personality, 70,* 661-694.

McGlashan, T.H., Grilo, C.M., Sanislow, C.A., et al. (2005). Two-year prevalence and stability of individual DSM-1V criteria for schizotypal, borderline, avoidant, and obsessive-compulsive personality disorders: Toward a hybrid model of Axis II disorders. *American Journal of Psychiatry, 162,* 883-889.

Oldham, J.M. (2005). *Guidelines watch: Practice guideline for the treatment of patients with borderline personality disorder.* Arlington: American Psychiatric Association.

Paris, J. (2006). Personality disorders: psychiatry's stepchildren come of age. Program and abstracts of the 159th Annual Meeting of the American Psychiatric Association, May 20-25, 2006, Toronto, Ontario, Canada.

Sadock, B.J., & Sadock, V.A. (2004). *Concise textbook of clinical psychiatry* (2nd ed.). Philadelphia: Lippincott Williams & Wilkins

Zimmerman, M., Rothschild, L., & Chelminski, I. (2005). The prevalence of DSM-1V personality disorders in psychiatric outpatients. *American Journal of Psychiatry, 162,* 1911-1918.

CHAPTER 11

Eating Disorders

Kathleen Ibrahim

Key Terms and Concepts

anorexia nervosa, p. 196
binge eating disorder, p. 208
bulimia nervosa, p. 196
cachectic, p. 197
cognitive distortions, p. 202

ideal body weight, p. 200
lanugo, p. 200
purging, p. 200
refeeding syndrome, p. 201

Objectives

1. Compare and contrast the signs and symptoms of anorexia nervosa and bulimia nervosa.
2. Discuss the causes and treatment for at least two life-threatening conditions that may develop for a patient with anorexia, and at least two for a patient with bulimia.
3. Give examples of therapeutic interventions that are appropriate for the acute phase of anorexia nervosa and those that are appropriate for the long-term phase of treatment.
4. Understand the effectiveness of cognitive-behavioral therapy in the treatment of anorexia nervosa and bulimia nervosa.
5. Distinguish between the needs of and treatment(s) for patients with acute bulimia and individuals in long-term therapy for bulimia.
6. Differentiate between the long-term prognosis of anorexia nervosa, bulimia nervosa, and binge eating disorder.

evolve

For additional resources related to the content of this chapter, visit the Evolve website at http://evolve.elsevier.com/Varcarolis/essentials.

- Chapter Outline
- Chapter Review Answers
- Case Studies and Nursing Care Plans

- Nurse, Patient, and Family Resources
- Concept Map Creator

For the majority of people, eating provides nourishment for the body as well as the soul. Families and friends gather around the table to break bread as they celebrate, mourn, laugh, cry, share, and demonstrate love. However, for some individuals, eating loses its communal value and becomes hidden and shrouded in secrecy and shame. People with eating disorders experience severe disruptions in normal eating patterns and a significant disturbance in the perception of body shape and weight.

Diagnostic categories include anorexia nervosa, bulimia nervosa, and eating disorders not otherwise specified. Individuals with **anorexia nervosa** engage in self-starvation, express intense fear of gaining weight, and have a disturbance in self-evaluation of weight and its importance; females with anorexia often experience amenorrhea. There are two subtypes of anorexia—those with one subtype restrict their intake of food, while those with the other subtype engage in binge eating and/or purging.

Individuals with **bulimia nervosa** engage in repeated episodes of binge eating followed by inappropriate *compensatory* behaviors such as self-induced vomiting; misuse of laxatives, diuretics, or other medications; fasting; or excessive exercise.

Individuals with eating disorders may display a mixture of anorectic and bulimic behaviors. **Eating disorders not otherwise specified (EDNOS)** is a category that includes disorders of eating that do not meet all the criteria for either anorexia nervosa or bulimia nervosa. For example, if a college-age woman exhibits every criterion for anorexia nervosa, but continues to menstruate, she would be diagnosed with EDNOS. Also considered in this category is **binge eating disorder** in which individuals engage in repeated episodes of binge eating after which they experience significant distress. These individuals do not regularly use the compensatory behaviors seen in patients with bulimia nervosa. See the discussion of binge eating disorder on pages 208-209 in this chapter.

PREVALENCE AND COMORBIDITY

Eating disorders are culturally influenced disorders with varying prevalence depending on the culture and its social norms. The actual number of individuals with eating disorders is not known because these disorders may exist for a long time before the person seeks help or is brought in for medical treatment.

The estimated lifetime prevalence rate among women for developing anorexia nervosa is about 1% and the rate among men is 0.3%. For bulimia nervosa, the lifetime prevalence rate for women is 1.5% and for men it is 0.5%

(Hudson et al., 2007). Female as well as male athletes demonstrate an increased incidence of eating disorders.

The course for anorexia seems to be shorter, lasting an average of a year and a half, whereas bulimia usually lasts more than 8 years. One out of two people with anorexia will go on to develop bulimia or bulimia patterns.

Eating disorders are almost always comorbid with other psychiatric illnesses. More than 50% of people with anorexia have one other concurrent psychiatric disorder, and almost 95% of people with bulimia have another psychiatric disorder. For example, anorexia nervosa is associated with social phobia (34% of cases), depression (65% of cases), and obsessive-compulsive disorder (26% of cases) (Sadock & Sadock 2007). There is a significant comorbidity with mood and anxiety disorders, substance abuse, body dysmorphic disorders, impulse control disorders, and personality disorders, especially borderline and obsessive-compulsive personality disorders.

A history of sexual abuse is more common in those with eating disorders than in the general population. Women with a history of eating disorders and sexual abuse have a higher rate of other comorbid psychiatric illnesses than women diagnosed solely with eating disorders (APA, 2000b).

THEORY

The etiology of eating disorders is varied and complex. It appears that these disorders include a biological vulnerability or predisposition that is activated by psychological, environmental, and cultural factors.

Neurobiological and Neuroendocrine Models

Neuroendocrine abnormalities are noted in both anorexia nervosa and bulimia nervosa (Brambilla & Monteleone, 2003). These abnormalities are of the "the chicken or the egg" quality because we are not certain if they cause the eating disorder or if the eating disorder causes them. There is some support for a primary pathology because people with active illness and people who have recovered have exactly the same abnormalities. Brain imaging studies demonstrate unusual activity in various regions of the brain including the frontal, cingulate, temporal, and parietal areas. In both anorexia nervosa and bulimia nervosa, serotonin pathways are abnormal (Kaye et al., 2005). Researchers believe that this altered serotonin pathway may be key to anxiety responses, inhibition, and even distortions in body image. Brain scans also reveal altered serotonin receptors and transporters. This may be the basis for mood problems, reduced impulse control, and the motivation for eating and enjoying food.

Genetic Models

There is strong evidence that suggests a genetic vulnerability to eating disorders and refutes the notion that these problems are simply self-inflicted. Up to 56% of the risk of developing these disorders may be genetic (Bulik et al., 2006). Female relatives of people with eating disorders are up to 12 times more likely to have them. By comparing monozygotic (identical) and dizygotic (fraternal) twins, it is possible to differentiate genetic from environmental influences. A variety of studies document monozygotic twins to have a 50% to 80% concordance rate for an eating disorder (Anderson & Yager, 2005). What is inherited is not clear. Genetic vulnerability might stem from an underlying neurotransmitter dysfunction, or perhaps the vulnerability is one of inherited temperament, cognitive style, mood-regulating tendencies, and unique weight set point.

Psychological Models

Although biology may create a predisposition for eating disorders, psychological determinants may play a role in setting them off. Anorexia nervosa results in amenorrhea in females and physiological changes that interfere with the development of an age-appropriate sexual role. Psychoanalytical theorists long believed that fear of sexual maturity and the need to maintain a childlike body were primary for people with anorexia. The "core psychopathology" in both anorexia and bulimia is thought to be low self-esteem and self-doubts about personal worth. These feelings produce harsh self-judgment focused solely on the issue of weight. The overvalued ideas about weight, shape, and control are critical to maintaining the eating-disordered behaviors (Fairburn, 2002).

Family theorists believe that specific dynamics converge to create individuals with eating disorders. For anorexia, these families are seen as controlling, emphasizing perfection, achievement, and compliance. Bulimic families are seen as chaotic and emotionally expressive, particularly in terms of conflict and negativity. Critics of these theories point out that these characteristics may not be the cause of the problem, but rather part of the genetic makeup related to the disorder. For example, the perfectionist and controlling tendencies qualities of anorectic families may be a result of obsessive genetic tendencies.

CULTURAL CONSIDERATIONS

Western women at risk for eating disorders are driven by the ideal to be competent in traditional as well as nontraditional ways, such as being an ideal homemaker while being a successful businesswoman. It is interesting to note that eating disorders do not flourish in male-dominated societies in which women are socialized into a stereotypical nurturing role; rather, the incidence of eating disorders increases in societies in which women have a choice in social roles (Miller & Pumariega, 2001).

Although the number of individuals who are overweight continues to increase, many individuals with eating disorders have internalized the societal ideal to be thin (Sypeck et al., 2004). In some Asian countries anorectic behavior does not include the pursuit of thinness or fear of being fat. In these countries the self-imposed weight restriction may represent control over one's life circumstances or grow out of spiritual or ascetic values (Miller & Pumariega, 2001).

CLINICAL PICTURE

Figure 11-1 identifies the *Diagnostic and Statistical Manual of Mental Disorders (DSM-IV-TR)* diagnostic criteria for anorexia nervosa, bulimia nervosa, and EDNOS.

Anorexia nervosa and bulimia nervosa are two separate syndromes and as such they present two clinical pictures. Box 11-1 identifies the signs and symptoms of these disorders.

Eating disorders are serious and in extreme cases can lead to death. Box 11-2 identifies a number of complications that can occur and the laboratory findings that may result in individuals with eating disorders. Because the eating behaviors in these conditions are so extreme, hospitalization may become necessary. Box 11-3 identifies when an individual should be hospitalized; often hospitalization is via the emergency department (ED).

In treating patients who have been sexually abused or who have otherwise been the victim of boundary violations, it is critical that the nurse and other health care workers maintain and respect clear boundaries (APA, 2000b).

Fundamental to the care of individuals with eating disorders is the establishment and maintenance of a therapeutic alliance. This will take time as well as diplomacy on the part of the nurse.

evolve

For comprehensive case studies and associated nursing care plans for patients experiencing anorexia nervosa, bulimia, EDNOS, visit the Evolve website at http://evolve.elsevier.com/Varcarolis/essentials.

Application of the Nursing Process: Anorexia Nervosa

ASSESSMENT

The nurse assessing a patient with anorexia observes a **cachectic** (severely underweight with muscle wasting) male

DSM-IV-TR CRITERIA FOR EATING DISORDERS

EATING DISORDERS

Anorexia Nervosa

A. Refusal to maintain body weight at or above a minimally normal weight for age and height (e.g., weight loss leading to maintenance of body weight less than 85% of that expected) or failure to make expected weight gain during period of growth, leading to body weight less than 85% of that expected.

B. Intense fear of gaining weight or becoming fat, even though underweight.

C. Disturbance in the way in which one's body weight or shape is experienced, undue influence of body weight or shape on self-evaluation, or denial of the seriousness of the current low body weight.

D. In females, postmenarcheal amenorrhea (i.e., the absence of at least three consecutive menstrual cycles). (A woman is considered to have amenorrhea if her periods occur only after hormone [e.g., estrogen] administration.)

Specify type:
Binge eating/purging type: During the episode of anorexia nervosa, the person engages in recurrent episodes of binge eating or purging behaviors.
Restricting type: During the episode of anorexia nervosa, the person does *not* engage in recurrent episodes of binge eating or purging behaviors.

Bulimia Nervosa

A. Recurrent episodes of binge eating. An episode of binge eating is characterized by both of the following:

(1) Eating in a discrete period (e.g., within any 2-hour period) an amount of food that is definitely larger than most people would eat during a similar period and under similar circumstances.
(2) A sense of lack of control over eating during the episode (e.g., a feeling that one cannot stop eating or control what or how much one is eating).

B. Recurrent inappropriate compensatory behavior to prevent weight gain such as self-induced vomiting; misuse of laxatives, diuretics, enemas, or other medications; fasting; or excessive exercise.

C. The binge eating and inappropriate compensatory behavior both occur on average at least twice a week for 3 months.

D. Self-evaluation is unduly influenced by body shape and weight.

E. The disturbance does not occur exclusively during episodes of anorexia nervosa.

Specify type:
Purging type: During the current episode of bulimia nervosa, the person has regularly engaged in self-induced vomiting or the misuse of laxatives, diuretics, or enemas.
Nonpurging type: During the current episode of bulimia nervosa, the person has used other inappropriate compensatory behaviors such as fasting or excessive exercise but has not regularly engaged in self-induced vomiting or the misuse of laxatives, diuretics, or enemas.

Eating Disorder Not Otherwise Specified (NOS)

The eating disorder not otherwise specified category is for disorders of eating that do not meet the criteria for any specific eating disorder. Examples include:

1. For females, all the criteria for anorexia nervosa are met except that the individual has regular menses.

2. All the criteria for anorexia nervosa are met except that despite significant weight loss, the individual's current weight is in the normal range.

3. All the criteria for bulimia nervosa are met except that the binge eating and inappropriate compensatory mechanisms occur at a frequency of less than twice a week for a duration of less than 3 months.

4. The regular use of inappropriate compensatory behavior by an individual of normal body weight after eating small amounts of food (i.e., self-induced vomiting after the consumption of two cookies).

5. Repeatedly chewing and spitting out, but not swallowing, large amounts of food.

6. Binge eating disorder: recurrent episodes of binge eating in the absence of the regular use of inappropriate compensatory behaviors characteristic of bulimia nervosa.

Figure 11-1 ■ Diagnostic criteria for eating disorders. (Adapted from American Psychiatric Association. [2000]. *Diagnostic and statistical manual of mental disorders* [4th ed., text rev.]. Washington, DC: Author.)

BOX 11-1

Possible Signs and Symptoms of Anorexia Nervosa and Bulimia Nervosa

Anorexia Nervosa

- Terror of gaining weight
- Preoccupation with thoughts of food
- View of self as fat even when emaciated
- Peculiar handling of food:
  - Cutting food into small bits
  - Pushing pieces of food around plate
- Possible development of rigorous exercise regimen
- Possible self-induced vomiting; use of laxatives and diuretics
- Cognition is so disturbed that the individual judges self-worth by his or her weight
- Controls what they eat to feel powerful to overcome feelings of helplessness

Bulimia Nervosa

- Binge eating behaviors
- Often self-induced vomiting (or laxative or diuretic use) after bingeing
- History of anorexia nervosa in one fourth to one third of individuals
- Depressive signs and symptoms
- Problems with:
  - Interpersonal relationships
  - Self-concept
  - Impulsive behaviors
- Increased levels of anxiety and compulsivity
- Possible chemical dependency
- Possible impulsive stealing
- Controls/undoes weight after bingeing, which is motivated by feelings of emptiness

BOX 11-2

Some Medical Complications of Anorexia Nervosa and Bulimia Nervosa

Anorexia Nervosa

- Bradycardia
- Orthostatic changes in pulse or blood pressure
- Cardiac murmur—one-third with mitral valve prolapse
- Sudden cardiac arrest caused by profound electrolyte disturbances
- Prolonged QT interval on electrocardiogram
- Acrocyanosis
- Symptomatic hypotension
- Leukopenia
- Lymphocytosis
- Carotenemia (elevated carotene levels in blood), which produces skin with yellow pallor
- Hypokalemic alkalosis (with self-induced vomiting or use of laxatives and diuretics)
- Elevated serum bicarbonate levels, hypochloremia, and hypokalemia
- Electrolyte imbalances, which lead to fatigue, weakness, and lethargy
- Osteoporosis, indicated by decrease in bone density
- Fatty degeneration of liver, indicated by elevation of serum enzyme levels
- Elevated cholesterol levels
- Amenorrhea
- Abnormal thyroid functioning
- Hematuria
- Proteinuria

Bulimia Nervosa

- Cardiomyopathy from ipecac intoxication (medical emergency that usually results in death)
- Cardiac dysrhythmias
- Sinus bradycardia
- Sudden cardiac arrest as a result of profound electrolyte disturbances
- Orthostatic changes in pulse or blood pressure
- Cardiac murmur; mitral valve prolapse
- Electrolyte imbalances
- Elevated serum bicarbonate levels (although can be low, which indicates a metabolic acidosis)
- Hypochloremia
- Hypokalemia
- Dehydration, which results in volume depletion, leading to stimulation of aldosterone production, which in turn stimulates further potassium excretion from kidneys; thus there can be an indirect renal loss of potassium as well as a direct loss through self-induced vomiting
- Severe attrition and erosion of teeth producing irritating sensitivity and exposing the pulp of the teeth
- Loss of dental arch
- Diminished chewing ability
- Parotid gland enlargement associated with elevated serum amylase levels
- Esophageal tears caused by self-induced vomiting
- Severe abdominal pain indicative of gastric dilation
- Russell's sign (callus on knuckles from self-induced vomiting)

Data from Halmi, K.A. (2004). Eating disorders. In R.E. Hales & S.C. Yudofsky (Eds.), *Essentials of clinical psychiatry* (2nd ed., pp. 762, 769-770). Washington, DC: American Psychiatric Publishing; Dixon-Works, D., Nenstiel, R.O., & Aliabadi, Z. (2003). Common eating disorders: A primer for primary care physicians. *Clinical Reviews, 13*(9), 45-51.

BOX 11-3

Criteria for Hospital Admission of Individuals with Eating Disorders

Physical Criteria
- Weight loss more than 30% over 6 months
- Rapid decline in weight
- Inability to gain weight with outpatient treatment
- Severe hypothermia caused by loss of subcutaneous tissue or dehydration (temperature lower than 36° C or 96.8° F)
- Heart rate less than 40 beats per minute
- Systolic blood pressure less than 70 mm Hg
- Hypokalemia (less than 3 mEq/L) or other electrolyte disturbances not corrected by oral supplementation
- Electrocardiographic changes (especially dysrhythmias)

Psychiatric Criteria
- Suicidal or severely out-of-control, self-mutilating behaviors
- Out-of-control use of laxatives, emetics, diuretics, or street drugs
- Failure to comply with treatment contract
- Severe depression
- Psychosis
- Family crisis or dysfunction

or female who may have **lanugo** (a growth of fine, downy hair on the face and back); mottled, cool skin on the extremities; and low blood pressure, pulse, and temperature readings. All of these findings are consistent with a malnourished and dehydrated state.

Clinicians base a diagnosis of anorexia nervosa in part on being 85% less than the **ideal body weight**, the weight considered appropriate and normal for a specific age, height, body type, and even waist circumference. Various standards define this ideal, including pediatric growth tables and Metropolitan Life Insurance tables. However, calculations based on body mass index (BMI) (weight in kilograms divided by height in meters squared) are more precise. Ideal BMIs are thought to be between 19 and 25. Automatic calculators of BMI are widely available on the Internet.

Individuals with the binge-purge type of anorexia nervosa may have prominent parotid glands—the largest of the salivary glands, located in each cheek in front of the ears—because of hyperstimulation from repeated vomiting. Furthermore, they may present with severe electrolyte imbalance as a result of **purging**, which may be in the form of vomiting, abusing laxatives or diuretics, or using enemas. These individuals may be dangerously ill and often begin treatment in an intensive care unit.

As with any comprehensive psychiatric nursing assessment, a complete evaluation of biopsychosocial function is mandatory. The areas to be covered include the following patient characteristics:
- Perception of the problem
- Eating habits
- History of dieting
- Methods used to achieve weight control (restricting, purging, exercising)
- Value attached to a specific shape and weight
- Interpersonal and social functioning
- Mental status and physiological parameters

Assessment Guidelines

Anorexia Nervosa

1. Determine if medical or psychiatric condition warrants hospitalization (see Box 11-3).
2. Assess level of family understanding about the disease and where to get support.
3. Assess acceptance of therapeutic modalities.
4. Perform a thorough physical examination with appropriate bloodwork.
5. Check for other medical conditions.
6. Determine the family and patient's need for teaching or information regarding the treatment plan (e.g., psychopharmacological interventions, behavioral therapy, cognitive therapy, family therapy, individual psychotherapy).
7. Assess the patient's and family's desire to participate in a support group.

VIGNETTE

Tina, a 16-year-old at 60% of ideal body weight, is cachectic on admission to an inpatient psychiatric unit. She has lanugo over most of her body and prominent parotid glands. She is further assessed to be hypotensive (86/50 mm Hg) and dehydrated. In addition, she has a low serum potassium level and dysrhythmias that appear on an electrocardiogram (ECG). A decision is made to transfer her to the intensive care unit until she is medically stabilized. As an intravenous catheter is inserted, her severe weight phobia and fear of being overweight are underscored when she cries, "There's not going to be sugar in the IV, is there?" The nurse responds, "I hear how frightened you are. We need to do what's necessary to get you past this crisis."

DIAGNOSIS

Imbalanced nutrition: less than body requirements is usually the most compelling nursing diagnosis initially for individuals with anorexia. It generates further nursing diagnoses; for example, *Decreased cardiac output, Risk for injury* (electrolyte imbalance), and *Risk for imbalanced fluid volume,* which would have first priority when problems are addressed. Other nursing diagnoses include *Disturbed body image, Anxiety, Chronic low self-esteem, Deficient knowledge, Ineffective coping, Powerlessness,* and *Hopelessness.*

OUTCOMES IDENTIFICATION

Outcomes need to be measurable and include a time estimate for attainment (ANA, 2007). Some common outcome criteria for patients with anorexia nervosa include the following (fill in the appropriate time [e.g., within 3 weeks, by discharge, etc.]); the patient will:

- Refrain from self-harm
- Normalize eating patterns, as evidenced by eating 75% of three meals per day plus two snacks
- Achieve 85% to 90% of ideal body weight
- Be free of physical complications
- Demonstrate two new, healthy eating habits
- Demonstrate improved self-acceptance, as evidenced by verbal and behavioral data
- Address maladaptive beliefs, thoughts, and activities related to the eating disorder
- Participate in treatment of associated psychiatric symptoms (defects in mood, self-esteem)
- Demonstrate at least one behavior and interest that are appropriate to age
- Participate in long-term treatment to prevent relapse

PLANNING

Planning is affected by the acuity of the patient's situation. In the case of a patient with anorexia who is experiencing extreme electrolyte imbalance or whose weight is less than 75% of ideal body weight, the plan is to provide immediate stabilization, most likely in an inpatient unit (APA, 2000b). Inpatient hospitalization is usually brief, attempts limited weight restoration, and addresses only acute complications, such as electrolyte imbalance and dysrhythmias and acute psychiatric symptoms, such as significant depression. Some hospitalized patients experience **refeeding syndrome**, a potentially catastrophic treatment complication in which the demands of a replenished circulatory system overwhelm the capacity of a nutritionally depleted cardiac muscle, which results in cardiovascular collapse (APA, 2000b).

Once a patient is medically stable, the plan begins to address the issues underlying the eating disorder. These issues are usually treated on an outpatient basis and will include individual, group, and family therapy as well as psychopharmacological therapy during different phases of the illness. The nature of the treatment is determined both by the inten-

sity of the symptoms—which may vary over time—and by the experienced disruption in the patient's life.

IMPLEMENTATION

See Table 11-1 for specific interventions regarding anorexia nervosa.

Acute Care

Patients with eating disorders may be admitted to intensive care, coronary care, and medical and special eating disorders units. Typically when an individual with an eating disorder is admitted to any of these units, the person is in a crisis state. The nurse is challenged to establish trust and monitor the eating pattern. Weight restoration and weight monitoring create opportunities to counter the distorted ideas that maintain the illness. Nurses provide milieu therapy, counseling, health teaching, and medication management. Within special eating disorder units and general psychiatric units, patient privileges may be linked to weight gain and treatment plan compliance.

Communication Guidelines

The nurse on a behavioral health inpatient unit may have to operate as both primary nurse and group leader. The initial focus depends on the results of a comprehensive assessment. Interventions include milieu therapy, teaching, and psychotherapy. Any acute psychiatric symptoms, such as suicidal ideation are addressed immediately. At the same time, a patient with anorexia begins a weight restoration program that allows for incremental weight gain. Based on the patient's height, a treatment goal is set at 90% of ideal body weight, the weight at which most women are able to menstruate.

In the effort to motivate the patient and take advantage of the decision to seek help and be healthier, the nurse must avoid authoritarianism and assumption of a parental role. As the nurse struggles to build a therapeutic alliance and be empathic, the patient's terror at gaining weight and resistance to nursing interventions may engender significant frustration. Nurses must appreciate the compelling force of this illness and be aware that one of the primary goals of treatment—weight gain—is the very thing the patient fears. Frequent acknowledgment of the difficulty of the situation for the patient and of the constant struggle that characterizes the treatment will help during times of extreme resistance.

Establishing a therapeutic alliance with a person with anorexia is challenging because the compelling force of the illness runs counter to therapeutic interventions. As patients begin to refeed, ideally they begin to participate in milieu

TABLE 11-1	Interventions for Anorexia Nervosa

Intervention	Rationale
1. Acknowledge the emotional and physical difficulty the patient is experiencing.	1. A first priority is to establish a therapeutic alliance.
2. Assess for suicidal thoughts/self-injurious behaviors.	2. The potential for a psychiatric crisis is always present.
3. Monitor physiological parameters (vital signs, electrolyte levels) as needed.	3. The life-threatening effect of weight restriction and/or purging needs to be monitored.
4. Weigh patient wearing only bra and panties/underwear only on a routine basis (same time of day after voiding and before drinking/eating). Some protocol includes weighing with the patient's back to the scale.	4. Weights are a high anxiety time. The underweight patient might try to manipulate the weight with drinking fluids or placing heavy objects in clothing before weighing in. Discussion of weight gain (or loss) may be postponed for the primary therapist.
5. Monitor patient during and after meals to prevent throwing away food and/or purging.	5. The compelling force of the illness makes it difficult to stop certain behaviors.
6. Recognize the patient's distorted image/overvalued ideas of body shape and size without minimizing or challenging patient's perceptions.	6. A matter-of-fact statement that the nurse's perceptions are different will help to avoid a power struggle. Arguments and power struggles intensify the patient's need to control.
7. Educate the patient about the ill effects of low weight and resultant impaired health.	7. The treatment goal of gaining weight is what the patient most resists. Focus on the benefits of improved health and increased energy at a more normalized weight.
8. Work with patient to identify strengths.	8. When patients are feeling overwhelmed, they no longer view their lives objectively.

BOX 11-4

Cognitive Distortions Related to Eating Disorders

Overgeneralization: A single event affects unrelated situations.
- "He didn't ask me out. It must be because I'm fat."
- "I was happy when I wore a size 6. I must get back to that weight."

All-or-nothing thinking: Reasoning is absolute and extreme, in mutually exclusive terms of black or white, good or bad.
- "If I have one Popsicle, I must eat five."
- "If I allow myself to gain weight, I'll blow up like a balloon."

Catastrophizing: The consequences of an event are magnified.

- "If I gain weight, my weekend will be ruined."
- "When people say I look better, I know they think I'm fat."

Personalization: Events are overinterpreted as having personal significance.
- "I know everybody is watching me eat."
- "People won't like me unless I'm thin."

Emotional reasoning: Subjective emotions determine reality.
- "I know I'm fat because I feel fat."
- "When I'm thin, I feel powerful."

Adapted from Bowers, W.A. (2001). Principles for applying cognitive-behavioral therapy to anorexia nervosa. *Psychiatric Clinics of North America, 24*(2), 293-303.

therapy, in which the **cognitive distortions** that perpetuate the illness are consistently confronted by all members of the interdisciplinary team. Box 11-4 identifies some common types of cognitive distortion characteristic of people with eating disorders. Although the eating behavior is targeted, the underlying emotions of anxiety, dysphoria, low self-esteem, and feelings of lack of control are also addressed through counseling.

Health Teaching and Health Promotion

Self-care activities are an important part of the treatment plan. These activities include learning more constructive coping skills, improving social skills, and developing problem-solving and decision-making skills. The skills become the focus of therapy sessions and supervised food

APPLYING THE ART   A Person with an Eating Disorder: Anorexia

SCENARIO: I met 15-year-old Stacie on the eating disorders unit. A straight A student, Stacie was 5 feet 7 inches and weighed 90 pounds. Her mother was a physician and her father a college professor. Her older brother quarterbacked his college team. We'd set up the contract that morning and she'd just finished the post-lunch focus group.

THERAPEUTIC GOAL: By the end of this interaction, Stacie will express at least one painful feeling directly instead of acting out with self-destructive behavior.

Student-Patient Interaction	Thoughts, Communication Techniques, and Mental Health Nursing Concepts
Stacie: "They think we're going to all go and vomit after lunch so they keep us talking. Like that's going to help." **Student's feelings:** *I am feeling a bit overwhelmed. Where to start! She looks like a skeleton, and here I am always struggling with my own weight.*	I should *clarify indefinite pronouns.* She used "they" a lot but I'm guessing she means the staff. Her feelings take precedence right now.
Student: "You sound pretty frustrated." **Student's feelings:** *Her thinness scares me.*	*Reflection* rarely fails to keep the interaction going. I am aware of my own potential for *countertransference* in this situation.
Stacie: "I am! Sometimes I feel like a piece of taffy being pushed and pulled and stretched by everyone else." **Student's feelings:** *I'm feeling some anxiety about being able to figure this out. She shares how controlled she feels by making an analogy to candy. Is her whole life about food?*	Control sounds like a key issue. She's revisiting *autonomy versus shame and doubt.* I remember that adolescents re-encounter all of Erikson's earlier stages as part of *identity versus role confusion.*
Student: "Pushed and pulled?"	*Restatement* and *encouraging her to elaborate.* I hope this shows Stacie I'm really listening by using her exact words.
Stacie: "Try being in that family of mine! You can't stay unless you're at the top of your game." **Student's feelings:** *I am feeling drawn into her story. How overwhelming for her.*	I wonder which carries the most emotional impact for her: achievement or staying in the family.
Student: "You feel a lot of pressure to excel . . . at everything?" **Student's feelings:** *I feel uncertain here. I probably should have focused first on the family part. Hope we can get back to her family stuff, too.*	I *restate* again. *Love and belonging* precedes *self-esteem needs.* Still, I do need to assess further with my *direct question* about how high she sets the bar for herself. If she sees herself as a constant failure and food becomes the only area she can control, then despair, even suicide, becomes a possibility.
Stacie: "My mom would say, 'Honey, just be yourself,' but she'd really mean, 'as long as you get straight A's and make the family proud, like your brother does' "! **Student's feelings:** *I kind of feel intimidated by her straight A's. She accomplishes more than I do in my own studies. Why can't that be enough? I feel sad that she never feels good enough.*	
Student: "Somehow you never quite feel good enough." *Concerned look, leaning toward her.*	I reflect back her feelings. I hope to convey *empathy* with my nonverbal behavior.
Stacie: "That's it, exactly." *Eyes fill with tears.*	

Continued

APPLYING THE ART   A Person with an Eating Disorder: Anorexia—cont'd

Student-Patient Interaction	Thoughts, Communication Techniques, and Mental Health Nursing Concepts
I pause to let her cry some. **Student's feelings:** *I want to comfort her but I stop myself because the tears are healthy. She actually lets herself feel frustration and now sadness.*	When a person is crying, feelings are very close to the surface. Saying comforting things might help her push her feelings down. Expressing emotions directly is much healthier for her than using food to *displace* feelings.
Stacie: *Crying.* "I can't tell you how long it's been since I actually cried." **Student's feelings:** *I'm glad she could unbottle some of her feelings and that she felt safe to do so with me.*	
Student: "Maybe crying is not such a bad thing."	I ask an *indirect question.* Maybe she will see that she can let out some of her painful feelings and that it is okay.
Stacie: "It's not done in my family." **Student's feelings:** *Seems like she never lets go of the pressures she feels from her family. In some ways I understand that with all my family does to keep me plugging through nursing, I feel like I'd really let them down if I failed.*	The family theme pervades her thoughts.
Student: "I wonder if a person can stay in the family yet still feel and do things a little differently than everyone else." **Student's feelings:** *I feel like Stacie really made some progress and we can build a foundation for the next time we talk. I feel more hopeful for her.*	Again, an *indirect question* asks Stacie to ponder without feeling interrogated. The work of *identity versus role confusion* means separating and *individuating* oneself as distinct from one's family.
Stacie: "Maybe. I never thought of it that way." *Takes the tissue I offer, looking thoughtful.*	I'll report this to my instructor and chart about her being able to cry.

shopping trips. As patients approach their goal weight, they are encouraged to expand the repertoire to include eating out in a restaurant, preparing a meal, and eating forbidden foods.

Discharge planning is a critical component in treatment. Often family members benefit from counseling. The discharge planning process must address living arrangements, school, and work, as well as the feasibility of independent financial status, applications for state and/or federal program assistance (if needed), and follow-up outpatient treatment.

Milieu Therapy

Individuals admitted to an inpatient unit designed to treat eating disorders participate in a program provided by an interdisciplinary team and consisting of a combination of therapeutic modalities. These modalities are designed to normalize eating patterns and to begin to address the issues raised by the illness. The milieu of an eating disorder unit is purposefully organized to assist the patient in establishing more adaptive behavioral patterns, including normalization of eating.

The highly structured milieu includes precise mealtimes, adherence to the selected menu, observation during and after meals, and regularly scheduled weighings. Close monitoring of patients includes monitoring of all trips to the bathroom after eating to ensure that there is no self-induced vomiting. Patients may also need monitoring on bathroom trips after seeing visitors and after any hospital pass. The latter is to ensure that the patient has not had access to and ingested any laxatives or diuretics.

Therapy groups are led by nurses and other interdisciplinary team members (especially dietitians) and are tailored to the issues of patients with eating disorders.

Psychotherapy

The patient may be involved in a variety of therapies as a multimodal approach to address different issues. According to Bremer and associates (2004), the following therapies are used in all of the eating disorders and are geared to the recovery point of the patient:

- **Cognitive-behavioral therapy** is used to diminish errors in the patient's thinking and perceptions that result in distorted attitudes and eating-disordered behaviors. The patient practices new ways of examining cognitions and self-monitors behaviors.
- **Psychodynamic therapy** explores the underpinnings of the disorder.
- **Group therapy** offers support to patients who feel isolated while offering an arena in which to explore the eating disorder.
- **Family therapy** is especially efficacious in early-onset and short-duration anorexia. It supports parent refeeding of children and identifies family dynamics that may be contributing to the problem.

These therapies may take place in a variety of settings, including a partial hospitalization program, community mental health center, psychiatric home care program, or more traditional outpatient treatment. Regardless of the setting, the goals of treatment remain the same: weight restoration with normalization of eating habits and initiation of the treatment of the psychological, interpersonal, and social issues that are integral to the experience of the patient.

Often the nurse and other health care workers might contract with the patient regarding the terms of treatment. For example, outpatient treatment can continue only if the patient maintains an agreed-on weight. If weight falls below the goal, other treatment arrangements must be made until the patient returns to the goal weight. This highly structured approach to treatment of patients whose weight is less than 75% of ideal body weight is essential. Techniques such as assisting the patient with a daily meal plan, reviewing a journal of meals and dietary intake, and providing for weekly weighing (ideally two or three times a week) are essential in order to reach a medically stable weight.

Families often report feeling powerless in the face of such mystifying behavior. For instance, patients are often unable to experience compliments as supportive and therefore are unable to internalize the support. They often seek attention from others but feel scrutinized when they receive it. Patients express that they want their families to care for and about them but are unable to recognize expressions of care. When others do respond with love and support, patients do not perceive this as positive. Consequently, families experience the tension of saying or doing the wrong thing and then feeling responsible if a setback occurs. Psychiatric nurse clinicians have an important role in assisting families and significant others to develop strategies for improved communication and to search for ways to be comfortably supportive to the patient.

Pharmacological, Biological, and Integrative Therapies

According to Anderson and Yager (2005), medications seem to be most helpful only after weight has been restored. The selective serotonin reuptake inhibitors (SSRIs), such as fluoxetine (Prozac) are useful in reducing the occurrence of relapse in anorexia nervosa when the patient has reached a maintenance weight and is taking in adequate dietary tryptophan, the precursor for serotonin (Mitchell et al., 2001). Atypical antipsychotic agents such as olanzapine (Zyprexa) are helpful in improving mood and in decreasing obsessional behaviors and resistance to weight gain (Attia & Schroeder, 2005; Mitchell et al., 2001).

Long-Term Treatment

Anorexia nervosa is a chronic illness that waxes and wanes. Recovery is evaluated as a stage in the process rather than a fixed event. Factors that influence the stage of recovery include percentage of ideal body weight that has been achieved, the extent to which self-worth is defined by shape and weight, and the amount of disruption existing in the patient's personal life. The patient will require long-term treatment that might include periodic brief hospital stays, outpatient psychotherapy, and pharmacological interventions. The combination of individual, group, couples, and family therapy (especially for the younger patient) provides a patient with anorexia with the greatest chance for a successful outcome.

EVALUATION

The process of evaluation is built into the outcomes specified by the goals. Evaluation is ongoing, and short-term and intermediate goals are revised as necessary to achieve the treatment outcomes established. The goals provide a daily guide for evaluating success and must be continually reevaluated for their appropriateness. Generally the long-term outcome for anorexia nervosa in terms of symptom recovery is less favorable than that for bulimia nervosa.

> ### *Application of the Nursing Process: Bulimia Nervosa*

ASSESSMENT

People with bulimia nervosa may not initially appear to be physically or emotionally ill. They are often at or slightly above or below ideal body weight. However, as the assessment continues and the nurse makes further observations, physical and emotional problems become apparent. On inspection, the patient may demonstrate enlargement of the parotid glands and dental erosion and caries if the patient has been inducing vomiting. The history may reveal difficulties with impulsivity as well as compulsivity. Family relationships may be chaotic and reflect a lack of nurturing. These individuals' lives reflect instability and troublesome interpersonal relationships as well. It is not uncommon for patients to have a history of impulsive stealing of items such as food, clothing, or jewelry (Halmi, 2003). Refer back to Box 11-1 for a listing of the characteristics of bulimia nervosa and anorexia nervosa

Assessment Guidelines

Bulimia Nervosa

1. Medical stabilization is the first priority. Problems resulting from purging are disruptions in electrolyte and fluid balance and cardiac function. Therefore a thorough medical examination is vital.
2. Medical evaluation usually includes a thorough physical examination as well as pertinent laboratory testing of the following:
   * Electrolyte levels
   * Glucose level
   * Thyroid function tests
   * Complete blood count
   * Electrocardiogram (ECG)
3. Psychiatric evaluation is advised because treatment of psychiatric comorbidity is important to outcomes (depression and suicide are concerns).

VIGNETTE

I was a three-sport athlete throughout high school and then played volleyball in college. How did the bingeing and purging start, and how did it happen to me? I began to down thousands of calories at my parents' house and secretly go to the bathroom and purge, and then start all over again. By the time I went to college, I would go to several fast-food restaurants and order cheeseburgers, french fries, tacos, and milkshakes; consume them all by the time I got home; and then induce vomiting the minute I walked through the door. As time went by, the cycles became worse. I despised what I was doing and what it was doing to me, breaking blood vessels in my face, causing my eyes to swell, and causing me to deceive everyone. I hated it so much that each time I binged and purged, I swore to myself that it would never happen again.—Carly

DIAGNOSIS

Assessment of the patient with bulimia nervosa may reveal the need for multiple potential nursing diagnoses as a result of a number disordered eating and weight control behaviors. Problems resulting from purging are a first priority because electrolyte and fluid balance and cardiac function are affected. Common nursing diagnoses include *Decreased cardiac output, Disturbed body image, Powerlessness, Chronic low self-esteem, Anxiety,* and *Ineffective coping* (substance abuse, impulsive responses to problems).

OUTCOMES IDENTIFICATION

Some useful measurable outcome criteria for patients with bulimia nervosa follow (fill in the timeframe [e.g., in 1 week, by discharge, etc.]); the patient will:
   * Refrain from binge-purge behaviors
   * Demonstrate at least two new skills for managing stress/anxiety/shame (triggers to binge-purge behaviors)
   * Obtain and maintain normal electrolyte balance
   * Be free of self-directed harm
   * Express feelings in a non–food-related way
   * Verbalize desire to participate in ongoing treatment
   * State feels good about self and about who he or she is as a person
   * Name two personal strengths

PLANNING

The criteria for inpatient admission of a patient with bulimia nervosa are included in the criteria for inpatient admission of a patient with an eating disorder presented in Box 11-3. As with anorexia nervosa, the patient with bulimia may be treated for life-threatening complications, such as gastric rupture (rare), electrolyte imbalance, and cardiac dysrhythmias, in an acute care unit of a hospital. If the patient is admitted to a general inpatient psychiatric unit because of acute suicidal risk, only the acute psychiatric manifestations are addressed short term. Planning will also include appropriate referrals for continuing outpatient treatment.

IMPLEMENTATION

See Table 11-2 for intervention guidelines for a patient with bulimia nervosa.

Acute Care

A patient who is medically compromised as a result of bulimia nervosa is referred to an inpatient unit for comprehensive treatment of the illness. The cognitive-behavioral model of treatment is highly effective and frequently serves as the cornerstone of the therapeutic approach. Inpatient

TABLE 11-2   Interventions for Bulimia Nervosa

Intervention	Rationale
1. Assess mood and presence of suicidal thoughts/behaviors.	1. Emotional dysregulation is at the core of bulimic behaviors and there is always the risk for self-destructive behaviors.
2. Monitor physiological parameters (vital signs, electrolyte levels) as needed.	2. The life-threatening effect of weight restriction and/or purging needs to be monitored.
3. Explore dysfunctional thoughts that maintain the binge/purge cycle.	3. Nonjudgmental reframing can balance and combat distorted thinking and challenge automatic behaviors.
4. Educate the patient that fasting sets one up to binge, the binge/purge cycle and its self-perpetuating nature.	4. The binge/purge cycle is maintained by the pattern of restricting, hunger, bingeing and purging accompanied by feelings of shame, then repetition of the cycle.
5. Monitor patient during and after meals to prevent throwing away food and/or purging.	5. A matter-of-fact statement that the nurse's perceptions are different will help avoid a power struggle. Arguments and power struggles intensify the patient's need to control.
6. Acknowledge the patient's overvalued ideas of body shape and size without minimizing or challenging patient's perceptions.	6. Cognitive-behavioral approaches can be very effective in helping the patient identify irrational beliefs about self and body image.
7. Encourage patient to keep a journal of thoughts and feelings.	7. The journal can provide information to identify irrational thinking and identify triggers that induce disordered eating behaviors. Reframing distorted beliefs and thinking can lead to healthier behaviors.

units designed to treat eating disorders are especially structured to interrupt the cycle of binge eating and purging and to normalize eating habits. Therapy is begun to examine the underlying conflicts and distorted perceptions of shape and weight that sustain the illness. Evaluation for treatment of comorbid disorders, such as major depression and substance abuse, is also undertaken. In most cases of substance dependence, the treatment of the eating disorder must occur after the substance dependence is treated.

Communication Guidelines

Compared with the food-restricting patient with anorexia, the patient with bulimia nervosa often more readily establishes a therapeutic alliance with the nurse because the eating behaviors are so ego-dystonic, or against what they want. The therapeutic alliance allows the nurse, along with other members of the interdisciplinary team, to provide counseling that gives useful feedback regarding the distorted beliefs held by the patient. See Box 11-4 for a list of common cognitive distortions.

In working with a patient who has bulimia, the nurse needs to be aware that the patient is sensitive to the perceptions of others. The patient may feel significant shame and totally out of control. In building a therapeutic alliance, the nurse needs to empathize with feelings of low self-esteem,

unworthiness, and dysphoria (sadness or unease). The nurse may suspect dishonesty when the patient does not report bingeing or purging. An accepting, nonjudgmental approach, along with a comprehensive understanding of the subjective experience of the patient, will help to build trust.

Milieu Therapy

The highly structured milieu of an inpatient unit has as its primary goals the interruption of the binge-purge cycle and the prevention of the disordered eating behaviors. Interventions such as observation during and after meals to prevent purging, normalization of eating patterns, and maintenance of appropriate exercise are integral elements of treatment. The interdisciplinary team uses a comprehensive approach to address the emotional and behavioral problems that arise when the patient is no longer binge eating or purging. The interruption of the binge-purge pattern allows underlying feelings to come to the surface and to be examined.

Health Teaching and Health Promotion

Health teaching focuses not only on the eating disorder but also on meal planning, use of relaxation techniques, maintenance of a healthy diet and exercise, coping skills, the physical and emotional effects of bingeing and purging, and the effect of cognitive distortions. This preparation lays the foundation for the second phase of treatment, in which there are carefully planned challenges to the patient's newly developed skills. For instance, the patient is expected to have a meal while on pass outside the hospital. On return to the unit, the patient can share the experience.

On discharge from the hospital, the individual is referred for long-term care to solidify the goals that have been achieved, address the attitudes and the perceptions that maintain the eating disorder, and deal with the psychodynamic issues that attend the illness. The patient and family could benefit from connecting with a national network that addresses eating disorders, Anorexia Nervosa and Related Eating Disorders (ANRED; www.anred.com).

Psychotherapy

A cognitive-behavioral approach is the most effective treatment for bulimia nervosa. Patients with bulimia nervosa, because of possible coexisting depression, substance abuse, and personality disorders, often undergo various therapies. Although the specific eating-disordered behaviors may not be targeted in some therapies, it is those very behaviors that are responsible for much of the patient's emotional distress. It is imperative that irrational attitudes and perceptions of weight and shape be addressed. Therefore restructuring faulty perceptions and helping individuals develop accepting attitudes toward themselves and their bodies is a primary focus of therapy. When patients do not indulge in these bulimic behaviors, issues of self-worth and interpersonal functioning become more prominent.

Pharmacological, Biological, and Integrative Therapies

Antidepressant medication along with psychotherapy has been shown to bring about improvement in bulimic symptoms. The use of the SSRI fluoxetine, in addition to cognitive-behavioral treatment, produces a modest gain in the treatment benefit. Fluoxetine treatment reduces the number of binge eating and vomiting episodes in patients with and without comorbid depression (Anderson & Yager, 2005).

EVALUATION

The process of evaluation is built into the outcomes specified by the goals. Evaluation is ongoing, and short-term and intermediate goals are revised as necessary to achieve the treatment outcomes established. The goals provide a daily guide for evaluating success and must be continually re-evaluated for their appropriateness.

BINGE EATING DISORDER

Binge eating disorder is a variant of compulsive overeating. Although considerable controversy exists over whether this proposed diagnosis constitutes a separate eating disorder, 20% to 30% of obese individuals seeking treatment report binge eating as a pattern of overeating.

Overeating is frequently noted as a symptom of a depression (i.e., atypical depression). High rates of mood disorders and personality disorders are found among binge eaters. Binge eaters report a history of major depression significantly more often than non-binge eaters. They further report that binge eating is soothing and helps to regulate their moods. Although dieting is almost always an antecedent of binge eating in bulimia nervosa, in approximately 50% of a sample of obese binge eaters, no attempt to restrict dietary intake occurred prior to bingeing (APA, 2000a).

In the *DSM-IV-TR* appendix, research criteria are listed for further study of binge eating disorders. Because the individual engages in no compensatory behaviors (purging, exercise) in an attempt to control weight in this disorder, it is currently diagnosed as an EDNOS.

An effective program for those with binge eating disorder must integrate modification of the disordered eating and the depressive symptoms with the ultimate goal of a more appropriate weight for the individual. Fairburn and associates (2000) found the course of binge eating disorder to be different from that of bulimia nervosa and the outcome to be better. The overwhelming majority of individuals with binge eating disorder recover. Peterson and colleagues (2000) found that the frequency of binge eating episodes prior to intervention was predictive of treatment outcome.

The use of SSRIs to treat binge eating disorder has been studied. The use of sertraline (Zoloft) reduced the frequency of binges and the overall severity of the illness (Mitchell et al., 2001). However, cognitive-behavioral therapy programs are at present the most effective treatment for individuals with binge eating disorders (Wilson, 2003).

EXAMINING THE EVIDENCE Binge Eating Disorder: The Development of a Diagnosis

How does a psychiatric problem like binge eating become a formal disorder in the *Diagnostic and Statistical Manual (DSM)*?

The *DSM* lists categories of psychiatric diagnoses and criteria for assigning those diagnoses. It is a work in progress. When first published in 1952, the *DSM* identified about 60 different disorders. The latest version, the *DSM-IV-TR* which was published in 2000, identifies about 300 disorders. One of the most infamous revisions to the *DSM* was in 1973 when the American Psychiatric Association voted to have homosexuality stricken from the text and replaced with "sexual orientation disturbance."

Binge eating disorder (BED), which is characterized by impaired control over eating, rapid ingestion of large amounts of food without compensatory behaviors (e.g., fasting or purging), being overweight or obese, was not listed as a separate *DSM-IV-TR* disorder along with its own criteria. Instead it is listed in the back of the manual under the heading of "Criteria Sets and Axes Provided for Further Study." Opponents to a stand-alone category argue that it is actually bulimia, a subtype of obesity, or a special psychopathology among the obese (Devlin, et al., 2003).

Should it become a bona fide disorder? If its inclusion is based on sheer numbers of people affected, then it certainly should. According to a large national survey of 9282 American adults, the reported lifetime prevalence for BED is about 3%, whereas bulimia is 1%, and anorexia is 0.6% (Kessler et al., 2005). Likely, the problem is underreported because, according to the Centers for Disease Control and Prevention (2007), about 33% of the population is overweight or obese. It should be noted that being obese doesn't mean a person has BID—the key feature of this disorder is bingeing, or the rapid consumption of a large amount of food.

Although prevalence may influence its status as a disorder, the American Psychiatric Association's task force for the development of the *DSM-IV-TR* identified BED as a proposal for which there was insufficient scientific evidence to support its inclusion. Researchers have risen to this challenge to uncover scientific evidence. A new *DSM-V* workgroup is examining the literature in order to provide a recommendation for this diagnosis's future (Bender, 2007).

Stay tuned for the fifth installment of the *DSM!*

Bender, E. (2007). Eating-disorder data show extensive comorbidities. *Psychiatry News, 42*(5), 23.

Centers for Disease Control and Prevention. (2007). Overweight and obesity. Available at www.cdc.gov/nccdphp/dnpa/obesity/index.htm. Washington, DC: Author.

Devlin, M.J., Goldfein, J.A., & Dobrow, I. (2003). What is this thing called BED? Current status of binge eating disorder nosology. *International Journal of Eating Disorders, 34*(S1), S2-S18.

Kessler, R.C., Chiu, W.T., Demler, O., & Walters, M.S. (2005). Prevalence, severity, and comorbidity of 12-month *DSM-IV* disorders in the National Comorbidity Survey Replication. *Archives of General Psychiatry, 62,* 617-627.

KEY POINTS TO REMEMBER

- A number of theoretical models help explain risk factors for the development of eating disorders.
- Neurobiological theories identify an association between eating disorders, depression, and neuroendocrine abnormalities.
- Psychological theories explore issues of control in anorexia and affective instability and poor impulse control in bulimia.
- Genetic theories postulate the existence of vulnerabilities that may predispose people toward eating disorders, and increasingly twin studies confirm genetic liability, which perhaps interacts with environmental mechanisms.
- Sociocultural models look at both our present societal ideal of being thin and the ideal feminine role model in general.
- In populations in which eating disorders had been rare and are now appearing, the dynamics—the stress of acculturation versus identification with the new culture—are being examined.
- Anorexia nervosa is a possibly life-threatening eating disorder that includes severe underweight; low blood pressure, pulse, and temperature; dehydration; and low serum potassium level and dysrhythmias.
- Anorexia may be treated in an inpatient treatment setting, in which milieu therapy, psychotherapy (cognitive), development of self-care skills, and psychobiological interventions can be implemented.
- Long-term treatment is provided on an outpatient basis and aims to help patients maintain healthy weight; it includes treatment modalities such as individual therapy, family therapy, group therapy, psychopharmacology, and nutrition counseling.
- Individuals with bulimia nervosa are typically within the normal weight range, but some may be slightly below or above ideal body weight.

KEY POINTS TO REMEMBER—cont'd

- Assessment of a patient with bulimia may show enlargement of the parotid glands, dental erosion, and caries if the patient has induced vomiting.
- Acute care may be necessary when life-threatening complications are present, such as gastric rupture (rare), electrolyte imbalance, and cardiac dysrhythmias.
- The primary goal of interventions for a patient with bulimia is to interrupt the binge-purge cycle.
- Psychotherapy as well as self-care skill training is included.
- Long-term treatment focuses on therapy aimed at addressing any coexisting depression, substance abuse, and/or personality disorders that are causing the patient distress and interfer-

ing with quality of life. Self-worth and interpersonal functioning eventually become issues that are useful to target.
- Eating disorders not otherwise specified (EDNOS) include a variety of patterns (binge eating disorder was introduced in this chapter).
- Binge eaters report a history of major depression significantly more often than non–binge eaters.
- Effective treatment for obese binge eaters integrates modification of the disordered eating, improvement of depressive symptoms, and achievement of an appropriate weight for the individual.

CRITICAL THINKING

1. Tom Shift, a 19-year-old model, has experienced a rapid decrease in weight over the past 4 months, after his agent told him he would have to lose some weight or lose a coveted account. Tom is 6 feet 2 inches tall and weighs 132 pounds, down from his usual 176 pounds. He is brought to the emergency department with a pulse of 40 beats per minute and severe dysrhythmias. His laboratory workup reveals severe hypokalemia. He has become extremely depressed, saying, "I'm too fat . . . I won't take anything to eat. If I gain weight my life will be ruined. There is nothing to live for if I can't model." Tom's parents are startled and confused, and his best friend is worried and feels powerless to help Tom. "I tell Tom he needs to eat or he will die. I tell him he is a skeleton, but he refuses to listen to me. I don't know what to do."
   A. Which physical and psychiatric criteria suggest that Tom should be immediately hospitalized? What other physical signs and symptoms may be found on assessment?
   B. What are some of the questions you would eventually ask Tom when evaluating his biopsychosocial functioning?
   C. What are your feelings toward someone with anorexia? Can you make a distinction between your thoughts and feelings toward women with anorexia and toward men with anorexia?
   D. What are some things you could do for Tom's parents and Tom's friend in terms of offering them information, support, and referrals? Identify specific referrals.
   E. Explain the kinds of interventions or restrictions that may be used while Tom is hospitalized (e.g., weighing,

observation after eating or visits, exercise, therapy, self-care).
   F. How would you describe partial hospitalization programs or psychiatric home care programs when asked if Tom will have to be hospitalized for a long time?
   G. What are some of Tom's cognitive distortions that would be a target for therapy?
   H. Identify at least five criteria that, if met, would indicate that Tom was improving.

2. You and your close friend Mary Alice have been together since nursing school and you are now working on the same surgical unit. Mary Alice told you that in the past she has made several suicide attempts. Today you accidentally come upon her bingeing off unit, and she looks embarrassed and uncomfortable when she sees you. Several times you notice that she spends time in the bathroom and you hear sounds of retching. In response to your concern, she admits that she has been binge-purging for several years but that now she is getting out of control and feels profoundly depressed.
   A. Although Mary Alice doesn't show any physical signs of bulimia nervosa, what would you look for when assessing an individual with bulimia?
   B. What kinds of emergencies could result from bingeing and purging?
   C. What would be the most useful type of psychotherapy for Mary Alice initially and what issues would need to be addressed?
   D. What kinds of new skills does a person with bulimia need to learn to lessen the compulsion to binge and purge?
   E. What would be some signs that Mary Alice is recovering?

CHAPTER REVIEW

Choose the most appropriate answer.

1. Which of the following is an example of all-or-nothing thinking, which is a frequent cognitive distortion of patients with an eating disorder?
    1. "If I allow myself to gain weight, I'll become immense."
    2. "I'm unpopular because I'm fat."
    3. "When I'm thin, I'm powerful."
    4. "When people say I look better, they're really thinking I look fat."

2. Typical goals of inpatient hospitalization for an anorexic patient do not include:
    1. stabilization of the patient's immediate condition.
    2. limited weight restoration.
    3. determination of the causes for the eating disorder.
    4. restoration of normal electrolyte balance.

3. Which patient with an eating disorder would be at greatest risk for hypokalemia? A patient with:
    1. anorexia who loses weight by restricting food intake.
    2. anorexia or bulimia who purges to promote weight loss.
    3. bulimia whose predominant pathological behavior is excessive nocturnal eating.

4. an eating disorder who exercises intensely more than 4 hours per day but maintains a normal electrolyte balance.

4. Which medication is likely to be used in the treatment of patients with eating disorders? An:
    1. SSRI such as fluoxetine.
    2. antipsychotic such as risperidone.
    3. anxiolytic such as alprazolam.
    4. anticonvulsant such as carbamazepine.

5. Which of the following is least likely to contribute to building an effective therapeutic alliance between the nurse and an anorexic patient?
    1. Establishing disciplined eating through the nurse's authoritarian approach with the patient
    2. Avoiding the stance of a parental role in order to foster a sense of empowerment
    3. Offering a highly structured approach in treating severely underweight patients
    4. Contracting with the outpatient person about treatment terms

REFERENCES

American Nurses Association, American Psychiatric Nurses Association, & International Society of Psychiatric-Mental Health Nurses. (2007). *Psychiatric-mental health nursing: Scope and standards of practice.* Silver Springs, MD: Nursesbooks.org.

American Psychiatric Association (APA). (2000a). *Diagnostic and statistical manual of mental disorders (DSM-IV-TR)* (4th ed., text rev.). Washington, DC: Author.

American Psychiatric Association (APA). (2000b). *Practice guidelines for the treatment of psychiatric disorders: Compendium 2000.* Washington, DC: Author.

Anderson, A.F., & Yager, J. (2005). Eating disorders. In B.J. Sadock & V.A. Sadock (Eds.), *Comprehensive textbook of psychiatry* (8th ed, pp. 2002-2062). Philadelphia: Lippincott Williams & Wilkins.

Attia, E., & Schroeder, L. (2005) Pharmacologic treatment of anorexia nervosa: Where do we go from here? *International Journal of Eating Disorders, 37*(S1), S60-S63.

Bowers, W.A. (2001). Principles for applying cognitive-behavioral therapy to anorexia nervosa. *Psychiatric Clinics of North America, 24*(2), 293-303.

Brambilla, F., & Monteleone, P. (2003). Physical complications and physiological aberrations in eating disorders: A review. In M. Maj, Halmi, K., Lopez-Ibor, J.J. et al. (Eds.), *Eating disorders* (pp. 139-192). West Sussex, England: Wiley.

Bremer, J., Herzog, D.B., & Beresin, E.V. (2004). The patient with anorexia or bulimia. In T.A. Stern, J.B. Herman, & P.L. Slavin

(Eds), *Massachusetts General Hospital guide to primary care psychiatry* (2nd ed.). New York: McGraw-Hill.

Fairburn, C.G. (2002). Cognitive-behavioral therapy for bulimia nervosa. In C.G. Fairburn & K.D. Brownell (Eds.), *Eating disorders and obesity* (2nd ed., pp. 302-333). New York: Guilford Press.

Halmi, K.A. (2003). Classification, diagnosis and comorbidities of eating disorders. In M. Maj Halmi, K., Lopez-Ibor, J.J. et al. (Eds.), *Eating disorders* (pp. 315-338). West Sussex, England: Wiley.

Hudson, J.I., Hiripi, E., Harrison, G.P., & Kessler, R.C. (2007). The prevalence and correlates of eating disorders in the national comorbidity survey replication. *Biological Psychiatry, 61,* 348-358.

Kaye, W.H., Frank, G.K., Bailer, U.S., et al. (2005). Serotonin alterations in anorexia and bulimia nervosa: New insights from imaging studies. *Physiology and Behavior, 85*(1), 73-81.

Miller, M.N., & Pumariega, A.J. (2001). Culture and eating disorders: A historical and cross-cultural review. *Psychiatry, 64*(2), 93-110.

Sadock, J.B., & Sadock, V.A. (2007). *Kaplan's and Sadock's Synopsis of psychiatry* (10th ed.). Philadelphia: Wolters/Lippincott Williams & Wilkins.

Wilson, G.T. (2003). Psychological interventions for eating disorders: A review. In M. Maj, Halmi, K., Lopez-Ibor, J.J. et al. (Eds.), *Eating disorders* (pp. 315-338). West Sussex, England: Wiley.

CHAPTER 12

Mood Disorders: Depression

Elizabeth M. Varcarolis

Key Terms and Concepts

Objectives

1. Compare and contrast major depressive disorder (MDD) with dysthymia.
2. Discuss the links between the stress model of depression and the biological model of depression.
3. Be able to assess behaviors in a depressed individual with regard to each of the following areas: (a) affect, (b) thought processes, (c) feelings, (d) physical characteristics, and (e) communication.
4. Discuss some communication strategies that are useful for depressed patients.
5. Evaluate the advantages of the selective serotonin reuptake inhibitors (SSRIs) over the tricyclic antidepressants.
6. Explain the unique attributes of two of the newer atypical antidepressants for use in specific circumstances.
7. Explain why special dietary/medication restrictions have to be maintained with the use of a monoamine oxidase inhibitor (MAOI).
8. Discuss why the selegiline transdermal system (STS) is such a breakthrough MAOI.
9. Identify potential adverse reactions to the SSRIs.
10. Describe the types of depression for which electroconvulsive therapy is most helpful.

evolve

For additional resources related to the content of this chapter, visit the Evolve website at
http://evolve.elsevier.com/Varcarolis/essentials.

- Chapter Outline
- Chapter Review Answers
- Case Study and Nursing Care Plans

- Nurse, Patient, and Family Resources
- Concept Map Creator

No amount of information can adequately convey the personal pain and suffering experienced by the individual with depression (Young et al., 2001). All races, all ages, and males as well as females are susceptible to depressive episodes, although some individuals are more susceptible than others.

PREVALENCE AND COMORBIDITY

Depression is the fourth leading cause of disability in the United States, and it is projected to be the second leading cause of disability by 2020 (Montano, 2003). The lifetime prevalence of a major depressive episode is 16.6%, with a projected lifetime risk at age 75 being 23.2% (Kessler et al., 2005). Lifetime prevalence for females is 21% (Oquendo & Liebowitz, 2005).

Most studies find that major depressive disorder (MDD) is twice as common in women (12.0%) than in men (6.6%). Dysthymic disorder (DD) (chronic mild depression) occurs in about 2.5% of the population over a lifetime (Kessler et al., 2005). About 40% of people with DD also meet the criteria for MDD or bipolar disorder (BD) in any given year (NIMH, 2001b).

A depressive syndrome frequently accompanies other psychiatric disorders such as anxiety disorders, schizophrenia, substance abuse, eating disorders, and schizoaffective disorder. People with anxiety disorders (e.g., panic disorder, generalized anxiety disorder, obsessive-compulsive disorder) commonly present with depression, as do people with personality disorders (particularly borderline personality disorder), adjustment disorder, and brief depressive reactions.

Mixed anxiety–depression is perhaps one of the most common psychiatric presentations. Symptoms of anxiety occur in an average of 70% of cases of major depression. The presence of comorbid anxiety disorder and depression has a negative effect on the disease course. Comorbidity has been shown to result in a higher rate of suicide, greater severity of depression, greater impairment in social and occupational functioning, and poorer response to treatment (Simon & Rosenbaum, 2003).

The incidence of major depression greatly increases among people with a medical disorder. People with chronic medical problems are at a higher risk for depression than those in the general population. Depression is often secondary to a medical condition. Depression also may be secondary to use of substances such as alcohol, cocaine, marijuana, heroin, and even anxiolytics and other prescription medications. Depression also can be a sequela of bereavement and grief (Chapter 22).

Children and Adolescents

Children as young as 3 years of age have been diagnosed with depression. MDD is said to occur in as many as 18% of preadolescents, which is perhaps a low estimate because depression in this age-group is often underdiagnosed. Children at 10 years have a lifetime prevalence of 14%, and by age 25, a person has a 19% chance of having an MDD (Kessler et al., 2005). Girls 15 years and older are twice as likely to experience a major depressive episode as boys (NIMH, 2000a). Major depression among adolescents is often associated with substance abuse and antisocial behavior, both of which can obscure accurate diagnosis (Dubovsky et al., 2004).

MDD in children has a high recurrence rate of up to 70% within 5 years. The appearance of MDD in adolescence heralds a severe disorder with a recurrent course (Gruenberg & Goldstein, 2003). Children in families with other depressed members seem to become depressed earlier (ages 12 to 13 years) than children in families with no other depressed members (16 to 17 years). Even before adolescence, girls are more vulnerable to depression than boys.

Older Adults

Depression among older adults (65 or older) is approximately 6% to 9% for major depression and 17% to 18% for minor depression. In fact, a disproportionate number of depressed older Americans are likely to die by suicide, accounting for 25% of all suicides, and the incidence appears to increase with age (Rosenbaum & Covino, 2006). The symptoms of geriatric depression often go unrecognized because many masquerade as medical symptoms. Depression in older adults is often associated with chronic illnesses, and depression can go undiagnosed 50% of the time. The good news is that efforts to improve recognition of depression and education have led to positive treatment response among older adults.

THEORY

Although many theories attempt to explain the cause of depression, the many psychological, biological, and cultural variables make identification of any one cause difficult. It is unlikely that there is a single cause for depression. It is becoming evident that depression is a heterogeneous, systemic illness involving an array of different neurotransmitters, neurohormones, and neuronal pathways. The idea that depression is the result of a simple hereditary process or traumatic life event that ultimately leads to a single neurotransmitter deficiency is simply unsubstantiated by the evidence (Dubovsky et al., 2004).

EXAMINING THE EVIDENCE   The Talking Treatment

If depression is a real illness with chemical causation (like diabetes), how does talking help a person get better? After all, I don't think it would be very helpful to try to talk a person's blood sugar down.

Depression is caused by a combination of neural vulnerability and environmental factors. Some people may possess highly vulnerable chemistry and spontaneously or with little provocation develop depression, whereas others who are not genetically predisposed to depression may develop it only when exposed to sufficient stress. Considering the role of a hostile environment in the development of depression in many people, it stands to reason that a therapeutic environment would be helpful in alleviating depression.

What do we know? Let's start with sea slugs, creatures whose brains have been well mapped out. Dr. Eric Kandel, a neurobiologist and psychiatrist, is famous for studying the slugs' brains and demonstrating that learning actually remodels neurons (Friedman, 2002). The implication is that if psychotherapy is a form of learning, then it causes changes to brain structure and function.

Researchers have been hard at work to objectively measure, mainly through neuroimaging, the effects of psychotherapy. Roffman and colleagues (2005) critically reviewed investigations of the effect of psychotherapy on brain function. They found that cognitive behavioral therapy and interpersonal therapy resulted in cortical-subcortical changes; these changes also occur with antidepressant medications. Another group of researchers, Etkin and colleagues (2005), also conducted an integrated literature review with similar results.

What is interesting is that the imaging changes associated with psychotherapy occur mainly in different areas (with some overlap) than changes associated with psychopharmacological treatments. In fact, researchers have found that people respond best when they receive a combination of talking and medication treatment (Schram et al., 2007).

Etkin, A., Phil, M., Pittenger, C., et al. (2005). Toward a neurobiology of psychotherapy: Basic science and clinical applications. *Journal of Neuropsychiatry and Clinical Neuropsychiatry, 17,* 145-158.

Friedman, R.A. (2002). Like drugs, talk therapy can change brain chemistry. *Forensic Psychiatry and Medicine.* Available at www.forensic-psych.com/articles/artNYTTalkTherapy8.27.02.html

Roffman, J.L., Marci, C.D., Gloick, D.M., et al. (2005). Neuroimaging and the functional neuroanatomy of psychotherapy. *Psychological Medicine, 35,* 1385-1398.

Schramm, E., van Calker, D., Dykierek, P., et al. (2007). An intensive treatment program of interpersonal psychotherapy plus pharmacotherapy for depressed inpatients: Acute and long-term results. *American Journal of Psychiatry, 164*(5), 768-777.

The high variability in symptoms, response to treatment, and course of the illness supports the supposition that depression may result from a complex interaction of causes. For example, genetic predisposition to the illness combined with childhood stress may lead to significant changes in the central nervous system (CNS) that result in depression. However, there are common risk factors for depression that may signal the presence of this common and serious psychiatric illness (Gruenberg & Goldstein, 2003) (Box 12-1).

Biological Theories

Genetic Factors

Twin studies consistently show that genetic factors play a role in the development of depressive disorders. Various studies reveal that the average concordance rate for unipolar depression mood disorders among monozygotic twins (twins sharing the same genetic constitution) is 50%. That is, if one twin is affected, the second has a 50% chance of being affected. The percentage for dizygotic twins (different genetic complement) is 20%. Thus identical twins (mono-

BOX 12-1

Primary Risk Factors for Depression

- History of prior episodes of depression
- Family history of depressive disorder, especially in first-degree relatives
- History of suicide attempts or family history of suicide
- Female gender
- Age 40 years or younger
- Postpartum period
- Medical illness
- Absence of social support
- Negative, stressful life events
- Active alcohol or substance abuse
- History of sexual abuse

From Gruenberg, A.M., & Goldstein, R.D. (2003). Mood disorders: Depression. In A. Tasman, J. Kay, & J.A. Lieberman (Eds.). *Psychiatry* (2nd ed., p. 1210). West Sussex, England: Wiley.

zygotic) have a greater concordance rate than dizygotic twins (Gelder et al., 2006). However, because concordance rates in monozygotic twins are only 50%, it appears that other factors also must be involved.

Adoptive studies also have pointed to genetic contribution for the development of depression. For example, children born to a parent or parents with a depressive illness have the same risk of depression if adopted to a nondepressive family as those children who are not adopted away (Sadock & Sadock, 2007). Therefore mood disorders are heritable for some people. Increased heritability is associated with an earlier age of onset, greater rate of comorbidity, and increased risk of recurrent illness. However, any genetic factors that are present must interact with environmental factors for depression to develop.

Biochemical Factors

The brain is a highly complex organ that contains billions of neurons. There is much evidence to support the concept that depression is a biologically heterogeneous disorder; that is, many CNS neurotransmitter abnormalities can probably cause clinical depression. These neurotransmitter abnormalities may be the result of inherited or environmental factors, or even of other medical conditions, such as cerebral infarction, hypothyroidism, acquired immunodeficiency syndrome, or drug use. Whatever the etiologic contributions of depression for an individual might be, depression is ultimately mediated through changes in the brain's neurochemistry and the circuitry involved in emotional regulations (Gelder et al., 2006).

Neurobiological investigations in depression have focused on the monoamine neurotransmitters (serotonin, noradrenaline, and dopamine). Specific neurotransmitters in the brain are believed to be related to altered mood states. **Serotonin** (5-hydroxytryptamine or 5-HT) **and norepinephrine are two major neurotransmitters involved in depression.** Serotonin is an important regulator of sleep, appetite, and libido. A serotonin circuit dysfunction can result in poor impulse control, low sex drive, decreased appetite, and irritability (Sadek & Nemeroff, 2000). Decreased levels of norepinephrine in the medial forebrain bundle may account for **anergia** (reduction in or lack of energy), **anhedonia** (an inability to find meaning or pleasure in existence), decreased concentration, and diminished libido in depression.

Serotonin and norepinephrine are also involved in the perception of pain by modifying the effects of substance P, glutamate, γ-aminobutyric acid (GABA), and other pain mediators (Montano, 2003). In fact, one study demonstrated that 43% of people with major depression had at least one chronic painful condition. This was four times the rate in those without MDD (Montano, 2003). There is considerable evidence of overlap in the physiology of pain and mood disorders (Kramer, 2004).

Current research suggests that depression results from the dysregulation of a number of other neurotransmitter systems in addition to serotonin and norepinephrine. The dopamine, acetylcholine, and GABA systems are believed to be involved in the pathophysiology of a major depressive episode (APA, 2000). Dopamine neurons in the mesolimbic system are thought to play a role in the reward and incentive behavior processes that are disrupted in depression. This is particularly true in melancholic states (severe MDD) (Gelder et al., 2006). It is now considered unlikely that a catecholamine deficiency alone is the actual cause of depression (Gruenberg & Goldstein, 2003).

It is important to keep in mind that the neurotransmitters specific to depression (norepinephrine, serotonin, and dopamine) each have many subtypes, thus the complexity in treatment and varied patient responses to attempts to increase these neurotransmitters through medications.

Stressful life events, especially losses, seem to be a significant factor in the development of depression. According to Gelder and colleagues (2006), research has shown the following:

- There is a sixfold excess of adverse life events in the months before the onset of a depressive disorder.
- "Loss" events are associated more with depression, whereas "threat" events seem to be associated more with anxiety.
- The importance of stressful adverse life events in the onset of depression decreases once depressive disorder is clearly established. Then depressive episodes continue in the absence of adverse stressful life events.

Norepinephrine, serotonin, and acetylcholine play a role in stress regulation. When these neurotransmitters become overtaxed through stressful events, neurotransmitter depletion may occur. There is evidence that people who possess a "short" gene, or stress-sensitive version of the serotonin transporter gene, are at a higher risk of depression if they have been abused as children or if they have been exposed to multiple stressful life events. However, people with the "long" or protected version of the gene who underwent multiple life stressors experienced no more depression than people who were totally spared life stressors (NIMH, 2003a).

No unitary mechanism of depressant action has been found. The relationships among the serotonin, norepinephrine, dopamine, acetylcholine, and GABA systems are complex and need further assessment and study. However, medication that helps regulate these neurotransmitters has proved empirically successful in the treatment of many patients. Figure 12-1 shows a positron emission tomogra-

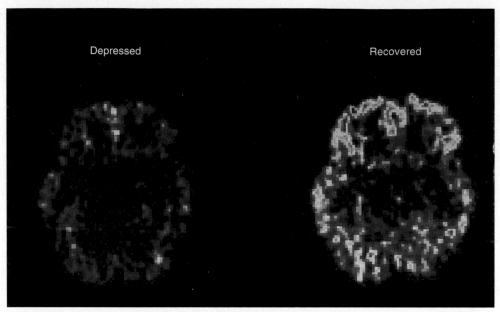

Figure 12-1 ■ Positron emission tomography (PET) scans of a 45-year-old woman with recurrent depression. The scan on the left was taken when the patient was on no medication and very depressed. The scan on the right was taken several months later when the patient was well, after she had been treated with medication for her depression. Note that her entire brain, particularly the left prefrontal cortex, is more active when she is well. (Courtesy Mark George, MD, Biological Psychiatry Branch, National Institute of Mental Health.)

phy (PET) scan of the brain of a woman with depression before and after taking medication.

Neuroendocrine Factors

The neuroendocrine characteristic most widely studied in relation to depression has been hyperactivity of the hypothalamic-pituitary-adrenal cortical axis. Evidence of increased cortisol secretion is apparent in 20% to 40% of depressed outpatients and 40% to 60% of depressed inpatients. This increase was once thought to be the result of depression, but research indicates that excess cortisol may in fact be causative (Ardayfio & Kim, 2006).

The dexamethasone suppression test (DST) is used to determine if cortisol is being inhibited properly by adrenocorticotropic hormone (ACTH) feedback. Dexamethasone, a synthetic steroid, is administered, and in about 50% of people with depression, it fails to suppress serum cortisol. Significantly, patients with severe and psychotic unipolar MDD have rates of nonsuppression of 80% to 90% (Dubovsky et al., 2004).

Image Findings

Computed axial tomography (CAT) and magnetic resonance imaging (MRI) scans show ventricular enlargement, cortical atrophy, and sulcal widening in many studies (Sadock & Sadock, 2007). Other areas that have shown consistent changes are decreased size of the caudate,

putamen, and possibly the cerebellum (Dubovsky et al., 2004). PET scans have repeatedly revealed reduced metabolic activity in the frontal lobes (Sadock & Sadock, 2007).

Psychodynamic Influences and Life Events

The stress-diathesis model of depression is a psychological theory that explains depression from an environmental and life-events perspective (stress) combined with biological vulnerability or predisposition (diathesis). What is certain is that psychosocial stressors and interpersonal events trigger certain neurophysical and neurochemical changes in the brain (NIMH, 2002). Early life trauma may result in long-term hyperactivity of the CNS corticotropin-releasing factor (CRF) and norepinephrine systems with a consequent neurotoxic effect on the hippocampus that leads to neuronal loss. These changes could cause sensitization of the CRF circuits to even mild stress in adulthood, leading to an exaggerated stress response (Heim & Nemeroff, 1999). With exposure to repeated stress in adulthood, these already stress-sensitive pathways become "markedly hyperactive leading to a persistent increase in CRF and cortisol secretion, which causes alterations in the glucocorticoid receptors and thus forms the basis for the development of mood and anxiety disorders" (Sadek & Nemeroff, 2000).

These stressors and life events may lead to a depressive syndrome in some individuals, particularly those who are biologically vulnerable to depression, such as those with the short or stress-sensitive version of the serotonin transporter gene mentioned earlier. Therefore life events (psychosocial stressors and interpersonal events) may influence the development and recurrence of depression through the psychological and biological experience of stress in some people, which results in changes in the connections among nerve cells in the brain.

Cognitive Theory

Aaron T. Beck, one of the early proponents of cognitive therapy, applied cognitive-behavioral theory to depression. Beck proposed that people acquire a psychological predisposition to depression through early life experiences. These experiences contribute to negative, illogical, and irrational thought processes that may remain dormant until they are activated during times of stress (Beck & Rush, 1995).

Beck found that depressed people process information in negative ways, even in the midst of positive factors that affect the person's life. Beck believed that three automatic negative thoughts—called **Beck's cognitive triad**—are responsible for the development of depression:

1. *A negative, self-deprecating view of self:* "I really never do anything well; everyone else seems smarter."
2. *A pessimistic view of the world:* "Once you're down, you can't get up. Look around, poverty, homelessness, sickness, war, and despair are every place you look."
3. *The belief that negative reinforcement (or no validation for the self) will continue:* "It doesn't matter what you do; nothing ever gets better. I'll be in this stupid job the rest of my life."

The phrase *automatic negative thoughts* refers to thoughts that are repetitive, unintended, and not readily controllable. This cognitive triad seems to be consistent in all types of depression, regardless of clinical subtype.

The goal of cognitive-behavioral therapy (CBT) is to change the way a patient thinks, which will in turn help relieve the depressive syndrome. This is accomplished by assisting the patient in the following:

1. Identifying and testing negative cognition
2. Developing alternative thinking patterns
3. Rehearsing new cognitive and behavioral responses

Learned Helplessness

One of the most popular theories of the cause of depression is Martin Seligman's theory of learned helplessness. Seligman (1973) stated that although anxiety is the initial response to a stressful situation, anxiety is replaced by depression if the person feels no control over the outcome of a situation. A person who believes that an undesired event is his or her fault and that nothing can be done to change it is prone to depression. The theory of learned helplessness has been used to explain the development of depression in certain social groups, such as older adults, people living in impoverished areas, and women.

CULTURAL CONSIDERATIONS

According to the Cross-National Collaborative Group, the prevalence rate of depressive disorders in Asian Americans was the lowest in comparison to whites, African Americans, and Hispanics (Rihmer & Angst, 2005). Prevalence rates for MDD in whites are significantly higher than in African Americans and Mexican Americans, although the opposite is true for DD (Riolo et al., 2005).

CLINICAL PICTURE

Figure 12-2 presents diagnostic criteria for MDD and DD, the two depressive disorders defined by the *Diagnostic and Statistical Manual of Mental Disorders (DSM-IV-TR)* (APA, 2000a). Depression can be manifested in a variety of other symptoms that are called specifiers. Other subgroups are being researched as well (Table 12-1).

Major Depressive Disorder

Patients with a **major depressive disorder (MDD)** experience substantial pain and suffering, as well as psychological, social, and occupational disability. A patient with MDD presents with a history of one or more major depressive episodes and no history of manic or hypomanic episodes. In MDD, the symptoms often interfere with the person's social or occupational functioning and in some cases may include psychotic features. Psychotic major depression is a severe form of **mood** disorder that is characterized by delusions or hallucinations. For example, patients might have delusional thoughts that interfere with their nutritional status (e.g., "God put snakes in my stomach and told me not to eat.").

The emotional, cognitive, physical, and behavioral symptoms an individual exhibits during a major depressive episode represent a change in the person's usual functioning.

The course of MDD is variable. An average episode may last about 9 months, although it has been shown that 20% of individuals will not have recovered by that time. Long-term studies indicate that after 5 years there is a 70% recurrence rate, and an 80% recurrence rate after 8 years (Psychdirect.com, 2006).

DSM-IV-TR CRITERIA FOR DEPRESSIVE DISORDERS

DEPRESSIVE DISORDERS

Major Depressive Disorder

1. Represents a change in previous functions.

2. Symptoms cause clinically significant distress or impair social, occupational, or other important areas of functioning.

3. **Five or more** of the following occur nearly every day for most waking hours over the same 2-week period:
   • Depressed mood most of day, nearly every day
   • Anhedonia
   • Significant weight loss or gain (more than 5% of body weight in 1 month)
   • Insomnia or hypersomnia
   • Increased or decreased motor activity
   • Anergia (fatigue or loss of energy)
   • Feelings of worthlessness or inappropriate guilt (may be delusional)
   • Decreased concentration or indecisiveness
   • Recurrent thoughts of death or suicidal ideation (with or without plan)

Dysthymia

1. Occurs over a 2-year period (1 year for children and adolescents), depressed mood.

2. Symptoms cause clinically significant distress in social, occupational, and other important areas of functioning.

3. **Two or more** of the following are present:
   • Decreased or increased appetite
   • Insomnia or hypersomnia
   • Low energy or chronic fatigue
   • Decreased self-esteem
   • Poor concentration or difficulty making decisions
   • Feelings of hopelessness or despair

Specifiers Describing Most Recent Episode

1. Chronic

2. Atypical features

3. Catatonic features

4. Melancholic features

5. Postpartum onset

Specify If

1. Early onset (before 21 years of age)

2. Late onset (21 years of age or older)

3. Atypical features

Figure 12-2 ■ Diagnostic criteria for major depression and dysthymia. (Adapted from American Psychiatric Association. [2000]. *Diagnostic and statistical manual of mental disorders* [4th ed., text rev.]. Washington, DC: Author.)

VIGNETTE

Sally, a bright, successful, 24-year-old businessperson, finds her world is changing. Over the past few weeks she has become more and more withdrawn. Her life has become empty of meaning. She has great difficulty getting out of bed in the mornings, but finds it hard to sleep more than 3 to 4 hours a night, waking at 2 or 3 AM. She is constantly exhausted.

Sally finds it impossible to concentrate at work and has called in sick the past 2 days, unable to find the energy to dress, bathe, groom, or even eat. She hasn't eaten for 3 days except for some water and a few glasses of milk and a few crackers she found in a neglected box tucked away in the pantry. She has lost considerable weight.

continued

TABLE 12-1	Depressive Disorders: Specifiers and Clinical Phenomena	
Disorder	***DSM-IV-TR* Status**	**Symptoms and Comments**
Major depressive disorder (MDD)	Disorder	Specific *DSM-IV-TR* criteria are outlined in Figure 12-2. Symptoms represent a change from usual functioning. Associated with high mortality rate. Impairment in physical, social, and role functioning, as well as increased potential for pain and physical illness.
With psychotic features	Specifier	Indicates the presence of delusions (e.g., delusions of guilt or being punished for sins, somatic delusions of horrible disease or body rotting, delusions of poverty or going bankrupt) or hallucinations (usually auditory, voices berating person for sins or shortcomings).
With postpartum onset	Specifier	Indicates onset within 4 weeks after childbirth. Can present with or without psychotic features. **Severe ruminations or delusional thoughts about infant signify increased risk of harm to infant.**
With seasonal characteristics; seasonal affective disorder (SAD)	Specifier	Indicates that episodes mostly begin in fall or winter and remit in spring. Characterized by anergia, hypersomnia, overeating, weight gain, and a craving for carbohydrates. Responds to light therapy.
With chronic features	Specifier	Indicates MDD lasting 2 years or longer.
Dysthymic disorder (DD)	Disorder	Specific *DSM-IV-TR* criteria are presented in Figure 12-2. Has an early and insidious onset (childhood to early adulthood). Shows a chronic course. Some 75% of people with DD go on to develop MDD. When dysthymia is superimposed on a major depression, it is called **double depression**.
With **atypical** features	Specifier	Indicates mood reactivity (can be cheered with positive events) and rejection sensitivity (pathological sensitivity to perceived interpersonal rejection) that are present through life and result in functional impairment. Other symptoms include hypersomnia, hyperphagia (overeating), leaden paralysis (feeling weighed down in extremities).
Mixed anxiety–depression	RDC	Prevalence of 5%. Characterized by significant functional disability. Criteria include at least 1 month of persistent dysphoric mood, with possible hypervigilance, difficulty concentrating, fatigue, low self-esteem, irritability, and more, all causing **significant distress or impairment in functioning**.
Recurrent brief depression	RDC	Meets criteria for depressive episode, but episodes last 1 day to 1 week. Depressive episode must recur at least once per month over 12 months or more. **Carries a high risk for suicide.**
Premenstrual dysphoric disorder	RDC	Characterized by more severe symptoms than premenstrual syndrome. Symptoms begin toward last week of luteal phase and are absent in the week following menses. Symptoms include depressed mood, anxiety, affective lability, or persistent and marked anger or irritability. Other symptoms include anergia, overeating, difficulty concentrating, feeling of being out of control or overwhelmed, and more.
Minor depression	RDC	Characterized by sustained depressed mood without the full depressive syndrome. Pessimistic attitude and self-pity are required for the diagnosis (Dubovsky & Buzan, 1999). May be chronic and may be complicated by a superimposed major depressive episode.

RDC, Research diagnostic category.

When her best friend calls to find out why she hasn't shown up for work, Sally tells her, "I don't know . . . I just can't concentrate; I can't focus on anything. Nothing seems to be worth doing. I feel so heavy and empty inside. I don't see things getting any better." When her friend tries to coax her out of her mood, Sally snaps at her and tells her to mind her own business and leave her alone. Later, Sally is filled with remorse, telling herself she is a horrible person and doesn't deserve her friend's concern and loyalty. She wonders what it would be like if she no longer had to deal with all this pain; could she take this much longer?

Subtypes Seen in MDD

The diagnosis for MDD may include a specifier in patients with specific symptoms. Specifiers include the following:

- **Psychotic feature:** breaks with reality (e.g., hallucinations, delusions)
- **Catatonic features:** such as peculiar voluntary movement, echopraxia or echolalia, and negativism
- **Melancholic features:** such as anorexia or weight loss, diurnal variations with symptoms worse in the morning, early morning awakening)
- **Postpartum onset:** within 4 weeks postpartum (e.g., severe anxiety, possible psychotic features)
- **Seasonal features (seasonal affective disorder, or SAD):** for example, generally occurring in fall or winter and remitting in the spring
- **Atypical features:** such as appetite changes or weight gain, hypersomnia, extreme sensitivity to perceived interpersonal rejection, high levels of anxiety

evolve

For a comprehensive case study and associated nursing care plans for a patient experiencing depression, visit the Evolve website at http://evolve.elsevier.com/Varcarolis/essentials.

Dysthymia

Dysthymic disorder (DD) often has an early and insidious onset and is characterized by a chronic depressive syndrome that is usually present for most of the day, more days than not, for at least 2 years (APA, 2000b). The depressive mood disturbance, because of its chronic nature, cannot be distinguished from the person's usual pattern of functioning ("I've always been this way") (APA, 2000b). Although people with dysthymia suffer from social and occupational distress, it is not usually severe enough to warrant hospitalization unless the person becomes suicidal. The age of onset

is usually from early childhood and teenage years to early adulthood. Patients with DD are at risk for developing MDD as well as other psychiatric disorders. This may be referred to as double depression.

Differentiating MDD from DD can be difficult because the disorders have similar symptoms. The main differences are in the severity of the symptoms; a DD is much less severe than an episode of MDD.

VIGNETTE

Sam has had another bad week at work. He just can't seem to perform the way he thinks he should—he never gets things right. Although his work seems acceptable to others, he constantly puts himself down. He wanted to take a class to improve his computer skills, but can't seem to find the energy or the time. His weekends are filled with hanging around his apartment, nothing much going on . . . there is never much going on. Life is dull; has it ever been otherwise? His brother is always telling him that he has a face as long as a football field. "What's the matter with you, bro? You're good looking, smart. Go find a girl and have some fun in life. Why can't you just enjoy anything?" Sam just sighs. Who could be interested in him? He gets a cold beer from the fridge and watches reruns on TV.

Application of the Nursing Process
ASSESSMENT

Undiagnosed and untreated depression is often associated with more severe presentation of depression, greater suicidality, somatic problems, and severe anxiety or anxiety disorders. Depression in older adults is often missed, especially if there are coexisting medical problems. Depression in children and adolescents may go undiagnosed when attention is focused on behavioral problems ("just a stage"). Racial disparities in health care, among other things, allow for underdiagnosing and undertreating African Americans, Hispanics, and other minorities (AHRQ, 2004).

A study by Bijl and associates (2004) concluded that depressed individuals who sought treatment manifesting psychological symptoms were recognized as depressed 90% of the time, in contrast with those who showed somatic symptoms (e.g., chronic pain, insomnia), who were recognized as depressed 50% of the time. In those who had a medical disorder, depression was identified 20% of the time.

Assessment Tools

Numerous standardized screening tools can help the clinician assess the type of depression a person may be

ZUNG'S SELF-RATING DEPRESSION SCALE	None or Little of the Time	Some of the Time	A Good Part of the Time	Most or All of the Time
1. I feel down-hearted, blue, and sad.	1	2	3	4
2. Morning is when I feel the best.	4	3	2	1
3. I have crying spells or feel like it.	1	2	3	4
4. I have trouble sleeping through the night.	1	2	3	4
5. I eat as much as I used to.	4	3	2	1
6. I enjoy looking at, talking to, and being with attractive women/men.	4	3	2	1
7. I notice that I am losing weight.	1	2	3	4
8. I have trouble with constipation.	1	2	3	4
9. My heart beats faster than usual.	1	2	3	4
10. I get tired for no reason.	1	2	3	4
11. My mind is as clear as it used to be.	4	3	2	1
12. I find it easy to do the things I used to do.	4	3	2	1
13. I am restless and can't keep still.	1	2	3	4
14. I feel hopeful about the future.	4	3	2	1
15. I am more irritable than usual.	1	2	3	4
16. I find it easy to make decisions.	4	3	2	1
17. I feel that I am useful and needed.	4	3	2	1
18. My life is pretty full.	4	3	2	1
19. I feel that others would be better off if I were dead.	1	2	3	4
20. I still enjoy the things I used to do.	4	3	2	1

* A raw score of 50 or above is associated with depression requiring hospital treatment.

Figure 12-3 ■ Nursing assessment: Zung's Self-Rating Depression Scale. (From Zung, W.K. [1965]. A self-rating depression scale. *Archives of General Psychiatry, 12,* 63.)

experiencing. For example, the Beck Depression Inventory, the Hamilton Depression Scale, and the Geriatric Depression Scale all are valuable tools. The Zung Self-Rating Depression Scale is a short inventory that highlights predominant symptoms seen in depressed individuals; it is presented here because of its ease of use and summation of depressive symptoms (Figure 12-3).

The National Mental Health Association (NMHA) has a website (www.depression-screening.org) that enables people to take a confidential screening test for depression online and find reliable information on the illness.

Assessment of Suicide Potential

The patient should be evaluated for suicidal or homicidal ideation. Between 10% and 15% of depressed people eventually commit suicide (Fuller & Sajatovic, 2000). Initial suicide evaluation might include the following statements or questions:

* "You have said you are depressed. Tell me what that is like for you."

* "When you feel depressed, what thoughts go through your mind?"
* "Have you ever thought about taking your own life in the past? Now? Do you have a plan? Do you have the means to carry out your plan? Is there anything that would prevent you from carrying out your plan?"

Refer to Chapter 20 for more on suicide prevention and intervention.

Areas to Assess

Mood

A depressed mood and **anhedonia** (lack of enjoyment in life) are the key symptoms in depression. Nearly 97% of people with depression have **anergia** (lack of energy). **Anxiety**, a common symptom in depression, is seen in about 60% to 90% of depressed patients. Some feelings that may be inherent in a depressed mood are as follows:

* Feelings of **worthlessness** range from feeling inadequate to having an unrealistic evaluation of self-worth.

These feelings reflect the low self-esteem that is a painful partner to depression. Statements such as "I am no good, I'll never amount to anything" are common. Themes of one's inadequacy and incompetence are repeated relentlessly.

- **Guilt** is a common accompaniment to depression. A person may ruminate over present or past failings. Extreme guilt can assume psychotic proportions: "I have committed terrible sins," "I have caused terrible pain and destruction to everyone I have ever known and now I'm paying for it."

- **Helplessness** is evidenced by everything believed too difficult to accomplish (e.g., grooming, housework, working, caring for children). With feelings of helplessness come feelings of **hopelessness**. Even though most depressive states are usually time limited, during a depressed period, people believe that things will never change, which leads some to look at suicide as a way out of constant mental pain. Hopelessness is one of the core characteristics of depression and suicide, as well as a characteristic of schizophrenia, alcoholism, and physical illness. Hopelessness results in negative expectations for the future and loss of control over future outcomes.

- **Anger** and **irritability** are natural outcomes of profound feelings of helplessness. Anger in depression is often expressed inappropriately. For example, anger may be expressed in destruction of property, hurtful verbal attacks, or physical aggression toward others. Anger may also be directed toward the self in the form of suicidal or self-destructive behaviors (alcohol abuse, substance abuse, overeating, smoking, etc.). These behaviors often result in feelings of low self-esteem and worthlessness.

Physical Changes

A person who is depressed sees the world through gray-colored glasses. Posture is poor, and the patient may look older than the stated age. Facial expressions convey sadness and dejection, and the patient may have frequent bouts of weeping. Conversely, the patient may say that he or she is unable to cry. Feelings of **hopelessness** and **despair** are readily reflected in the person's affect. For example, the patient may not make eye contact, may speak in a monotone, may show little or no facial expression (flat affect), and may make only yes or no responses. Frequent sighing is common.

People who are depressed often complain of lack of energy (**anergia**). Lethargy and fatigue can result in psychomotor retardation. Movements are slow, facial expressions are decreased, and gaze is fixed. The continuum in **psychomotor retardation** may range from slowed and dif-

ficult movements to complete inactivity and incontinence. At other times the nurse may note **psychomotor agitation**. For example, patients may constantly pace, bite their nails, smoke, tap their fingers, or engage in some other tension-relieving activity. At these times, patients feel fidgety and unable to relax.

Grooming, dress, and personal hygiene are markedly neglected. People who usually take pride in their appearance and dress may be poorly groomed and allow themselves to look shabby and unkempt.

Vegetative signs of depression are universal. Vegetative signs refer to alterations in those activities necessary to support physical life and growth (eating, sleeping, elimination, sex). For example, **changes in eating patterns** are common. About 60% to 70% of people who are depressed report having anorexia; overeating occurs more often in dysthymia.

Changes in sleep patterns are a cardinal sign of depression. Often, people have **insomnia,** waking at 3 or 4 AM and staying awake, or sleeping only for short periods. The light sleep of a depressed person tends to prolong the agony of depression over a 24-hour period. For some, sleep is increased (**hypersomnia**) and provides an escape from painful feelings. This is more common in young depressed individuals or those with bipolar tendencies. In any event, sleep is rarely restful or refreshing.

Changes in bowel habits are common. Constipation is seen most frequently in patients with psychomotor retardation. Diarrhea occurs less frequently, often in conjunction with psychomotor agitation. **Interest in sex declines** (loss of libido) during depression. Some men experience impotence, and a declining interest in sex often occurs among both men and women, which can further complicate marital and social relationships.

Stuart (2003) reports that more than two thirds of people suffering from depression complain of **pain** with or without reporting psychological symptoms. People who suffer from **chronic pain** need careful assessment for possible depression.

Cognition

When people are depressed, their thinking is slow and their memory and concentration are usually affected. Depressed people dwell on and exaggerate their perceived faults and failures and are unable to focus on their strengths and successes. As mentioned, identifying the presence of suicidal thoughts and suicide potential has the highest priority in the initial assessment. Approximately two thirds of depressed people contemplate suicide, and up to 15% of untreated or inadequately treated patients give up hope and actually follow through with the suicide (see Chapter 20).

When depressed, a person's ability to solve problems and think clearly is negatively affected. Judgment is poor, and indecisiveness is common. The individual may claim that the mind is slowing down. Evidence of delusional thinking may be seen in a person with major depression. Common statements of delusional thinking are "I have committed unpardonable sins," and "I am wicked and should die."

Assessment Guidelines

Depression

1. Always evaluate the patient's risk of harm to self or others. Overt hostility is highly correlated with suicide (see Chapter 20).
2. A thorough medical and neurological examination helps determine if the depression is primary or secondary to another disorder. Depression can be secondary to a host of medical or other psychiatric disorders, as well as medications. Essentially, evaluate whether:
   • The patient is psychotic
   • The patient has taken drugs or alcohol
   • Medical conditions are present
   • The patient has a history of a comorbid psychiatric syndrome (eating disorder, borderline or anxiety disorder)
3. Assess history of depression and determine what happened as well as what worked and did not work.
   • "Have you ever gone through or felt anything like this before?"
   • "What seemed to help you at that time?"
4. Assess support systems, family, and significant others and the need for information and referrals.
   • "With whom do you live?"
   • "Whom do you trust?"
   • "To whom do you talk when you are upset?"
5. Assess for any events that might have "triggered" a depressive episode.
   • "Has anything happened recently to upset you?"
   • "Have you had any major changes in your life?"
   • "Have you had any recent losses: job, divorce, loss of partner, child moving away, deaths?"
6. Include a psychosocial assessment that includes cultural beliefs related to mental health and treatment, and spiritual practices and how the depression is affecting the patient's beliefs and practice.
   • "How do you view depression?"
   • "Have you tried taking any over-the-counter remedies [e.g., herbs] to help with your depression?"
   • "Do you find solace in spiritual activities or find in a place of worship [e.g., church, temple, mosque]?"

DIAGNOSIS

Depression is complex, depressed individuals have a variety of needs, and nursing diagnoses are many. However, during the initial assessment, a high priority for the nurse is identification of the presence of suicide potential. Therefore the nursing diagnosis of *Risk for suicide* is always considered. Other key targets for nursing interventions are represented by the diagnoses of *Hopelessness, Ineffective coping, Social isolation, Spiritual distress*, and one or more of the *Self-care deficits (bathing/hygiene, dressing/grooming, feeding, toileting)*. Table 12-2 identifies signs and symptoms commonly experienced in depression and offers possible nursing diagnoses.

OUTCOMES IDENTIFICATION

Outcomes should include goals for safety. Even if the patient is not having self-destructive thoughts, one goal should be to name a person that the patient will contact if such thoughts arise. Goals for the outcomes of the vegetative or physical signs of depression (e.g., *reports adequate sleep*) are formulated to show, for example, evidence of weight gain, return to normal bowel activity, sleep of 6 to 8 hours per night, or return of sexual desire.

PLANNING

The planning of care for patients with depression is geared toward the phase of depression the person is in and the particular symptoms the person is exhibiting. At all times the nurse and members of the health care team are cognizant of the potential for suicide, and assessment of risk for self-harm (or harm to others) is ongoing during the care of the depressed person. There is evidence that a combination of therapy (cognitive, behavioral, interpersonal) and psychopharmacology can be an effective approach in treating depression.

Nurses and clinicians need to assess and plan for any vegetative signs of depression, as well as changes in concentration, activity level, social interaction, personal appearance, and so on. Therefore the planning of care for a patient who is depressed is based on the individual's symptoms and attempts to encompass a variety of areas in the person's life. Safety is always the highest priority.

IMPLEMENTATION
Communication Guidelines

A person who is depressed may speak and comprehend very slowly. The lack of an immediate response by the patient

TABLE 12-2   Potential Nursing Diagnoses for Depression

Signs and Symptoms	Nursing Diagnoses
Previous suicidal attempts, putting affairs in order, giving away prized possessions, suicidal ideation (has plan, ability to carry it out), overt or covert statements regarding killing self, feelings of worthlessness, hopelessness, helplessness	*Risk for suicide* *Risk for self-mutilation*
Lack of judgment, memory difficulty, poor concentration, inaccurate interpretation of environment, negative ruminations, cognitive distortions	*Disturbed thought processes*
Difficulty with simple tasks, inability to function at previous level, poor problem solving, poor cognitive functioning, verbalizations of inability to cope	*Ineffective coping* *Interrupted family processes* *Risk for impaired parent/infant/child attachment* *Ineffective role performance*
Difficulty making decisions, poor concentration, inability to take action	*Decisional conflict*
Feelings of helplessness, hopelessness, powerlessness	*Hopelessness*
Feelings of inability to make positive change in one's life or have a sense of control over one's destiny.	*Powerlessness*
Questioning meaning of life and own existence, inability to participate in usual religious practices, conflict over spiritual beliefs, anger toward spiritual deity or religious representatives	*Spiritual distress* *Impaired religiosity* *Risk for impaired religiosity*
Feelings of worthlessness, poor self-image, negative sense of self, self-negating verbalizations, feeling of being a failure, expressions of shame or guilt, hypersensitivity to slights or criticism	*Chronic low self-esteem* *Situational low self-esteem*
Withdrawal, noncommunicativeness, speech that is only in monosyllables, avoidance of contact with others	*Impaired social interaction* *Social isolation* *Risk for loneliness*
Vegetative signs of depression: changes in sleeping, eating, grooming and hygiene, elimination, sexual patterns	*Self-care deficit (bathing/hygiene, dressing/grooming)* *Imbalanced nutrition: less than body requirements* *Disturbed sleep pattern* *Constipation* *Sexual dysfunction*

to a remark does not mean that the patient has not heard or chooses not to reply; rather, the patient just needs a little more time to compose a reply. In extreme depression, however, a person may be mute.

Some depressed patients are so withdrawn that they are unwilling or unable to speak. Nurses may feel uncomfortable with silence and not be able to "do anything" to effect immediate change. However, just sitting with a patient in silence may be a valuable intervention. It is important to be aware that this time spent together can be meaningful to the depressed person, especially if the nurse has a genuine interest in learning about the depressed individual.

VIGNETTE

Doris, a senior nursing student, is working with a depressed, suicidal, withdrawn woman. The instructor notices in the second week that Doris spends a lot of time talking with other students and their patients and little time with her own patient. In postconference, Doris acknowledges feeling threatened and useless and says that she wants a patient who will interact with her. After reviewing the symptoms of depression, its behavioral manifestations, and the needs of depressed individuals, Doris turns her attention back to her patient and spends time rethinking her plan of care. After 4 weeks of sharing her feelings in postconfer-

continued

TABLE 12-3	Interventions for Severely Withdrawn Individuals: Communication
Intervention	**Rationale**
1. When a patient is mute, use the technique of *making observations:* "There are many new pictures on the wall" or "You are wearing your new shoes."	1. When a patient is not ready to talk, direct questions can raise the patient's anxiety level and frustrate the nurse. Pointing to commonalities in the environment draws the patient into, and reinforces, reality.
2. Use simple, concrete words.	2. Slowed thinking and difficulty concentrating impair comprehension.
3. Allow time for the patient to respond.	3. Slowed thinking necessitates time to formulate a response.
4. Listen for covert messages and ask about suicide plans, e.g., "Have you had thoughts of harming yourself in any way?"	4. People often experience relief and decrease in feelings of isolation when they share thoughts of suicide.
5. Avoid platitudes, such as, "Things will look up" or "Everyone gets down once in a while."	5. Platitudes tend to minimize the patient's feelings and can increase feelings of guilt and worthlessness because the patient cannot "look up" or "snap out of it."

ences, working with her instructor, and trying a variety of approaches with her patient, Doris is rewarded. On the day of discharge, the patient tells Doris how important their time together was for her: "I actually felt someone cared."

It is difficult to say when a withdrawn or depressed person will be able to respond. However, certain techniques are known to be useful in guiding effective nursing interventions. Some communication interventions to use with a severely withdrawn patient are listed in Table 12-3. Communication interventions for work with depressed patients are offered in Table 12-4.

Health Teaching and Health Promotion

It is important for patients and their families to understand that depression is a legitimate medical illness over which the patient has no voluntary control. Depressed patients and their families need to learn about the biological symptoms of depression, as well as the psychosocial and cognitive changes. Families need to know about the overt and covert signs of suicidal ideation, and know what to do and who to contact should warning signs of suicidal thinking or planning occur (see Chapter 20). Review of the medications and their adverse reactions helps families evaluate clinical changes and stay alert for reactions that might affect patient compliance. The section on psychopharmacology provides information on adverse effects to antidepressants and specific areas to be covered in patient and family teaching.

Early in hospitalization, predischarge counseling should be carried out with the patient and the patient's significant others. One purpose of this counseling is to clarify the interpersonal stresses and discuss steps that can alleviate tension in the family system. Including significant others in discharge planning facilitates progress in the following ways:

- Increases the understanding and acceptance of the depressed family member during the aftercare period
- Increases the patient's use of aftercare facilities in the community
- Contributes to higher overall adjustment in the patient after discharge
- Increases understanding of symptoms that signal the need for relapse prevention.

Health teaching also may include teaching and interventions for self-care deficits. In addition to experiencing intense feelings of hopelessness, despair, low self-worth, and fatigue, the depressed person also may have physical deficits related to the depression. Some effective interventions targeting the physical needs of the depressed patient are listed in Table 12-5 on page 229.

Milieu Therapy

When a person is acutely and severely depressed, the structure of the hospital setting may be necessary. The depressed person needs protection from suicidal acts in a supervised environment for regulating antidepressant medications. If a patient is thought to be suicidal, finding a safe environment may be the first action taken. Hospitals have protocols for suicidal observation and protection. If a patient is highly suicidal, not eating, becoming debilitated, or has a psy-

TABLE 12-4	Interventions for Depression: Communication

Intervention	Rationale
1. Help the patient question underlying assumptions and beliefs and consider alternate explanations to problems.	1. Reconstructing a healthier and more hopeful attitude about the future can alter depressed mood.
2. Work with the patient to identify cognitive distortions that encourage negative self-appraisal. For example:	2. Cognitive distortions reinforce a negative, inaccurate perception of self and world.
a. Overgeneralizations	a. The patient takes one fact or event and makes a general rule out of it ("He always . . ."; "I never . . .").
b. Self-blame	b. The patient consistently blames self for everything perceived as negative.
c. Mind reading	c. The patient assumes others don't like him or her, and so forth, without any real evidence that assumptions are correct.
d. Discounting of positive attributes	d. The patient focuses on the negative.
3. Encourage activities that can raise self-esteem. Identify need for (a) problem-solving skills, (b) coping skills, and (c) assertiveness skills.	3. Many depressed people, especially women, are not taught a range of problem-solving and coping skills. Increasing social, family, and job skills can change negative self-assessment.
4. Encourage exercise, such as running and/or weightlifting. Initially walking 10 to 15 minutes a day 3 or 4 times a week has short-term benefits.	4. Exercise can help alleviate depression and anxiety, improve self-concept, and shift neurochemical balance.
5. Encourage formation of supportive relationships, such as through support groups, therapy, and peer support.	5. Such relationships reduce social isolation and enable the patient to work on personal goals and relationship needs.
6. Provide information referrals, when needed, for spiritual/religious information (e.g., readings, programs, tapes, community resources).	6. Spiritual and existential issues may be heightened during depressive episodes—many people find strength and comfort in spirituality or religion.

APPLYING THE ART   A Person with Depression

SCENARIO: After a medical workup revealed no physical problems, Nadia, a 39-year-old mother of three, admitted herself voluntarily to the inpatient psychiatric unit, stating she no longer had the energy to care for her children, her marriage, saying, "I am not fit to be a mother or wife." I saw Nadia 3 days later and set up a contract with her for after breakfast, expecting that later we would attend group therapy, then meet for one-to-one. Instead Nadia, after missing group, reluctantly met with me in the day room.

THERAPEUTIC GOAL: By the conclusion of this interaction, Nadia will state she understands that depression is a treatable disorder and that her symptoms were the cause of her despondent behavior.

Student-Patient Interaction	Thoughts, Communication Techniques, and Mental Health Nursing Concepts
Nadia: *Speaking slowly, eyes downcast.* "I couldn't face all those people."	
Student: "You're looking down like you are sad." *No response from Nadia.* "I wonder what facing the group means to you." **Student's feelings:** *I should have stayed with "sad." I aimed for her feelings, then did not wait for her to share any feelings.*	Depression slows everything: thoughts, feelings, and responses to others. I *make an observation* and *attempt to translate into feelings*, then shift to an *indirect question*. Because depression hinders Nadia's processing of information, I need to slow my pace. Allow more silence.
Nadia: *Slowly shakes her head back and forth. Silent for 3 minutes. No eye contact.*	

APPLYING THE ART   A Person with Depression—cont'd

Student-Patient Interaction	Thoughts, Communication Techniques, and Mental Health Nursing Concepts
Student: *With a concerned look.* "You shake your head as if you are saying no." **Student's feelings:** *I know it's the right thing to do, but waiting during the silence makes me so anxious. I need to stay mindfully alert and attentive. I can endure the silence for Nadia's sake.*	I use *silence* along with attending behavior. I *make an observation* and then use *restatement*.
Nadia: "Everybody in group makes progress. I just keep sinking deeper."	
Student: "Sinking deeper?"	Nadia has just begun antidepressant medication. Most affect *serotonin or norepinephrine neurotransmitter levels*, but therapeutic effectiveness takes 2 to 3 weeks. I use *restatement* to encourage Nadia to say more.
Nadia: "Into depression. I can't pull it together even though I know my kids need me." *Makes eye contact.* **Student's feelings:** *I know from experience that it's hard to pull anything together when you feel depressed.*	Depression erodes self-esteem, and low self-esteem in turn exacerbates depression.
Student: "You care about your children." *She nods.* "Sounds like you find it difficult at this time to care about yourself very much." **Student's feelings:** *I've noticed that sometimes, like Nadia, nurses find it easier to care for others than take care of self, even basic self-care or prevention measures.*	I *attempt to translate into feelings* adding "at this time" to imply a temporary state, e.g., she will again find self-caring as she heals.
Nadia: *Sustaining eye contact.* "I can't do anything right. I have nothing to show for my life."	
Student: "Think about what you've accomplished! You have your children, your marriage, your teaching career." *Nadia shrugs, eyes downcast.* **Student's feelings:** *She has so much going for her. Why can't she see that?* *My response causes Nadia to pull away by withdrawing eye contact. When I deliver positives about Nadia before she feels more positive about herself, I discount her experience, which interferes with trust.* *I need to remember that support and nonjudgmental acceptance provide the foundation for the nurse-patient relationship.*	I inadvertently minimized her feelings by giving *approval* and *advice,* which is *nontherapeutic.* Even though all the things I pointed out may be valid, none of it rings true for Nadia right now. One step that helps with depression would be for Nadia to problem-solve and work through any cognitive distortions, e.g., "I can't do anything right." *Cognitive behavioral therapy,* like the antidepressant medication takes time, but depression is a treatable disorder.
Student: *After waiting for 2 minutes.* "Nadia, I am here to be with you right where you are at this moment. No pressure."	I *offer self* and *acceptance.*
Nadia: *Looking up.* "Thank you. You don't know how much that means. I do want to get better and not feel like depression consumes who I am."	

Continued

APPLYING THE ART   A Person with Depression—cont'd

Student-Patient Interaction	Thoughts, Communication Techniques, and Mental Health Nursing Concepts
Student: *Nods.* "You want to get better. You were able to take the first courageous step. In deciding to get admitted, you acknowledge that your symptoms are a problem, and they are the symptoms of depression, a disorder." **Student's feelings:** *Nadia feels swallowed up (consumed) by the depression. I want her to know that depression need not be her life.*	I *give support.* Separating out oneself as distinct from the disorder of depression restores some sense of control to Nadia.
Nadia: "Oh, I never thought of it that way . . . as a first step, not a sign of failure. My symptoms are from the depression." **Student's feelings:** *As a nurse, my belief in Nadia's ability to battle the depression offers hope.*	
Student: *Nods.* "A treatable disorder." I continue to sit with Nadia in silence for a short while.	At some level, Nadia acknowledges a self not fully consumed by depression.
Nadia: "Yes, depression is a disorder, not all that I am."	Hope will grow as Nadia begins to take charge of her disorder through active investment in treatment.

chotic depression, then electroconvulsive therapy (ECT) may be administered.

Psychotherapy

CBT, interpersonal therapy (IPT), and behavioral therapy have been proven effective in the treatment of depression. However, only CBT and IPT demonstrate superiority in the maintenance phase. CBT helps people change their negative styles of thinking and behaving, whereas IPT focuses on working through personal relationships that may contribute to depression. Outcome research has consistently found that CBT and medication are largely comparable, but CBT is more effective in protecting against relapse than medications (Feldman, 2007).

Some studies indicate that psychotherapy alone (CBT or IPT), especially in individuals with early life traumas (child abuse), is more effective than pharmacology alone (Nemeroff et al., 2007). CBT combined with medications is proven effective in people with chronic depressions (Feldman, 2007).

Group Therapy

Group therapy is a widespread modality for the treatment of depression; it increases the number of people who can receive treatment at a decreased cost per individual. Another advantage is that groups offer patients an opportunity to socialize and to share common feelings and concerns as well as provide patients with the opportunity to reach out to others and support others. Belonging to a group can help decrease feelings of isolation, hopelessness, helplessness, and alienation. Medication groups for patients and families can increase understanding of medications, how to handle various side effects, and compliance.

Pharmacological, Biological, and Integrative Therapies
Antidepressant Medication Therapy

Antidepressant therapy benefits about 65% to 80% of people with nondelusional unipolar depression. ECT has a 75% to 85% efficacy rate for those patients who are delusional or melancholic (Maxmen & Ward, 2002). It should be noted, however, that the combination of specific psychotherapies (e.g., CBT, IPT, behavioral) and antidepressant therapy is superior to either psychotherapy or psychopharmacological treatment alone (Sutherland et al., 2003). In fact, it is believed that the combination and continuation of at least two of these therapies may reduce the risk of recurrence or relapse of MDD and DD (Dubovsky et al., 2004). Essentially, the core symptoms of depression improve with antidepressant therapy, and quality-of-life measures improve with certain psychotherapies (Culpepper et al., 2003).

Antidepressant drugs can positively alter poor self-concept, degree of withdrawal, vegetative signs of depression, and activity level. Target symptoms include the following:

- Sleep disturbance
- Appetite disturbance (decreased or increased)

TABLE 12-5   Interventions Targeting the Physical Needs of the Depressed Patient

Intervention	Rationale
Nutrition—Anorexia	
1. Offer small high-calorie and high-protein snacks frequently throughout the day and evening.	1. Low weight and poor nutrition render the patient susceptible to illness. Small, frequent snacks are more easily tolerated than large plates of food when the patient is anorexic.
2. Offer high-protein and high-calorie fluids frequently throughout the day and evening.	2. These fluids prevent dehydration and can minimize constipation.
3. When possible, encourage family or friends to remain with the patient during meals.	3. This strategy reinforces the idea that someone cares, can raise the patient's self-esteem, and can serve as an incentive to eat.
4. Ask the patient which foods or drinks he or she likes. Offer choices. Involve the dietitian.	4. The patient is more likely to eat the foods provided.
5. Weigh the patient weekly and observe the patient's eating patterns.	5. Monitoring the patient's status gives the information needed for revision of the intervention.
Sleep—Insomnia	
1. Provide periods of rest after activities.	1. Fatigue can intensify feelings of depression.
2. Encourage the patient to get up and dress and to stay out of bed during the day.	2. Minimizing sleep during the day increases the likelihood of sleep at night.
3. Encourage the use of relaxation measures in the evening (e.g., tepid bath, warm milk).	3. These measures induce relaxation and sleep.
4. Reduce environmental and physical stimulants in the evening—provide decaffeinated coffee, soft lights, soft music, quiet activities.	4. Decreasing caffeine and epinephrine levels increases the possibility of sleep. music, and quiet activities.
Self-Care Deficits	
1. Encourage the use of toothbrush, washcloth, soap, makeup, shaving equipment, and so forth.	1. Being clean and well groomed can temporarily increase self-esteem.
2. When appropriate, give step-by-step reminders such as, "Wash the right side of your face, now the left."	2. Slowed thinking and difficulty concentrating make organizing simple tasks difficult.
Elimination—Constipation	
1. Monitor intake and output, especially bowel movements.	1. Many depressed patients are constipated. If the condition is not checked, fecal impaction can occur.
2. Offer foods high in fiber and provide periods of exercise.	2. Roughage and exercise stimulate peristalsis and help evacuation of fecal material.
3. Encourage the intake of fluids.	3. Fluids help prevent constipation.
4. Evaluate the need for laxatives and enemas.	4. These measures prevent fecal impaction.

- Fatigue
- Decreased sex drive
- Psychomotor retardation or agitation
- Diurnal variations in mood (often worse in the morning)
- Impaired concentration or forgetfulness
- Anhedonia (loss of ability to experience joy or pleasure in living)

One drawback to the use of antidepressant medication is that improvement in mood may take 1 to 3 weeks or longer. If a patient is acutely suicidal, this may be too long to wait. At these times, ECT may be a consideration in some facilities.

A Note About Safety

The possibility that antidepressant medication might contribute to suicidal behavior has been well covered in the media and caused grave concerns among the professional community and general public. However, there has not been any conclusive evidence to support this concern. To the contrary, the review of the use of selective serotonin reuptake inhibitors (SSRIs) in 27 countries over time saw a strong association with increased antidepressant prescribing and a reduction in suicide (Ludwig & Marcotte, 2005).

All treatments have potential risks. At present, there is no conclusive evidence that either the newer or the older antidepressants precipitate suicide (Goldberg et al., 2006). The U.S. Food and Drug Administration (FDA) is still evaluating data from numerous studies and recommends that all consumers of antidepressants be observed carefully for worsening of depression and suicidal thoughts. This is especially true for children, adolescents, and older adults.

Choosing an Antidepressant

All antidepressants work equally well, although they certainly do not all work well for all individuals. Because the complex interplay of neurotransmitters responsible for depression is unique for different individuals, a variety of antidepressants or a combination of antidepressants may need to be tried before the most effective regimen is found. Each antidepressant has adverse effects as well as cost, safety, and maintenance considerations. The following are some of the primary and secondary considerations when choosing a specific antidepressant:

Primary considerations
- Side effect profile (e.g., sexual dysfunction, weight gain)
- Ease of administration
- Past response
- Safety and medical considerations
- Specific depressive symptoms (e.g., anxiety, irritability, hyposomnia, insomnia)
- Medical considerations (diabetes, high cholesterol, cardiac disease)

Secondary considerations
- Neurotransmitter specificity
- Family history of response
- Cost

The neurotransmitters and receptor sites in the brain are the targets of pharmacological intervention (Table 12-6). While reading the following section, see if you can identify potential side effects caused by the blockage of the given neurotransmitter.

Studies that compare the newer SSRIs to the older tricyclic antidepressants (TCAs) fail to find support for one group over the other (U.S. Dept. of Veterans Affairs, 2006). The difference lies in the quality and quantity of adverse effects and complications. Basic antidepressant classes include the following:

First-line agents
- Cyclic antidepressants (e.g., TCAs)
- SSRIs
- The newer atypical antidepressants

TABLE 12-6   Potential Effects of Receptor Blockade

	Receptor Blocked	Potential Effects
NE	Norepinephrine	Decreased depression Tremors Tachycardia Erectile and/or ejaculatory dysfunction
α_1	Specific receptor for epinephrine	Antipsychotic effect Postural hypotension Dizziness Reflux tachycardia Ejaculatory dysfunction and/or impotence Memory dysfunction
α_2	Specific receptor for norepinephrine	Priapism
5-HT	Serotonin	Decreased depression Antianxiety effects Gastrointestinal disturbance Sexual dysfunction
5-HT$_2$	Serotonin	Decreased depression Decreased suicidal behavior Antipsychotic effects Hypotension Ejaculatory dysfunction Weight gain and carbohydrate craving
DA	Dopamine reuptake blocked	Decreased psychosis Psychomotor agitation Parkinsonian effect
ACh **H$_1$**	Acetylcholine Histamine	Anticholinergic effects Sedation Weight gain Cognitive impairment

Second-line agents
- Monoamine oxidase inhibitors (MAOIs)

Tricyclic Antidepressants

The **tricyclic antidepressants (TCAs)** inhibit the reuptake of norepinephrine and serotonin by the presynaptic neurons in the CNS. Therefore the amount of time that norepinephrine and serotonin are available to the postsynaptic receptors is increased. This increase in norepinephrine and serotonin in the brain is believed to be responsible for mood elevations when TCAs are given to depressed people.

The sedative effects of the TCAs are attributed to antihistamine (H_1 receptor) actions and somewhat to anticholinergic actions (Maxmen & Ward, 2002). Patients must take therapeutic doses of TCAs for 10 to 14 days or longer before they begin to work. The full effects may not be seen for 4 to 8 weeks. An effect on some symptoms of depression, such as insomnia and anorexia, may be noted sooner. A person who has had a positive response to TCA therapy would probably be maintained on that medication for 6 to 12 months to prevent an early relapse. Choice of TCA is based on the following:

- What has worked for the patient or a family member in the past
- The drug's adverse effects

For example, a patient who is lethargic and fatigued may have the best results with a more stimulating TCA, such as desipramine (Norpramin) or protriptyline (Vivactil). If a more sedating effect is needed for agitation or restlessness, drugs such as amitriptyline (Elavil) and doxepin (Sinequan) may be more appropriate choices. **Regardless of which TCA is given, the dosage should always be low initially and should be increased gradually.** Caution should be used, especially in older adults because slow drug metabolism may be a problem. The rule of thumb for older adults is always, **"Start low, go slow."**

Common Adverse Reactions. The chemical structure of the TCAs is similar to that of the antipsychotic medications. Therefore the **anticholinergic** actions (e.g., dry mouth, blurred vision, tachycardia, constipation, urinary retention, and esophageal reflux) are similar. These side effects are more common and more pronounced in patients taking antidepressants. These adverse effects are usually not serious and are often transitory, but **urinary retention and severe constipation warrant immediate medical attention**.

The α-adrenergic blockade of the TCAs can produce postural orthostatic hypotension and tachycardia. Postural hypotension can lead to dizziness and increase the risk of falls.

Administering the total daily dose of TCA at night is beneficial for two reasons. First, most TCAs have sedative effects and thereby aid sleep. Second, the minor side effects occur during sleep, which increases compliance with drug therapy. Table 12-7 reviews TCAs in common use, their common side effects, and dosage ranges.

Potential Toxic Effects. The most serious effects of the TCAs are cardiovascular: dysrhythmias, tachycardia, myocardial infarction, and heart block. Because the cardiac side effects are so serious, TCA use is considered a risk in patients with cardiac disease and in older adults. Patients should have a thorough cardiac workup before beginning TCA therapy. The risk of a lethal overdose with a TCA slould always be taken into consideration when choosing an antidepressant.

Drug Interactions. Individuals taking TCAs can have adverse reactions to numerous other medications. A few of the more common medications usually *not* given while TCAs are being used are listed in Box 12-2. A patient who is taking any of these medications along with a TCA should have a medical clearance beforehand because some of the reactions can be fatal.

Use of antidepressants may precipitate a psychotic episode in a person with schizophrenia. An antidepressant can precipitate a manic episode in a patient with bipolar disorder (BD). Depressed patients with BD often receive lithium along with the antidepressant.

Contraindications. People who have recently had a myocardial infarction (or other cardiovascular problems), those with narrow-angle glaucoma or a history of seizures, and pregnant women should not be treated with TCAs, except with extreme caution and careful monitoring.

Patient Teaching. Teaching patients and one or more of their significant others about medications is an expected nursing responsibility. Medication teaching is begun in the hospital. The nurse or another qualified health care provider must review the medications, possible side effects, and necessary patient precautions. Areas for the nurse to discuss when teaching patients and their families about TCA therapy are presented in Box 12-3. Patients and significant others need to have written information for all medications that will be taken at home.

BOX 12-2

Drugs to Be Used with Caution in Patients Taking a Tricyclic Antidepressant

- Phenothiazines
- Barbiturates
- Monoamine oxidase inhibitors
- Disulfiram (Antabuse)
- Oral contraceptives (or other estrogen preparations)
- Anticoagulants
- Some antihypertensives (clonidine, guanethidine, reserpine)
- Benzodiazepines
- Alcohol
- Nicotine

TABLE 12-7   Tricyclic Antidepressants (TCAs): Overview of Adverse Reactions and Dosage Range

	Sedation	Weight Gain	Sexual Dysfunction	Other Key Adverse Reactions
TCAs	Common	Common	Yes	• Anticholinergic side effects* • Orthostasis • CHF effects (tachycardia, dysrhythmias, ECG changes, heart failure) • Lethal in overdose

Specific Medications

Generic Name	Trade Name	Initial Dosage (mg/Day)	Therapeutic Dosage Range (mg/Day)	Maximum Dosage (mg/Day)
Amitriptyline	Elavil, Endep	25-50	100-200	300
Amoxapine	Asendin	50-100	150-400	400
Desipramine	Norpramin, Pertofrane	25-50	75-200	300
Doxepin	Adapin, Sinequan	25-50	75-150	300
Imipramine	Tofranil	25-50	75-150	300
Nortriptyline	Aventyl, Pamelor	10-25	75-100	125
Protriptyline	Vivactil	10	15-40	60
Trimipramine	Surmontil	25-50	100-200	300
Maprotiline	Ludiomil	25-50	100-150	225

*Anticholinergic side effects include dry mouth, blurred vision, constipation, urinary retention, tachycardia, and possible confusion.
CHF, Congestive heart failure; *ECG*, electrocardiogram.

Selective Serotonin Reuptake Inhibitors

The introduction of Prozac, the first **selective serotonin reuptake inhibitor (SSRI)** in 1988 heralded an important advance in pharmacotherapy. Essentially, the SSRIs selectively block the neuronal uptake of serotonin (e.g., 5-HT, 5-HT$_1$ receptors) thereby leaving more serotonin available at the synaptic site. (See Chapter 4 for detailed information on how the SSRIs work.)

SSRI antidepressant drugs have a lower incidence of anticholinergic side effects (e.g., dry mouth, blurred vision, urinary retention), less cardiotoxicity, and faster onset of action than the TCAs. Patients are more likely to comply with a regimen of SSRIs than of TCAs because of the more favorable side effect profile, and compliance is a crucial step toward recovery or remission. The SSRIs seem to be effective in depression with anxiety features as well as in depression with psychomotor agitation.

Because the SSRIs cause fewer adverse effects and have low cardiotoxicity, they are less dangerous when they are taken in overdose. The SSRIs, serotonin-norepinephrine reuptake inhibitors (SNRIs), and newer atypical antidepressants have a low lethality risk in suicide attempts compared with the TCAs, which have a very high potential for lethality with overdose.

Indications. The SSRIs have a broad base of clinical use. In addition to their use in treating depressive disorders, the SSRIs have been prescribed with success to treat some of the anxiety disorders, in particular, obsessive-compulsive disorder and panic disorder (see Chapter 8). Fluoxetine has been found to be effective in treating some women who suffer from late luteal phase dysphoric disorder and bulimia nervosa.

Common Adverse Reactions. Agents that selectively enhance synaptic serotonin within the CNS may induce agitation, anxiety, sleep disturbance, tremor, sexual dysfunction (primarily anorgasmia), or tension headache. The effect of the SSRIs on sexual performance may be the most significant undesirable outcome reported by patients.

Autonomic reactions (e.g., dry mouth, sweating, weight change, mild nausea, and loose bowel movements) also may be experienced with the SSRIs. See Table 12-8 for a general side effect profile of the SSRIs, specific SSRIs, and dosage.

Potential Toxic Effects. One rare and life-threatening event associated with the SSRIs is **serotonin syndrome**. This is thought to be related to overactivation of the central

BOX 12-3

Patient and Family Teaching About Tricyclic Antidepressants

- The patient and family should be told that mood elevation may take from 7 to 28 days. Up to 6 to 8 weeks may be required for the full effect to be reached and for major depressive symptoms to subside. The family should reinforce this frequently to the depressed family member because depressed people have trouble remembering and respond to ongoing reassurance.
- The patient should be reassured that drowsiness, dizziness, and hypotension usually subside after the first few weeks.
- When the patient starts taking tricyclic antidepressants (TCAs), the patient should be cautioned to be careful working around machines, driving cars, and crossing streets because of possible altered reflexes, drowsiness, or dizziness.

- Alcohol can block the effects of antidepressants. The patient should be told to refrain from drinking.
- If possible, the patient should take the full dose at bedtime to reduce the experience of side effects during the day.
- If the patient forgets the bedtime dose (or the once-a-day dose), the next dose should be taken within 3 hours; otherwise the patient should wait until the usual medication time the next day. The patient should *not* double the dose.
- Suddenly stopping TCAs can cause nausea, altered heartbeat, nightmares, and cold sweats in 2 to 4 days. The patient should call the physician or take one dose of TCA until the physician can be contacted.

TABLE 12-8	Selective Serotonin Reuptake Inhibitors (SSRIs): Overview of Adverse Reactions and Dosage Range			
	Sedation	**Weight Gain**	**Sexual Dysfunction**	**Other Key Adverse Reactions**
SSRIs	Minimal	Rare	Yes	• Initial: nausea, loose bowel movements, headache, insomnia • Toxic effects (rare): serotonin syndrome • Concern regarding increased suicidal potential as yet unproven through long-term studies

Specific Medications

Generic Name	Trade Name	Initial Dosage (mg/Day)	Dosage After 4 to 8 Weeks (mg/Day)	Maximum Dosage (mg/Day)
Citalopram	Celexa	10-20	20-60	60
Fluoxetine	Prozac	10-20	20-80	80
Fluvoxamine*	Luvox	50-100	50-300	300
Paroxetine	Paxil	10-20	20-50	50
Sertraline	Zoloft	50	50-150	200
Escitalopram[†]	Lexapro	10	10-20	20

*Older adult patients and those with hepatic disease should start at 50% less than the standard dosages listed in the table. This applies to patients with coexisting panic or anxiety symptoms.
[†]Escitalopram is the single active isomer of citalopram, which gives it some advantages in the treatment of depression.

---

serotonin receptors, caused by either too high a dose or interaction with other drugs. Symptoms include abdominal pain, diarrhea, sweating, fever, tachycardia, elevated blood pressure, altered mental state (delirium), myoclonus (muscle spasms), increased motor activity, irritability, hostility, and mood change. Severe manifestation can induce hyperpy-

rexia (excessively high fever), cardiovascular shock, or death.

The risk of this syndrome seems to be the greatest when an SSRI is administered in combination with a second serotonin-enhancing agent, such as an MAOI. For example, a person taking fluoxetine would have to be off this medica-

BOX 12-4

Symptoms and Interventions for Serotonin Syndrome

Symptoms

- Hyperactivity or restlessness
- Tachycardia → cardiovascular shock
- Fever → hyperpyrexia
- Elevated blood pressure
- Altered mental states (delirium)
- Irrationality, mood swings, hostility
- Seizures → status epilepticus
- Myoclonus, incoordination, tonic rigidity
- Abdominal pain, diarrhea, bloating
- Apnea → death

Emergency Measures

1. Discontinue offending agent(s)
2. Initiate symptomatic treatment:
   - Serotonin receptor blockade: cyproheptadine, methysergide, propranolol
   - Cooling blankets, chlorpromazine for hyperthermia
   - Dantrolene, diazepam for muscle rigidity or rigors
   - Anticonvulsants
   - Artificial ventilation
   - Paralysis

BOX 12-5

Patient and Family Teaching About Selective Serotonin Reuptake Inhibitors

- Selective serotonin reuptake inhibitors (SSRIs) may cause sexual dysfunction or lack of sex drive. Inform nurse or physician.
- SSRIs may cause insomnia, anxiety, and nervousness. Inform nurse or physician.
- SSRIs may interact with other medications. Be sure physician knows other medications patient is taking (digoxin, warfarin). SSRIs should not be taken within 14 days of the last dose of a monoamine oxidase inhibitor (MAOI).
- No over-the-counter drug should be taken without first notifying physician.
- Common side effects include fatigue, nausea, diarrhea, dry mouth, dizziness, tremor, and sexual dysfunction or lack of sex drive.
- Because of the potential for drowsiness and dizziness, patient should not drive or operate machinery until these side effects are ruled out.
- Alcohol should be avoided. SSRIs may act synergistically, and people report increased effects of alcohol, e.g., one drink can seem like two. Alcohol is also a central nervous system (CNS) depressant that may work against the desired effect of the SSRI.
- Liver and renal function tests should be performed and blood counts checked periodically.
- Medication should not be discontinued abruptly. People report such effects as dizziness, nausea, diarrhea, muscle jerkiness, and tremors. If side effects from the SSRIs become bothersome, patient should ask physician about changing to a different drug. Abrupt cessation can lead to serotonin withdrawal.
- Any of the following symptoms should be reported to a physician immediately:
  - Increase in depression or suicidal thoughts
  - Rash or hives
  - Rapid heartbeat
  - Sore throat
  - Difficulty urinating
  - Fever, malaise
  - Anorexia and weight loss
  - Unusual bleeding
  - Initiation of hyperactive behavior
  - Severe headache

tion for a full 5 weeks before being switched to an MAOI (5 weeks is the half-life for fluoxetine). If a patient is already taking an MAOI, the person should wait at least 2 weeks before starting fluoxetine therapy. Other SSRIs have shorter periods of activity; for example, sertraline and paroxetine have half-lives of 2 weeks, so there would need to be a 2-week gap between different medications.

Box 12-4 lists the symptoms of serotonin syndrome and gives emergency treatment guidelines. Box 12-5 is a useful tool for patient and family teaching about the SSRIs.

New Atypical (Novel) Antidepressants

Most newly released antidepressants affect a variety of neurotransmitters. These **novel antidepressants** are all effective agents. Table 12-9 introduces these newer atypical antidepressants and identifies the main neurotransmitters involved. Each of these agents blocks different neurotransmitters and transmitter subtypes, which accounts for their strengths in targeting unique populations of depressed

TABLE 12-9 Newer Atypical (Novel) Antidepressants

Agent	Neurotransmitters Affected	May Help People With:
Bupropion (Wellbutrin, Zyban)	Blocks norepinephrine (NE) and dopamine (DA) reuptake (NDRI)	• ADHD • Chronic fatigue syndrome • Rapid cycling bipolar II disorder • Sexual side effects from use of other antidepressants • Anxiety disorders (GAD, OCD, phobic disorders, PTSD, panic disorders) • Nicotine addiction (Zyban)
Trazodone (Desyrel)	Shows selective but moderate blockage of serotonin (5-HT$_2$ receptor) (only used in conjunction with other drugs)	• Older adult patients • SSRI-induced insomnia
Dual-Action Reuptake Inhibitors—SNRIs (Serotonin and Norepinephrine)		
Venlafaxine (Effexor)	Inhibits reuptake of serotonin (5-HT) and NE Inhibits DA to a lesser extent	• Treatment-resistant depression • Chronic depression • Bipolar depression • Depression with ADHD • Medical illness and depression • Anxiety • Geriatric depression
Mirtazapine (Remeron)	Blocks serotonin (5-HT, 5-HT$_2$, 5-HT$_3$, 5-HT$_4$ receptors), is an α_2-adrenoreceptor antagonist (ACh), and blocks histamine (H$_1$) (enhances both nonadrenergic and serotonergic transmitters)	• Sleep disturbances • Poor appetite • Pain • Medical illness with depression • Anxiety • SSRI-induced sexual dysfunction
Duloxetine (Cymbalta)	Inhibits reuptake of serotonin (5-HT) and NE (SNRI) Inhibits DA to a lesser extent	• Major depression • Geriatric depression

ACh, Acetylcholine; *ADHD*, attention deficit hyperactivity disorder; *GAD*, generalized anxiety disorder; *OCD*, obsessive-compulsive disorder; *PTSD*, posttraumatic stress disorder; *SSRI*, selective serotonin reuptake inhibitor.

individuals as well as for their efficacy in treating other conditions. Table 12-10 lists the usual maintenance daily dose and presents some of the advantages and disadvantages of each of these atypical agents.

Monoamine Oxidase Inhibitors

MAOIs demonstrate proven benefits for patients who have not responded to other medication or ECT treatment. They also have been found useful in re-refractory anxiety states. In particular, MAOIs have established efficacy in depression in people with **atypical depression** (see Table 12-1).

In addition to being effective with atypical depression and MDD, MAOIs can be useful in treating other disorders such as panic disorder, social phobia, generalized anxiety disorder, obsessive-compulsive disorder, posttraumatic stress disorder, and bulimia. Essentially, MAOIs prevent the breakdown of norepinephrine, serotonin, and dopamine in the brain, thereby increasing the levels of these brain amines and resulting in increased mood. (See Chapter 4 for detailed information on how the MAOIs work.) Common adverse reactions and potential toxic effects of MAOIs are outlined in Table 12-11.

Unfortunately, the MAOIs also inhibit the breakdown of tyramine in the liver. Increased levels of tyramine can

TABLE 12-10 Newer Atypical Agents: Dosages and Effects

Agent (Trade Name)	Usual Dosage (mg/Day)	Advantages	Adverse Effects
Bupropion (Wellbutrin)	50-300	• Sexual dysfunction rare • No weight gain • Stimulant properties • Antianxiety properties	• Medication-induced seizures if more than 300 mg • High seizure risk in at-risk individuals • Some nausea
(Zyban)	150-300		
Trazodone (Desyrel)	150-400	• No anticholinergic side effects,* low potential for cardiac effects • In conjunction with other antidepressants, can aid sleep	• Possible priapism[†] • Postural hypotension • Weight gain • Memory dysfunction
Dual-Action Reuptake Inhibitors—SNRIs (Serotonin and Norepinephrine)			
Venlafaxine (Effexor)	75-225	• Useful for treatment-resistant chronic depression • Low potential for drug interaction	• Risk of sustained hypertension for some people • Possible somnolence, dry mouth, and dizziness • Rapid discontinuation can cause withdrawal symptoms
Mirtazapine (Remeron)	15-45	• Antidote to SSRI sexual dysfunction • Noninterference with sleep • Low interference with metabolism of other drugs • Anxiolytic properties	• Strong sedating effect • Possible increased appetite, weight gain, and cholesterol elevation
Duloxetine (Cymbalta)	20-30 mg bid	• Response to medication within 1 to 4 weeks • Mild side effects	• Nausea • Somnolence • Dry mouth • Constipation • Decreased appetite • Increased sweating • Fatigue • Twice-a-day dosing

*Anticholinergic side effects include dry mouth, blurred vision, constipation, urinary retention, tachycardia, and possible confusion.
[†]Priapism is prolonged painful penile erection that may warrant surgery.
[§]Catalepsy is characterized by a trancelike state of consciousness and a posture in which the limbs hold any position (waxy flexibility). An anticataleptic agent helps minimize or prevent this phenomenon in patients with schizophrenia.

lead to high blood pressure, hypertensive crisis, and eventually cerebrovascular accident and death. Therefore people taking MAOIs must restrict their intake of tyramine so that their blood pressure does not rise to dangerous levels. See Table 12-12 for a list of foods that are high on tyramine and other vasopressors.

Until 2006, the MAOIs commonly used in the United States were phenelzine (Nardil) and tranylcypromine sulfate (Parnate). In 2006 the FDA approved an MAOI that is delivered transcutaneously by way of a patch called the *selegiline transdermal system (STS)*. STS is able to inhibit monamine oxidase in the central nervous system, increasing the availability of norepinephrine, serotonin, and dopamine, while at the same time avoiding the breakdown of tyramine in the liver and digestive tract. When STS is applied in doses of 6 mg over 24 hours by way of a skin patch, it does **not** require a tyramine-restricted diet (Nemeroff et al., 2007). At higher doses (9 or 12 mg), dietary restrictions must be observed.

See Table 12-13 for an overview of MAOIs in current use, their adverse effects, and dosage ranges. Patients who do not improve with initial therapy often show improvement when switched to another class of antidepressants or when a drug from another class is added to the therapy.

TABLE 12-11 Common Adverse Reactions to and Toxic Effects of Monoamine Oxidase Inhibitors

Adverse Reactions	Comments
• Hypotension • Sedation, weakness, fatigue • Insomnia • Changes in cardiac rhythm • Muscle cramps • Anorgasmia or sexual impotence • Urinary hesitancy or constipation • Weight gain	Hypotension is the most critical side effect (10%); older adults, especially, may sustain injuries from it.

Toxic Effects	Comments
Hypertensive crisis* • Severe headache • Stiff, sore neck • Flushing, cold, clammy skin • Tachycardia • Severe nosebleeds, dilated pupils • Chest pains, stroke, coma, death • Nausea and vomiting	1. Patient should go to local emergency department immediately—blood pressure should be checked. 2. One of the following may be given to lower blood pressure: • 5 mg intravenous phentolamine (Regitine) *or* • Oral chlorpromazine *or* • Nifedipine (Procardia) (calcium channel blocker), 10 mg sublingually

*Related to interaction with foodstuffs and cold medication.

TABLE 12-12 Foods That Can Interact with Monoamine Oxidase Inhibitors

Foods That Contain Tyramine

Category	Unsafe Foods (High Tyramine Content)	Safe Foods (Little or No Tyramine)
Vegetables	Avocados, especially if overripe; fermented bean curd; fermented soybean; soybean paste	Most vegetables
Fruits	Figs, especially if overripe; bananas, in large amounts	Most fruits
Meats	Meats that are fermented, smoked, or otherwise aged; spoiled meats; liver, unless very fresh	Meats that are known to be fresh (exercise caution in restaurants; meats may not be fresh)
Sausages	Fermented varieties; bologna, pepperoni, salami, others	Nonfermented varieties
Fish	Dried, pickled, or cured fish; fish that is fermented, smoked, or otherwise aged; spoiled fish	Fish that is known to be fresh; vacuum-packed fish, if eaten promptly or refrigerated only briefly after opening
Milk, milk products	Practically all cheeses	Milk, yogurt, cottage cheese, cream cheese
Foods with yeast	Yeast extract (e.g., Marmite, Bovril)	Baked goods that contain yeast
Beer, wine	Some imported beers, Chianti	Major domestic brands of beer; most wines
Other foods	Protein dietary supplements; soups (may contain protein extract); shrimp paste; soy sauce	

Foods That Contain Other Vasopressors

Food	Comments
Chocolate	Contains phenylethylamine, a pressor agent; large amounts can cause a reaction.
Fava beans	Contain dopamine, a pressor agent; reactions are most likely with overripe beans.
Ginseng	Headache, tremulousness, and mania-like reactions have occurred.
Caffeinated beverages	Caffeine is a weak pressor agent; large amounts may cause a reaction.

From Lehne, R.A. (2007). *Pharmacology for nursing care* (6th ed.). St. Louis: Saunders.

TABLE 12-13 Monoamine Oxidase Inhibitors (MAOIs): Overview of Adverse Reactions and Dosage Range

	Sedation	Weight Gain	Sexual Dysfunction	Other Key Adverse Reactions
MAOIs	Yes	Yes	Yes	• Orthostatic hypotension • Insomnia • Peripheral edema (avoid use in patients with CHF) • Avoid phenelzine in patients with hepatitis • Potential life-threatening drug interactions • Strict dietary and medication restrictions (see Table 12-12 and Box 12-7)

Specific Medications

Generic Name	Trade Name	Initial Dosage (mg/Day)	Dosage After 4 to 8 Weeks (mg/Day)	Maximum Dosage (mg/Day)
Phenelzine	Nardil	45	45-60	90
Tranylcypromine	Parnate	20-30	30-40	60
Selegiline transdermal system (STS)	EMSAM	6 Via skin patch	6-9	12

Reversible Inhibitors of MAO Not Yet Available in the United States

| Moclobemide | Manerix, Aurorix | 300 | 300-600 | 900 |

BOX 12-6

Patient and Family Teaching About Monoamine Oxidase Inhibitors

• Tell the patient and the patient's family to avoid certain foods and all medications (especially cold remedies) unless prescribed by and discussed with the patient's physician (see Table 12-12 and Box 12-7 for specific food and drug restrictions).
• Give the patient a wallet card describing the monoamine oxidase inhibitor (MAOI) regimen.
• Instruct the patient to avoid Chinese restaurants (where sherry, brewer's yeast, and other contraindicated products may be used).

• Tell the patient to go to the emergency department immediately if he or she has a severe headache.
• Ideally, monitor the patient's blood pressure during the first 6 weeks of treatment (for both hypotensive and hypertensive effects).
• Instruct the patient that after the MAOI is stopped, dietary and drug restrictions should be maintained for 14 days.

Box 12-6 can be used as a teaching guide for patients and their families regarding MAOIs.

Contraindications. Use of MAOIs may be contraindicated when one of the following is present:
• Cerebrovascular disease
• Hypertension and congestive heart failure
• Liver disease
• Consumption of foods containing tyramine, tryptophan, and dopamine (see Table 12-12)
• Use of certain medications (see Box 12-7)
• Recurrent or severe headaches
• Surgery in the previous 10 to 14 days
• Age younger than 16 years

BOX 12-7

Drugs That Can Interact with Monoamine Oxidase Inhibitors

Use of the following drugs should be restricted in patients taking monoamine oxidase inhibitors (MAOIs):

- Over-the-counter medications for colds, allergies, or congestion (any product containing ephedrine, phenylephrine hydrochloride, or phenylpropanolamine)
- Tricyclic antidepressants (imipramine, amitriptyline)
- Narcotics
- Antihypertensives (methyldopa, guanethidine, reserpine)
- Amine precursors (levodopa, L-tryptophan)
- Sedatives (alcohol, barbiturates, benzodiazepines)
- General anesthetics
- Stimulants (amphetamines, cocaine)

Somatic Treatments
Electroconvulsive Therapy

Electroconvulsive therapy (ECT) remains one of the most effective treatments for major depression and life-threatening psychiatric conditions (e.g., self-harm). Unfortunately, it is also one of the most stigmatized treatments for depression (NIMH, 2000a). During the early years of ECT, methods were primitive and unrefined, but today ECT is considered safe and effective.

ECT can achieve a higher than 90% remission rate in depressed patients within 1 to 2 weeks. Because 20% to 30% of depressed individuals do not respond to antidepressants, ECT remains an effective treatment particularly for depressions with psychotic features or those refractory to other treatments. ECT is indicated when:

- There is a need for a rapid, definitive response when a patient is suicidal or homicidal.
- The patient is in extreme agitation or stupor.
- The patient develops a life-threatening illness because of refusal of foods and fluids.
- The patient has a history of poor drug response, a history of good ECT response, or both.

ECT is useful in treating patients with major depressive and bipolar depressive disorders, especially when psychotic symptoms are present (e.g., delusions of guilt, somatic delusions, or delusions of infidelity). Patients who have depression with marked psychomotor retardation and stupor also respond well. However, ECT is not necessarily effective in patients with DD, atypical depression, personality disorders, drug dependence, or depression secondary to situational or social difficulties. The usual course of ECT for a depressed patient is two or three treatments per week to a total of 6 to 12 treatments.

Procedure. The procedure is explained to the patient, and informed consent is obtained if the patient is being treated voluntarily. When informed consent cannot be obtained from a patient treated involuntarily, permission may be obtained from the next of kin, although in some states treatment must be court ordered. Use of a general anesthetic and muscle-paralyzing agents has revolutionized the comfort and safety of ECT.

Potential Adverse Reactions. On awakening from ECT, the patient may be confused and disoriented. The nurse and significant others may need to orient the patient frequently during the course of treatment. Many patients state that they have memory deficits for the first few weeks after treatment. Memory usually, although not always, recovers. ECT is not a permanent cure for depression, and maintenance treatment with TCAs or lithium decreases the relapse rate. Maintenance ECT (once a week to once a month) may also help to decrease relapse rates for patients with recurrent depression.

Vagus Nerve Stimulation

Vagus nerve stimulation (VNS) is an FDA-approved, adjunctive, long-term treatment for patients with **treatment resistant depression (TRD)** (those with chronic or recurrent MDD who have failed a minimum of four antidepressant medication trials) (Sadock & Sadock, 2007). ECT is considered by many the most effective acute intervention for TRD, but TRD patients often relapse during the first year following ECT.

The exact method of therapeutic action of VNS is not totally understood. VNS does affect blood flow to different parts of the brain and affects neurotransmitters including serotonin and norepinephrine, which are implicated in depression. A 2-year study by Sackeim and associates (2007) of the efficacy of VNS demonstrated a 50% improvement for people with severe chronic depression that was resistant to other therapies. Between 61% and 79% sustained this response for 24 months (Grohol, 2007).

VNS involves a surgically implanted device (upper left chest) that sends electric impulses to the left vagus nerve in the neck at regular intervals. "Wearable" devices are being developed and tested. Because the vagus nerve affects many functions of the brain, VNS is being studied for other conditions as well (e.g., anxiety disorder, Alzheimer's disease, migraines, and fibromyalgia) (Grohol, 2007).

Integrative Therapies
Light Therapy

Light therapy is the first-line treatment for seasonal affective disorder (SAD) (see Table 12-1). People with SAD often live in climates in which there are marked seasonal differences in the amount of daylight. Seasonal variations in mood disorders in the Southern Hemisphere are the reverse of those in the Northern Hemisphere. Light therapy also may be useful as an adjunct in treating chronic MDD or dysthymia with seasonal exacerbations (APA, 2000b).

Light therapy is thought to be effective because of the influence of light on melatonin. Melatonin is secreted by the pineal gland and is necessary for maintaining and shifting biological rhythms. Exposure to light suppresses the nocturnal secretion of melatonin, which seems to have a therapeutic effect on people with SAD (Zahourek, 2000). Treatments consist of exposure to light balanced to replicate the effects of sunlight for 30 to 60 minutes a day.

St. John's Wort

St. John's wort *(Hypericum perforatum)* is a whole plant product with antidepressant properties that is not regulated by the FDA. St. John's wort has superior efficacy compared with placebo and was generally comparable in effect to low-dose TCAs, and less so to SSRIs (Mischoulon, 2007). The herb is not to be taken in certain situations (e.g., MDD, pregnancy, age younger than 2 years) (Fuller & Sajatovic, 2000). Nor should St. John's wort be taken with certain substances, such as amphetamines or other stimulants, other antidepressants (MAOIs, SSRIs), warfarin, theophylline, or digoxin (Fuller & Sajatovic, 2000; Mischoulon, 2007). Research suggests that St. John's wort may be less effective in cases of severe or chronic depression and that people who have the milder forms of depression are the best candidates (Mischoulon, 2007).

Exercise

There is substantial evidence that exercise can enhance mood and reduce symptoms of depression and anxiety (Mayo Foundation for Medical Education and Research, 2005). It may take at least 30 minutes a day for at least 3 to 5 days a week in order to reduce the symptoms of depression and anxiety; however, shorter periods of time (10 to 15 minutes) have shown to reduce depression and anxiety in the short term (Mayo Foundation for Medical Education and Research, 2005).

The Future of Treatment

There is a great need for earlier detection and intervention, achievement of remission, prevention of progression, and integration of neuroscience and behavioral science in the treatment of depression (Greden, 2004). High-risk ages and groups, including the following, are in need of screening:

- Individuals in late adolescence and early adulthood
- Women in their reproductive years
- Adults and older adults with medical problems
- People with a family history of depression

There is also a need for education, particularly about the linkage between physical symptoms and depression. Psychopharmacological treatment should be augmented with cognitive-behavioral therapies, and there is need for more supplementary strategies, such as the following:

- Promotion of sleep hygiene
- Increase in exercise
- Better total health care

Continual research will bring more genetic screening tools and pharmacogenetics understanding; the use of neuroimaging will become a common diagnostic tool and will not be restricted to research. These and other advances are consistent with the goals of the President's New Freedom Commission on Mental Health (2003) for transforming mental health care in America. (www.mentalhealthcommission.gov/reports/finalreport/toc.html).

Transcranial Magnetic Stimulation

Transcranial magnetic stimulation (TMS) applies the principles of electromagnetism to deliver an electrical field to the cerebral cortices, but unlike ECT, the waves do not result in generalized seizure activity (Rosenbaum, 2004). Early studies of this technique support further research into its use in the treatment of serious, relapsing, medication-resistant depression. Whereas some studies of TMS find significant antidepressant effect in individuals with medication-resistant major depression (Avery et al., 2006). There is still some question as to its efficacy, and more research is needed.

Brain Imaging

A study from the University of Wisconsin–Madison (Johnstone et al., 2007), perhaps the first study to use brain imaging, revealed a breakdown in normal patterns of emotional processing in people who are depressed. Using a functional magnetic resonance imaging scanner, the researchers found that healthy people are able to regulate their negative emotions through conscious efforts, such as envisioning a more positive outcome or reframing a negative situation. The scan revealed that high levels of regulatory activity correlated with low levels of activity in the emotional response centers. They found that some depressed individuals lacked the ability to regulate emotions. In these individuals, high levels of regulatory activity did not change the levels of activity in the emotional centers, demonstrating the neural circuits regulating emotion in some depressed individuals are dysfunctional.

EVALUATION

Short-term indicators and outcome criteria are frequently evaluated. For example, if the patient comes into the unit with suicidal thoughts, the nurse evaluates whether the patient still has suicidal thoughts, is able to state alternatives to suicidal impulses in the future, and is able to explore thoughts and feelings that precede suicidal impulses. Outcomes relating to thought processes, self-esteem, and social interactions are frequently formulated because these areas are often problematic in people who are depressed.

Physical needs warrant nursing or medical attention. If a person has lost weight because of anorexia, is the appetite returning? If a person was constipated, are the bowels now functioning normally? If the person was suffering from insomnia, is he or she now getting 6 to 8 hours of sleep per night? If the indicators have not been met, an analysis of the data, nursing diagnoses, goals, and planned nursing interventions is made. The patient should be reassessed and the care plan reformulated when necessary.

KEY POINTS TO REMEMBER

- Depression is the most commonly seen psychiatric disorder in the health care system.
- There are a number of subtypes of depression and depressive clinical phenomena. The two primary depressive disorders are major depressive disorder (MDD) and dysthymic disorder (DD).
- The symptoms in major depression are usually severe enough to interfere with a person's social or occupational functioning (inability to experience pleasure [anhedonia], significant weight loss, insomnia or hypersomnia, extreme fatigue [anergia], psychomotor agitation or retardation, diminished ability to think or concentrate, feelings of worthlessness, recurrent thoughts of death).
- A person with MDD may or may not have psychotic symptoms, and the symptoms a person usually exhibits during a major depression are different from the characteristics of the normal premorbid personality.
- In DD, the symptoms are often chronic (lasting at least 2 years) and are considered mild to moderate. Usually, a person's social or occupational functioning is not as greatly impaired as they are in MDD, although they may cause significant distress or some impairment in these areas. The symptoms in a dysthymic depression are often congruent with the person's usual pattern of functioning.
- Many theories exist about the cause of depression. The most accepted is the psychophysiological theory; however, cognitive theory, learned helplessness theory, and psychodynamic and life events issues help explain triggers to depression and maintenance of depressive thoughts and feelings.

- Nursing assessment includes the evaluation of affect, thought processes (especially suicidal thoughts), feelings, physical behavior, and communication. The nurse also needs to be aware of the symptoms that mask depression.
- Nursing diagnoses can be numerous. Depressed individuals are always evaluated for *Risk for suicide*. Some other common nursing diagnoses are *Disturbed thought processes*, *Chronic low self-esteem*, *Imbalanced nutrition*, *Constipation*, *Disturbed sleep pattern*, *Ineffective coping*, and *Disabled family coping*.
- Interventions with patients who are depressed involve several approaches, including using specific principles of communication, planning activities of daily living, administering or participating in psychopharmacological therapy, maintaining a therapeutic environment, and teaching patients about the biochemical aspects of depression and medication teaching.
- Several short-term psychotherapies are effective in the treatment of depression, including IPT, CBT, and some forms of group therapy.
- Electroconvulsive therapy (ECT) is an effective treatment for people with major depression with psychotic features and patients refractory to other treatments. Vagus nerve stimulation (VNS) can be a valuable adjunctive treatment in treatment-resistant depression. Light therapy is the first line of treatment for seasonal effective disorders (SAD).
- Evaluation is ongoing throughout the nursing process, and patients' outcomes are compared with the stated outcome criteria and short-term and intermediate goals. The care plan is revised by use of the evaluation process when desired outcomes are not being met.

CRITICAL THINKING

1. You are spending time with Mr. Plotsky, who is being given a workup for depression. He hardly makes eye contact and slouches in his seat, and his expression appears blank, but sad. Mr. Plotsky has had numerous bouts of major depression in the past and says to you, "This will be my last depression. I will never go through this again."

   A. If safety is the first concern, what are the appropriate questions to ask Mr. Plotsky at this time?

   B. Give an example of the kinds of signs and symptoms you might find when you assess a patient with depression in terms of behaviors, thought processes, activities of daily living, and ability to function at work and at home?

   C. Mr. Plotsky tells you that he has been on every medication there is but that none have worked. He asks you about the herb St. John's wort. What is some

CRITICAL THINKING—cont'd

information he should have about its effectiveness for severe depression, its interactions with other antide-pressants, and its regulatory status?

D. What might be some somatic options for a person who is resistant to antidepressant medications?

E. Mr. Plotsky asks what causes depression. In simple terms, how might you respond to his query?

F. Mr. Plotsky tells you that he has never tried therapy because he thinks it is for babies. What information

could you give him about various therapeutic modali-ties that have proven effective for some other depressed patients?

2. When you are teaching Ms. Mac about her SSRI sertraline (Zoloft), she asks you, "What makes this such a good drug?"

A. What are some of the positive attributes of SSRIs? What is one of the most serious, although rare, side effects of the SSRIs?

B. Devise a teaching plan for Ms. Mac.

CHAPTER REVIEW

Choose the most appropriate answer.

1. If a nurse subscribes to the theory that learned helplessness is a major factor in the development of depression, which statement best represents her belief?

1. TCAs, MAOIs, and SSRIs are the most useful tools to combat depression.

2. Depression develops when a person believes he or she is powerless to effect change in a situation.

3. Depressive symptoms result from experiencing signifi-cant loss and turning aggression against the self.

4. Psychosocial stressors and interpersonal events trigger neurophysical and neurochemical changes in the brain.

2. Which response to a patient experiencing depression would be helpful from the nurse?

1. "Don't worry, we all get down once in a while."

2. "Don't consider suicide. It's an unacceptable option."

3. "Try to cheer up. Things always look darkest before the dawn."

4. "I can see you're feeling down. I'll sit here with you for a while."

3. Which of the following is considered a vegetative symptom of depression?

1. Sleep disturbance

2. Trouble concentrating

3. Neglected grooming and hygiene

4. Negative expectations for the future

4. For a person with severe depression, which statement about cognitive functioning is true?

1. Reality testing remains intact.

2. Concentration is unimpaired.

3. Repetitive negative thinking is noted.

4. Ability to make decisions is improved.

5. When the nurse is caring for a depressed patient, the problem that should receive the highest nursing priority is:

1. powerlessness.

2. suicidal ideation.

3. inability to cope effectively.

4. anorexia and weight loss.

REFERENCES

Agency for Healthcare Research and Quality (AHRQ). (2004). *Improving depression care has long-lasting benefits for African Americans and Hispanics* [Press release]. Retrieved April 5, 2004, from www.ahrq.gov/news/press/pr2004/depminpr.htm.

American Psychiatric Association (APA). (2000a). *Diagnostic and statistical manual of mental disorders (DSM-IV-TR)* (4th ed., text rev.). Washington, DC: Author.

American Psychiatric Association (APA). (2000b). *Practice guidelines for the treatment of psychiatric disorders: Compendium 2000.* Washington, DC: Author.

Ardayfio, P., & Kim, K.S. (2006). Anxiogenic-like effect of chronic corticosterone in the light-dark emergence task in mice. *Behavioral Neuroscience, 120*(2), 249-256.

Avery, D.H., (2006). A controlled study of repetitive transcranial magnetic stimulation in medication-resistant major depression. *Biological Psychiatry, 59*(2), 187-194.

Beck, A.T., & Rush, A.J. (1995). Cognitive therapy. In H.I. Kaplan & B.J. Sadock (Eds.), *Comprehensive textbook of psychiatry/VI* (6th ed., vol. 2, pp. 1847-1856). Baltimore: Williams & Wilkins.

Bijl, D., van Marwijk, H.W., de Haan, M., et al. (2004). Effectiveness of disease management programs for recognition, diagnosis and treatment of depression in primary care. *European Journal of General Practice, 10*(1), 6-12. Abstract.

Culpepper, L., Krishman, R.R., Kroenke, K., et al. (2003). *Spotlight on remission: Achieving an evidence-based goal in depression and anxiety.* Retrieved January 13, 2004, from www.medscape.com/viewprogram/2544.

Dubovsky, S.L., & Buzan, R. (1999). Mood disorders. In R.E. Hales, S.C. Yudofsky, & J.A. Talbott (Eds.), *Textbook of psychiatry* (pp. 479-566). Washington, DC: American Psychiatric Publishing.

Dubovsky, S.L., Davies, R., & Dubovsky, A.N. (2004). Mood disorders. In R.E. Hales, & S.C. Yudofsky (Eds.), *Essentials of clinical psychiatry* (2nd ed., pp. 273-274). Washington, DC: American Psychiatric Publishing.

Feldman, G. (2007). Cognitive and behavioral therapies for depression: Overview, new directions and practical recommendations for dissemination. *Psychiatric Clinics of North America, 30*(1), 39-50.

Gelder, M., Harrison, P., & Cowen, P. (2006). *The shorter Oxford textbook of psychiatry* (5th ed.). Oxford: Oxford University Press.

Golden, R.N., Dawkins, K., Nicholas, L. (2006). Trazodone and mefazodone. In A.F. Schatzberg & C.B. Nemeroff (Eds.), Essentials of clinical psychopharmacology. Washington, DC: American Psychiatric Publishing, p. 127.

Greden, J.F. (2004). *Best practices for achieving remission in depression with physical symptoms: Current and future trends.* Paper presented in symposium 10E conducted at the American Psychiatric Association Annual Meeting, May 1-6, New York.

Grohol, J.M. (2007). VNS for treatment resistant depression. Retrieved March 30, 2007, from www.psychocentral.com/news/2007/03/30/vns-for-treatment-resistant-depression.

Gruenberg, A.M., & Goldstein, R.D. (2003). Mood disorders: Depression. In A. Tasman, J. Kay, & J.A. Lieberman (Eds.), *Psychiatry* (2nd ed.). West Sussex, England: Wiley.

Heim, C., & Nemeroff, C.B. (1999). The impact of early adverse experiences on brain systems involved in the pathophysiology of anxiety and affective disorders. *Social Biology and Psychiatry, 46*, 1-15.

Jain, R., & Russel, N. (2003). *Addressing both the emotional and physical symptoms in depression.* Retrieved March 21, 2003, from www.medscape.com/viewprogram/2240.

Johnstone, T., van Reekum, C.M., & Urry, H.L. (2007). Failure to regulate: Counterproductive recruitment of top-down prefrontal-subcortical circuitry in major depression. *Journal of Neuroscience, 27*(33), 8877-8884.

Kessler, R.C., Berglund, P., Demler, O., et al. (2005). Lifetime prevalence and age of onset distributions of DSM-IV disorders in the national comorbidity survey replication. *Archives of General Psychiatry, 62*(6): 592-602.

Kramer, T.A.M. (2004). *The relationship between depression and physical symptoms.* Paper presented at the American Psychiatric Association Annual Meeting, May 1-6, New York.

Lenze, E.J., Molsant, B.H., Shear, M.K., et al. (2003). Comorbidity of depression and anxiety in the elderly. *Current Psychiatric Reports, 5*, 62-67.

Ludwig, J., & Marcotte, D.E. (2005). Antidepressants, suicide and drug regulation. *Journal of Policy, Analysis and Management, 24*, 249-272.

Marangell, L.B., Yudofsky, S.C., Silver, J.M., et al. (2004). Psychopharmacology and electroconvulsive therapy. In R.E. Hales, & S.C. Yudofsky (Eds.), *Essentials of clinical psychiatry* (4th ed.). Washington, DC: American Psychiatric Publishing.

Martin, J.L.R., Barbanoj M.J., Schlaepfer T.E., et al. (2007). Transcranial magnetic stimulation for treating depression (abstract). Retrieved January 22, 2008, from www.medscape.com/viewarticle/486646.

Maxmen, J.S., & Ward, N.G. (2002). *Psychotropic drugs: Fast facts* (2nd ed.). New York: Norton.

Mayo Clinic Staff. (2005). *Depression and anxiety: Exercise eases symptoms.* Retrieved August 21, 2007, from http://mayoclinic.com/health/depression-and-exercise/MH00043.

Mischoulon, D. (2007). Update and critique of natural remedies as antidepressant treatments. *Psychiatric Clinics of North America, 30*(1), 51-68.

Montano, C.B. (2003). *New frontiers in the treatment of depression.* Retrieved September 30, 2003, from www.medscape.com/viewprogram/2689.

National Institute of Mental Health (NIMH). (2000). *Depression: What every woman should know* (NIH Publication No. 004779). Washington, DC: Author. Retrieved February 28, 2005, from www.nimh.nih.gov/publicat/depwomenknows.cfm.

National Institute of Mental Health (NIMH). (2001b). *The numbers count: Mental disorders in America* (NIH Publication No. 01-4584). Retrieved January 16, 2005, from www.nimh.nih.gov/publicat/numbers.cfm.

National Institute of Mental Health (NIMH). (2002). *Depression research at the National Institute of Mental Health* (NIH Publication No. 004501). Bethesda, MD: National Institutes of Health.

National Institute of Mental Health (NIMH). (2003). *NIH News: Gene more than doubles risk of depression following life stresses.* Retrieved January 16, 2005, from www.nih.gov/news/pr/jul2003/nimh-17.htm.

Nemeroff, C, DeVane, L., Lydiard, B. (2007). *Emerging trends for monoamine oxidase inhibition in the management of depression: A patient-focused, interactive program.* CME. Office of Continuing Education, Medical University of South Carolina (MUSC).

Oquendo, M., & Liebowitz, M. (2005). *The diagnosis and treatment of depression in primary care: An evidence-based approach.* Retrieved August 7, 2006, from www.medscape.com/viewprogram/4571.

President's New Freedom Commission on Mental Health (2003). Retrieved January 23, 2008 from http://www.mentalhealthcommission.gov/.

Psych Direct Evidenced Based Mental Health Education and Information (2006). *Mood disorders: Professional audiences.* Retrieved August 8, 2006, from www.psychdirect.com/depression/depression_pro,htm#Anchor-DOES-49425.

Rihmer, Z., & Angst, J. (2005). Mood disorders: Epidemiology. In B.J. Sadock & V.A. Sadock, (Eds.), *Kaplan and Sadock's comprehensive textbook of psychiatry* (8th ed., vol. 1). Philadelphia: Lippincott Williams & Wilkins.

Riolo, S., Nguyen, T.A, Greden, J.F. (2005). Prevalence of depression by race/ethnicity: Findings from the National Health and Nutrition Examination survey. *American Journal of Public Health, 95*(6), 998-1000.

Rosenbaum, J.F. (2004). *New brain stimulation therapies for depression.* Paper presented at the American Psychiatric Association Annual Meeting, May 1-6, New York. Retrieved January 16, 2005, from www.medscape.com/viewarticle/480897.

Rosenbaum, J.F., & Covino, J.M. (2006). Depression in geriatric patients. *Medscape Psychiatry and Mental Health.* Retrieved August 6, 2006, from www.medscape.com/viewarticle/520524.

Sackheim, H.A., Brannan, S.K., Rush, A.J., et al. (2007). Durability of antidepressant response to vagus nerve stimulation (VNS). *The International Journal of Neuropsychopharmacology, 9*: 1-10.

Sadek, N., & Nemeroff, C.B. (2000). *Update on the neurobiology of depression.* Retrieved January 16, 2005, from www.medscape.com/viewprogram/142.

Sadock, B.J., & Sadock, V.A. (2007). *Kaplan & Sadock's synopsis of psychiatry* (10th ed.). Philadelphia: Lippincott Williams & Wilkins.

Seligman, M.E. (1973). Fall into hopelessness. *Psychology Today, 7*, 43.

Serby, M., & Yu, M. (2003). There is good news about depression in the elderly. *Clinical Advisor*, 64-75.

Simon, N.M., & Rosenbaum, J.F. (2003). *Anxiety and depression comorbidity: Implications and intervention.* Retrieved January 16, 2005, from www.medscape.com/viewarticle/451325.

Stuart, D.E. (2003). Physical symptoms of depression: Emerging needs in special populations. *Journal of Clinical Psychiatry, 64*(7), 12-16.

Sutherland, J.E., Sutherland, S.J., & Hoehns, J.D. (2003). Achieving the best outcome in treatment of depression. *Journal of Family Practice, 52*(3), 201-209.

U.S. Department of Veterans Affairs (2006). *Evidence-based depression treatment.* Retrieved August 8, 2006, from www.va.gov/tides_waves/page.cfm?pg = 20.

Young, J.E., Weinberger, A.D., & Beck, A.T. (2001). Cognitive therapy for depression. In D.H. Barlow (Ed.), *Clinical handbook of psychological disorders* (3rd ed.). New York: Guilford Press.

Zahourek, R. (2000). Alternative, complementary, or integrative approaches to treating depression. *Journal of the American Psychiatric Nurses Association, 6*(3), 77-86.

CHAPTER 13

Mood Disorders: Bipolar

Elizabeth M. Varcarolis

Key Terms and Concepts

acute phase, p. 256
antiepileptic drugs (AEDs), p. 262
bipolar I disorder, p. 246
bipolar II disorder, p. 246
clang associations, p. 252
continuation phase, p. 256
cyclothymia, p. 246
electroconvulsive therapy (ECT), p. 265
finger foods p. 260

flight of ideas, p. 252
hypomania, p. 247
lithium carbonate, p. 261
maintenance phase, p. 256
mania, p. 247
psychoeducation, p. 265
rapid cycling, p. 246
seclusion protocol, p. 259

Objectives

1. Describe the progression of behaviors, speech patterns, and thought process of a person escalating from hypomania to mania to delirious mania.
2. Discuss the physical, safety, personal, and legal considerations a nurse must be aware of during a patient's manic phase.
3. Explain the rationale for the communication strategies that are effective with patients in acute mania.
4. Describe a safe milieu for a patient in acute mania.
5. Identify expected side effects of lithium therapy.

6. Distinguish between signs of early and severe lithium toxicity.
7. Compare and contrast basic clinical conditions that may respond better to anticonvulsant therapy with those that may respond better to lithium therapy.
8. Identify important areas of a teaching plan for a patient with bipolar disorder.
9. Distinguish between the focus of treatment for a person in the acute manic phase and that for a person in the continuation or maintenance phase of a bipolar I disorder.

evolve

For additional resources related to the content of this chapter, visit the Evolve website at
http://evolve.elsevier.com/Varcarolis/essentials.

- Chapter Outline
- Chapter Review Answers
- Case Study and Nursing Care Plans

- Nurse, Patient, and Family Resources
- Concept Map Creator

Bipolar disorder, formerly called manic-depressive illness, is characterized by two opposite poles. One pole is mania, an exaggerated euphoria or irritability, and the other pole is depression. Bipolar disorder is not a unitary illness, but a group of disorders with different courses and treatments (Dubovsky, 2005). Alternating mood episodes are characterized by mania, hypomania, depression, and concurrent mania and depression (mixed episodes in which depressive symptoms occur during a manic attack). Periods of normal functioning may alternate with periods of illness (highs, lows, or mixed highs and lows). However, only 37% to 40% of individuals with bipolar disorder regain full occupational and social functioning even though 97% appear to recover clinically within a 2-year period (Spollen, 2003). Indeed, many individuals with bipolar disorder experience chronic interpersonal or occupational difficulties during remission (Blairy et al., 2004). The morbidity rate is not only high but also severe: bipolar disorder is associated with the highest lifetime rate of suicide of any psychiatric illness (Jamison, 2000).

Bipolar disorders are chronic, recurrent, and life-threatening illnesses that require lifetime monitoring; unfortunately, they frequently go undiagnosed and people go for years without obtaining proper treatment.

Bipolar disorders are identified based on severity and patterns, listed from most to least severe:

- **Bipolar I disorder:** At least one episode of mania alternating with major depression. Psychosis may accompany the manic episode.
- **Bipolar II disorder:** Hypomanic episode(s) alternating with major depression. Psychosis is not present in bipolar II. The hypomania of bipolar II tends to be euphoric and the depression tends to put people at particular risk for suicide.
- **Cyclothymia:** Hypomanic episodes alternating with minor depressive episodes (at least 2 years in duration). Individuals with cyclothymia tend to have irritable hypomanic episodes.

The specifier **rapid cycling** (four or more mood episodes in a 12-month period) is used to indicate more severe symptoms such as poorer global functioning, high recurrence risk, and resistance to conventional somatic treatments (Schneck et al., 2003).

PREVALENCE AND COMORBIDITY

The lifetime prevalence of bipolar disorder in the U.S. population is estimated to be 3.9% (Kessler, 2005). Whereas major depression usually starts between 25 and 30 years of age, bipolar disorders emerge between the ages of 18 and 30. Mean age of the first episode of the disorder appears lower for people with a family history of the disease (Dubovsky et al., 2004). The first episode in males is likely to be a manic episode, whereas in females the disease usually presents with a depressive episode. During the course of the illness, the episodes increase in number and severity as the person gets older.

Cyclothymia usually begins in adolescence or early adulthood and has a lifetime prevalence of 2.5% (Kessler, 2005). There is a 15% to 50% risk that an individual with cyclothymia will subsequently develop bipolar I or bipolar II disorder.

Substance use disorders are exceptionally common in individuals with a bipolar disease. This may be caused, in part, by an attempt to self-medicate. Substance-abusing patients seem to experience more rapid cycling and more mixed or dysphoric mania (anger and irritability) and report more hospitalizations. Other associated disorders include personality disorders, anxiety disorders (panic disorder and social phobia), anorexia nervosa, bulimia nervosa, and attention deficit hyperactivity disorder (APA, 2000a). Men are more apt to present with comorbid substance use disorder, whereas women present more frequently with comorbid anxiety disorders and eating disorders. Comorbid substance and anxiety disorders worsen the prognosis and greatly increased the risk of suicide (Sadock & Sadock, 2007). Also, there seem to be high rates of *medical* comorbidity as well, especially cardiovascular, cerebrovascular, and metabolic diseases.

THEORY

Phillips and Frank (2006) state that because of increasingly sophisticated neuroimaging and genetic research, our knowledge of the neurobiology of bipolar disorder is one of complexity. It is a disorder involving complex disturbances in relationships and marked disruption in sleep patterns, linking environment, genes, neural systems and behaviors, and high rates of certain psychological and medical comorbidities. Defining bipolar as solely a disorder of episodic mood disturbances is too simplistic. There seems to have been a shift to defining bipolar disorder as a multisystem disorder involving disturbances in all of these aforementioned domains (Phillips & Frank, 2006). For this reason, a biopsychosocial approach is likely the most successful approach to treatment (Bauer, 2003).

Biological Theories
Genetic Factors
Twin, family, and adoption studies provide significant evidence to support the view that bipolar disorders have a strong

genetic component. The inheritance of the bipolar disorders is not a matter of "one gene, one illness" but an expression of multiple genes and chromosomes. Increasingly, researchers are finding evidence that there is a genetic link for susceptibility to both bipolar disorder I and schizophrenia, disorders that frequently run in the same family (Craddock et al., 2005). An early age of onset is associated with hereditability, which increases with the amount of shared genetic material. Therefore, identical twins have greater heritable risk (60% to 80%) than fraternal twins (20%). Fraternal twins have about the same risk as first-degree relatives (5.4% to 14%) (Dubovsky et al., 2004; Thase, 2004).

Because the concordance rates for most disorders in twins is not 100%, it is strongly accepted that any genetic basis for bipolar disorder most likely involves multiple genes interacting with each other in, as yet, unknown ways (Payne et al., 2005). Researchers have, however, identified two specific genes (*G72* and *G30*) located on the long arm of chromosome 13 that are associated with bipolar disorder as well as schizophrenia (Hattori et al., 2003).

Neurobiological Factors

Neurotransmitters (norepinephrine, serotonin, and dopamine) have been studied since the 1960s as causal factors in mania and depression. For example, during a manic episode, patients with bipolar disorder demonstrate significantly higher plasma levels of norepinephrine and epinephrine than they do when they are depressed or *euthymic* (have normal mood) (Freedman & McElroy, 1999; Nathan et al., 1995). Other research has found that the interrelationships in the neurotransmitter system are complex.

More elaborate theories have been developed since the amine hypotheses were originally proposed. Mood disorders are most likely a result of complex interactions among various chemicals, including neurotransmitters and hormones. One study reported that people with bipolar disorder have 30% more neurotransmitters in two major areas of the brain, which may cause an overstimulation in the brain (Zubieta et al., 2000). Neuroreceptor oversensitivity also has been identified as a cause of bipolar disorder symptoms.

Neuroendocrine Factors

The hypothalamic-pituitary-thyroid-adrenal (HPA) axis has been closely scrutinized in people with mood disorders for decades. The severity of manic episodes seems to be highly correlated to the degree of neuroendocrine alteration (Daban et al., 2005). Bipolar individuals exhibit significantly higher cortisol contractions than do unipolar patients in acute episodes as well as in remission. Therefore, it appears that a higher degree of HPA dysfunction is present (Daban et al., 2005).

Neuroanatomical Factors

Brain pathways implicated in the pathophysiology of bipolar disorder are in subregions of the prefrontal cortex (PFC) and medial temporal lobe (MTL). Dysregulation in the neurocircuits surrounding these areas has been viewed through functional imaging (e.g., positron emission tomography, magnetic resonance imaging) (Pollock & Kuo, 2004).

Psychological Influences

Although there is increasing evidence for genetic and biological vulnerabilities in the etiology of the mood disorders, stressful life events can trigger symptoms of bipolar disorder. Two studies of family atmosphere suggest an association between high expressed emotion and relapse. Another study of bipolar patients who suffered abuse as children revealed earlier onset of bipolar disorder, faster cycling frequencies, and an increase in comorbid disorders such as substance abuse (Leverich et al., 2002).

CULTURAL CONSIDERATIONS

Some evidence suggests that the bipolar disorders may be more prevalent in the upper socioeconomic classes. The exact reason for this is unclear; however, people with bipolar disorders appear to achieve higher levels of education and higher occupational status than nonbipolar depressed individuals. The educational levels of individuals with nonbipolar depressive disorders, on the other hand, appear to be no different from those of nondepressed individuals within the same socioeconomic class. Also, the proportion of bipolar patients among creative writers, artists, highly educated men and women, and professional people is higher than in the general population.

CLINICAL PICTURE

The *Diagnostic and Statistical Manual of Mental Disorders (DSM-IV-TR)* (APA, 2000a) makes a distinction between **mania** and **hypomania** for diagnostic purposes, as shown in Figure 13-1.

Individuals with bipolar disorder are often misdiagnosed or underdiagnosed. On average, people spend 8 years seeking treatment before receiving a correct diagnosis. Early diagnosis and proper treatment can help people avoid the following:

- Suicide (one out of five patients with bipolar disorder)
- Alcohol or substance abuse (50% abuse alcohol or drugs, which signals a worse outcome)
- Marital or work problems
- Development of medical comorbidity

DSM-IV-TR CRITERIA FOR BIPOLAR DISORDER

1. A distinct period of abnormality and persistently elevated, expansive, or irritable mood for at least:
   - 4 days for hypomania
   - 1 week for mania

2. During the period of mood disturbance, **three or more** of the following symptoms have persisted (four if the mood is only irritable) and have been present to a significant degree:
   - Inflated self-esteem or grandiosity
   - Decreased need for sleep (e.g., the person feels rested after only 3 hours of sleep)
   - More talkative than usual or pressure to keep talking
   - Flight of ideas or subjective experience that thoughts are racing
   - Distractibility (i.e., the person's attention is too easily drawn to unimportant or irrelevant external stimuli)
   - Increase in goal-directed activity (either socially, at work or school, or sexually) or psychomotor agitation
   - Excessive involvement in pleasurable activities that have a high potential for painful consequences (e.g., the person engages in unrestrained buying sprees, sexual indiscretions, or foolish business investments)

Hypomania

1. The episode is associated with an unequivocal change in functioning that is uncharacteristic of the person when not symptomatic.

2. The disturbance in mood and the change in functioning are observed by others.

3. Absence of marked impairment in social or occupational functioning.

4. Hospitalization is not indicated.

5. Symptoms are not due to direct physiological effects of substance (e.g., drug abuse, medication, or other medical conditions).

Mania

1. Severe enough to cause marked impairment in occupational activities, usual social activities, or relationships.

   or

2. Necessitate hospitalization to prevent harm to self or others, or there are psychotic features.

3. Symptoms are not due to direct physiological effects of substance (drug abuse, medication) or general medical condition (e.g., hyperthyroidism).

Figure 13-1 ■ Diagnostic criteria for bipolar disorder. (Adapted from American Psychiatric Association. [2000a]. *Diagnostic and statistical manual of mental disorders* [4th ed., text rev.]. Washington, DC: Author.)

evolve

For a comprehensive case study and associated nursing care plans for a patient experiencing bipolar disorder, visit the Evolve website at http://evolve. elsevier.com/Varcarolis/essentials.

Application of the Nursing Process

ASSESSMENT

Figure 13-2 presents the Mood Disorder Questionnaire (MDQ). This is *not* a diagnostic test; rather, it is a helpful screening device for assessment purposes.

MOOD DISORDER QUESTIONNAIRE

Instructions: Please answer each question as best you can.

	Yes	No
1. Has there ever been a period of time when you were not your usual self and....		
you felt so good or so hyper that other people thought you were not your normal self or you were so hyper that you got into trouble?	○	○
you were so irritable that you shouted at people or started fights or arguments?	○	○
you felt much more self-confident than usual?	○	○
you got much less sleep than usual and found you didn't really miss it?	○	○
you were much more talkative or spoke much faster than usual?	○	○
thoughts raced through your head or you couldn't slow down your mind?	○	○
you were so easily distracted by things around you that you had trouble concentrating or staying on track?	○	○
you had much more energy than usual?	○	○
you were much more active or did many more things than usual?	○	○
you were much more social or outgoing than usual; for example, you telephoned friends in the middle of the night?	○	○
you were much more interested in sex than usual?	○	○
you did things that were unusual for you or that other people might have thought were excessive, foolish, or risky?	○	○
spending money got you or your family into trouble?	○	○
2. If you answered "Yes" to more than one of the above, have several of these ever happened during the same period of time?	○	○

3. How much of a problem did any of these cause you — like being unable to work; having family, money, or legal troubles; or getting into arguments or fights? Please select one response only.

○ No problem   ○ Minor problem   ○ Moderate problem   ○ Serious problem

4. Have any of your blood relatives (children, siblings, parents, grandparents, aunts, uncles) had manic-depressive illness or bipolar disorder?	○	○
5. Has a health care professional ever told you that you have manic-depressive illness or bipolar disorder?	○	○

Criteria for Results: Answering "Yes" to 7 or more of the events in question 1, answering "Yes" to question 2, and answering "Moderate problem" or "Serious problem" to question 3 is considered a positive screen result for bipolar disorder.

Figure 13-2 ■ The Mood Disorder Questionnaire. (From Hirschfeld, R.M.A., et al. [2000]. Development and validation of a screening instrument for bipolar spectrum disorder: The Mood Disorder Questionnaire, *American Journal of Psychiatry, 157*[11], 1873-1875. © 2004 Eli Lilly and Company.)

Level of Mood

The euphoric mood associated with a bipolar illness is unstable. During euphoria patients may state they are experiencing an intense feeling of well-being, are "cheerful in a beautiful world," or are becoming "one with God." This mood may change to irritation and quick anger when the elated person is thwarted. The irritability and belligerence may be short-lived, or it may become the prominent feature of a person's manic illness. When the person is elated, the overjoyous mood may seem out of proportion to what is going on, and a cheerful mood may be inappropriate to the circumstances.

People in a manic state may laugh, joke, and talk in a continuous stream, with uninhibited familiarity. Manic people demonstrate boundless enthusiasm, treat everyone with confidential friendliness, and incorporate everyone into their plans and activities. They know no strangers. Energy and self-confidence seem boundless.

Elaborate schemes to get rich and famous and acquire unlimited power may be frantically pursued, despite objections and realistic constraints. Excessive phone calls and e-mails are made, often to famous and influential people all over the world. People in the manic phase are busy all hours of the day and night furthering their grandiose plans and wild schemes. To the manic person, no aspirations are too high and no distances are too far. No boundaries exist in reality to curtail the elaborate schemes.

In the manic state, a person often gives away money, prized possessions, and expensive gifts. The manic person throws lavish parties, frequents expensive nightclubs and restaurants, and spends money freely on friends and strangers alike. This spending, excessive use of credit cards, and high living continue even in the face of bankruptcy. Intervention is often needed to prevent financial ruin.

As the clinical course progresses, sociability and euphoria are replaced by a stage of hostility, irritability, and paranoia. The following is a patient's description of this experience (Jamison, 1995b, p. 67):

VIGNETTE

At first when I'm high, it's tremendous . . . ideas are fast, like shooting stars you follow until brighter ones appear. All shyness disappears; the right words and gestures are suddenly there. Uninteresting people and things become intensely interesting. Sensuality is pervasive; the desire to seduce and be seduced is irresistible. Your marrow is infused with unbelievable feelings of ease, power, well-being, omnipotence, euphoria . . . you can do anything. But somewhere this changes.

The fast ideas become too fast and there are far too many. Overwhelming confusion replaces clarity. You stop keeping up with it—memory goes. Infectious humor ceases to amuse—your friends become frightened . . . everything now is against the grain. You are irritable, angry, frightened, uncontrollable, and trapped in the blackest caves of the mind—caves you never knew were there. It will never end. Madness carves its own reality.

Refer to Table 13-1 for further description of hypomania, acute mania, and delirious mania.

Behavior

During Mania

When in full-blown mania, a person constantly goes from one activity to another, one place to another, and one project to another. Many projects may be started, but few, if any, are completed. Inactivity is impossible, even for the shortest period of time. Hyperactivity may range from mild, constant motion to frenetic, wild activity. The writing of flowery and lengthy letters and the making of excessive long-distance telephone calls are accentuated. Individuals become involved in pleasurable activities that can have painful consequences. For example, spending large sums of money on frivolous items, giving money away indiscriminately, or making foolish business investments can leave a family penniless. Sexual indiscretion can dissolve relationships and marriages.

Bipolar individuals can be manipulative, profane, fault finding, and adept at exploiting others' vulnerabilities. They constantly push limits. These behaviors often alienate family, friends, employers, health care providers, and others.

When people are hypomanic they have voracious appetites for food as well as for indiscriminate sex. Although the constant activity of the hypomanic prevents proper sleep, short periods of sleep are possible. However, all patients experiencing mania sleep less, and some patients may not sleep for several days in a row. The person is too busy to eat, sleep, or engage in sexual activity. **This nonstop physical activity and the lack of sleep and food can lead to physical exhaustion and even death if not treated and therefore constitutes an emergency.**

Modes of dress often reflect the person's grandiose yet tenuous grasp of reality. Dress may be described as outlandish, bizarre, colorful, and noticeably inappropriate. Makeup may be garish or overdone. Manic people are highly distractible. Concentration is poor, and individuals go from one activity to another without completing anything. Judgment is poor, and impulsive marriages and divorces often take place.

TABLE 13-1   Mania on a Continuum

Hypomania	Acute Mania	Delirious Mania
Communication		
1. Talks and jokes incessantly, is the "life of the party," gets irritated when not center of attention.	1. May go suddenly from laughing to anger or depression. *Mood is labile.*	1. Totally out of touch with reality.
2. Treats everyone with familiarity and confidentiality; often borders on crude.	2. Becomes inappropriately demanding of people's attention, and intrusive nature repels others.	—
3. Talk is often sexual—can reach obscene, inappropriate propositions to total strangers.	3. Speech may be marked by profanities and crude sexual remarks to everyone (nursing staff in particular).	—
4. Talk is fresh; flits from one topic to the next. Marked by *pressure of speech.*	4. Speech marked by *flight of ideas,* in which thoughts race and fly from topic to topic. May have *clang associations.*	4. Most likely has clang associations.
Affect and Thinking		
1. Full of pep and good humor, feelings of euphoria and sociability; may show inappropriate intimacy with strangers.	1. Good humor gives way to increased irritability and hostility, short-lived period of rage, especially when not getting his or her way or when controls are set on behavior. May have quick shifts of mood from hostility to docility.	1. May become destructive or aggressive—totally out of control.
2. Feels boundless self-confidence and enthusiasm. Has elaborate schemes for becoming rich and famous. Initially, schemes may seem plausible.	2. Grandiose plans are totally out of contact with reality. Thinks he or she is a musician, prominent businessman, great politician, or religious figure, without any basis in fact.	2. May experience undefined hallucinations and delirium.
3. Judgment often poor. Gets involved with schemes in which job, marriage, or financial status may be destroyed.	3. Judgment is extremely poor.	—
4. May write large quantities of letters to rich and famous people regarding schemes or may make numerous worldwide telephone calls.	—	—
5. Decreased attention span to internal and external cues.	5. Decreased attention span and distractibility are intensified.	—
Physical Behavior		
1. Overactive, distractible, buoyant, and busily occupied with grandiose plans (not delusions); goes from one action to the next.	1. Extremely restless, disorganized, and chaotic. Physical behavior may be difficult to control. May have outbursts, such as throwing things or becoming briefly assaultive when crossed.	1. *Dangerous state.* Incoherent, extremely restless, disoriented, and agitated. Hyperactive. Motor activity is totally aimless (must have physical or chemical restraints to prevent exhaustion and death).

Continued

TABLE 13-1   Mania on a Continuum—cont'd

Hypomania	Acute Mania	Delirious Mania
2. Increased sexual appetite; sexually irresponsible and indiscreet. Illegitimate pregnancies in hypomanic women and venereal disease in both men and women are common. Sex used for escape, not for relating to another human being.	2. No time for sex—too busy. Poor concentration, distractibility, and restlessness are severe.	2. Same as in acute mania but in the extreme.
3. May have voracious appetite, eat on the run, or gobble food during brief periods.	3. No time to eat—too distracted and disorganized.	3. Same as acute mania but in the extreme.
4. May go without sleeping; unaware of fatigue. However, may be able to take short naps.	4. No time for sleep—psychomotor activity too high; if unchecked, can lead to exhaustion and death.	—
5. Financially extravagant, goes on buying sprees, gives money and gifts away freely, can easily go into debt.	5. Same as in hypomania but in the extreme.	5. Too disorganized to do anything.

After Mania

People often emerge from a manic state startled and confused by the shambles of their lives. The following description conveys one patient's experience (Jamison, 1995b, p. 68):

VIGNETTE

Now there are only others' recollections of your behavior—your bizarre, frenetic, aimless behavior. At least mania has the grace to dim memories of itself . . . now it's over, but is it? Incredible feelings to sort through. Who is being too polite? Who knows what? What did I do? Why? And most hauntingly, will it, when will it, happen again? Medication to take, resist, resent, forget . . . but always to take. Credit cards revoked . . . explanations at work . . . bad checks and apologies overdue . . . memory flashes of vague men (what did I do?) . . . friendships gone, a marriage ruined.

Thought Processes

Flight of ideas is a nearly continuous flow of accelerated speech with abrupt changes from topic to topic that are usually based on understandable associations or plays on words. At times the attentive listener can keep up with the changes, even though direction changes from moment to moment. Speech is rapid, verbose, and circumstantial (including minute and unnecessary details). When the condition is severe, speech may be disorganized and incoherent. The incessant talking often includes joking, puns, and teasing:

How are you doing, kid, no kidding around, I'm going home . . . home sweet home . . . home is where the heart is . . . the heart of the matter is I want out, and that ain't hay . . . hey, Doc . . . get me out of this place.

The content of speech is often sexually explicit and ranges from grossly inappropriate to vulgar. Themes in the communication of the manic individual may revolve around extraordinary sexual prowess, brilliant business ability, or unparalleled artistic talents (e.g., writing, painting, and dancing). The person may actually have only average ability in these areas.

Speech is not only profuse but also loud, bellowing, or even screaming. One can hear the force and energy behind the rapid words. As mania escalates, flight of ideas may give way to clang associations. **Clang associations** are the stringing together of words because of their rhyming sounds, without regard to their meaning:

Cinema I and II, last row. Row, row, row your boat. Don't be a cutthroat. Cut your throat. Get your goat. Go out and vote. And so I wrote.

Grandiosity (inflated self-regard) is apparent in both the ideas expressed and the person's behavior. People with mania may exaggerate their achievements or importance, state that they know famous people, or believe that they

EXAMINING THE EVIDENCE   Sleep Disruption and the Manic Switch

My patient is diagnosed with bipolar disorder and has been awake for 3 days. What is the connection between sleep and bipolar disorder?

You're caring for a person who is experiencing one of the most striking features of mania—severe sleep disruption. People in a manic phase may not sleep at all, or sleep a few hours a night, for days on end. Intriguingly, although most of us would become quite alarmed if we quit sleeping, this sleeplessness isn't troubling to the person experiencing mania (Riemann et al., 2002). Altered sleep patterns are symptoms of the disorder as well as causative for other troubling symptoms of the disorder.

It seems that the disorder itself predisposes people to poor sleep. Research demonstrates a measurable disruption in circadian rhythms that is an essential characteristic of people with bipolar disorder even when they are not acutely ill or experiencing a sleep disturbance (Jones et al., 2005). Millar and colleagues (2004) also report that bipolar outpatients in remission sleep longer, complain of difficulty initiating sleep, and have variable quality of sleep compared with people without bipolar disorder.

In what often becomes a vicious cycle, these sleep disturbances bring on manic episodes (rather than depressive ones) in vulnerable people (Malkoff-Schwartz et al., 1998). Even in healthy individuals, we know that intense sleep deprivation results in delusions (false thoughts), illusions (false interpretation of real objects), and hallucinations (hearing or seeing things that are not there) in healthy individuals (Turkington et al., 2006). For those experiencing mania, this sleeplessness leads to the psychotic symptoms associated with the disorder.

Treating the problem should address the disorder itself and the environment. You'll likely be giving antimanic agents, as well as a short-term benzodiazepine (clonazepam or lorazepam) to promote sleep (Goodwin, 2003). External stressors lead to sleep pattern disturbances and should be addressed and minimized. Psychoeducation will include balancing levels of activities, monitoring sleep patterns, and increases in activity, and protecting the sleep/wake cycle (Otto et al., 2003). As your patient stabilizes, you'll shift your focus to prevention, particularly on developing a diurnal routine; although a daily cycle is helpful for anybody's mental performance and emotional stability, it is particularly important for those prone to mania (Frank et al., 2006).

Frank, E., Gonzalez, J., & Fagiolini, A. (2006). The importance of routine for preventing recurrence in bipolar disorder. *American Journal of Psychiatry, 163,* 981-985.

Goodwin, G.M. (2003). Evidence-based guidelines for treating bipolar disorder: Recommendations from the British Association for Psychopharmacology. *Journal of Psychopharmacology, 17,* 149-173.

Jones, S.H., Hare, D.J., & Evershed, K. (2005). Actigraphic assessment of circadian activity and sleep patterns in bipolar disorder. *Bipolar Disorders, 7*(2), 176-186.

Malkoff-Schwartz, S.F., Frank, E., Anderson, B., et al. (1998). Stressful life events and social rhythm disruption in the onset of manic and depressive bipolar episodes: A preliminary investigation. *Archives of General Psychiatry, 55,* 702-707.

Millar, A., Espie, C.A., & Scott, J. (2004). The sleep of remitted bipolar outpatients: A controlled naturalistic study using actigraphy. *Journal of Affective Disorders, 80,* 145-153.

Otto, M.W., Reilly-Harrington, N., Sachs, & Gary, S. (2003). Psychoeducational and cognitive-behavioral strategies in the management of bipolar disorder. *Journal of Affective Disorders, 73,* 171-181.

Riemann, D., Voderholzer, U., & Berger, M. (2002). Sleep and sleep-wake manipulations in bipolar depression. *Neuropsychobiology, 45,* 7-12.

Turkington, D., Kingdon, D., & Weiden, P.J. (2006). Cognitive behavior therapy for schizophrenia. *American Journal of Psychiatry, 163,* 365-373.

A special thanks to Carly Albert-Kiber, graduate student at the University of Akron, for her research assistance.

have great powers. The boast of exceptional powers and status can take delusional proportions in mania.

Grandiose persecutory delusions are common. For example, manic people may think that God is speaking to them or that the FBI is out to stop them from saving the world. Sensory perceptions may become altered as the mania escalates, and hallucinations may occur. However, in hypomania, no evidence of delusions or hallucinations is present.

Cognitive Function

The onset of bipolar disorder is often preceded by comparatively high cognitive function. However, there is growing evidence that about one third of patients who are bipolar display significant and persistent cognitive difficulties that include problems with verbal memory, sustained attention, and occasionally executive functioning (Spollen, 2003). These deficits persist even in remission. Cognitive impairment appears to be a core feature of bipolar disorder and a contributing factor to poor psychosocial outcomes (Robinson & Ferrier, 2006).

According to Spollen (2003), the potential cognitive dysfunction among a large subgroup of patients with bipolar disorder has specific clinical implications.

- Cognitive function greatly affects overall function.
- Cognitive deficits correlate with greater number of manic episodes, history of psychosis, chronicity of illness, and poor functional outcome.

- Early diagnosis and treatment are crucial to prevent illness progression, cognitive deficits, and poor outcome.
- Medication selection should consider not only the efficacy of the drug in reducing mood symptoms but also the cognitive effect of the drug on the patient.

Assessment Guidelines

Bipolar Disorder

1. Assess whether the patient is a danger to self and others:
   - Manic patients can exhaust themselves to the point of death.
   - Patients may not eat or sleep, often for days at a time.
   - Poor impulse control may result in harm to others or self.
   - Uncontrolled spending may occur.
2. Assess for need for controls. Controls may be needed to protect patient from bankruptcy because manic patients may give away all of their money or possessions.
3. Assess for need for hospitalization to safeguard and stabilize the patient.
4. Assess medical status:
   - A person in acute untreated mania may become dehydrated or exhausted, which has led to severe dehydration and cardiac collapse. Therefore cardiac status, signs of dehydration (poor skin turgor, dark and scant urinary output), and poor skin integrity—which may develop into infections—should be assessed.
   - A thorough medical examination helps to determine whether mania is primary (bipolar disorder or cyclothymia) or secondary to another condition.
     - Mania can be secondary to a general medical condition (e.g., brain disease, certain infections including human immunodeficiency virus [HIV], and endocrine disorders) (Gelder et al., 2006). Disorders secondary to medical conditions are known as organic mood disorders.
     - Mania can be substance induced (caused by use or abuse of a drug or substance, or by toxin exposure).
5. Assess for any coexisting medical or other condition that warrants special intervention (e.g., substance abuse, anxiety disorder, metabolic disease, cardiac problems, legal or financial crises).
6. Assess the patient's and family's understanding of bipolar disorder, knowledge of medications, and knowledge of support groups and organizations that provide information on bipolar disorder.

DIAGNOSIS

Nursing diagnoses vary for a patient with a bipolar disorder. A primary consideration for a patient in acute mania is the prevention of exhaustion and death from cardiac collapse. Because of the patient's poor judgment, excessive and constant motor activity, probable dehydration, and difficulty evaluating reality, *Risk for injury* is a likely and appropriate diagnosis if the patient's activity level is dangerous to his or her health. During the continuation phase, such areas as compliance to medication, risk for suicide, optimizing family support, social support, and such go a long way for securing relapse prevention. Refer to Table 13-2 for a list of potential nursing diagnoses for bipolar disorders.

OUTCOMES IDENTIFICATION
Phase I: Acute Phase (Acute Mania)

The overall goal during the acute manic phase is to prevent injury. Outcomes in phase I reflect physiological as well as psychiatric issues (stated in measurable terms within safe timeframes). For example, the patient will:
- Be well hydrated within 24 hours—as evidenced by good skin turgor—and within normal limits of urinary output, concentration, and dilution.
- Maintain stable cardiac status, as evidenced by stable vital signs staying within normal limits (by *date*).
- Maintain or obtain tissue integrity, as evidenced by absence of infection or absence of untreated cuts or abrasions (by *date*).
- Get sufficient sleep and rest while in the hospital, as evidenced by 4 to 6 hours sleep at night and 10-minute rest periods every hour.
- Demonstrate self-control with aid of staff or medication, as evidenced by absence of harm to others *(state the behaviors)* (by *date*).
- Make no attempt at self-harm with aid of staff or medication, as evidenced by physical safety checked with regularity throughout period of acute mania.

Phase II: Continuation of Treatment Phase

The continuation phase lasts for approximately 2 to 6 months. Although the overall outcome of this phase is relapse prevention, many other outcomes must be accomplished to achieve relapse prevention. These outcomes include the following:
- Patient and family will attend psychoeducational classes that discuss a variety of topics and give directions to patients and families to help prevent relapse:

TABLE 13-2	Potential Nursing Diagnoses for Bipolar Disorders
Signs and Symptoms	**Nursing Diagnoses**
Excessive and constant motor activity Poor judgment Lack of rest and sleep Poor nutritional intake (excessive or relentless mix of above behaviors can lead to cardiac collapse)	*Risk for injury*
Loud, profane, hostile, combative, aggressive, demanding behaviors	*Risk for other-directed violence* *Risk for self-directed violence* *Risk for suicide*
Intrusive and taunting behaviors Inability to control behavior Rage reaction	*Ineffective coping*
Manipulative, angry, or hostile verbal and physical behaviors Impulsive speech and actions Property destruction or lashing out at others in a rage reaction	*Defensive coping* *Ineffective coping*
Racing thoughts, grandiosity, poor judgment	*Disturbed thought processes* *Ineffective coping*
Giving away of valuables, neglect of family, impulsive major life changes (divorce, career changes)	*Interrupted family processes* *Caregiver role strain*
Continuous pressured speech jumping from topic to topic *(flights of ideas)*	*Impaired verbal communication*
Constant motor activity, going from one person or event to another Annoyance or taunting of others; loud and crass speech Provocative behaviors	*Impaired social interaction*
Failure to eat, groom, bathe, dress self because too distracted, agitated, and disorganized	*Imbalanced nutrition: less than body requirements* *Deficient fluid volume* *Self-care deficit (bathing/hygiene, dressing/grooming)*
Inability to sleep because too frantic and hyperactive (sleep deprivation can lead to exhaustion and death)	*Disturbed sleep pattern*

- Knowledge of disease process
- Knowledge of early signs of relapse
- Knowledge of medication
- Consequences of substance addictions for predicting future relapse
- Knowledge of early signs and symptoms of relapse
- Support groups or therapy (psychoeducational groups and cognitive-behavioral [CBT], interpersonal social rhythm [IPSRT], and family-focused [FFT] therapies are all evidence-based treatment modalities)
- Communication and problem-solving skills training

Phase III: Maintenance Treatment Phase

The overall outcomes for the maintenance phase continue to focus on prevention of relapse and to limit the severity and duration of future episodes.

- Participation in learning interpersonal strategies related to work, interpersonal, and family problems
- Participation in psychotherapy group or other ongoing supportive therapy modality that has evidence-based support.
- Relapse prevention
- Medication compliance
- Family psychoeducation or therapy
- Increased social support

PLANNING

The planning of care for an individual with bipolar disorder usually is geared toward the particular phase of mania (acute mania, continuation of treatment, or maintenance treatment) as well as any other co-occurring issues identified in the assessment (e.g., risk of suicide, risk of violence to person or property, family crisis, legal crises, substance abuse, risk-taking behaviors, issues of medical compliance).

Acute Phase

During the **acute phase** (0 to 2 months), planning focuses on medically stabilizing the patient while maintaining safety. When mania is acute, hospitalization is usually the safest place for a patient. Nursing care is often geared toward decreasing physical activity, increasing food and fluid intake, ensuring at least 4 to 6 hours of sleep per night, alleviating any bowel or bladder problems, and intervening to see that self-care needs are met. Some patients may require seclusion or even electroconvulsive therapy, and they certainly need careful medication management.

Continuation Phase

During the **continuation phase** (2 to 6 months), planning focuses on maintaining compliance with the medication regimen and preventing relapse. Interventions are planned in accordance with the assessment data regarding the patient's interpersonal and stress reduction skills, cognitive functioning, employment status, substance-related problems, social support systems, and such. During this time, psychoeducational teaching is a must for patient and family. The need for referrals to community programs, groups, and support for any co-occurring disorders or problems (e.g., substance abuse, family problems, legal issues, and financial crises) is evaluated.

Evaluation of the need for communication skills training and problem-solving skills training is important. People with bipolar disorders often have interpersonal problems that affect their work, family, and social lives, as well as other emotional problems. Residual problems resulting from reckless, violent, withdrawn, or bizarre behavior that may have occurred during a manic episode often leave lives shattered and family and friends hurt and distant. For some patients, specific psychotherapy (in addition to medication management) is needed to address these issues, although the focus of psychotherapeutic treatment will vary over time for each person.

Maintenance Phase

The **maintenance phase** begins at about 6 months, and planning focuses on preventing relapse and limiting the severity and duration of episodes. Patients with bipolar disorders require medications over long periods of time, if not a lifetime. Specific psychosocial therapies, support or psychoeducational groups, and periodic evaluations all help patients maintain their family and social lives, continue employment, and minimize relapse rates.

IMPLEMENTATION

Patients with bipolar disorders are often ambivalent about treatment. They may minimize the destructive consequences of their behaviors or deny the seriousness of the disease. Some are reluctant to give up the increased energy, euphoria, and heightened sense of self-esteem of hypomania, before the devastating features of full-blown mania commence (Hirschfeld et al., 2000). Unfortunately, nonadherence to the regimen of mood-stabilizing medication is a major cause of relapse. Therefore establishing a therapeutic alliance with the bipolar individual is crucial.

Acute Phase

Hospitalization provides safety for a patient in acute mania (bipolar I disorder), imposes external controls on destructive behaviors, and provides medical stabilization.

Communication Guidelines

Communicating with a patient who is acutely manic can be challenging, but there are some unique and effective approaches for communicating with a person in the manic phase of bipolar disorder (Table 13-3).

Milieu Therapy
Seclusion

Control during the acute phase of hyperactive behavior almost always includes immediate treatment with an antipsychotic. However, when a patient is dangerously out of control, seclusion or restraints also may be indicated. Seclusion provides comfort and relief to many patients who can no longer control their own behavior and serves the following purposes:

- Reduces overwhelming environmental stimuli
- Protects a patient from injuring self, others, or staff
- Prevents destruction of personal property or property of others

Seclusion is warranted when documented data collected by the nursing and medical staff reflect the following points:

- Substantial risk of harm to others or self is clear.
- The patient is unable to control his or her actions.
- Problematic behavior has been sustained (continues or escalates despite other measures).
- Other measures (e.g., setting limits beginning with verbal de-escalation or using chemical restraints) have failed.

The use of seclusion or restraints is associated with complex therapeutic, ethical, and legal issues. Most state laws prohibit the use of unnecessary physical restraint or isolation. Barring an emergency, the use of seclusion and

APPLYING THE ART   A Person with Bipolar Disorder

SCENARIO: I approached Gloria, a 33-year-old woman, who had seemed edgy and distracted when we'd talked earlier. She'd been admitted to the hospital for the third time angry, and threatening suicide over losing a job she'd loved of exercising and caring for the animals at a pet store. She is on suicide precautions.

THERAPEUTIC GOAL: By the end of this session, Gloria will show increased ability to problem solve as evidenced by insight that stopping medication exacerbates the disorder.

Student-Patient Interaction	Thoughts, Communication Techniques, and Mental Health Nursing Concepts
Student: *Smiling.* "Hi, Gloria. Would you talk some more about your feelings when you heard you were going to be fired from your job?"	I know that "could" or "would" acts like an *indirect question* rather than a *direct question* meaning I'll get more than a yes or no answer.
Gloria: "Get the _____ away from me! I'm sick of you people asking about that _____ job." *Clenching fists, practically yelling.*	
Student's feelings: *I forgot to tune in to Gloria as a person before I jumped in with questions. She's loud, but I'm okay. Her fear and loss fuel all that anger. Okay, self, mindfully breathe.*	I forgot to *assess* first! I must remember, she's afraid and *displacing* her frustration onto me. Each time she gets admitted means starting over. If only she'd kept taking her Depakote and Abilify.
Student: *Quiet and concerned.* "Gloria, I'm _____, your nursing student. You've been through such a rough time. You feel upset at the job and anyone that asks you about it." **Student's feelings:** *I can do this. I'll step back a little, slow things down, and keep telling myself that her anger is not really about me. I care about Gloria so I'm not going to be pushed away that easily.*	Using *reflection* makes sense because I hope that reflecting the feelings lets my *empathy* get through to her.
Student's feelings: *I'm struggling with anxiety, too.*	I remember now. *Anxiety is communicated interpersonally.*
Gloria: "I need to walk." Starts pacing quickly down the hall. **Student's feelings:** *I hope she'll let me walk with her. Walking will help my anxiety, too!*	Gloria's using walking as a healthy relief behavior for her anxiety.
Student: "Good idea. Let's walk together. Tell me what's happening inside." We quickly walk down the hall. **Student's feelings:** *As she responds while we walk, I'm feeling calmer, too.*	I'm offering myself by walking with her. Using an indirect question often helps the patient talk without feeling interrogated.
Gloria: "I feel like, why even try anymore? While I worked at the pet store, I felt like my life meant something. Then I go and stop taking my medicine. It's just so expensive. I'm such a loser." Eyes fill with tears. **Student's feelings:** *I feel so sad for her. She struggles so hard, and then seems to give in by quitting her medication. Sometimes I feel like a loser. Sometimes I feel like nursing school pressures me too much, especially when I bomb a test. I need to put my own "failure worries" on hold to handle later and refocus to fully tune in to Gloria.*	

Continued

Student-Patient Interaction	Thoughts, Communication Techniques, and Mental Health Nursing Concepts
Student: "Sounds like right now you're blaming yourself for what you've lost." *I pause, handing her a tissue.* "Gloria, I care about what happens to you. When you say, 'why even try' you mean . . . ?"	By saying "right now" I plant the idea that she may not always choose to see herself as a failure. I must stay alert for countertransference. Using Gloria's name and reminding her who I am factors in that she's probably experiencing moderate anxiety, so her *perceptual field* of what she's able to take in decreases. I need to assess even a *covert reference* to *suicide*, especially with Gloria's history.
Gloria: "Don't worry. I don't want to kill myself anymore. But I just keep screwing up! I even let my animals down." *Glancing at me.* **Student's feelings:** *I wish she could see the survivor I see when I'm with her. I'm relieved Gloria recognizes she wants to live now. I have so much hope inside for her.*	When Gloria tells me not to worry she may be using *projection* in that she may still have some latent concern about her suicide potential. She is still on *15-minute checks*, which continues to be necessary, and I'll report and chart about all this.
Student: "Talk some more about your animals."	By using a *focusing* approach, I remind her of what she values. She may also remember what she was able to do well, which may help her *self-esteem*. She said, "my animals," so I deliberately *restated*, "your animals" because they are so important to her.
Gloria: "I loved caring for all of the animals, but especially the puppies. One little beagle had such sad eyes, I took him home. That's when I got in trouble. I know I wouldn't have done that if I'd kept taking my meds.	Was Gloria using *identification*? The beagle's "sad" eyes may have resonated with Gloria's own sadness.
Student: "So you recognize a link between stopping your meds and doing some things you wouldn't usually do when you take charge of your bipolar disorder by staying on your meds?" **Student's feelings:** *I feel kind of proud of myself for knowing to praise her about the meds.*	I'm using the *behavior modification technique of positive reinforcement* by *attending* to Gloria's insight when she connects her impulsive behavior with stopping her psychotropics. I'm also empowering her by deliberately associating taking her medications with taking charge of her disorder.
Gloria: "I still get mad too easily, but I'm starting to think more clearly since my Abilify's been upped. I've been wondering if my boss would give me a second chance. I did well with the animals. My boss said so before I got sick again. My case manager made sure the beagle pup got back okay.	Gloria's actually able to problem solve now, so that means her anxiety has *decreased to mild.*
Student: "I hear you reminding yourself that your skills in pet care endure even through this bout in the hospital."	I think the animals provide some of Gloria's *love and belonging needs*, which precede *self-esteem* needs. I *validate* with Gloria about her pet care skills.
Gloria: "I really love those animals. I'm going to run this idea past the nurse and work out when and how to phrase things to call my boss." **Student's feelings:** *She's taking charge of this. Wow! I feel honored that Gloria trusted me. I'm beginning to trust myself some, too.*	The treatment team will be doing discharge planning.
Student: "You are able to find a goal to work toward, maybe even begin to believe in yourself a little." **Gloria:** *Nods.*	I give Gloria *support* by naming her mentally healthy verbalizations as a goal. I am careful to add qualifiers— "maybe," "begin to," and "a little"—to insert the idea about believing in herself without overwhelming her.

TABLE 13-3 Interventions for Acute Mania: Communication

Intervention	Rationale
1. Use firm and calm approach: "John, come with me. Eat this sandwich."	1. Structure and control are provided for patient who is out of control. Feelings of security can result: "Someone is in control."
2. Use short and concise explanations or statements.	2. Short attention span limits comprehension to small bits of information.
3. Remain neutral; avoid power struggles and value judgments.	3. Patient can use inconsistencies and value judgments as justification for arguing and escalating mania.
4. Be consistent in approach and expectations.	4. Consistent limits and expectations minimize potential for patient's manipulation of staff.
5. Have frequent staff meetings to plan consistent approaches and to set agreed-on limits.	5. Consistency of all staff is needed to maintain controls and minimize manipulation by patient.
6. With other staff, decide on limits, tell patient in simple, concrete terms with consequences; for example, "John, do not yell at or hit Peter. If you cannot control yourself, we will help you" or "The seclusion room will help you feel less out of control and prevent harm to yourself and others."	6. Clear expectations help patient experience outside controls as well as understand reasons for medication, seclusion, or restraints (if unable to control behaviors).
7. Hear and act on legitimate complaints.	7. Underlying feelings of helplessness are reduced, and acting-out behaviors are minimized.
8. Firmly redirect energy into more appropriate and constructive channels.	8. Distractibility is the nurse's most effective tool with the manic patient.

restraints warrants the patient's consent; therefore, most hospitals have well-defined protocols for treatment with seclusion. **Seclusion protocol** includes a proper reporting procedure through the chain of command when a patient is to be secluded. Refer to Chapter 21 for more on seclusion and restraint and accepted protocols and to Chapter 26 for more on the legal parameters.

Safety and Physical Needs

Unique strategies can help maintain the safety of the patient during the hospitalized period. Staff members continually set limits in a firm, nonthreatening, and neutral manner to prevent further escalation of mania and to provide safe boundaries for the patient and others (Table 13-4).

Pharmacological, Biological, and Integrative Therapies

During the acute phase, medications are vital to bring the patient to a safe physical and level of functioning. However, medications are pivotal and vital through all phases of treatment and for many patients, they are a lifelong protection against the pain and destruction of relapse.

Mood Stabilizers

Individuals with bipolar disorder often require multiple medications. There may be times when an antianxiety agent can help reduce agitation or anxiety or an antipsychotic agent can reduce psychomotor activity and delusions or hallucinations. Antidepressants are prescribed for reducing bipolar depression, but their use for targeting bipolar depression is somewhat controversial (Sachs et al., 2007). Antianxiolytics, antipsychotics, or even antidepressants may be used for a limited time, but mood stabilizers are considered lifetime maintenance therapy for bipolar patients (Preston et al., 2005). Most treatment guidelines advocate lithium and divalproex (Depakote) as first-line mood-stabilizing agents (Preston et al., 2005).

For individuals whose recent episode was manic or hypomanic, lithium and olanzapine seem to have the largest body of evidence to help stabilize their mood. For those with recent episodes of depression, lamotrigine (Lamictal) is more appropriate. Lithium is particularly effective for preventing mania and lamotrigine is particularly effective for preventing depression (Expert Interview, 2007).

TABLE 13-4   Interventions for Acute Mania: Safety and Physical Needs

Intervention	Rationale
Structure in a Safe Milieu	
1. Maintain low level of stimuli in patient's environment (e.g., away from bright lights, loud noises, and people).	1. Decrease escalating anxiety.
2. Provide structured solitary activities with nurse or aide.	2. Structure provides security and focus.
3. Provide frequent high-calorie fluids.	3. Prevent dangerous levels of dehydration.
4. Provide frequent rest periods.	4. Prevent exhaustion.
5. Redirect violent behavior through physical exercise (e.g., walking)	5. Physical exercise can decrease tension and provide focus.
6. When warranted in acute mania, use antipsychotics and seclusion to minimize physical harm via physician's order.	6. Exhaustion and death can result from dehydration, lack of sleep, and constant physical activity.
7. Observe for signs of lithium toxicity.	7. There is a small margin of safety between therapeutic and toxic doses.
8. Protect patient from giving away money and possessions. Hold valuables in hospital safe until rational judgment returns.	8. Patient's "generosity" is in fact a symptom of the disease and can lead to catastrophic financial ruin for patient and family.
Nutrition	
1. Monitor intake, output, and vital signs.	1. Adequate fluid and caloric intake are ensured; development of dehydration and cardiac collapse is minimized.
2. Offer frequent high-calorie protein drinks and finger foods (e.g., sandwiches, fruit, milkshakes).	2. Constant fluid and calorie replacement are needed. Patient may be too active to sit at meals. **Finger foods** allow "eating on the run."
3. Frequently remind patient to eat. "Tom, finish your milkshake." "Sally, eat this banana."	3. The manic patient is unaware of bodily needs and is easily distracted. Needs supervision to eat.
Sleep	
1. Encourage frequent rest periods during the day.	1. Lack of sleep can lead to exhaustion and death.
2. Keep patient in areas of low stimulation.	2. Relaxation is promoted and manic behavior is minimized.
3. At night, provide warm baths, soothing music, and medication when indicated. Avoid giving patient caffeine.	3. Promote relaxation, rest, and sleep.
Hygiene	
1. Supervise choice of clothes; minimize flamboyant and bizarre dress (e.g., garish stripes or plaids and loud, unmatching colors).	1. The potential is decreased for ridicule, which lowers self-esteem and increases the need for manic defense. The patient is helped to maintain dignity.
2. Give simple step-by-step reminders for hygiene and dress. "Here is your razor. Shave the left side . . . now the right side. Here is your toothbrush. Put the toothpaste on the brush."	2. Distractibility and poor concentration are countered through simple, concrete instructions.
Elimination	
1. Monitor bowel habits; offer fluids and foods that are high in fiber. Evaluate need for laxative. Encourage patient to go to the bathroom.	1. Fecal impaction resulting from dehydration and decreased peristalsis is prevented.

Lithium Carbonate

Lithium carbonate ($LiCO_3$) is effective in the acute treatment of mania and depressive episodes and the prevention of recurrent mania and depressive episodes. Once primary acute mania has been diagnosed, lithium is most often the first choice of treatment.

Lithium aborts 60% to 80% of acute manic and hypomanic episodes within 10 to 21 days; within these cases, 65% to 70% of patients experience a full initial response, 20% experience a partial initial response, and 10% have no initial response (Maxmen & Ward, 2002). Lithium is less effective in people with mixed mania (elation and depression), those with rapid cycling, and those with atypical features. Lithium is particularly effective in reducing the following:

- Elation, grandiosity, and expansiveness
- Flight of ideas
- Irritability and manipulativeness
- Anxiety

To a lesser extent, lithium controls:

- Insomnia
- Psychomotor agitation
- Threatening or assaultive behavior
- Distractibility
- Hypersexuality
- Paranoia

Initially in the treatment of acute mania, an antipsychotic or benzodiazepine can help calm symptoms. Antipsychotics act promptly to slow speech, inhibit aggression, and decrease psychomotor activity. The immediate action of the antipsychotic or benzodiazepine medication serves to prevent exhaustion, coronary collapse, and death until lithium reaches therapeutic levels.

Lithium must reach therapeutic levels in the patient's blood to be effective. This usually takes from 7 to 14 days, or longer for some patients. As lithium becomes effective in reducing manic behavior, the antipsychotic drugs are usually discontinued. Although lithium is an effective intervention for treating the manic phase of a bipolar disorder, it is not a cure. Many patients receive lithium for maintenance indefinitely and experience manic and depressive episodes if the drug is discontinued.

Trade names for lithium carbonate include Lithane, Eskalith, and Lithonate. During the *active phase*, 300 to 600 mg by mouth is given two or three times a day to reach a clear therapeutic result, or a lithium level of 0.8 to 1.4 mEq/L. **The actual maintenance blood levels should range between 0.4 and 1.3 mEq/L.** However, levels of 0.6 to 0.8 mEq/L may be effective for many. To avoid serious toxicity, lithium levels should *not* exceed 1.5 mEq/L (Hopkins & Gelenberg, 2000). At serum levels greater than 1.5 mEq/L, early signs of toxicity can occur; at 1.5 to

2 mEq/L, advanced signs of toxicity may be seen; and at 2 to 2.5 mEq/L or more, severe toxicity can occur, and emergency measures should be taken immediately.

Cases of severe lithium toxicity with levels of 2 mEq/L or greater constitute a life-threatening emergency. In such cases, gastric lavage and treatment with urea, mannitol, and aminophylline can hasten lithium excretion. Hemodialysis also may be used in extreme cases.

Adverse Reactions. A small increment exists between the therapeutic and the toxic dosage of lithium. Initially, blood levels are measured weekly or biweekly until the therapeutic level has been reached. After therapeutic levels have been reached, blood levels are determined every month. After 6 months to a year of stability, measurement of blood levels every 3 months may suffice (Freeman et al., 2004). Blood should be drawn 8 to 12 hours after the last dose of lithium is taken. Refer to Table 13-5 for side effects, signs of lithium toxicity, and interventions.

For older adult patients, the principle of **"start low and go slow"** still applies. Levels are often monitored every 3 or 4 days. Some older patients may respond to a dose as low as 0.3 to 0.4 mEq/L (Maxman & Ward, 2002). As mentioned, toxic effects are usually associated with lithium levels of 2 mEq/L or higher, but they can occur at much lower levels (even within a therapeutic range).

Maintenance Therapy. Some clinicians suggest that patients with bipolar disorder need to be given lithium for 9 to 12 months, and some patients may need lifelong lithium maintenance to prevent further relapses. Many patients respond well to lower dosages during maintenance or prophylactic lithium therapy.

Lithium is unquestionably effective in preventing both manic and depressive episodes in patients with bipolar disorder. However, complete suppression occurs in only 50% or fewer patients, even with compliance with the maintenance therapy regimen. Therefore both the person with a bipolar disorder and his or her significant other should be given careful instructions about (1) the purpose and requirements of lithium therapy, (2) its adverse effects, (3) its toxic effects and complications, and (4) situations in which the physician should be contacted. The patient and family also should be advised that suddenly stopping lithium can lead to relapse and recurrence of mania. Box 13-1 outlines patient and family teaching regarding lithium therapy.

Patients need to know that **two major long-term risks of lithium therapy are hypothyroidism and impairment of the kidneys' ability to concentrate urine**. Therefore a person receiving lithium therapy must have periodic follow-ups to assess thyroid and renal function. Health care providers need to stress to patients with bipolar disorder and

TABLE 13-5 Lithium Side Effects and Signs of Lithium Toxicity

Level	Signs	Interventions
Expected Side Effects		
<0.4 to 1 mEq/L (therapeutic level)	Fine hand tremor, polyuria, and mild thirst Mild nausea and general discomfort Weight gain	Symptoms may persist throughout therapy. Symptoms often subside during treatment. Weight gain may be helped with diet, exercise, and nutritional management.
Early Signs of Toxicity		
<1.5 mEq/L	Nausea, vomiting, diarrhea, thirst, polyuria, slurred speech, muscle weakness	Medication should be withheld, blood lithium levels measured, and dosage reevaluated.
Advanced Signs of Toxicity		
1.5 to 2 mEq/L	Coarse hand tremor, persistent gastrointestinal upset, mental confusion, muscle hyperirritability, electroencephalographic (ECG) changes, incoordination	Interventions outlined above or below should be used, depending on severity of circumstances.
Severe Toxicity		
2 to 2.5 mEq/L	Ataxia, serious ECG changes, blurred vision, clonic movements, large output of dilute urine, tinnitus, blurred vision, seizures, stupor, a severe hypotension, coma. Death is usually secondary to pulmonary complications.	There is no known antidote for lithium poisoning. The drug is stopped, and excretion is hastened. If patient is alert, an emetic is administered. Otherwise, gastric lavage and treatment with urea, mannitol, and aminophylline hasten lithium excretion.
>2.5 mEq/L	Symptoms may progress rapidly. Coma, cardiac dysrhythmia, peripheral circulatory collapse, proteinuria, oliguria, and death.	In addition to the interventions above, hemodialysis may be used in severe cases.

Data from Lehne, R.A. (2007). *Pharmacology for nursing care* (6th ed.). St. Louis: Saunders; Skidmore-Roth, L. (2008). *Mosby's nursing drug reference* (21st ed). St. Louis: Mosby.

their families the importance of discontinuing maintenance therapy gradually.

Contraindications. Before lithium is administered, a medical evaluation is performed to assess the patient's ability to tolerate the drug. In particular, baseline physical and laboratory examinations should include assessment of renal function; determination of thyroid status, including levels of thyroxine and thyroid-stimulating hormone; and evaluation for dementia or neurological disorders, which presage a poor response to lithium. Other clinical and laboratory assessments, including an electrocardiogram, are performed as needed depending on the individual's physical condition.

Lithium therapy is generally contraindicated in people with cardiovascular disease and in those who have brain damage, renal disease, thyroid disease, or myasthenia gravis. Lithium also may harm a fetus and, whenever possible, is not given to women who are pregnant. Both the fear of pregnancy and the wish to become pregnant are major concerns for many bipolar women taking lithium. Lithium use is also contraindicated in mothers who are breast-feeding and in children younger than 12 years of age.

Antiepileptic Drugs

As many as 20% to 40% of bipolar patients may not respond or respond insufficiently to lithium, or they may not tolerate it. Some subgroups of bipolar patients may not respond well to lithium but may do well when treated with **antiepileptic drugs (AEDs)**. These include patients with the following (Hopkins & Gelenberg, 2000):

BOX 13-1

Patient and Family Teaching About Lithium Therapy

The patient and the patient's family should receive the following teaching. (They should be encouraged to ask questions and given the material in written form as well.)

- Lithium can treat your current emotional problem and helps prevent relapse. Therefore it is important to continue taking the drug after the current episode is over.
- Because therapeutic and toxic dosage ranges are so close, it is important to monitor lithium blood levels very closely—more frequently at first, then once every several months after that.
- Lithium is not addictive.
- It is important to eat a normal diet with normal salt and fluid intake (1500-3000 mL/day or six 12 ounce glasses of fluid). Lithium decreases sodium reabsorption in the kidneys, which could lead to a sodium deficiency.
- Watch sodium levels. A low sodium intake leads to a relative increase in lithium retention, which could produce toxicity.
- You should stop taking lithium if you have excessive diarrhea, vomiting, or sweating. All of these symptoms can lead to dehydration. Dehydration can raise lithium levels in the blood to toxic levels. **Inform your physician if you have any of these problems**.

- Do not take diuretics (water pills) while you are taking lithium.
- Lithium is irritating to the lining in your stomach. It helps to take lithium with meals.
- Lithium can cause renal damage. Kidney function should be assessed prior to treatment and once a year thereafter.
- Lithium can promote goiter (thyroid enlargement) and frank hypothyroidism. Plasma levels of T_3, T_4, and thyroid-stimulating hormone (TSH) should be measured prior to treatment and yearly thereafter.
- Don't take any over-the-counter medicines without checking first with your physician.
- If you find that you are gaining a lot of weight, you may need to talk this over with your physician or nutritionist.
- Many self-help groups are available to provide support for people with bipolar disorder and their families. The local self-help group is (give name and telephone number).
- You can find out more information by calling (give name and telephone number).
- Keep a list of side effects and toxic effects handy (see Table 13-5) along with the name and number of a contact person.
- If lithium is to be discontinued, your dosage will be tapered gradually to minimize risk of early relapse.

- Dysphoric mania (depressive thoughts and feelings during manic episodes)
- Rapid cycling (four or more episodes a year)
- Electroencephalographic abnormalities
- Substance abuse not associated with mood episodes
- Progression in the frequency and severity of symptoms
- No family history of bipolar disorder among first-degree relations

Three AEDs have demonstrated efficacy for the treatment of mood disorders: carbamazepine (Tegretol), divalproex (Depakote), and lamotrigine (Lamictal) (Preston et al., 2005). Newer anticonvulsants seem to be effective in some cases of refractory bipolar disease (those cases not responding to traditional approaches). AEDs are thought to be:

- Superior for continually cycling patients
- More effective when there is no family history of bipolar disease
- Effective at dampening affective swings in schizoaffective patients
- Effective at diminishing impulsive and aggressive behavior in some nonpsychotic patients

- Helpful in cases of alcohol and benzodiazepine withdrawal
- Beneficial in controlling mania (within 2 weeks) and depression (within 3 weeks or longer)

Divalproex (Depakote)

Valproic acid is useful in treating lithium nonresponders who are in acute mania, who experience rapid cycles, who are in dysphoric mania, or who have not responded to carbamazepine. It is also helpful in preventing manic episodes. As with carbamazepine, it is important to monitor liver function and platelet count periodically, although serious complications are rare.

Carbamazepine (Tegretol)

Some patients with treatment-resistant bipolar disorder improve after taking carbamazepine and lithium or carbamazepine and an antipsychotic. Carbamazepine seems to work better in patients with rapid cycling and in severely paranoid and angry manic patients than in euphoric, overactive, and overfriendly manic patients. It is also thought to be more effective in dysphoric manic patients.

TABLE 13-6 Antiepileptic Drugs (AEDs)

Drug	Dosage Range	Major Adverse Effects
Carbamazepine (Tegretol)	800-1200 mg/day	• **Agranulocytosis** and **aplastic anemia** are most serious side effects. • Blood levels should be monitored throughout first 8 weeks because drug induces liver enzymes that speed its own metabolism. Dosage may need to be adjusted to maintain serum level of 6-8 mg/L. • Sedation is most common problem; tolerance usually develops. • Diplopia, incoordination, and sedation can signal excessive levels.
Valproate (Depakene)	750-1500 mg/day	• **Baseline liver function tests should be performed and results monitored** at regular intervals. Hepatitis, although rare, has been reported, with fatalities in children. • Signs and symptoms to watch for include fever, chills, right upper quadrant pain, dark urine, malaise, and jaundice. • Common side effects include tremors, gastrointestinal upset, weight gain, and, rarely, alopecia.
Lamotrigine (Lamictal)	50-400 mg/day	• **Life-threatening rash** reported in 3 out of every 1000 individuals (Steven-Johnson syndrome). • Use caution when renal, hepatic, or cardiac function is impaired. • Dizziness, diplopia, headache, ataxia, and somnolence are among frequent side effects.
Gabapentin (Neurontin)	300-1800 mg/day	• Most serious adverse effects are difficulty in breathing, swelling of the lips, rash, slurred speech, drowsiness, and diarrhea. • Fatigue, somnolence, dizziness, ataxia, diplopia, hypertension are the more frequent side effects. • Used off label; not presently FDA approved for bipolar disorder.
Topiramate (Topamax)	50-300 mg/day	• Used in acute mania or in combination with other drugs. • Adverse effects include weight loss, cognitive side effects, fatigue, dizziness, and paresthesia. • Used off label; not presently FDA approved for bipolar disorder

Blood levels of carbamazepine should be monitored at least weekly for the first 8 weeks of treatment because the drug can increase the levels of liver enzymes that can speed its own metabolism. In some instances this can cause bone marrow suppression and liver inflammation.

Lamotrigine (Lamictal)

Lamotrigine is a first-line treatment for bipolar depression and is approved for acute and maintenance therapy. It is generally well tolerated, but there is one serious but rare dermatological reaction: a potentially life-threatening rash. Patients should be instructed to seek immediate medical attention if a rash appears, although most are likely benign (Preston et al., 2005).

Newer Antiepileptic Drugs

Other popular AEDs that may be used in the treatment of refractory bipolar disorder are gabapentin (Neurontin) and topiramate (Topamax). Gabapentin is effective in targeting anxiety and is unlikely to interact with other medications. Topiramate is helpful in mania and does not appear to

cause weight gain. See Table 13-6 for commonly prescribed AEDs, their adverse reactions, and dosage ranges.

Anxiolytics
Clonazepam (Klonopin) and Lorazepam (Ativan)

Clonazepam and lorazepam are useful in the treatment of acute mania in some patients with treatment-resistant mania. These drugs are also effective in managing the psychomotor agitation seen in mania. They should be avoided, however, in patients with a history of substance abuse.

Antipsychotics

In addition to showing sedative properties during the early phase of treatment, which may help with insomnia, anxiety, and agitation, the newer atypical antipsychotics seem to have mood-stabilizing properties. For example, an initial study showed that olanzapine (Zyprexa) is better tolerated and prevents mania relapse more effectively than lithium (Tohen, 2003). Quetiapine (Seroquel) is also effective in treating the anxiety symptoms and acute mania in bipolar depression (Moyer, 2004). In 2006, the U.S. Food and

Drug Administration (FDA) approved this drug for targeting the depressive phase of bipolar disorder as well. The other antipsychotics out of the five now approved for early treatment bipolar disorder are risperidone (Risperdal), aripiprazole (Abilify), and ziprasidone (Geodon) (Lehne, 2007).

Electroconvulsive Therapy

Electroconvulsive therapy (ECT) is used to subdue severe manic behavior, especially in patients with treatment-resistant mania and patients with rapid cycling (i.e., those who experience four or more episodes of illness a year). ECT is effective in patients with bipolar disorder who experience rapid cycling, those with paranoid-destructive features who often respond poorly to lithium therapy, and in acutely suicidal patients (Chapter 12).

Continuation Phase

The treatment continuation phase is a crucial one for patients and their families. The outcome for this phase is to prevent relapse. Community resources are chosen based on the needs of the patient, the appropriateness of the referral, and the availability of resources. Frequently, it is a case manager who evaluates appropriate follow-up care for patients and their families.

Medication compliance during this phase is perhaps the most important treatment outcome. This follow-up is frequently handled in a mental health center. However, adherence to the medication regimen is also addressed in day hospitals and in psychiatric home care visits. Some patients may attend day hospitals if they are not too excitable and are able to tolerate a certain level of stimuli. In addition to medication oversight, day hospitals offer structure, decrease social isolation, and help patients channel their time and energy. If a patient is homebound and unable to get to a mental health center or day hospital, then psychiatric home care is the appropriate modality for follow-up care.

Health Teaching and Health Promotion

Patients and families need information about bipolar illness with particular emphasis on the chronic and highly recurrent nature of the illness. They also need to be taught the symptoms of impending episodes. For example, changes in sleep patterns are especially important because they usually precede, accompany, or precipitate mania. Even a single night of unexplainable sleep loss can be taken as an early warning of impending mania. Health teaching stresses the importance of establishing regularity in sleep patterns, meals, exercise, and other activities.

Psychoeducation includes a rich combination of tools to improve functional outcomes for patients and their families (Box 13-2) (Gutman & Gutman, 2006). At the very least, psychoeducation increases compliance and improves the regularity of daily life and sleep habits.

BOX 13-2

Psychoeducation for Patients with Bipolar Disorder and Their Families

Patients with bipolar disorder and their families need to know the following:

1. The chronic and episodic nature of bipolar disorder.
2. The fact that bipolar disorder is long term and that maintenance treatment therefore will require that one or more mood-stabilizing agents be taken for a long time.
3. The expected side effects and toxic effects of the prescribed medication, as well as whom to call and where to go in case of a toxic reaction.
4. The signs and symptoms of relapse that may "come out of the blue."
5. The role of family members and others in preventing a full relapse.
6. The phone numbers of emergency contact people, which should be kept in an easily accessed place.
7. The use of alcohol, drugs of abuse, even small amounts of caffeine, and over-the-counter medications can produce a relapse.
8. Good sleep hygiene is critical to stability. Frequently, the prodrome of a manic episode is lack of sleep. In some cases, mania may be averted by the use of sleep medications (e.g., temazepam [Restoril]).
9. Psychosocial strategies are important for dealing with work, interpersonal, and family problems; lowering stress; enhancing a sense of personal control; and increasing community functioning.
10. Group and individual psychotherapy is invaluable for gaining insight as well as skills in relapse prevention, providing social support, increasing coping skills in interpersonal relations, improving compliance with the medication regimen, reducing functional morbidity, and decreasing rehospitalizations.

Health care workers need to remember the following:

1. Minimization and denial are common defenses that require gradual introduction of facts.
2. Anger and abusive remarks, although aimed at the health care provider, are symptoms of the disease and are not personal.

Adapted from Zerbe, K.J. (1999). *Women's mental health in primary care.* Philadelphia: Saunders; Milkowitz, D.J. (2003). Bipolar disorder. In D.H. Barlow (Ed.), *Clinical handbook of psychological disorders* (pp. 523-560). New York: Guilford Press.

Maintenance Phase

Maintenance therapy is aimed at preventing recurrence. Not only are some of the community resources cited earlier helpful, but patients and their families often greatly benefit from mutual support and self-help groups.

Psychotherapy

Pharmacotherapy and psychiatric management are essential in the treatment of acute manic attacks. Individuals with bipolar disorder suffer from the psychosocial consequences of their past episodes and their vulnerability to experiencing future episodes. People who have bipolar disease also have to face the burden of long-term treatments that may involve some unpleasant side effects.

During the course of their illness, many patients have sustained strained interpersonal relationships, marriage and family problems, academic and occupational problems, and legal or other social difficulties. Psychotherapy can help people work through these difficulties and decrease some of the psychic distress and increase self-esteem. Psychotherapeutic treatments in conjunction with psychopharmacology also can help patients improve their functioning between episodes and attempt to decrease the frequency of future episodes.

A recent study report by Miklowitz and colleagues (2007) demonstrated that intensive psychotherapy given weekly and biweekly for up to 30 sessions in 9 months using cognitive-behavioral therapy (CBT), interpersonal and social rhythm therapy (IPSRT), and family-focused therapy (FFT) was far superior in higher year-end recovery rates and resulted in shorter recovery times than those in a control group. The control, called "collaborative therapy," consisted of brief psychoeducational intervention consisting of three sessions in 6 weeks. CBT, IPSTR, and FFT are three very effective psychosocial therapies used in conjunction with medication that can greatly benefit individual suffering from bipolar conditions.

Psychotherapy is an important treatment in bipolar illness and results in greater compliance with the lithium regimen (Jamison, 1995a). Often patients receiving medication and psychotherapy place more value on psychotherapy than do clinicians. Moreover, patients treated with cognitive therapy are more likely to take their medications as prescribed than patients who do not participate in therapy (Jamison, 1995a; Lam et al., 2003).

One patient describes her feelings about drug therapy and psychotherapy as follows (Jamison, 1995b):

> I cannot imagine leading a normal life without lithium. From starting and stoppings of it, I now know it is an essential part of my sanity. Lithium prevents my seductive but disastrous highs, diminishes my depressions, clears out the weaving of my disordered thinking, slows me, gentles me out, keeps me in my relationships, in my career, out of a hospital, and in psychotherapy. It keeps me alive, too.
>
> But psychotherapy heals, it makes some sense of the confusion, it reins in the terrifying thoughts and feelings, it brings back hope and the possibility of learning from it all. Pills cannot, do not, ease one back into reality. They bring you back headlong, careening, and faster than can be endured at times. Psychotherapy is a sanctuary, it is a battleground, and it is where I have come to believe that someday I may be able to contend with all of this. No pill can help me deal with the problem of not wanting to take pills, but no amount of therapy alone can prevent my manias and depressions. I need both.

Cognitive-Behavioral Therapy

Cognitive-behavioral techniques for bipolar disorder are an adaptation of Beck's cognitive therapy treatment for depressive disorders and later bipolar disorder. **Cognitive-behavioral therapy (CBT)** has been found valuable in helping patients with bipolar disorder accept their illness and the need for medical treatment. Cognitive techniques have also been shown to be effective in decreasing affective symptoms, increasing social functioning, reducing the rate of relapse, and reducing the number of hospital admissions (Gelder et al., 2006; Lam et al., 2003). A follow-up study by Lam and associates demonstrated continued benefits 2 years after treatment (2005).

CBT focuses mainly on medication adherence, early detection and intervention, and stress and lifestyle management using a variety of CBT techniques (Lam et al., 2003; Otto et al., 2003). These interventions have been found most effective with patients who have bipolar I disorder (www.PsychEducation.org, updated 2007). CBT is typically used as an adjunct to pharmacotherapy and involves identifying maladaptive cognitions and behaviors that may be barriers to a person's recovery and ongoing mood stability (Fredman & Rosenbaum, 2004). It is also being used for bipolar disorder in children (Barclay, 2003).

Interpersonal and Social Rhythm Therapy

Interpersonal and social rhythm therapy (IPSRT), a formalized psychotherapy, is based on the idea that problems in interpersonal relationships and disruptions in daily routines can contribute to the recurrence of manic and depressive episode in an individual with a bipolar disorder. IPSRT has been found effective in shortening a depressive episode in bipolar I patients (Scott & Colom, 2005). The interpersonal aspects of IPSRT derive from interpersonal psychotherapy and focus on resolutions of interpersonal problems (e.g., unresolved grief, disputes, role transitions) and prevention of further disputes. IPSRT is effective in the acute as well as the maintenance phases of treatment.

Family Focused Therapy

Behavioral family management, family therapy, and psychoeducation help families to stay together, lead to lower rates of rehospitalization, and improve family functioning (APA, 2000b; Miklowitz et al., 2000). Family-focused therapy (FFT) combines many of the key target areas of CBT and IPSRT (PsychEducation, revised 2007), including:

- Psychoeducation
- Relapse drill (prevention)
- Ways to make the diagnosis of bipolar disorder more acceptable to the patient

FFT is different from CBT and IPSRT in that it includes the family in therapy. FFT focuses on communication within the family, teaches communications skills, and prepares the entire family for relapse episodes (PsychEducation, revised 2007).

Support Groups

Patients with bipolar disorder, as well as their friends and families, benefit from forming mutual support groups, such as those sponsored by the Depression and Bipolar Support Alliance (DBSA), the National Alliance for the Mentally Ill (NAMI), the National Mental Health Association, and the Manic-Depressive Association.

EVALUATION

Outcome criteria often dictate the frequency of evaluation of short-term and intermediate indicators. For example, are the patient's vital signs stable, and is he or she well hydrated within safe time limits? Is the patient able to control own behavior or respond to external controls? Is the patient able to sleep for 4 or 5 hours per night or take frequent short rest periods during the day? Does the family have a clear understanding of the patient's disease and need for medication? Do the patient and family know which community agencies may help them?

If outcomes or related indicators are not achieved satisfactorily, the preventing factors are analyzed. Were the data incorrect or insufficient? Were nursing diagnoses inappropriate or outcomes unrealistic? Was intervention poorly planned? After the outcomes and care plan are reassessed, the plan is revised if indicated. Longer-term outcomes include compliance with the medication regimen; resumption of functioning in the community; achievement of stability in family, work, and social relationships and in mood; and improved coping skills for reducing stress.

KEY POINTS TO REMEMBER

- Biological factors appear to play a role in the etiology of the bipolar disorders. Strong genetic correlates have been revealed especially through twin studies.
- Little doubt exists that an excess of, and imbalance in, neurotransmitters is also related to bipolar mood swings, which supports the existence of neurobiological influences.
- Neuroendocrine and neuroanatomical findings support evidence for biological influences.
- Bipolar disorder often goes unrecognized, and early detection can help diminish comorbid substance abuse, suicide, and decline in social and personal relationships, and may help promote more positive outcomes.
- The nurse assesses the patient's level of mood (hypomania, acute mania, delirious mania), behavior, and thought processes and is alert to cognitive dysfunction.
- Some nursing diagnoses appropriate for a patient who is manic are *Risk for violence, Defensive coping, Ineffective coping, Disturbed thought processes,* and *Situational low self-esteem.*
- During the acute phase of mania, physical needs often take priority and demand nursing interventions. Therefore deficient fluid volume and imbalanced nutrition or elimination, as well as disturbed sleep pattern, are usually addressed in the nursing plan.
- The diagnosis *Interrupted family processes* is vital. Support groups, psychoeducation, and guidance for the family can greatly affect the patient's compliance with the medication regimen.
- Planning nursing care involves identifying the specific needs of the patient and family during the three phases of mania.
- Antimanic medications are available. Lithium has a narrow therapeutic index, which necessitates thorough patient and family teaching and regular follow-up. AEDs such as carbamazepine and valproic acid are useful, especially in treating people with disease refractory to lithium therapy; newer AEDs are also useful in treating patients who need rapid de-escalation and do not respond to other treatment approaches.
- Antipsychotic agents may be needed because of their sedating and mood-stabilizing properties, especially during initial treatment.
- For some patients, ECT may be the most appropriate medical treatment.
- Patient and family teaching takes many forms and is most important in encouraging compliance with the medication regimen and reducing the risk of relapse.
- Evaluation includes examining the effectiveness of the nursing interventions, changing the outcomes as needed, and reassessing the nursing diagnoses. Evaluation is an ongoing process and is part of each of the other steps in the nursing process.

CRITICAL THINKING

1. Kioshi Sung is taken into the emergency department after threatening in a loud voice to "blow up the world to save the poor, and many more, where's the door? No more, no more . . . Let me loose." He had attacked a bartender who wouldn't give him any more to drink. He has not eaten or slept for more than a week, only taking sips of fluids when offered. He talks nonstop, moving constantly, flailing his arms, and bumping into objects as he speeds by.
   A. Identify Mr. Sung's immediate needs (in terms of a nursing diagnosis). Describe the interventions you would plan for his physiological safety and his milieu (safe environment).
   B. Discuss the most appropriate communication techniques and approaches for Mr. Sung at this time. Give examples of what you would say and how you would say it.
   C. What possible medications would Mr. Sung most likely be given immediately? Long term?
   D. Write a medication treatment plan for Mr. Sung and his family.
   E. Describe at least four evidence-based therapeutic modalities for a bipolar patient.

CHAPTER REVIEW

Choose the most appropriate answer.

1. In communicating with a patient who is experiencing elated mood, which of the following interventions by the nurse is most appropriate?
   1. Use a calm, firm approach.
   2. Give expanded explanations.
   3. Make use of abstract concepts.
   4. Encourage lighthearted optimism.
2. For a person in the "continuation of treatment" phase of bipolar disorder, which of the following is an appropriate nursing outcome? Patient will:
   1. avoid involvement in self-help groups.
   2. adhere to medication regimen.
   3. demonstrate euphoric mood.
   4. maintain normal weight.
3. When a patient has been prescribed lithium, the medication teaching plan should include which information?
   1. The importance of periodic monitoring of renal and thyroid function
   2. Dietary teaching to restrict daily sodium intake
   3. The importance of blood draws to monitor serum potassium level
   4. Discontinuing the drug if weight gain and fine hand tremors are noticed
4. For a patient with mania, which symptom related to communication is likely to be present?
   1. Mutism
   2. Verbosity
   3. Poverty of ideas
   4. Confabulation
5. When a patient is experiencing a severe manic episode, which bodily system is most at risk for decompensation?
   1. Renal
   2. Cardiac
   3. Endocrine
   4. Pulmonary

REFERENCES

American Psychiatric Association. (2000a). *Diagnostic and statistical manual of mental disorders (DSM-IV-TR)* (4th ed., text rev.). Washington, DC: Author.

American Psychiatric Association. (2000b). *Practice guidelines for the treatment of psychiatric disorders: Compendium 2000.* Washington, DC: Author.

Barclay, L. (2003). *Cognitive behavioral therapy useful for bipolar disorder in children* [Abstract C6]. Paper presented at the 50th Annual Meeting of the American Academy of Child and Adolescent Psychiatry, October 20, 2003, Miami.

Bauer, M.S. (2003). Mood disorders: Bipolar (manic depression) disorders. In A. Tasman, J. Kay, & J.A. Lieberman (Eds.), *Psychiatry* (2nd ed.). West Sussex, England: Wiley.

Blairy, S., Linotte, S., Sovery, D., et al. (2004). Social adjustment and self-esteem of bipolar patients: A multicentric study. *Journal of Affective Disorders, 79,* 97-103.

Craddock, N., Donovan, M.C., & Owen, M.J. (2005). The genetics of schizophrenia and bipolar disorder: Dissecting psychosis. *Journal of Medical Genetics, 42*(3), 193-204.

Daban, C., Vieta, E., & Young (2005). Hypothalmic-pituitary-adrenal axis and bipolar disorder. In E. Sherwood Brown (Ed.), *Psychiatric Clinics of North America, 28*(2), 469-480.

Dubovsky, S.L. (2005). Treatment in bipolar depression. In E. Sherwood Brown (Ed.), *Psychiatric Clinics of North America, 28*(2), 349-370.

Dubovsky, S.L., Davies, R., & Dubovsky, A.N. (2004). Mood disorders. In R.E. Hales & S.C. Yudofsky (Eds.), *Essentials of clinical psychiatry* (2nd ed.). Washington, DC: American Psychiatric Publishing.

Expert Interview. (2007). *Maintenance treatment of bipolar disorder: An expert interview with Trisha Suppes.* Retrieved March 20, 2007, from www.medscape.com/viewarticle/552834.

Fredman, S.J., & Rosenbaum, J.F. (2004). *Psychosocial intervention for bipolar disorder.* Paper presented at the 157th Annual Meeting of the American Psychiatric Association, New York.

Freedman, M.P., & McElroy, S.L. (1999). Clinical picture and etiologic models of mixed states. *Psychiatric Clinics of North America, 22*(3), 535-546.

Freeman, M.P., Wiegand, C., & Gelenberg, A.J. (2004). Lithium. In A.F. Schatzberg & C.B. Nemeroff (Eds.), *The American Psychiatric Publishing textbook of psychopharmacology* (3rd ed., pp. 547-568). Washington, DC: American Psychiatric Publishing.

Gelder, M., Harrison, P., & Cowen, P. (2006). *Shorter Oxford textbook of psychiatry.* Oxford, England: Oxford University Press

Ginns, E.I., et al. (1996). A genome-wide search for chromosomal loci linked to bipolar affective disorder in the Old Order Amish. *National Genetics, 12*(4), 431.

Gutman, D.A., & Gutman, A.R. (2006). *Emerging therapies for bipolar disorders: A clinical update.* American Psychiatric Association 2006 annual meeting, May 20-25, 2006, Toronto, Canada. Retrieved August 12, 2006, from www.medscape.com/viewarticle/537392.

Hattori, E.,(2003). Polymorphisms at the G72/G30 gene locus, on L13q33, are associated with bipolar disorder in two independent pedigree series. *American Journal of Human Genetics, 72*(5), 1131-1140.

Hirschfeld R.M.A. (2000). Practice guidelines for the treatment of patients with bipolar disorder. In American Psychiatric Association, *Practice guidelines for the treatment of psychiatric disorders: Compendium 2000.* Washington, DC: Author.

Hopkins, H.S., & Gelenberg, A.J. (2000). Mood stabilizers. In J.A. Lieberman & A. Tasman (Eds.), *Psychiatric drugs.* Philadelphia: Saunders.

Jamison, K.R. (1995a, November 18). *Psychotherapy of bipolar patients.* Paper presented at the U.S. Psychiatric and Mental Health Congress, November 18, 1995, New York.

Jamison, K.R. (1995b). *An unquiet mind.* New York: Knopf.

Jamison, K.R. (2000). Suicide and bipolar disorder [Abstract]. *Journal of Clinical Psychiatry, 61*(Suppl. 19), 47-51.

Kessler, R.C., Berglund, P. Dember, O., et al. (2005). Lifetime prevalence and age-of-onset distributions of DSM-IV disorders in the National Comorbidity Survey Replication. *Archives of General Psychiatry, 62*(6): 593-602.

Lam, D.H., Watkins, ER, Hayward, P., et al. (2003). A randomized controlled study of cognitive therapy for relapse prevention for bipolar affective disorder: Outcome of the first year. *Archives of General Psychiatry, 60*, 145-152.

Lam, D.H., Hayward, P., Watkins, E.R., et al. (2005). Relapse prevention in patients with bipolar disorder: Cognitive therapy outcomes after 2 years. *American Journal of Psychiatry, 162*, 324-329.

Lehne, R.A. (2007). *Pharmacology for nursing care* (6th ed.). St. Louis: Saunders.

Maxmen, J.S., & Ward, N.G. (2002). *Psychotropic drugs: Fast facts* (3rd ed.). New York: Norton.

Miklowitz, D.J., Simponeau, T.L., George, E.R., et al. (2000). Family-focused treatment of bipolar disorder: 1-year effects of a psychoeducational program in conjunction with pharmacotherapy. *Biological Psychiatry, 48*(6), 582-592.

Miklowitz, M.J., Otto, M.W., Frank, E., et al. (2007). Psychosocial treatments for bipolar depression: A 1-year randomized trial from the systemic treatment enhancement program. *Archives of General Psychiatry, 64*(4), 419-426.

Moyer, P. (2004). *Quetiapine effective against anxiety in bipolar depression* [Abstract NR743]. Paper presented at the 157th Annual Meeting of the American Psychiatric Association, May 5, 2004, New York.

Nathan, K.I., & Schatzberg, A.F. (1995). Biology of mood disorders. In A.F. Schatzberg & C.B. Nemeroff (Eds.), *The American Psychiatric Publishing textbook of psychopharmacology* (pp. 439-477). Washington, DC: American Psychiatric Publishing.

Otto, M.W., Reilly-Harrington, N., & Sachs, G.S. (2003). Psychoeducational and cognitive-behavioral strategies in the management of bipolar disorder [Abstract]. *Journal of Affective Disorders, 73*, 171-181.

Payne, J.L., Potash, J.B., & DePeulo (2005). Recent findings in the genetic basis of bipolar disorder. In E. Sherwood Brown (Ed.), *Psychiatric Clinics of North America, 28*(2), 481-497.

Phillips, M.L., & Frank, E. (2006). Redefining bipolar disorder: Toward DSM-V. *American Journal of Psychiatry, 163*, 1135-1136.

Pollock, R., & Kuo, I. (2004). *Neuroimaging in bipolar disorder.* Paper presented at the 5th Invitational Congress of Biological Psychiatry, February 9-13, 2004, Sydney, Australia.

Preston, J.D., O'Neal, J.H., & Talaga, M. C. (2005). *Handbook of clinical psychopharmacology for therapists* (4th ed.). Oakland, CA: New Harbinger Publications.

PsychEducation (revised 2007). Psychotherapy for bipolar disorder. Retrieved August 28, 2007, from www.psycheducation.org/depression/Psychotherapy.htm.

Robinson, L.J., & Ferrier, I.N. (2006). Evolution of cognitive impairment in bipolar disease: A systematic review of cross-sectional evidence. *Bipolar Disorder, 8*(2), 103-116.

Sachs, G.S., Nierenberg, A.A., Calabrese, J.R., et al. (2007). Effectiveness of adjunctive antidepressant treatment of bipolar depression. *New England Journal of Medicine, 356*(17), 1711-1722.

Sadock, B.J., & Sadock, V.A. (2007). *Kaplan & Sadock's synopsis of psychiatry* (10th ed.) Philadelphia: Lippincott Williams & Wilkins.

Schneck, C.D., Allen, M.H., & Shelton, M.D. (2003). Current concepts in rapid cycling-bipolar disorder [Abstract]. *Current Psychosis and Therapeutics Reports, 1*, 72-78.

Scott, J., & Colom, F. (2005). Psychosocial treatments for bipolar disorders. In E. Sherwood Brown (Ed.). *Psychiatric Clinics of North America, 28*(2), 371-384.

Skidmore-Roth, L. (2008). *Mosby's nursing drug reference* (21st ed.). St. Louis: Mosby.

Spollen, J. (2003). Impaired cognition in bipolar disorder: Something to think about. Paper presented at the American Psychiatric Association 156th Annual Meeting, May 17-22, 2003, San Francisco, CA.

Thase, M.E. (2004). Mood disorders: Neurobiology. In B.J. Sadock & V.A. Sadock (Eds.), *Kaplan and Sadock's comprehensive textbook of psychiatry* (8th ed., vol. 1, pp. 1594-1602). Philadelphia: Lippincott Williams & Wilkins.

Tohen, M. (2003). *Olanzapine more effective for preventing mania relapse.* Paper presented at the 5th International Congress of Bipolar Disorders, June 18, 2003, Pittsburgh, PA.

Zerbe, K.J. (1999). *Women's mental health in primary care.* Philadelphia: Saunders.

Zubieta, J.K., Huguelet, P., Ohl, L.H., et al. (2000). High vesicular monoamine transporter binding in asymptomatic bipolar I disorder: Sex differences and cognitive correlates. *American Journal of Psychiatry, 157*, 1619-1628.

CHAPTER 14

The Schizophrenias

Elizabeth M. Varcarolis

Key Terms and Concepts

Objectives

1. Describe symptoms (prodromal) that a person with schizophrenia may exhibit during the prepsychotic phase.
2. Discuss the neurobiological-anatomical-nongenetic findings that indicate that schizophrenia is a neurological disease.
3. Differentiate between the positive and negative symptoms of schizophrenia with regard to (a) their effect on quality of life, (b) their significance for the prognosis of the disease, and (c) their side effect profile.
4. Explain how the cognitive symptoms of schizophrenia affect a person's prognosis and quality of life.
5. Identify nursing interventions for a patient who is (a) hallucinating, (b) paranoid, and (c) experiencing a delusion.
6. Understand the properties of typical and atypical antipsychotic drugs regarding the following: (a) target symptoms, (b) indications for use, (c) adverse effects and toxic effects, (d) need for patient and family teaching and follow-up, and (e) potential for medical compliance.
7. Identify evidence-based psychosocial therapies for patients with schizophrenia and their families.
8. Differentiate among the three phases of schizophrenia in terms of symptoms, focus of care, and intervention needs using Table 14-5 as a guide.

continued

Schizophrenia is a devastating brain disease that affects thinking, language, emotions, social behavior, and ability to perceive reality accurately. Unfortunately, people with this disease are often misunderstood and stigmatized not only by the general population but even by the medical community (Moller & Murphy, 2002). Schizophrenia is described as a psychotic disorder. The term *psychotic* refers to "delusions, any prominent hallucinations, disorganized speech, or disorganized catatonic behavior" (APA, 2004). Other psychotic disorders are identified in Box 14-1.

Many people with schizophrenia function well with the aid of medications and social supports. Others are more disabled, and need a higher level of support in terms of housing, health maintenance, monetary aid, and more. Although schizophrenia is treatable, it is not curable and is a severe mental illness (SMI). Refer to Chapter 24 for a broader understanding of all people with a severe mental illness.

PREVALENCE AND COMORBIDITY

The lifetime prevalence of schizophrenia is 1% worldwide with no differences related to race, social status, culture, gender, or environment (APA, 2004). A premorbid condition can be an indication of the potential complexity and eventual outcome for an individual who is later diagnosed with schizophrenia. For example, individuals with an early age of onset (18 to 25 years) are more often male, have poorer premorbid adjustment, more evidence of structural brain abnormalities, and more prominent negative symptoms. Individuals with a later onset (25 to 35 years) are more likely to be female, have less evidence of structural brain abnormalities, and have better outcomes (APA, 2000). The younger the patient is at the onset of schizophrenia, the more discouraging the prognosis.

An abrupt onset of symptoms with good premorbid functioning is usually a favorable prognostic sign. A slow, insidious onset over a period of 2 or 3 years is more ominous. Those whose prepsychotic personalities show good social, sexual, and occupational functioning have a greater chance for remission or complete recovery. A childhood history of withdrawn, reclusive, eccentric, and tense behavior is an unfavorable diagnostic sign.

Substance abuse disorders occur in approximately 40% to 50% of individuals with schizophrenia (Kirkpatrick & Tek, 2005). They are associated with a variety of negative outcomes, including incarceration, homelessness, violence, suicide, and infection with human immunodeficiency virus (HIV) and linked with a poorer prognosis.

Nicotine dependence is very common in people with schizophrenia, and 75% to 85% people with schizophrenia smoke (Evins et al., 2005). Smoking results in significant morbidity and mortality and is linked with a high rate of emphysema and other pulmonary and cardiac problems. These risks are even greater in people with schizophrenia because they tend to smoke two to three times more than the average smoker.

Contrary to some earlier studies, Barnes and colleagues (2006) found that smoking did not mediate nor was it associated with positive, negative, cognitive, or mood symptoms among people with schizophrenia. They did find, however, that smoking is associated with lower levels of akathisia brought on by the use of antipsychotic medications. Akathisia may emerge after the cessation of smoking in these patients.

Depressive symptoms occur frequently in schizophrenia. **Suicide** is the leading cause of premature death in this population and is 20 times more prevalent in people with schizophrenia than in the general population (Butcher, 2007). The rate of comorbid **anxiety disorders** in individuals with schizophrenia also has been found to be higher than the rate of anxiety disorders in the general population.

BOX 14-1

Psychotic Disorders Other Than Schizophrenia

Schizophreniform Disorder

The essential features of schizophreniform disorder are exactly those of schizophrenia except that:

- The total duration of the illness is at least 1 month but less than 6 months.
- Impaired social or occupational functioning during some part of the illness may not be apparent (although it may appear).

This disorder may or may not have a good prognosis.

Brief Psychotic Disorder

Brief psychotic disorder is characterized by a sudden onset of psychotic symptoms (delusions, hallucinations, disorganized speech) or grossly disorganized or catatonic behavior. The episode lasts at least 1 day but less than 1 month, following which the individual returns to his or her premorbid level of functioning. Brief psychotic disorders are often precipitated by extremely stressful life events.

Schizoaffective Disorder

Schizoaffective disorder is characterized by an uninterrupted period of illness during which time there is a major depressive, manic, or mixed episode, concurrent with symptoms that meet the criteria for schizophrenia. The symptoms must not be a result of any substance use or abuse or to a general medical condition.

Delusional Disorder

Delusional disorder involves non-bizarre delusions (situations that occur in real life, such as being followed, infected, loved at a distance, deceived by a spouse, or having a disease) of at least 1 month's duration. The person's ability to function is not markedly impaired, nor is the person's behavior obviously odd or bizarre. Common types of delusions seen in this disorder are of grandeur, persecution, or jealousy, somatic delusions, and mixed delusions.

Shared Psychotic Disorder *(Folie à Deux)*

A shared psychotic disorder is a condition in which one individual who is in a close relationship with another individual who has a psychotic disorder with a delusion eventually comes to share the delusional beliefs either in total or in part. Apart from the shared delusion, the behavior of the person who takes on the other's delusional behavior is not odd or unusual. Impairment of the person who shares the delusion is usually much less than that of the person who has the psychotic disorder with the delusion. The cult phenomenon is an example, as was demonstrated at Waco and Jonestown.

Induced or Secondary Psychosis

Psychosis may be induced by substances (drugs of abuse, alcohol, medications, or toxins) or caused by the physiological consequences of a general medical condition (delirium, neurological conditions, metabolic conditions, hepatic or renal diseases, and many others). Medical conditions and substances of abuse must always be ruled out before a primary diagnosis of schizophrenia or other psychotic disorder can be made.

Psychosis-induced polydipsia is the compulsive drinking of water (between 4 and 10 L/day). Polydipsia is associated with psychological disturbances and occurs in some people with chronic or SMI. There are clearly increased rates of polydipsia in people with schizophrenia, which may result in severe hyponatrenemia, cerebral edema, and even death.

THEORY

Determining the causes of schizophrenia is clearly a complicated matter. What is known is that brain chemistry and brain activity are different in a person with schizophrenia than in a person without schizophrenia. Schizophrenia most likely occurs as a result of a combination of **inherited genetic factors** and extreme **nongenetic factors** (e.g., virus infection, birth injuries, nutritional factors), which can affect the genes governing the brain or injure the brain directly. These factors may alter the structures of the brain, affect the brain's neurotransmitter system, and disrupt the neural circuits, resulting in impairment in cognition.

Neurobiological Factors

For many years the most widely accepted explanation for the biochemical pathophysiology in schizophrenia was the **dopamine theory.** This theory is derived from the study of the action of the antipsychotic drugs that block the activity of dopamine (D_2) and in doing so, reduce some of the symptoms of schizophrenia. Amphetamines, cocaine, methylphenidate (Ritalin), and levodopa are drugs that increase the activity of dopamine in the brain. These drugs can exacerbate the symptoms of schizophrenia in psychotic patients and simulate symptoms of paranoid schizophrenia in a person without schizophrenia.

More recent hypotheses postulate a role for other neurotransmitter systems (e.g., norepinephrine, serotonin,

EXAMINING THE EVIDENCE   Combating the Stigma of Mental Illness

During my medical-surgical rotation I was caring for a person with a diagnosis of pneumonia and schizophrenia. The nurse who gave me report said, "Good luck working with Mr. Crazy." I was shocked that a health care provider would talk like that!

This is a real problem, especially because people with psychiatric disorders have enough challenges and we would expect health care professionals (including nurses) to be the most understanding. Although polite people would not dream of using racial slurs or disparaging terms for racial groups or for people with physical handicaps, they seem to accept terms such as crazy, psycho, schizo, mental, nut, and wacko. These result from the stigma that stems from the belief that a person is somehow flawed and that flaw is brought about by such things as weakness of character or lack of spiritual strength.

How can the stigma be stopped? Research demonstrates that there are three broad approaches to dispelling stigma: protest, education, and contact (Corrigan & Gelb, 2006). Protest focuses on the wrongness or immorality of treating people badly. It can take the form of organized rallies with people carrying signs such as "See the person and not the illness," or boycotting businesses that use stigmatizing messages in their advertising: "We must be *crazy* to sell cars at these prices!" Corrigan and associates (2001) caution that this approach may backfire because we aren't really changing people's beliefs; we're just pushing them underground. Yet how we act may truly influence our thoughts. Try smiling, for example, when you're in a bad mood. Additionally, look at the successes of civil and gay rights protests as a model of what could be accomplished in mental health.

Education is the second strategy shown to be effective in reducing stigma and simply means presenting facts and debunking myths. This can be accomplished through a variety of media including the Internet, public service announcements, flyers, movies, and educational forums. A significant campaign was undertaken in the United Kingdom to address stigma, which relied heavily on educational strategies (Crisp et al., 2005). This campaign resulted in reductions in stigmatizing attitudes. However, one educational technique in this campaign, the use of fact sheets, did not result in people having kinder attitudes toward those with mental illness (Luty et al., 2007).

How about contact? If you've known someone with a mental illness are you more likely to respond favorably to all people with a like diagnosis? Corrigan and associates (2001) found that face-to-face contact helps and reports that it works better than protest or education. Subjects who were exposed to someone with mental illness were more likely to donate the $20 given to them for being in the study to the National Alliance for the Mentally Ill as compared to members of the control (no contact) group.

We have work to do in developing evidence based interventions to combat stigma. When considering the strategies of both education and contact, we have to ask how nurses (like the one talking about "Mr. Crazy") who are both educated and come into routine contact with people who have mental illness, could maintain the same stereotypes as the general public.

Corrigan, P., & Gelb, B. (2006). Three programs that use mass approaches to challenge the stigma of mental illness. *Psychiatric Services, 57*, 393-398.

Corrigan, P.W., River, P., Lundin, R.K., et al. (2001). Three strategies for changing attributions about severe mental illness. *Schizophrenia Bulletin, 27*, 187-195.

Crisp, A., Gelder, M., Goddard, E., & Meltzer, H. (2005) Stigmatisation of people with mental illnesses: A follow-up study within the Changing Minds campaign of the Royal College of Psychiatrists. *World Psychiatry, 4*(2), 106-113.

Luty, J., Umoh, O., Sessay, M., & Sarkhel, A. (2007). Effectiveness of Changing Minds campaign factsheets in reducing stigmatised attitudes towards mental illness. *Psychiatric Bulletin, 31*, 377-381.

glutamate, γ-aminobutyric acid [GABA], neuropeptides, and neuromodulatory substances) in the pathophysiology of schizophrenia (Beng-Choon et al., 2004). The development of the atypical antipsychotic drugs that block serotonin as well as dopamine suggests that **serotonin** may play a role in causing some of the symptoms of schizophrenia.

Phencyclidine piperidine (PCP) induces a state that closely resembles schizophrenia. This observation led to sustained interest in the *N*-methyl-D-aspartate (NMDA) receptor complex and the possible role of **glutamate** in the pathophysiology of schizophrenia.

Genetic Factors

Although most people with schizophrenia do not have a family history of the disease, schizophrenia and schizophrenia-like symptoms occur at an increased rate in first-degree (parents, siblings, offspring) or second-degree relatives (grandparents, aunts, and uncles) (Beng-Choon et al., 2004; Mariani, 2004). Older fathers are more likely to have children with schizophrenia as a result of genetic mutations in aging sperm. Numerous studies of twins (fraternal and identical) and biological parents (one and both) bear out a significantly higher probability of susceptibility gene involvement with the risk of getting schizophrenia. For identical twins reared apart the concordance rate for schizophrenia is between 40% and 50%, a rate that indicates a strong genetic component. It also indicates that there must be environmental factors because if it were purely a genetic disease, both twins would be affected 100% of the time if one were affected.

It appears that schizophrenia is not a "one gene, one illness" disease like Huntington's, but rather caused by the involvement of multiple genes. Researchers have begun to identify regions on chromosomes that are probably related to the development of schizophrenia. In 2005 the National Institute of Mental Health established a Human Genetics Initiative for schizophrenia, its goal to create a national resource for research and publications related to the genetics of schizophrenia, to better understand the disorder, and ultimately to develop effective treatments.

Neuroanatomical Factors

Disruptions in the connections and communication within neural circuitry (communication pathways) are thought to be severe in schizophrenia. Therefore it is conceivable that structural cerebral abnormalities cause disruption to the entire circuitry of the brain. Brain-imaging techniques, such as computed tomography (CT), magnetic resonance imaging (MRI), and positron emission tomography (PET), provide substantial evidence that some people with schizophrenia have structural brain abnormalities. For example, MRI and CT scans demonstrate lower brain volume, larger lateral and third ventricles, atrophy in the frontal lobe, and more cerebrospinal fluid, among other findings, in people with schizophrenia. PET scans show a low rate of blood flow and glucose metabolism in the frontal lobes of the cerebral cortex, which govern planning, abstract thinking, social adjustment, and decision making.

Nongenetic Risk Factors

Infants for whom there is a history of pregnancy or birth complications are at increased risk for developing schizophrenia as adults. Prenatal risk factors include viral infection, poor nutrition or starvation, or exposure to toxins. Lack of oxygen during birth is also considered a risk factor for the development of schizophrenia. Cornblatt states that essentially any early insult to the brain of a developing fetus or child (e.g., viral infections, environmental toxins, presence of certain genes) can lead to brain abnormalities. These brain abnormalities can be biochemical, structural, or functional, which may lead to biological vulnerability (2005).

Stress (social, psychological, and physical), although not a cause of schizophrenia, may precipitate the illness in vulnerable individuals and play a role in the severity and course of the disease. The use of street drugs such as cannabis, methamphetamine, and lysergic acid diethylamide (LSD) increases the risk of developing schizophrenia, especially for those younger than age 21 whose brains are still developing.

CULTURAL CONSIDERATIONS

Different cultural groups may view and interpret symptoms seen in schizophrenia in entirely different ways. What is considered normal or acceptable in one culture may be seen as pathological in another. In some subculture groups "visions" or "voices" are an integral and expected part of various religious experiences (USDHHS, 1999). In some cultural settings, people who experience hallucinations may be perceived as gifted or special. A person from another cultural setting experiencing the same phenomena may be perceived as being possessed or evil and is therefore taunted, isolated, or punished. In either of these two scenarios, effective treatment may be prolonged or never obtained.

Another consideration is that people from different cultural backgrounds who are eventually diagnosed with schizophrenia may present with very different sets of symptoms. The reason for this is that a person's cultural background can influence the content and form of the positive and negative symptoms of schizophrenia (USDHHS, 1999). Therefore it is important to understand how family groups from different subcultures view a family member's "voices" or "visions." Knowing how the family views these symptoms and how they treat such phenomena in their cultural group can provide important information as to how mental health professions can best approach and reframe treatment to the family and patient to make it more acceptable.

CLINICAL PICTURE

Refer to Figure 14-1 for the *Diagnostic and Statistical Manual of Mental Disorders (DSM-IV-TR)* criteria for schizophrenia.

Application of the Nursing Process

ASSESSMENT

Subtypes of Schizophrenia

Figure 14-2 shows the diagnostic criteria for the five *DSM-IV-TR* subtypes of schizophrenia: paranoid, catatonic, disorganized, undifferentiated, and residual.

DSM-IV-TR Criteria for Schizophrenia

A. Characteristic Symptoms
Two or more of the following during a 1-month period (or less if successfully treated)
1. Delusions
2. Hallucinations
3. Disorganized speech (e.g., LOA)
4. Grossly disorganized or catatonic behavior
5. Negative symptoms (e.g., affective flattening, avolition, alogia)

If delusions bizarre or auditory hallucinations and
a. voices keep a running commentary about person's thoughts/behaviors **or**
b. two or more voices converse with each other

Then only one criterion is needed.

B. Social/Occupational Dysfunction
If one or more major areas of the person's life are markedly below premorbid functioning (work, interpersonal relationships, or self-care) **or**

If childhood or adolescence failure to achieve expected level of interpersonal, academic, or occupational achievement

Then meets criteria of **B**.

C. Duration
Continuous signs persist for at least 6 months with at least 1 month that meets criteria of **A** (active phase) and may include prodromal or residual symptoms.

D.
1. **All other mental diseases** (e.g., schizoaffective/ mood disorder) have been ruled out.
2. **All other medical conditions** (substance use/ medications or general medical conditions) have been ruled out.
3. **If history of pervasive developmental disorders**, then prominent hallucinations or delusions for 1 month are needed to make the diagnosis of schizophrenia.

Figure 14-1 ■ Diagnostic criteria for schizophrenia. *LOA,* Looseness of association. (Adapted from American Psychiatric Association. [2000]. *Diagnostic and statistical manual of mental disorders* [4th ed., text rev.]. Washington, DC: Author.)

Paranoid

Any intense and strongly defended irrational suspicion can be regarded as **paranoia.** Paranoid ideas cannot be corrected by experiences and cannot be modified by facts or reality. **Projection** is the most common defense mechanism used by people who are paranoid. For example, when paranoid individuals feel self-critical, they experience others as being harshly critical toward them. When they feel angry, they experience others as being unjustly angry at them, as if to say, "I'm not angry, you are!"

Because people who are paranoid are unable to trust the actions of those around them, they are usually guarded, tense, and reserved. Although patients may keep themselves aloof from interpersonal contacts, impairment in actual functioning may be minimal. To ensure interpersonal distance, they may adopt a superior, hostile, and sarcastic attitude. A common defense used by paranoid individuals to maintain self-esteem is to disparage others and dwell on the shortcomings of others. The patient frequently misinterprets the messages of others or gives private meaning to the communications of others (**ideas of reference).** For example, a patient might see his or her nurse talking to the physician and believe that they are planning to harm him or her in some manner. Minor oversights are often interpreted as personal rejection.

People with paranoid schizophrenia usually have a later age of onset of the disease (late 20s to 30s). In some cases, the presence of paranoid schizophrenia is associated with a good outcome or with recovery.

VIGNETTE

Sam stares at the nurse as she explains how to replace a bandage after minor surgery on his face. He frequently looks at the door and places himself near it. His general demeanor is condescending, and he becomes sarcastic when the nurse drops a bandage asking, "Are you the best they could give me?" When the nurse answers the phone, he says, "So they got to you, too. You are all plotting against me again now" *(ideas of reference).* He starts to mutter to himself and look to his side as if he is talking to someone (auditory hallucinations).

Paranoid states may occur in numerous mental or organic disorders. For example, people experiencing psychotic depression, a manic episode, or certain physical conditions (e.g., organic brain disease, drug intoxications) also may exhibit paranoid symptoms.

evolve

For a comprehensive case study and associated nursing care plan for a patient experiencing paranoid schizophrenia, visit the Evolve website at http://evolve.elsevier.com/Varcarolis/essentials.

Catatonic

Although we tend to think of catatonia in terms of immobility, the essential feature of catatonic schizophrenia is extreme abnormal motor behavior. In fact, patients exhibit either extreme motor agitation or extreme psychomotor retardation (with mutism, or even stupor) in this *rare* form of schizophrenia. Other behaviors identified with catatonia include:

DSM-IV-TR CRITERIA FOR SCHIZOPHRENIA SUBTYPES

SCHIZOPHRENIC DISORDERS

Paranoid (Positive)

1. Dominant: hallucinations and delusions.

2. No disorganized speech, disorganized behavior, catatonia, or inappropriate affect present.

Disorganized

1. Dominant: disorganized speech and disorganized behavior and inappropriate affect.

2. Delusions and hallucinations, if present, are not prominent or fragmented.

3. Associated features include grimacing, mannerisms, and other oddities of behavior.

Catatonic

1. Motor immobility (waxy flexibility or stupor).

2. Excessive purposeless motor activity (agitation).

3. Extreme negativism or mutism.

4. Peculiar voluntary movement:
   • Posturing
   • Stereotyped movements
   • Prominent mannerisms
   • Prominent grimaces

5. Echolalia or echopraxis.

Residual

1. No longer has active-phase symptoms (e.g., delusions, hallucinations, or disorganized speech and behaviors).

2. However, persistence of some symptoms is noted, e.g.:
   • Marked social isolation or withdrawal
   • Marked impairment in role function (wage earner, student, or homemaker)
   • Markedly eccentric behavior or odd beliefs
   • Marked impairment in personal hygiene
   • Marked lack of initiative, interest, or energy
   • Blunted or inappropriate affect

Undifferentiated (Mixed Type)

1. Has active-phase symptoms (does have hallucinations, delusions, and bizarre behaviors).

2. No one clinical presentation dominates, e.g.:
   • Paranoid
   • Disorganized
   • Catatonic

Figure 14-2 ■ Diagnostic criteria for schizophrenia subtypes. (Adapted from American Psychiatric Association. [2000]. *Diagnostic and statistical manual of mental disorders* [4th ed., text rev.]. Washington, DC: Author.)

• Bizarre **posturing**—such as holding arms or legs rigidly or bent at severe angles for a long period of time
• **Waxy flexibility**—when placed in an awkward position by someone else, the position is held for an uncomfortable length of time.

• **Stereotyped behavior**—following a routine obsessively, continually arranging and rearranging objects
• **Extreme negativism and resistance** or **automatic obedience**

- **Echolalia**—persistently repeating the words of others
- **Echopraxia**—mimicking a movement or gesture of others

During the very withdrawn phase, the person does not move or eat, thus becoming vulnerable to body sores, contractures, and malnutrition. During the extreme motor activity phase, the patient may run about ceaselessly and without purpose with the result of exhaustion, cardiac difficulties, and collapse. The onset of catatonia is usually abrupt, and the prognosis is favorable. Fortunately, with pharmacotherapy and improved individual management, severe catatonic symptoms are rarely seen today.

VIGNETTE

Mary has been motionless and hasn't spoken for days. When her husband raises her arm to dress her and take her to the hospital, it stays raised in the air until he lowers it *(waxy flexibility)*. When she starts to move, she does everything she is told to do (get up, sit down) and only moves on command *(automatic obedience)*. When he speaks to her, she repeats everything he says (e.g., "Mary drink this water," "Mary drink this water" *(echolalia)*.

---

evolve

For a comprehensive case study of a patient experiencing catatonia, visit the Evolve website at http://evolve.elsevier.com/Varcarolis/essentials.

Disorganized

Disorganized (formerly *hebephrenic*) schizophrenia represents the most regressed and socially impaired of all the schizophrenias. A person diagnosed with disorganized schizophrenia may have marked looseness of associations, grossly inappropriate affect, bizarre mannerisms, and incoherence of speech, and may display extreme social withdrawal. Although delusions and hallucinations are present, they are fragmentary and poorly organized. Behavior may be considered odd, and giggling or grimacing in response to internal stimuli is common.

Disorganized schizophrenia has an earlier age of onset (early to middle teens) and often develops insidiously. It is associated with poor premorbid functioning, a significant family history of psychopathological disorders, and a poor prognosis. Often, these patients are in state hospitals and can live in the community safely only in a structured and well-supervised setting. Unfortunately a large portion of the homeless population consists of people with this disorder. Families living with a person with disorganized schizophrenia need significant community support, respite care, and day hospital affiliations.

VIGNETTE

Pete pushes his grocery cart down the street loaded with rags, bottles, bags, and such. He appears disheveled and dressed in a dirty plaid shirt, wears a dirty baseball hat and ragged jeans. He is giggling and laughing to himself. Once in a while he shouts out something, "Alms for the poor me . . . howdy to you all . . . Where is it? Where is it?" *(looseness of association)*. He goes from garbage can to garbage can rummaging for food.

---

evolve

For a comprehensive case study of a patient experiencing disorganized thinking, visit the Evolve website at http://evolve.elsevier.com/Varcarolis/essentials.

Undifferentiated

In the undifferentiated type of schizophrenia, active signs of the disorder (positive or negative symptoms) are present, but the individual does not meet the criteria for paranoid, catatonic, or disorganized type. As does disorganized schizophrenia, undifferentiated schizophrenia begins early and has an insidious onset (early to middle teens). However, the premorbid state is less predictable, and the disability remains fairly stable, although persistent, over time.

Residual

In the residual type of schizophrenia, active-phase symptoms are no longer present, but evidence of two or more residual symptoms persists. Residual symptoms include lack of initiative, social withdrawal, inability to work or study, vague or lack of content of speech, and magical thinking or odd beliefs.

Course of the Disease

The course of schizophrenia usually includes recurrent acute exacerbations of psychosis. However, what used to be thought of as disease with an unalterable march to progressive deterioration might not be quite accurate. A decade's worth of longitudinal studies demonstrated that early and aggressive treatment with antipsychotics may alter the course of the schizophrenias when given at the time of the first psychotic break (Perkins et al., 2006). Prevention of relapse can be more important than the risk of side effects from medications because most side effects are reversible, whereas the consequences of relapse may be irreversible. *With each relapse of psychosis, there is an increase in residual dysfunction and deterioration* (Lewis et al., 2005).

The following are the phases in the course of the disease:

- **Prodromal phase:** Signs and symptoms that precede the acute, fully manifested signs and symptoms of disease. In people with schizophrenia, prodromal symptoms occur in up to 80% to 90% of people before the emergence of frank psychosis (acute phase) (Addington, 2006). Early prodromal symptoms include social withdrawal and deterioration in function and depressive mood, followed by perceptual disturbances, magical thinking, and peculiar behavior, among others (Cornblatt, 2005). Prodromal symptoms may appear a month to a year before the first psychotic break and represent a clear deterioration in previous functioning. Essentially, the symptoms include perceptual difficulties, increased stress, depression, anxiety, sleep disturbance, and decline in ability to function (Addington, 2006). Speech may be characterized by obscure symbolism. Late in the phase, words and phrases may become indecipherable. Frequently, the history of a person with schizophrenia reveals that during adolescence the person was withdrawn from others, lonely, perhaps depressed, and expressed vague or unrealistic plans regarding the future.
- **Acute phase:** Periods of florid positive symptoms (more fully developed and flagrant) (e.g., hallucina-

tions, delusions) as well as negative symptoms (e.g., apathy, withdrawal, lack of motivation) and cognitive symptoms.
- **Maintenance phase:** Period in which acute symptoms decrease in severity, particularly the positive symptoms.
- **Stabilization phase:** Period in which symptoms are in remission, although there might be milder persistent symptoms.

Treatment-Relevant Dimensions of Schizophrenia

The major symptoms of schizophrenia can be grouped into positive, negative, and cognitive. Depression is a frequent comorbidity and can negatively affect the patient's future prognosis and the severity of emotional pain and confusion. Figure 14-3 presents an overview of these major symptom groups and the ways in which they can affect an individual's life.

Positive symptoms (e.g., hallucinations, delusions, bizarre behavior, and paranoia) are referred to as *florid psychotic symptoms;* they are the ones that capture our attention. Three decades of analysis of treatment and study findings indicate that perhaps these florid psychotic symp-

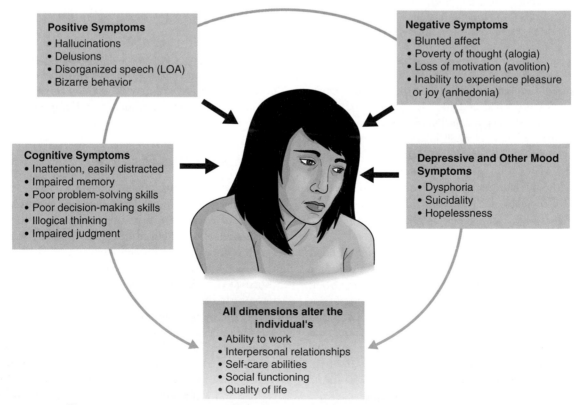

Figure 14-3 ■ Treatment-relevant dimensions of schizophrenia. *LOA,* Looseness of association.

BOX 14-2

Positive and Negative Symptoms of Schizophrenia

Positive Symptoms

Hallucinations
- Auditory
  - Voices commenting
  - Voices conversing
  - Voices commanding
- Somatic-tactile
- Olfactory
- Visual

Delusions
- Persecutory delusions
- Jealous delusions
- Grandiose delusions
- Religious delusions
- Somatic delusions
- Delusions of reference
- Delusions of being controlled
- Delusions of mind reading
- Thought broadcasting, insertion, withdrawal

Bizarre Behavior
- Clothing, appearance
- Social and sexual behavior
- Aggressive, agitated behavior
- Repetitive, stereotyped behavior

Positive Formal Thought Disorder and Speech Patterns
- Derailment
- Tangentiality
- Incoherence
- Illogicality
- Circumstantiality
- Pressure of speech
- Distractible speech
- Clang associations

Negative Symptoms

Affective Flattening
- Unchanging facial expression
- Decreased spontaneous movements
- Paucity of expressive gestures
- Poor eye contact
- Inappropriate affect
- Lack of vocal inflections

Alogia
- Poverty of speech
- Poverty of content of speech
- Blocking

Avolition, Apathy
- Impaired grooming and hygiene
- Lack of persistence at work or school
- Physical anergia

Anhedonia, Asociality
- Few recreational interests or activities
- Little sexual interest or activity
- Impaired intimacy and closeness
- Few relationships with friends or peers

Attention Deficits
- Social inattentiveness

---

toms may not be the core deficiency after all. Actually, the crippling negative symptoms (e.g., apathy, lack of motivation, anhedonia, and poor thought processes) persist and seem to be the most destructive because they render a person inert and unmotivated. The negative and cognitive symptoms are negatively related to a person's ability to function on a job, engage in social activities, and care for self adequately and safely. Refer to Box 14-2 for a list of positive and negative symptoms.

Positive Symptoms

Positive symptoms, such as hallucinations, delusions, bizarre behavior, and paranoia are associated with an acute onset, normal premorbid functioning, normal CT findings, normal neuropsychological test results, and favorable response to antipsychotic medications.

The positive symptoms appear early in the first phase of the illness and often precipitate hospitalization. They are, however, the least important prognostically and usually respond to antipsychotic medication. The positive symptoms are presented here in terms of alterations in thinking, speech, perception, and behavior.

Alterations in Thinking

Delusions. Alterations in thinking can take many forms. **Delusions** are most often defined as false fixed beliefs that cannot be corrected by reasoning. They may be simple beliefs or part of a complex delusional system. In schizophrenia, delusions are often loosely organized and may be bizarre. Most commonly, delusional thinking involves the following themes: ideas of reference, persecution, grandiosity, somatic sensations, jealousy, and

TABLE 14-1	Summary of Delusions*		
Type of Delusion	**Definition**		**Example**
Ideas of reference	Misconstruing trivial events and remarks and giving them personal significance		When Maria saw the doctor and nurse talking together, she believed they were plotting against her. When she heard on the radio that a hurricane was coming, she believed this was really a message that harm was going to befall her.
Persecution	The false belief that one is being singled out for harm by others; this belief often takes the form of a plot by people in power against the person, being followed, persecuted by friends or colleagues		Sam believed that the Secret Service was planning to kill him. He believed that the Secret Service was poisoning his food. Therefore he would only eat food that he was certain was safe.
Grandeur	The false belief that one is a very powerful and important person, having special abilities, possessing great wealth or beauty		Sally believed that she was Mary Magdalene and that Jesus controlled her thoughts and was telling her how to save the world.
Somatic delusions	The false belief that the body is changing in an unusual way (e.g., rotting inside, heart is no longer beating)		David told the doctor that his brain was rotting away.
Jealousy	The false belief that one's mate is unfaithful; may have so-called proof		Harry accused his girlfriend of going out with other men, even though this was not the case. His "proof" was that she came home from work late twice that week. He persisted in his belief, even when the girlfriend's boss explained that everyone had worked late.

*A false belief held and maintained as true, even with evidence to the contrary. This does not include unusual beliefs maintained by one's culture or subculture.

control. Table 14-1 provides definitions and examples of delusions.

About 75% of people with schizophrenia experience delusions at some time during their illness. The most common delusions are persecutory and grandiose, as well as those involving religious or hypochondriacal ideas. A person experiencing delusions is convinced that what he or she believes to be real *is* real. The person's thinking often reflects feelings of great fear and isolation: "I know the doctor talks to the FBI about getting rid of me" or "Everyone wants me dead." Delusions may reflect the person's feelings of low self-worth through the use of reaction formation (observed as grandiosity). "I'm the only one who can save the world, but they won't let me."

At times, delusions hold a kernel of truth. One patient came into the hospital acutely psychotic. He repeatedly told the staff that the mafia was out to kill him. Later, the staff learned that the patient had been selling drugs, had not paid his contacts, and gang members were trying to find him to hurt or even kill him.

Other common delusions observed in schizophrenia include the following:

- **Thought broadcasting**—belief that one's thoughts can be heard by others (e.g., "My brain is connected to the world mind. I can control all heads of state through my thoughts.")
- **Thought insertion**—belief that thoughts of others are being inserted into one's mind (e.g., "They make me think bad thoughts.")
- **Thought withdrawal**—belief that thoughts have been removed from one's mind by an outside agency (e.g., "The devil takes my thoughts away and leaves me empty.")
- **Delusion of being controlled**—belief that one's body or mind is controlled by an outside agency (e.g., "There is a man from darkness who controls my thoughts with electrical waves") and made to feel emotions or sensations (e.g., sexual) that are not one's own.

Concrete Thinking. **Concrete thinking** refers to an overemphasis on specific details and impairment in the ability to use abstract concepts. For example, during an assessment, the nurse might ask what brought the patient to the hospital. The patient might answer "a cab" rather than explaining the reason for seeking medical or psychiatric aid. When asked to give the meaning of the proverb "People in glass houses shouldn't throw stones," the person with schizophrenia might answer, "Don't throw stones or the windows will break." The answer is literal; the ability to use abstract reasoning is absent.

Alterations in Speech

Associative Looseness. Associations are the threads that tie one thought to another and one concept to another. In schizophrenia, these threads are missing, and connections are interrupted. In **associative looseness**, thinking becomes haphazard, illogical, and confused. Zelda Fitzgerald wrote her husband, the writer F. Scott Fitzgerald, an account of going mad:

> Then the world became embryonic in Africa—and there was no need for communication. . . . I have been living in vaporous places peopled with one-dimensional figures and tremulous buildings until I can no longer tell an optical illusion from a reality . . . head and ears incessantly throb and roads disappear. (Vidal, 1982)

Neologisms. **Neologisms** are made-up words that have special meaning for the person (e.g., "I was going to tell him the *mannerologies* of his hospitality just won't do." "I want all the *vetchkisses* to leave the room and let me be."). Children and creative writers often make up their own words, but their creation of neologisms is imaginative, constructive, and adaptive. Neologisms in people with schizophrenia represent a disruption in thought processes.

Echolalia. **Echolalia** is the pathological repeating of another's words by imitation and is often seen in people with catatonia. Echolalia is the counterpart of **echopraxia**, mimicking of the *movements* of another, which is also seen in catatonia.

Clang Association. **Clang association** is the meaningless rhyming of words, often in a forceful manner ("On the track . . . have a Big Mac . . . or get the sack"), in which the rhyming is often more important than the context of the word. This form of speech pattern may be seen in individuals with schizophrenia; however, it may also be seen in people in the manic phase of a bipolar disorder or in individuals with a cognitive disorder, such as Alzheimer's disease or HIV-related dementia.

Word Salad. **Word salad** is a term used to identify a jumble of words that is meaningless to the listener and perhaps to the speaker as well. It may include a string of neologisms. For example, "I sang out for my mother . . . for this to hell I went. How long is road? These little said three hills hop aboard, share the appetite of the Christmas mice spread . . . within three round moons the devil will be washed away."

Alterations in Perception

Hallucinations. Hallucinations, especially auditory hallucinations, are the major example of schizophrenic alteration in perception. **Hallucinations** can be defined as sensory perceptions for which no external stimulus exists. The most common types of hallucination are the following:

- Auditory—hearing voices or sounds
- Visual—seeing persons or things
- Olfactory—smelling odors
- Gustatory—experiencing tastes
- Tactile—feeling bodily sensations

Table 14-2 provides examples of these common types of hallucinations and describes the difference between hallucinations and **illusions.**

It is estimated that up to 90% of people with schizophrenia experience hallucinations at some time during their illness. Although manifestations of hallucination are varied, auditory hallucinations are most common in schizophrenia. Voices may seem to come from outside or inside the person's head. The voices may be familiar or strange, single or multiple. Voices speaking directly to the person or commenting on the person's behavior are most common. A person may believe that the voices are from God, the devil, deceased relatives, or strangers. The auditory hallucinations may occasionally take the form of sounds other than voices.

Command hallucinations must be assessed carefully because the voices may command the person to hurt self or others. For example, a patient might state that "the voices" are saying "jump out the window" or "take a knife and kill your child." Command hallucinations are often terrifying for the individual. Command hallucinations may signal a psychiatric emergency. Patients who can give an identity to the hallucinated voice are at somewhat greater risk of compliance with the hallucinated command than are those who cannot (Junginger, 1995).

Evidence of possible auditory hallucinatory behavior is turning or tilting of the head—as if the patient is listening to someone—or frequent blinking of the eyes and grimacing. Sometimes, patients verbally respond to "unseen others." Visual hallucinations occur less frequently in people with schizophrenia and are more likely to occur in organic disorders. Olfactory, tactile, or gustatory hallucinations account for about 10% of hallucinations in people with schizophrenia (Moller & Murphy, 2002).

Personal Boundary Difficulties. People with schizophrenia often lack a sense of where their bodies end in relationship to where others begin. Patients might say that they are

TABLE 14-2   Summary of Hallucinations*

Type of Hallucination	Definition	Example
Auditory	Hearing voices or sounds that do not exist in the environment but are projections of inner thoughts or feelings	Anna "hears" the voice of her dead mother call her a whore and a tramp.
Visual	Seeing a person, object, or animal that does not exist in the environment	Charles, who is experiencing alcohol withdrawal delirium, "sees" hungry rats coming toward him.
Olfactory	Smelling odors that are not present in the environment	Theresa "smells" her insides rotting.
Gustatory	Tasting sensations that have no stimulus in reality	Sam will not eat his food because he "tastes" the poison the FBI is putting in his food.
Tactile	Feeling strange sensations where no external objects stimulate such feelings; common in delirium tremens	Jack suffers from paranoid schizophrenia. He "feels" electrical impulses controlling his mind.

*A hallucination is a false sensory perception for which no external stimulus exists. Hallucinations are different from illusions in that illusions are misperceptions or misinterpretations of a real experience. For example, a man sees his coat hanging on a coat rack and believes it to be a bear about to attack him. He does see something real but misinterprets what it is.

merging with others or are part of inanimate objects. For example, **depersonalization** is a nonspecific feeling that a person has lost his or her identity; the self is different or unreal. People may be concerned that body parts do not belong to them, or they may have an acute sensation that the body has drastically changed. For example, a woman may see her fingers as snakes or her arms as rotting wood. A man may look in a mirror and state that his face is that of an animal. **Derealization** is the false perception by a person that the environment has changed. For example, everything seems bigger or smaller, or familiar surroundings have become somehow strange and unfamiliar.

Alterations in Behavior

Bizarre and agitated behaviors are associated with schizophrenia and may have a variety of manifestations. **Bizarre behavior** may take the form of a stilted, rigid demeanor and eccentric dress, grooming, and rituals. Many of these behaviors are associated with catatonic schizophrenia but may be seen in other conditions as well (e.g., brain damage, extreme manic phase of bipolar disorder).

- **Extreme motor agitation** is excited physical behavior, such as running about, in response to inner and outer stimuli, which can be harmful to self as well as to others.
- **Stereotyped behaviors** are motor patterns that originally had meaning to the person (e.g., sweeping the floor, washing windows) but are now mechanical and lack purpose.

- **Automatic obedience** is the performance by a catatonic patient of all simple commands in a robot-like fashion.
- **Waxy flexibility**, seen in catatonia, is evidenced by excessive maintenance of posture. Patients can hold unusual postures for long periods.
- **Stupor** refers to a state in which the catatonic patient is motionless for long periods and may even appear to be in a coma.
- **Negativism** is equivalent to resistance. In *active negativism,* the patient does the opposite of what he or she is told to do. When a person does not perform activities that are normal expectations, such as getting out of bed, dressing, and eating, the behavior is termed *passive negativism (catatonia).*

When patients with schizophrenia are acutely ill, impulse control is lacking. Frequently the lack of impulse control is expressed in socially inappropriate **agitated behaviors** such as grabbing another's cigarette, throwing food on the floor, and obtaining the television remote control and changing channels abruptly.

Negative Symptoms

Negative symptoms, such as apathy, anhedonia, poor social functioning, and poverty of thought, are most likely a result of the neurocognitive defects and are associated with an insidious onset, premorbid history of emotional problems, chronic deterioration, demonstration of atrophy on CT scans, abnormal results on neuropsychological tests, and poor response to antipsychotic therapy.

The negative symptoms of schizophrenia develop over a long period of time. These are the symptoms that most interfere with the individual's adjustment and ability to survive. The presence of negative symptoms impedes the person's ability to initiate and maintain relationships and conversations, hold a job, make decisions, and maintain adequate hygiene and grooming.

The presence of negative symptoms contributes to the person's poor social functioning and social withdrawal. During an acute psychotic episode, negative symptoms are difficult to assess because the positive and more florid symptoms, such as delusions and hallucinations, dominate. Some of the negative phenomena are outlined in Table 14-3.

Affect is the observable behavior that expresses a person's emotions. In people with schizophrenia, affect may not coincide with inner emotions. Affect can usually be categorized in one of three ways: flat or blunted, inappropriate, or bizarre. A **flat affect** (immobile facial expression or a blank look) or **blunted affect** (minimal emotional response) is commonly seen in schizophrenia. **Inappropriate affect** refers to an emotional response to a situation that is not congruent with the tone of the situation. For example, a young man breaks into laughter when told that his father has died. **Bizarre affect** is especially prominent in the disorganized form of schizophrenia and includes grimacing, giggling, and mumbling to oneself. Bizarre affect is marked when the patient is unable to relate logically to the environment.

Cognitive Symptoms

Cognitive symptoms represent the third dimension and affect at least 40% to 60% of people with schizophrenia. The degree of cognitive impairment is a better predictor of functional impairment than is the severity of psychosis (positive symptoms). Cognitive impairment involves difficulty with attention, memory, and executive functions (e.g., decision making and problem solving) and is evident when the patient is unable to manage his or her own health care, hold a job, initiate or maintain a social support system, or live alone.

The degree of cognitive deficit is associated with the severity of negative symptoms; **disorganized thinking** reflects the degree to which disorganized speech, disorganized behavior, or inappropriate affect is present (APA, 2000). Good verbal memory is one cognitive indicator that the individual eventually can function within the community because it helps with acquisition of psychosocial skills, learning, and retention of skills. These are all necessary for eventual rehabilitation (Beng-Choon et al., 2004).

Depressive and Other Mood Symptoms

Depressive symptoms increase the suffering of patients with schizophrenia and are all too common. Recognition of depression during assessment is crucial because it can increase the likelihood of suicide and substance abuse as well as impaired functioning.

Assessment Guidelines

Schizophrenia and Other Psychotic Disorders

1. Determine if the patient had a medical workup; if so, was medical or substance-induced psychosis ruled out?
2. Verify whether the patient is dependent on alcohol or drugs.
3. Assess for command hallucinations (e.g., voices telling the person to harm self or another). If present, ask the patient:
   - Do you plan to follow the command?
   - Do you believe the voices are real?
   - Do you recognize the voices?

TABLE 14-3	Negative Phenomena
Phenomenon	**Explanation**
Affective blunting	In *affective blunting*, severe reduction in the expression and range and intensity of affect occurs; in *flat affect* no facial expression of emotion is present.
Anergia	Lack of energy: passivity, lack of persistence at work or school.
Anhedonia	Inability to experience any pleasure in activities that usually produce pleasurable feelings; result of profound emotional barrenness.
Avolition	Lack of motivation: inability to initiate tasks, such as social contacts, grooming, and other aspects of activities of daily living.
Poverty of content of speech	Speech that is adequate in amount but conveys little information because of vagueness, empty repetitions, or use of stereotypes or obscure phrases.
Poverty of speech	Restriction in the amount of speech—answers range from brief to monosyllabic one-word answers.
Thought blocking	May be signaled when a patient stops talking in the middle of a sentence and remains silent. After a patient stops abruptly: *Nurse:* "What just happened now?" *Patient:* "I forgot what I was saying. Something took my thoughts away."

4. Review the patient's belief system. Is it fragmented? Poorly or well organized? Is it systematized? Is the system of beliefs unsupported by reality (delusion)? If yes, then find out if:
   • Delusions focus on someone trying to harm the patient
   • The patient is planning to retaliate against a person or organization
   • Precautions need to be taken
5. Assess for co-occurring disorders including:
   • Depression
   • Suicidality
   • Anxiety
   • Substance dependency
   • History of violence
6. Inventory the patient's medications and assess whether the patient is adhering to the medication regimen.
7. Determine the family's response to increased symptoms. Are they overprotective? Hostile? Suspicious?
8. Assess the manner in which family members and the patient relate.
9. Review the support system. Is the family well informed about the disease? Does the family understand the need for medication adherence? Is the family familiar with support groups available in the community or where to go for respite and family support? Have family members received or been referred for psychoeducation?
10. Assess the patient's global functioning (using the Global Assessment of Functioning [GAF] Scale (see Chapter 2).

DIAGNOSIS

People with schizophrenia have multiple disturbing and disabling symptoms that necessitate a multifaceted approach to care and treatment of the patient as well as the family. Table 14-4 lists potential nursing diagnoses for a person with schizophrenia.

OUTCOMES IDENTIFICATION
Phase I (Acute)

During the acute phase of the illness, the overall goal is **patient safety and medical stabilization.** Therefore if the patient is at risk for violence to self or others, initial outcome criteria should address safety issues (e.g., *patient consistently refrains from inflicting serious injury to self or others*). Another outcome might be *patient consistently refrains from acting on delusions or hallucinations*. Medication adherence is a vital

outcome for all phases of recovery. Ideally, outcomes should focus on enhancing the patient's strengths and minimizing the patient's deficits.

Phase II (Maintenance) and Phase III (Stabilization)

Outcome criteria during the maintenance and stabilization phases focus on helping the patient to adhere to medication regimens, understand schizophrenia, and participate in available psychoeducational activities for both the patient and the family.

During the stabilization phase, goals are directed toward continual recovery, improvement in functioning, and enhancement of the individual's quality of life. Improvement in functioning includes the ability to participate in social, vocational, or self-care skills training and involvement in socializing groups at various levels.

It is also important to include outcomes that address anxiety control and relapse prevention. Mills (2000) identifies desired outcomes to reduce the patient's vulnerability to psychosis: Maintain a regular sleep pattern; reduce alcohol, drug, and caffeine intake; keep in touch with supportive friends and family; stay active (engage in exercise, hobbies, employment); have a routine daily and weekly schedule including enjoyable activities; and take medication regularly.

PLANNING
Phase I (Acute)

During the acute phase of schizophrenia, brief hospitalization is frequently indicated if the patient is considered a danger to self or others, refuses to eat or drink, or is too disorganized to provide self-care. Another indication for hospitalization is the need for specific observation, neurological workup, or other medically related tests or treatments. The planning process focuses on the best strategies to ensure patient safety and provide symptom stabilization.

At this time the treatment team identifies aftercare needs for follow-up and support, as well as the appropriate referrals that will benefit the patient and family. Discharge planning considers not only external factors, such as the patient's living arrangement, economic resources, social supports, and family relationships but also the internal factor of the patient's vulnerability to stress. Because relapse can be devastating to long-term functioning, vigorous efforts are made to connect the patient with community agencies that provide social supports and programs designed to help the patient remain well.

TABLE 14-4   Potential Nursing Diagnoses for Schizophrenia

Symptom	Nursing Diagnoses
Positive Symptoms	
Hallucinations	
Hears voices that others do not	*Disturbed sensory perception:* auditory or visual
Hears voices telling him or her to hurt self or others *(command hallucinations)*	*Risk for self-directed/other-directed violence*
Distorted Thinking Not Based on Reality	
Persecution: Thinks that others are trying to harm self	*Disturbed thought processes*
Jealousy: Thinks that spouse or lover is being unfaithful, or thinks others are jealous of self when they are not	*Defensive coping*
Grandeur: Thinks he or she has powers and talents that are not possessed or is someone powerful or famous	
Reference: Believes that all events within the environment are directed at or hold special meaning for self	
Looseness of association: Shows loose association of ideas	*Impaired verbal communication*
Clang association: Uses words that rhyme in a nonsensical fashion	*Disturbed thought processes*
Echolalia: Repeats words that are heard	
Mutism: Does not speak	
Circumstantiality: Delays getting to the point of communication because of unnecessary and tedious details	
Concrete thinking: Unable to abstract; uses literal translations concerning aspects of the environment	
Negative Symptoms	
Uncommunicative, withdrawn, makes no eye contact	*Social isolation*
Preoccupied with own thoughts	*Impaired social interaction*
Expresses feelings of rejection or aloneness (lies in bed all day, positions back to door)	*Risk for loneliness*
Is stigmatized for diagnosis of schizophrenia	*Risk for compromised human dignity*
Talks about self as "bad" or "no good"	*Chronic low self-esteem*
Feels guilty because of "bad thoughts"; extremely sensitive to real or perceived slights	*Risk for self-directed violence*
Shows lack of energy (**anergia**)	*Ineffective coping*
Shows lack of motivation (**avolition**), unable to initiate tasks (social contact, grooming, and other aspects of daily living)	*Self-care deficit (bathing/hygiene, dressing/grooming)* *Constipation*
Other	
Families and significant others become confused or overwhelmed, have lack of knowledge about disease or treatment, feel powerless in coping with patient at home.	*Compromised family coping* *Impaired parenting* *Caregiver role strain* *Deficient knowledge*
Nonadherence to medication and treatment. Patient stops taking medication (often from side effects), stops going to therapy groups, family and significant others not aware of need for medications and treatments.	*Nonadherence*

Phase II (Maintenance) and Phase III (Stabilization)

Planning during the maintenance and stabilization phases of treatment focuses on strategies to provide patient and family education and skills training (psychosocial educa-tion). **Relapse prevention skills are vital.** Planning identi-fies the social, interpersonal, coping, and vocational skills needed, as well as how and where these needs can best be met within the community. **Interventions are always geared toward the patient's strengths and healthy func-tioning as well as areas of deficiency.**

IMPLEMENTATION

Phase I (Acute)

As with outcomes identification and planning, interventions are geared toward the phase of schizophrenia (Table 14-5). During phase I the clinical focus is on crisis intervention, acute symptom stabilization (medication), and safety. As a result of the recent trend toward decreasing the length of hospital stays, alternatives such as partial hospitalization, halfway houses, and day treatment centers are frequently used as cost-effective alternatives to hospitalization (Beng-Choon et al., 2004).

Acute phase interventions include acute psychopharmacological treatment (psychobiological intervention),

supportive and directive communications, limit setting (milieu management and counseling), and psychiatric, medical, and neurological evaluation.

Phase II (Maintenance) and Phase III (Stabilization)

Once the acute symptoms are somewhat stabilized, the hospitalized patient is discharged to the community, where appropriate treatment can be carried out during the maintenance and stabilization phases. Effective long-term care of an individual with schizophrenia relies on a three-pronged approach: medications, nursing interventions, and community support. **Family psychoeducation, as well as com-**

TABLE 14-5   Treatment Focus at Different Phases of Schizophrenia

Phase I		Phase II	Phase III
Acute: Onset, Exacerbation, or Relapse	**Subacute or Convalescent**	**Maintenance Adaptive Plateau**	**Stable Plateau**
Clinical Focus			
Crisis intervention	Social supports	Understanding and acceptance of illness	Social, vocational, and self-care skills
Safety	Stress and vulnerability assessment		Learning or relearning
Acute symptom stabilization	Living arrangements		Identification of realistic expectations
	Daily activities		Adaptation to deficits
	Economic resources		
Intervention			
Acute psychopharmacological treatment	Psychosocial evaluation	Support and teaching	Attention to details of self-care, social, and work functioning
Limit setting	Linkage with:	Medication teaching and side effect management	Direct intervention with family and/or employers
Supportive and directive care	• Social services	Direct assistance with situational problems	Cognitive and social skills enhancement
Psychiatric, medical, neurological evaluation	• Human services	Identification of prodromal and acute symptoms and signs of relapse	Medication maintenance
Meeting with family	• Community treatment agencies	Continued psychoeducational work with families as needed	Continued psychoeducational intervention with families as needed
	Psychoeducational interventions with families		
Professional Collaboration			
Inpatient treatment team	Social work department	Community support staff	Group therapists
Residential alternative to hospitalization	Health and human services	Family support groups	Social, vocational, and self-care providers
Community crisis intervention	Day treatment or a variety of community support	Group therapists and self-help groups	Family, employer, community support staff
Internist		Practitioners of behavioral therapies using educational models and cognitive restructuring.	
Neurologist			

Adapted from Gabbard, G.O. (2001). *Treatments of psychiatric disorders* (3rd ed.). Washington, DC: American Psychiatric Publishing.

munity support, is a key component of effective treatment.

Phase II and III interventions include the following:

Health teaching:

- For the patient and family about the disease
- For the patient and family about medication management
- In cognitive and social skills enhancement
- Of strategies to minimize stress and to control anxiety levels

Health promotion and maintenance:

- To identify signs of relapse and take preventive steps
- To improve deficits in self-care, social, and work functioning
- To encourage participation in nonthreatening activities
- To encourage social relationships
- To encourage family interaction

Communication Guidelines

Therapeutic strategies for communicating with patients with schizophrenia focus on lowering the patient's anxiety, decreasing defensive patterns, encouraging participation in therapeutic and social events, raising feelings of self-worth, and increasing medication compliance. Familiarity with the principles used for dealing with phenomena such as hallucinations, delusions, paranoia, and looseness of association is helpful for establishing rapport and being effective.

Hallucinations

Because hearing voices is the most common hallucinatory experience reported by patients, the nurse initially should try to understand what the voices are saying or telling the person to do. Suicidal or homicidal messages necessitate initiation of safety measures for all members of the health care team.

Hallucinations are real to the person who is experiencing them. Nurses should approach patients who are hallucinating in a nonthreatening and nonjudgmental manner (Moller & Murphy, 2002). Moller (1989) emphasizes that often when a person is hallucinating, the individual is experiencing anxiety, fear, loneliness, and low self-esteem, and the brain is not processing stimuli accurately.

During the acute phase of the illness, the nurse should maintain eye contact, call the patient by name, and speak simply but in a louder voice than usual.

Patient: "I hear my mother's voice saying terrible things about me. She says I am no good and should be punished."

Nurse: "That must be very upsetting, Tom. Are you feeling upset?" (*Nurse waits for a response.*)

Patient: "Yes, I feel bad."

Nurse: "Let's go over here and play gin. I hear you are a very good gin player."

Here the nurse tries to identify the feelings the patient is experiencing and then distract his attention to something he can do well. Table 14-6 lists interventions for hallucinations.

Delusions

Delusions reflect the misperception of cognitive stimuli. When the nurse attempts to see the world as it appears through the eyes of the patient, it is easier to understand the patient's delusional experience.

Patient: "I see now . . . you are in on the CIA plot to drain my brain . . . you all want me destroyed."

Nurse: "I don't want to hurt you, Tom. Thinking that everyone wants to destroy you must be very frightening."

In this example, the nurse clarifies the reality of the patient's experience and empathizes with the patient's apparent experience and feelings of fear. The nurse avoids being drawn into the conversation regarding the content of the delusion (CIA and plot to destroy) but attempts to identify the feelings that the patient is experiencing. Talking about the person's feelings is helpful; talking about delusional material is not.

It is *never* useful to argue with or try to "reason" with the patient regarding the content of the delusion. Doing so can intensify the patient's retention of irrational beliefs. However, it is helpful for the nurse to clarify misinterpretations of the environment.

Patient: "I see the doctor is here, and he is part of this plan to destroy me."

Nurse: "It is true the doctor wants to see you, but he wants to talk to you about your treatment. Would you feel more comfortable talking to him in the day room?"

Interacting with the patient about concrete realities in the environment helps minimize the time available for the patient to focus on delusional thoughts. Performance of specific manual tasks within the scope of the patient's abilities is also useful in distracting the patient from delusional thinking. The more time the patient spends engaged in reality-based activities or with people, the more opportunity the patient has to become comfortable with reality. Table 14-7 lists interventions for a patient experiencing delusions.

Paranoia

A paranoid patient may make offensive yet accurate criticisms of the nurse or the unit policies. It is important that the staff not react to these criticisms with anxiety or rejec-

TABLE 14-6 Interventions for Hallucinations

Intervention	Rationale
1. Watch patients for cues that they may be hallucinating, e.g., eyes darting to one side, muttering, or staring sideways, changes in facial expressions.	1. Patients are usually in high levels of anxiety at this time. Early intervention may help interrupt hallucinatory process and lessen patient's anxiety and potential for harm.
2. Ask patients directly if they are hallucinating. "Are you hearing voices?" "What are they saying to you?"	2. The content of the "voices" can help both you and the patient discover patient's feelings, e.g., fear, anger, worthlessness. The nurse can then address the feelings.
3. If voices are telling patient to harm self or others (command hallucinations): a. Notify appropriate authority, e.g., police, physician, administrator, according to unit protocols b. If in the community, evaluate need for hospitalization	3. People often obey hallucinatory commands to kill self or others. Early assessment and intervention could save lives.
4. **Document:** what patients say, if they are a threat to self or others, who was contacted and notified and when.	4. If patient threatens self or others, documentation shows that correct legal protocols were followed. Otherwise nurses, physicians, and institutions can be held legally responsible,
5. Accept the fact that the voices are real to the patient, but explain that you do not hear the voices. Refer to the voices as "your voices" or "the voices that you hear."	5. Validating that your reality does not include voices may help patients cast doubt on their voices.
6. Present a calm demeanor and stay with patient while he or she is hallucinating. At times you can tell the patient to tell the "voices they hear" to go away.	6. When patients feel comfortable with a nurse, they can sometimes learn to push the voices aside when given repeated instruction.
7. Keep patients focused on simple, basic, reality-based topics. Help patient focus on one idea at a time.	7. Hallucinating patients are confused and disorientated; helps patient focus on people and happenings in reality.
8. Help patient identify times and situations when hallucinations are the most prevalent and intense.	8. Helps nurse and patient identify situations and times that are the most threatening and find ways to mitigate perceived threats.
9. Assess for signs of increase in anxiety, fear, or agitation and intervene as soon as possible.	9. The earlier intervention takes place, the easier it is to calm patient down and prevent harm.

tion of the patient. Staff conferences, peer groups, and clinical supervision are effective ways of looking beyond the behaviors to the motivations of the patient. This provides the opportunity to reduce the patient's anxiety and increase staff effectiveness.

It is important to approach a patient who is paranoid in a nonjudgmental, respectful manner and use clear and simple language, which helps minimize the opportunity for the patient to misconstrue the meaning of a message. Be honest and consistent with the patient regarding expectations and in enforcing rules. Suspicious people are quick to discern dishonesty. Honesty and consistency increase stability and decrease tension. Explaining to the patient what you are going to do prepares the patient and minimizes the opportunity for misinterpreting your intent as hostile or aggressive. Avoid laughing, whispering, or talking quietly when the patient cannot hear what is being said. Suspicious

patients will automatically think that they are the target of the interaction and interpret it in a negative manner *(ideas of reference)*.

Associative Looseness

The symptom of associative looseness often mirrors the patient's autistic thoughts and reflects the person's poorly organized thinking. An increase in this type of communication often indicates that the patient is feeling increased anxiety and an inability to respond to internal and external stimuli. The patient's ramblings also may confuse and frustrate the nurse. The following communication guidelines are useful with a patient whose speech is confused and disorganized:

- Do not pretend that you understand the patient's communications when you are confused by words or meanings.

TABLE 14-7   Interventions for Delusions

Intervention	Rationale
1. Assess if external controls are needed, if agitated and believe someone is going to harm them or they have to harm someone else to survive; use safety measures	1. Beliefs are real for the patient and delusional thinking might dictate a need for self-defense. Evaluate least restrictive alternatives (confer with others if helpful).
2. Be aware that the patients' delusions represent the way that they are experiencing reality.	2. Identifying patient's experience helps the nurse to understand the patient's feelings.
3. Identify feelings: a. If belief is an attempt to "get" patient, then patient is experiencing *fear*. b. If belief is someone is controlling patient's thoughts, then the patient is experiencing *helplessness*.	3. The nurse can focus on feelings, not delusional content.
4. Do not argue with patient's beliefs or try to correct false beliefs with logic or facts.	4. Arguing will only increase patient's defensive position thereby reinforcing false beliefs.
5. Do not touch patient; use gestures very carefully, particularly if patient is paranoid	5. Give delusional patient lots of space. Touching may be perceived as an aggressive or sexual attempt; gestures may be misconstrued to support their delusional thinking.
6. A paranoid patient might not eat or drink, thinking the food is poisoned. Offer food and fluids in closed containers such as can soda, carton of yogurt, fruit in their skins, hard boiled egg, etc.	6. Food that hasn't "been tampered with" is "safe" to eat, and some nutritional intake is possible.
7. After understanding the patient's underlying feelings, e.g., fear, helplessness, engage patient in reality based activities such as cards or crafts. If patient is paranoid, often intellectual functions are higher and may respond better to more intellectually taxing noncompetitive activities.	7. When patients are focused on reality based activities, then their minds are not focused on their delusional thinking, thus the feelings that result with that thinking are momentarily lessened. The more a person is focused in reality, the healthier it is for that person
8. Observe for events that trigger delusions	8. Essentially, observe for events that make the patient anxious and fearful. Problem-solve ways to mitigate the effect of these situations or events.
9. If anxiety begins to escalate out of control use least restrictive interventions, one-to-one, prn medications, or seclusions. Always follow unit protocol and provide careful documentation.	9. The whole idea is to lower patients' anxiety. Usually a calm nonthreatening presence during high levels of anxiety help people lower their anxiety levels.

- Tell the patient that you are having difficulty understanding.
- Place the difficulty in understanding on yourself, *not* on the patient. For example, say, "I am having trouble following what you are saying," *not* "You are not making any sense."
- Look for recurring topics and themes in the patient's communications. For example, "You've mentioned trouble with your brother several times. Tell me about your brother and your relationship with him."
- Emphasize what is going on in the patient's immediate environment (here and now) and involve the patient in simple reality-based activities. These measures can help the patient better focus thoughts.

- Tell the patient what you do understand, and reinforce clear communication and accurate expression of needs, feelings, and thoughts.

Health Teaching and Health Promotion

The family needs to be included in any psychological strategies aimed at reducing exacerbation of psychotic symptoms. Education is an essential strategy and includes teaching the patient and family about the illness (causes, medications, medication side effects, prevention of relapse); helping the patient and family recognize the effect of stress; ensuring an understanding of the importance of medication to a

APPLYING THE ART   A Person with Schizophrenia

SCENARIO: I noticed Aaron standing barefooted in the hallway with both shoes in his outstretched hand. He almost looked like a statue with his blank, unaware demeanor. He deliberately picked up each foot then slowly rubbed the ball of one foot then the other against the carpet.

THERAPEUTIC GOAL: By the end of the present encounter, Aaron will demonstrate increased comfort with the student nurse as evidenced by voluntarily walking together in the hallways of the psychiatric unit.

Student-Patient Interaction	Thoughts, Communication Techniques, and Mental Health Nursing Concepts
Student: "Aaron, I am _____, one of the nursing students. Aaron, I'm standing next to you, on your right side." *Student's feelings: I'm kind of nervous. How scary and lonely his world must be.*	With *schizophrenia* it's important to say his name and say my own name to make clear our separateness.
Aaron: *Quietly murmuring.* "Don't know left, right, right, correct. I can't quite gather first one, last one. Can't last long . . . long . . . long lost soul. Soul train." *Student's feelings: I wonder why he rubs each foot against the floor like he really needs to feel where the floor is.*	He may have an *ego boundary* disturbance. He also holds his shoes far away from his body. What are the clues inside his *loose associations*? He looks stuck just standing there yet he holds his shoes like he's *ambivalent* about going somewhere.
Student's feelings: That part, "long lost soul" makes me feel sad. I felt lost when I first arrived here at school without a single friend. When I let myself know what I'm feeling, memories of the losses in my childhood begin to stir.	I need to focus on Aaron and deal with potential *countertransference* later. His most intense words are "lost soul." That phrase is near the end of his rambling associations. He may remember the last words he spoke at some level. I'll *restate* then use *reflection* of feelings.
Student: "Long lost soul. You're feeling kind of lost right now. It's hard to decide what to do next."	Maybe he wants to get away on his own "soul train." Is he an *elopement* risk? Probably not. He's too confused right now to plan anything, though he may follow easily. I'll give some structure to meet *safety needs*.
Student: "Aaron, it's _____. Come with me and we'll figure out how to help you. *I touch his arm to direct him toward the day area.*"	
Aaron: *Abruptly tilts his head toward opposite wall. He begins mumbling like he's responding back to an unseen other.* *Student's feelings: I'm so upset with myself. I acted without thinking about how threatening my touch would be without asking first. I so want to help him and now I've scared him. I want to say, "I'm sorry" but that's my need. I'll tell him later when he's able to process information. Okay, keep focused. He needs to feel safe more than anything.*	The touch violated his precarious *ego boundary*. He's *hallucinating*—my touch tipped him from *moderate to severe anxiety*. I need to speak in short sentences with lots of pauses to slow this down.
Student: "Aaron, I'm here. I'll stay with you."	I *offer self*.
Aaron: *Mumbles.* "The mistop . . . don't . . . can't . . ." *Looks panicked.*	He is approaching *panic level* anxiety. "Mistop." What's that? Is it a *neologism*?
Student: "Aaron, talk to me. What are the voices saying?" *Student's feelings: My first job is to stay calm myself. He looks terrified. I need to let him know he's safe. I am okay. Even if I don't say everything right, I do care.*	

APPLYING THE ART   A Person with Schizophrenia—cont'd

Student-Patient Interaction	Thoughts, Communication Techniques, and Mental Health Nursing Concepts
Aaron: *Shakes his head.* "Soul train, blame, shame, going to the end of the line . . . supine . . . surprise . . . demise."	He's making *clang associations.* I hear covert references maybe to suicide. I'll *restate* then ask a *direct question* to assess suicide potential.
Student: "The end of the line; demise. Aaron, are the voices telling you to hurt yourself or someone else?" **Student's feelings:** *Overwhelmed, I can't do this alone. Maybe medication will help. I hope at some level he will feel safer.*	He probably can't *reality test* enough to tell me whether the voices tell him to kill himself. I must report this now, but I also don't want to leave him alone if there's the slightest potential for suicide. He needs *close constant observation.*
Aaron: *Mumbles.* **Student:** *Without crowding him, I position myself so he can see my face. Quiet and concerned.* "Let's go together to talk to the nurse." **Aaron:** *Slowly walks with me.*	Before he did not come with me. Now he is walking beside me. He feels more comfortable with me now.

good outcome; encouraging involvement in psychosocial activities; and identifying sources for ongoing support in dealing with the illness. Some hospitals and clinics offer medication groups for patients (and sometimes family members as well). Medication groups can help patients deal more effectively with troubling side effects, alert the nurse to possible adverse or toxic reactions, and increase adherence to the medication regimen.

When people lack understanding of the disease and its symptoms, they may misinterpret the patient's apathy and lack of drive as laziness. This erroneous assumption can foster hostility by family members, caregivers, or others in the community. Thus further teaching about the negative and positive symptoms of schizophrenia can reduce these tensions.

It is vital that nurses, physicians, and social workers be aware of the community support resources and make this information available to discharged patients as well as their families. Examples of such resources include community mental health services, home health services, work support programs, day hospitals, social skills and support groups, family educational skills groups, and respite care.

Milieu Therapy

Effective hospital care involves more than protection from family, social, or work environments that are stressful or disruptive. Many patients need the structure provided by hospitalization. In fact, patients in the acute phase of

schizophrenia improve more on a unit with a structured milieu than on an open unit that allows greater freedom. Partial hospitalization programs, halfway houses, and day treatment centers also provide a structured milieu. A therapeutic milieu provides safety, useful activities, resources for resolving conflicts, and opportunities for learning social and vocational skills.

Safety

A schizophrenic patient, especially in the acute phase, is prone to physical violence, often in response to hallucinations or delusions. During this time, measures need to be taken to protect the patient and others. If verbal de-escalation efforts and chemical restraints (antipsychotic medication) fail to lessen the patient's aggression, physical restraints and seclusion may be indicated (see Chapters 13, 21, and 26).

With the shifting of care for the seriously mentally ill from inpatient to community-based treatment centers, the need for transitional care is heightened, and the role of the nurse in providing a therapeutic milieu is broadened. Alternatives to hospitalization include partial hospitalization, halfway houses, and day treatment programs:

- **Partial hospitalization:** Patients sleep at home and attend treatment sessions during the day or evening.
- **Halfway houses:** Patients live in the community with a group of other patients, sharing expenses and responsibilities. Staff are present in the house 24 hours a day, 7 days a week.

- **Day treatment programs:** Patients live in a halfway house or on their own, sometimes with home visits, or in residential programs. Patients attend a structured program during the day.

Some of these programs may include group therapy, supervised activities, individual counseling, or specialized training and rehabilitation.

Psychotherapy

Program for Assertive Community Treatment

Program for Assertive Community Treatment (PACT) is designed for the most marginally adjusted and poorly functioning patients. Its aim is to prevent relapse, maximize social and vocational functioning, and keep the individual in the community. It emphasizes the patient's strengths in adapting to the community, provides support and assertive outreach, and involves almost all aspects of the patient's life (e.g., food, shelter, schooling, grooming, budgeting, transportation, etc.). PACT is a 24-hour-a-day, 7-day-a-week team approach. Medication adherence is emphasized (APA, 2004).

Family Therapy

All evidence-based approaches emphasize the value of family participation in treatment. Families with members who are struggling with schizophrenia often endure considerable hardships while coping with the psychotic and residual symptoms of the illness. Often these families become isolated from their relatives and communities. Families are perhaps the most consistent factor in patients' lives. More than half of patients discharged from a psychiatric facility return to their family of origin. The following example shows how a family came to distinguish between "Martha's problem" and "the problem caused by schizophrenia."

> It was a good idea, us all meeting in the comfort of our own home to discuss my sister's illness. We were all able to say how it felt, and for the first time I realized that I knew very little about what she was suffering from or how much—the word *schizophrenia* meant nothing to me before but it's much clearer now. I used to think she was just being lazy until she told me in the meeting what it was really like. (Gamble & Brennan, 2000).

Programs that provide support, education, coping skills training, and social network development are extremely effective. This approach is called **psychoeducational,** and it brings educational and behavioral approaches into family treatment. The psychoeducational approach recognizes that families are secondary victims of a biological illness. In family therapy sessions, fears, faulty communication patterns, and distortions are identified. Improved problem-solving skills can be taught, and healthier alternatives to situations of conflict can be explored. Family guilt and anxiety can be lessened, which facilitates change.

Families that receive psychoeducational treatment in multiple-family groups do even better than those treated in single-family groups. Although single- and multiple-family treatments are cost effective, multiple-family groups are even more so and the most beneficial to families as well as the family members with schizophrenia. Improvement seems to stem from an expansion of the social network available to the family and patient as well as an expansion in problem-solving capacity afforded by a group. Multiple-family groups also decrease emotional overinvolvement while increasing the overall positive tone, which is characteristic of such groups. Box 14-3 gives psychoeducational strategies for the patient and family.

Cognitive-Behavioral Therapy

Data support the efficacy of cognitive-behavioral therapy (CBT) for reducing the frequency and intensity of delusions and hallucinations (positive symptoms). People with schizophrenia or delusional disorders that seem to benefit are usually chronic outpatients with treatment-resistant and often distressing delusions or hallucinations. Usually several months are required, although treatment can last up to years (see Chapters 3 and 12 for more on the use of CBT).

Social Skills Training

Social skills training (SST) can improve the level of social activity, foster new social contacts, improve quality of life, and help lower anxiety (Patel et al., 2003). Complex behaviors used in daily living are broken down into discrete behavioral techniques (e.g., how to properly answer the phone and take a message, how to initiate a social dialogue, how to order a meal, etc.).

Pharmacological, Biological, and Integrative Therapies

Drugs used to treat psychotic disorders are called *antipsychotic medications.* Although they may alleviate many of the symptoms of schizophrenia, they cannot cure the underlying psychotic processes. Therefore when patients stop taking their medications, psychotic symptoms usually return. An additional concern is that with each relapse following medication discontinuation, it takes longer to achieve remission after restarting medications. This leads to the possibility that the patient will eventually become unresponsive to treatment (Tsung-Ung et al., 2004).

BOX 14-3

Psychoeducational Strategies for Patient and Family

1. Learn all you can about the illness.
   - Attend psychoeducational groups.
   - Attend support groups.
   - Join the National Alliance for the Mentally Ill (NAMI).
   - Contact the National Institute of Mental Health (NIMH).
2. Develop a relapse prevention plan.
   - Know the early warning signs of relapse (e.g., social withdrawal, trouble sleeping, increased bizarre or magical thinking).
   - Know whom to call and where to go when early signs of relapse appear.
   - Relapse is part of the illness, not a sign of failure.
3. Take advantage of all psychoeducational tools.
   - Participate in family, group, individual therapy.
   - Learn new behaviors and cognitive coping skills to help handle intrafamily stress and interpersonal, social, and vocational difficulties. Get information from health care workers (nurse, case manager, physician), NAMI, community mental health groups, or a hospital.
   - Everyone needs a place to address their fears and losses, and to learn new ways of coping.

4. Comply with treatment.
   - Research has determined that people who do the best in coping with the disease comply with treatment that works for them.
   - Tell your health care worker (nurse, caseworker, physician, social worker) about troubling side effects (e.g., sexual problems, weight gain, "feeling funny"). Most side effects can be treated.
   - Keeping side effects a secret or stopping medication can prevent you from having the best quality of life. Share your concerns.
5. Avoid alcohol and drugs; they can act on the brain and precipitate a relapse.
6. Keep in touch with supportive people.
7. Keep healthy—stay in balance.
   - Self-care deficit is reflected in high rates of medical comorbidity.
   - Maintain a regular sleep pattern.
   - Maintain self-care (e.g., diet and hygiene).
   - Keep active (hobbies, friends, groups, sports, job, special interests).
   - Learn ways to reduce stress.

Patients and family members should be given telephone numbers and addresses of local support groups that are affiliated with NAMI (www.nami.org).

Data from Zerbe, K.J. (1999). *Women's mental health in primary care.* Philadelphia: Saunders; Baillière Tindall; Tandon, R., et al. (2003). *Beyond symptoms control: Moving towards positive patient outcomes.* Paper presented at the American Psychiatric Association 55th Institute on Psychiatric Services, October 31, 2003, Boston. Retrieved January 21, 2005, from www.medscape.com/viewprogram/2835_pnt.

There are two groups of antipsychotic drugs: conventional (traditional), the dopamine antagonists [D_2 receptor antagonists]) and atypical (second generation), the (serotonin-dopamine antagonists [$5\text{-}HT_{2A}$ receptor antagonists]). In addition, some drugs are used to augment the antipsychotic agents for treatment-resistant patients.

All antipsychotic drugs are effective for most acute exacerbations of schizophrenia and for preventing or mitigating relapse. The **conventional (first-generation) antipsychotics** target the positive symptoms of schizophrenia, and the newer **atypical (second-generation) antipsychotics** are thought to diminish some of the negative symptoms as well. The atypical agents have fewer side effects and thus are better tolerated. The newer atypical agents also help with symptoms of anxiety and depression, decrease suicidal behavior, and are thought to increase neurocognitive functioning.

Although most individuals prefer oral medications, those who are nonadherent to medication therapy and are prone to frequent relapse are candidates for long-lasting injectable formulations.

Antipsychotic agents usually take effect 3 to 6 weeks after the regimen is started. Most patients with schizophrenia respond at least partially to antipsychotic drug therapy. However, without drug treatment, 70% to 80% of individuals will relapse within a year (MMDT, 2002).

Because the newer atypical agents (except for clozapine) are generally the treatment of choice for patients experiencing their first episode of schizophrenia, these drugs are discussed first.

Atypical (Second-Generation) Antipsychotics

The atypical antipsychotics (AAPs) are a newer generation of antipsychotics that first emerged in the early 1990s with clozapine (Clozaril). Unfortunately, clozapine produces agranulocytosis in 0.8% to 1% of people who take it; the drug also increases the risk for seizures. However, clozapine remains the gold standard for treatment-refractory patients (Beng-Choon et al., 2004). The AAPs developed after clozapine do not share these same disadvantages.

The atypical antipsychotics permit more than just control of the most alarming symptoms of schizophrenia (e.g., hallucinations, delusions); they also allow for improvement in the quality of life. **These drugs are often chosen as first-line antipsychotics** because they have the following characteristics (Kuo, 2004). They:

- Produce minimal to no extrapyramidal symptoms (EPS) or tardive dyskinesia
- May improve the neurocognitive defects associated with schizophrenia
- May decrease affective symptoms (anxiety and depression)
- Decrease suicidal behavior
- Seem to target the neurocognitive symptoms
- Are associated with lower relapse rates

One significant disadvantage of the AAPs is that they all (with the exception of ziprasidone and aripiprazole) have a tendency to cause significant weight gain. Weight gain is a serious metabolic side effect and is associated with a cascade of additional side effects, including:

- Glucose dysregulation, which increases the propensity for diabetes
- Hypercholesterolemia, which increases the propensity for cardiovascular disease
- Hypertension
- Diminished self-esteem related to weight, which leads to problems in following the medication regimen

An additional disadvantage of the AAPs is that they are more expensive than the traditional antipsychotics. Table 14-8 lists the AAPs, their dosage ranges, some properties of these drugs, and comments.

Conventional (First-Generation) Antipsychotics

The typical antipsychotic agents are becoming much less widely used because of their troubling side effects, although they are being revisited because of the concern over the metabolic side effects of the AAPs. The National Institute of Mental Health has conducted groundbreaking clinical antipsychotic trials of intervention effectiveness (CATIE) studies to compare continuation rates of typical and atypical antipsychotics. Important findings so far are that people quit taking older medications because of side effects, and that they quit taking the newer ones because of weight gain (Lieberman et al., 2005).

Dopamine(D_2) neurotransmission plays a role in psychosis. The conventional antipsychotics are antagonists at the D_2 receptor site in both the limbic and motor centers. This blockage of D_2 receptor sites in the motor areas is responsible for some of the most troubling side effects of the conventional antipsychotics, namely, the **extrapyramidal symptoms (EPS)** of akathisia, dystonia, parkinsonism, and tardive dyskinesia. Other adverse reactions include anticholinergic effects, orthostasis, and lowered seizure threshold.

When these agents are used, the specific drug is often chosen for its side effects profile. For example, chlorpromazine (Thorazine) is the most sedating agent and has fewer EPS than do other antipsychotic agents, but it causes hypotension at large dosages. Haloperidol (Haldol) is the least sedating and is often used in large dosages to reduce assaultive behavior but has a high incidence of EPS. The value of haloperidol for treating violent behaviors is its effectiveness in controlling hallucinatory phenomena with a low incidence of hypotension. People who are functioning at work or at home may prefer less-sedating drugs; patients who are agitated or excitable may do better with a more sedating medication.

All of the traditional antipsychotic drugs can cause tardive dyskinesia, and should be used with caution in people who have seizure disorders because they can lower the seizure threshold. Table 14-9 identifies which drugs are low, medium, and high potency; gives dosages for treatment of acute symptoms and usual maintenance dosages; and lists other considerations.

Tardive dyskinesia (TD) is an EPS that usually appears after prolonged treatment, is more serious, and is not always reversible. Tardive dyskinesia consists of involuntary tonic muscular spasms that typically involve the tongue, fingers, toes, neck, trunk, or pelvis. This potentially serious EPS is most frequently seen in women and older patients, and affects up to 50% of individuals receiving long-term high-dose therapy. Tardive dyskinesia varies from mild to moderate and can be disfiguring or incapacitating.

Early symptoms of tardive dyskinesia are fasciculations of the tongue or constant lip smacking. These early oral movements can develop into uncontrollable biting, chewing, or sucking motions, an open mouth, and lateral movements of the jaw. In many cases, the early symptoms of tardive dyskinesia disappear when the antipsychotic medication is discontinued. In other cases, however, early symptoms are not reversible and may progress. No proven cure for advanced tardive dyskinesia exists. The National Institute of Mental Health developed a brief test for the detection of tardive dyskinesia referred to as the Abnormal Involuntary Movement Scale (AIMS).

Three of the more common EPS are **acute dystonia** (muscle cramps of the head and neck), **akathisia** (internal restlessness and external restless pacing or fidgeting), and **pseudoparkinsonism** (stiffening of muscular activity in the face, body, arms, and legs). The Abnormal Involuntary Movement Scale (AIMS) mentioned in Chapter 5 is one of

TABLE 14-8 Atypical (Second-Generation) Antipsychotic Agents (AAPs)

Drug	Route(s)	Maintenance Dosage Range (mg/Day)	EPS	ACh	OH	Sed	Comments/Notable Adverse Reactions
Clozapine (Clozaril)	Oral PO ODT*: FazaClo	300-900	No	High	High	High	• **Not first line;** refractory cases only • Agranulocytosis in 0.8%-1%; scheduled WBC required • High seizure rate • Significant weight gain (67%) • High lipid abnormalities • Excessive salivation • Tachycardia
Risperidone (Risperdal)	Oral ODT*: Risperdal M-TAB Consta Injectable (long-acting): Risperdal Consta	4-6	Mild	Very low	Moderate	Low	• Hypotension • Insomnia • Sedation • Rarely NMS, TD • Sexual dysfunction • Weight gain (18%) • Moderate lipid abnormalities
Olanzapine (Zyprexa)	Oral ODT*: Zyprexa *Injectable* (short acting)	5-20[†]	Low	Moderate	Moderate	Low	• Significant weight gain (34%) • High lipid abnormalities • Drowsiness • Agitation and restlessness • Insomnia • Possibly akathisia or parkinsonism
Quetiapine (Seroquel)	Oral	300-400[†]	Low	Mild	Moderate	Moderate	• Weight gain (23%) • Moderate lipid abnormalities • Headache • Drowsiness • Orthostasis
Ziprasidone (Geodon)	Oral Injectable (short acting)	80-120	Low	Mild	Mild	Low	• ECG changes[‡] • QT prolongation, not to be used with other drugs known to prolong QT interval • Low propensity for weight gain • No lipid abnormalities • Targets depressive symptoms
Aripiprazole (Abilify)	Oral/liquid IM	10-15	Low	Low-mild	Low-mild	Low	• New class of AAP • Little or no weight gain or increase in glucose, HDL, LDL, or triglyceride levels

*An orally disintegrating tablet (ODT) is a fast-disintegrating tablet or wafer that dissolves on the tongue.
[†]The safety of olanzapine at dosages of >20 mg/day and quetiapine at dosages of >800 mg/day has not been evaluated in clinical trials.
[‡]Ziprasidone use may carry a risk for QT prolongation in patients with preexisting cardiac disease, low electrolyte levels, or family history of QTc syndrome or in patients taking other drugs that cause long QTc profiles.
ACh, Anticholinergic side effects (dry mouth, blurred vision, urinary retention, constipation, agitation); *ECG,* electrocardiogram; *EPS,* extrapyramidal symptoms; *HDL,* high-density lipoprotein; *IM,* intramuscular; *LDL,* low-density lipoprotein; *NMS,* neuroleptic malignant syndrome; *ODT,* orally disintegrating tablet; *OH,* orthostatic hypotension; *PO,* by mouth; *Sed,* sedation; *TD,* tardive dyskinesia; *WBC,* white blood cell count.
Drug dosages from Lehne, R.A. (2007). *Pharmacology for nursing care* (6th ed.). St. Louis: Saunders; Preston, J.D., O'Neal, J.H., & Talaga, M.C. (2005). *Handbook of clinical psychopharmacology for therapists* (4th ed.). Oakland, CA: New Harbinger Publications.

TABLE 14-9   Typical (First-Generation) Antipsychotics

Drug	Route(s) of Administration	Acute Dosage (mg/Day)*	Maintenance Dosage (mg/Day)*	Special Considerations
High Potency				
Haloperidol (Haldol)	PO, IM	5-50	1-15	• Has low sedative properties; is used in large doses for assaultive patients to avoid the severe side effect of hypotension • Appropriate for older adults for the same reason; lessens the chance of falls from dizziness or hypotension • High incidence of extrapyramidal side effects
Haloperidol decanoate (Haldol)	IM, LAI	0	50-250	• Given deep muscle Z-track IM • **Given every 3-4 weeks**
Trifluoperazine (Stelazine)		5-35	5-30	• Low sedative effect—good for symptoms of withdrawal or paranoia • High incidence of extrapyramidal side effects • Neuroleptic malignant syndrome may occur
Fluphenazine (Prolixin)	PO, IM, subQ	5-30	1-15	• Among the least sedating
Fluphenazine decanoate (Prolixin)	IM	0	6.25-50	• Given deep muscle Z-track IM • **Effective when given every 2-4 weeks**
Thiothixene (Navane)	PO, IM	10-60	6-30	• High incidence of akathisia
Medium Potency				
Loxapine (Loxitane)	PO, IM	20-160	10-60	• Possibly associated with weight reduction
Molindone (Moban)	PO	40-225	15-100	• Possibly associated with weight reduction
Perphenazine (Trilafon)	PO, IM, IV	12-64	8-24	• Can help control severe vomiting
Low Potency				
Chlorpromazine (Thorazine)	PO, IM, R	200-1000	50-400	• Increases sensitivity to sun (as do other phenothiazines) • Highest sedative and hypotensive effects; least potent • May cause irreversible retinitis pigmentosa at 800 mg/day
Chlorprothixene (Taractan)	PO, IM	50-600	75-600	• Weight gain common
Thioridazine (Mellaril)	PO	200-800	50-400	• **Not recommended as first-line antipsychotic** • Dose-related severe ECG changes (prolonged QTc intervals), may cause sudden death

Drug dosages from Lehne, R.A. (2007). *Pharmacology for nursing care* (6th ed.). St. Louis: Saunders; Preston, J.D., Oneal, J.H., and Talaga, M.C. (2005). *Handbook for clinical psychopharmacology for therapists* (4th ed.). Oakland, CA: New Harbinger Publications.
*Dosages vary with individual response to the antipsychotic agent used.
IM, Intramuscular; *IV,* intravenous; *PO,* by mouth; *R,* rectal; *LAI,* long-acting injectable; *SubQ,* subcutaneous.

the tools nurses and physicians can use to detect these EPS.

Neuroleptic malignant syndrome (NMS) occurs in about 0.2% to 1% of patients who have taken antipsychotic agents. It is believed that the acute reduction in brain dopamine activity plays a role in the development of NMS, which is fatal in about 10% of cases. It usually occurs early in the course of therapy but has been reported in people after 20 years of treatment.

Neuroleptic malignant syndrome is characterized by decreased level of consciousness, greatly increased muscle tone, and autonomic dysfunction, including hyperpyrexia, labile hypertension, tachycardia, tachypnea, diaphoresis, and drooling. Treatment consists of early detection, discontinuation of the antipsychotic agent, management of fluid balance, reduction of temperature, and monitoring for complications. Mild cases of neuroleptic malignant syndrome are treated with bromocriptine (Parlodel), whereas more severe cases are treated with intravenous dantrolene (Dantrium) and even with electroconvulsive therapy in some cases (Wilkaitis et al., 2004). See Table 14-10 for the side effects, onset, and nursing measures for EPS and NMS.

Agranulocytosis is also a serious side effect and can be fatal. Liver involvement also may occur. Nurses need to be aware of the prodromal signs and symptoms of these side effects and teach them to their patients and patients' families.

Side effects often appear early in therapy and can be minimized with treatment. Treatment usually consists of lowering the dosage or prescribing antiparkinsonian drugs, especially centrally acting anticholinergic drugs. Commonly used drugs include trihexyphenidyl (Artane), benztropine mesylate (Cogentin), diphenhydramine hydrochloride (Benadryl), and amantadine hydrochloride (Symmetrel). However, treatment with antiparkinsonian drugs is not completely benign because the anticholinergic side effects of the antipsychotics may be intensified (e.g., urinary retention, constipation, failure of visual accommodation [blurred vision], cognitive impairment, and delirium).

Most patients develop tolerance to EPS after a few months. Effective nursing and medical management is important to encourage compliance with the medication regimen until the major side effects have been properly managed. Table 14-11 identifies some of the drugs most commonly used for the treatment of EPS.

Adjuncts to Antipsychotic Drug Therapy
Antidepressants
Antidepressants are added to antipsychotics when the symptoms meet the criteria for major depression, are severe, and cause severe distress, including suicidal thoughts or when depression is disabling (APA, 2004).

Other Drugs
Lithium. Lithium and other mood stabilizers help reduce aggressive behavior, but their effectiveness has not been determined adequately (Beng-Choon et al., 2004). The same is true of propranolol and other β-blockers. Randomized controlled studies did not find evidence to support their use as adjunctive treatment in schizophrenia (Beng-Choon et al., 2004).

Benzodiazepines. Benzodiazepine augmentation can improve positive and negative symptoms by about 50%. Use of clonazepam as an adjunct to antipsychotics may diminish anxiety, agitation, and possibly psychosis (Maxmen & Ward, 2002).

EVALUATION

Evaluation is always an important step in the planning of care and is especially important for people who have chronic psychotic disorders. Frequently, outcomes are too ambitious and serve only to discourage patient and staff alike. It is critical for staff to remember that change is a process that occurs over time; for a person diagnosed with schizophrenia, the period may be prolonged.

It is important to schedule regular evaluations for chronically ill patients so that new data can be considered and the patient's problems can be reassessed. Questions to be asked include the following:
- Is the patient not progressing because a more important need is not being met?
- Is the staff using the patient's strengths and interests to achieve the outcomes?
- Are more appropriate interventions available for this patient to facilitate progress?
- If a newer antipsychotic agent is being tried, is there evidence of improvement or a regression in functioning?
- Is the family involved? Are family members supportive? Do they understand the patient's disease and treatment issues?
- Are the patient and family aware of relapse issues (prodromal symptoms of relapse, medication compliance)?
- Are the patient and family hooked up with effective community supports and treatments?

Active staff involvement and interest in the patient's progress communicates concern, help the patient to form and sustain interest, and prevent feelings of helplessness and burnout. Input from the patient can offer valuable information about why a certain desired behavior or situation has not occurred.

TABLE 14-10 Nursing Measures for Extrapyramidal Symptoms and Neuroleptic Malignant Syndrome: Typical (First-Generation) Antipsychotics

Side Effect	Onset	Nursing Measures
Extrapyramidal Symptoms (EPS)		
1. **Pseudoparkinsonism:** masklike facies, stiff and stooped posture, shuffling gait, drooling, tremor, "pill-rolling" phenomenon	5 hours-30 days	1. Alert medical staff. An anticholinergic agent (e.g., trihexyphenidyl [Artane] or benztropine [Cogentin]) may be used.
2. **Acute dystonic reactions:** acute contractions of tongue, face, neck, and back (tongue and jaw first) • **Opisthotonos:** tetanic heightening of entire body, head and belly up • **Oculogyric crisis:** eyes locked upward	1-5 days	2. First choice: diphenhydramine hydrochloride (Benadryl) 25-50 mg IM/IV. Relief occurs in minutes. Second choice: benztropine, 1-2 mg IM/IV. Prevent further dystonias with any anticholinergic agent (see Table 14-11). Experience is very frightening. Take patient to quiet area and stay with him or her until medicated.
3. **Akathisia:** motor inner-driven restlessness (e.g., tapping foot incessantly, rocking forward and backward in chair, shifting weight from side to side)	2 hours-60 days	3. Physician may change antipsychotic agent or give antiparkinsonian agent. Tolerance does not develop to akathisia, but akathisia disappears when neuroleptic is discontinued. Propranolol (Inderal), lorazepam (Ativan), or diazepam (Valium) may be used.

4. **Tardive dyskinesia:**
• **Facial:** protruding and rolling tongue, blowing, smacking, licking, spastic facial distortion, smacking movements
• **Limbs:**
  • **Choreic:** rapid, purposeless, and irregular movements
  • **Athetoid:** slow, complex, and serpentine movements
• **Trunk:** neck and shoulder movements, dramatic hip jerks and rocking, twisting pelvic thrusts
	Months to years	4. No known treatment. Discontinuing the drug does not always relieve symptoms. Possibly 20% of patients taking these drugs for more than 2 years may develop tardive dyskinesia. Nurses and physicians should encourage patients to be screened for tardive dyskinesia at least every 3 months.

Neuroleptic Malignant Syndrome (NMS)		
Somewhat rare, potentially fatal. • **Severe extrapyramidal:** severe muscle rigidity, oculogyric crisis, dysphasia, flexor-extensor posturing, cogwheeling • **Hyperpyrexia:** elevated temperature (>103° F [39° C]) • **Autonomic dysfunction:** hypertension, tachycardia, diaphoresis, incontinence	Can occur in the first week of drug therapy but often occurs later. Rapidly progresses over 2 to 3 days after initial manifestation **Risk factors:** • **Concomitant use of psychotropics** • **Older age** • **Female gender (3 : 2)** • **Presence of a mood disorder (40%)** • **Rapid dose titration**	Stop neuroleptic. Transfer stat to medical unit. Bromocriptine (Parlodel) can relieve muscle rigidity and reduce fever. Dantrolene (Dantrium) may reduce muscle spasms. Cool body to reduce fever. Maintain hydration with oral and IV fluids. Correct electrolyte imbalance. Dysrhythmias should be treated. Small doses of heparin may decrease possibility of pulmonary emboli. Early detection increases patient's chance of survival.

Stat, Immediately.

TABLE 14-11 Treatment of Acute Extrapyramidal Side Effects

Drug	Oral Dose (mg)	Intramuscular or Intravenous Dose (mg)	Chemical Type
Trihexyphenidyl* (Artane)	5-15 in 3 to 4 divided doses	—	ACA
Benztropine mesylate* (Cogentin)	1-4 bid	1-2	ACA
Biperiden* (Akineton)	2 bid or tid	2	ACA
Diphenhydramine hydrochloride (Benadryl)	25-50 tid or qid	10-50	Antihistamine
Bromocriptine mesylate (Parlodel)	2-10 mg q8h	0.02-0.1/hr (per hr)	

*Antiparkinsonian drug.
ACA, Anticholinergic agent (after 1 to 6 months of long-term maintenance antipsychotic therapy, most ACAs can be withdrawn).
Drug dosages from Skidmore-Roth, L. (2008). *Mosby's nursing drug reference* (21st ed.). St. Louis: Mosby; Sadock, B.J., and Sadock, V.A. (2007). *Kaplan and Sadock's synopsis of psychiatry* (10th ed.). Philadelphia: Lippincott Williams & Wilkins.

KEY POINTS TO REMEMBER

• Schizophrenia is a biologically based disease of the brain. It is not one disorder but a group of disorders. Psychotic symptoms in schizophrenia are more pronounced and disruptive than are symptoms found in other disorders. The basic differences are in the degree of severity, withdrawal, alteration in affect, impairment of intellect, and regression.

• Neurochemical (catecholamines and serotonin), genetic, and neuroanatomical findings help explain the symptoms of schizophrenia. However, at present no one theory accounts for all phenomena found in schizophrenic disorders.

• When the nurse works with patients with schizophrenia, four specific groups of symptoms may be evident. No one symptom is found in all cases. The positive, negative, and cognitive symptoms of schizophrenia are three major categories of symptoms. Depression is almost always present.

• The positive symptoms are more florid (hallucinations, delusions, looseness of associations) and respond to antipsychotic drug therapy.

• The negative symptoms (poor social adjustment, lack of motivation, withdrawal) are more debilitating and do not respond as well to antipsychotic therapy.

• The cognitive degree of impairment warrants careful assessment and interventions to increase the person's quality of life and ability to function in the community.

• Comorbid depression needs to be identified and treated to lower the potential for suicide, substance abuse, and relapse.

• Some nursing diagnoses are offered for positive symptoms (delusions and hallucinations), negative symptoms (withdrawal, lack of energy), and some are family focused (see Table 14-4).

• Planning of outcomes proceeds by identifying the phase of schizophrenia and assessing the patient's individual needs based on functional ability and involves identifying short-term and intermediate indicators.

• Interventions for people with schizophrenia include communication guidelines, health teaching and health promotion, milieu management and strategies, psychotherapy, and pharmacological, biological, and integrative therapies.

• Specific communication strategies are necessary when dealing with a patient who is hallucinating, delusional, or paranoid.

• Because antipsychotic medication is essential, the nurse must understand the properties, adverse effects, toxic effects, and dosages of the traditional, atypical, and other medications used to treat schizophrenia. This information must be shared with the patient and family.

CRITICAL THINKING

1. Using Table 14-5, teach a group (study group, co-workers) about the acute and long-term needs of people with schizophrenia. Identify the basic focus and interventions for the different phases.

2. Jamie, a 29-year-old woman, is being discharged in 2 days from the hospital after her first psychotic break (paranoid schizophrenia). Jamie is recently divorced and has been working as a legal secretary, although her work had become erratic, and her suspicious behavior was calling attention to herself at work. Jamie will be discharged in her mother's care until she is able to resume working. Jamie's mother is overwhelmed and asks the nurse how she is going to cope. "Jamie has become so distant, and she always takes things the wrong way. I can hardly say anything to her without her misconstruing everything. She is very mad at me because I called 911 and had her admitted after she told me she was going to get justice back in the world by blowing up evil forces that have been haunting her life and then proceeded to try to run over her ex-husband, thinking he was the devil. She told me there is nothing wrong with her, and I am concerned she won't take her medication once she is discharged. What am I going to do?"

3. Answer the following questions related to the case study just given. It is best if you can discuss and analyze responses to such situations with your classmates or instructor.

A. What are some of the priority concerns that the nurse could address in the hospital setting before Jamie's discharge?

B. How would you explain to Jamie's mother some of the symptoms that Jamie is experiencing? What suggestions could you give her to handle some of her immediate concerns?

C. What issues could you bring up to the staff about Jamie's medication compliance? What would be some ways to deal with this issue?

D. What are some of the community resources that the case manager could contact to help support this family and increase the chances of continuity of care? Identify some useful community referrals that would be supportive for Jamie and her mother. Choose at least three and describe how they could be supportive to this family.

E. What do you think of the prognosis for Jamie? Support your hypothesis with data regarding influences on the course of schizophrenia.

CHAPTER REVIEW

Choose the most appropriate answer.

1. In which of the following situations can the nurse make the assessment that the patient is experiencing auditory hallucinations?
   1. Mrs. D. tells the nurse, "There are worms crawling on my arms and legs."
   2. Ms. E. states, "I have seen the Vorels who are planning to abduct me."
   3. Miss F. mentions, "The food on my plate is poisoned. Take it away immediately."
   4. Mr. G., who is seated by himself, pleads, "I am a good person. Stop shouting those bad things about me."

2. To plan appropriate interventions, the nurse must know that depersonalization and derealization are examples of:
   1. delusions.
   2. hallucinations.
   3. automatic obedience.
   4. personal boundary difficulties.

3. Which symptoms of schizophrenia are most amenable to treatment with both low- and high-potency antipsychotic medications?
   1. Hallucinations and delusions

   2. Lack of motivation and initiative
   3. Inadequate hygiene and grooming
   4. Social withdrawal and isolation

4. A nursing strategy that usually proves helpful when caring for a person with schizophrenia is:
   1. asking directly about hallucinations or asking the patient to describe a delusion he or she is experiencing.
   2. responding to the patient's hallucinations as if they are real.
   3. limiting contact to one or two short interactions daily.
   4. assuming knowledge of what is meant when the patient talks about "they," when "they" are the internal voices that are communicating with the patient during a hallucination.

5. Which nursing diagnosis is universally applicable to patients with schizophrenia?
   1. *Noncompliance*
   2. *Disturbed body image*
   3. *Disturbed thought processes*
   4. *Risk for other-directed violence*

REFERENCES

Addington, J. (2006). *An ounce of prevention: Identifying patients with prodromal symptoms*. Retrieved August 8, 2006, from www.medscap.com/viewprogram/5298_pnt.

American Psychiatric Association (APA). (2000). *Diagnostic and statistical manual of mental disorders (DSM-IV-TR)* (4th ed., text rev.). Washington, DC: Author.

American Psychiatric Association (APA). (2004). *Practice guidelines for the treatment of patients with schizophrenia* (2nd ed.). Washington, DC: Author.

Barnes, M., Lawford, B.R., Burton, S.C., et al. (2006). Smoking and schizophrenia: Is symptoms profile related to smoking and which antipsychotic medication is of benefit in reducing cigarette use? *Australian and New Zealand Journal of Psychiatry, 40*(6-7), 575-680.

Beng-Choon, H., Black, D.W., & Andreasen, N.C. (2004). Schizophrenia and other psychotic disorders. In R.E. Hales & S.C. Yudofsky (Eds.), *Essentials of clinical psychiatry* (2nd ed., p. 200). Washington, DC: American Psychiatric Publishing.

Bramon, E., & Sham, P.C. (2001). The common liability link between schizophrenia and bipolar disorder: A review. *Current Psychiatric Reports, 3*, 332.

Citrome, L. (2002). *Current treatments of agitation and aggression: CME. Medscape clinical update*. Retrieved February 14, 2005, from www.medscape.com/viewprogram/1866.

Cornblatt, B.A. (2005). Prevention and *early intervention for schizophrenia*. Presented at American Psychopathological Association 95th Annual Meeting on Prevention of Mental Illness, March 3-5, 2005, New York, NY. Retrieved August 19, 2006, from www.medscape.com/viewarticle/501648_2.

Evins, A.E., Cather, C., Deckersbach, T. (2005). A double-bind placebo-controlled trial of bupropion sustained-release for smoking cessation in schizophrenia. *Journal of Clinical Psychopharmacology, 25*(3), 218-225 (Abstract).

Gamble, C., & Brennan, G. (2000). Working with families and informed careers. In C. Gamble & G. Brennan (Eds.), *Working with serious mental illness: A manual for clinical practice*. London: Baillière Tindall.

Junginger, J. (1995). Common hallucinations and predictions of dangerousness. *Psychiatric Services, 46*(9), 911.

Kirkpatrick, B., & Tek Chen. (2005). Schizophrenia: Clinical features and psychopathology concepts. In B.J. Sadock & V.A. Sadock (Eds.), *Kaplan and Sadock's comprehensive textbook of psychiatry* (8th ed., vol. I). Philadelphia: Lippincott Williams & Wilkins.

Kuo, I. (2004). *Acute and long-term biological treatment of schizophrenia*. Paper presented at the International Congress of Biological Psychiatry, February 9-13, 2004, Sydney, Australia.

Lewis, M.M., & Lockwood, A. et al. (2005). Prognosis: Review: Longer duration of untreated psychosis is associated with worse outcome in people with first episode psychosis. *Archives of General Psychiatry, 62*, 975-983.

Lieberman, J.A., Stroup, T.S., McEvoy, J.P., et al. (2005). Effectiveness of antipsychotic drugs in patients with chronic schizophrenia. *New England Journal of Medicine, 353*, 1209-1223.

Marder, S.R. (2006). *Long-term effectiveness of antipsychotic therapy and overall patient health*. Retrieved July 27, 2006, from www.medscape.com/viewarticle/507858_10.

Marder, S.R. (2006). Advances in the pharmacological management of negative and positive symptoms: An expert interview with Stephen R. Marder, MD. *Medscape Psychiatry and Mental Health, 11*(1).

Mariani, S. (2004). Origin and neuropathology of schizophrenia. *Medscape Molecular Medicine, 6*(1).

Maxmen, J.S., & Ward, N.G. (2002). *Psychotropic drugs: Fast facts* (2nd ed.). New York: Norton.

MMDT. (2002). *The Merck manual of diagnosis and therapy schizophrenia*. Retrieved August 30, 2006, from www.merck.com/mrkshared/mmmanual/section15/chapter193/1936.jsp.

Mills, J. (2000). Dealing with voices and strange thoughts. In C. Gamble & G. Brennan (Eds.), *Working with serious mental illness: A manual for clinical practice*. London: Baillière Tindall.

Moller, M.D. (1989). Understanding and communicating with an individual who is hallucinating [Videotape]. Omaha, NE: NurScience.

Moller, M.D., & Murphy, M.F. (2002). *Recovering from psychosis: A wellness approach* (15th ed.). Nine Mile Falls, WA: Psychiatric Resource Network.

Patel, J.K., Pinals, D.A., & Breier, A. (2003). Schizophrenia and other psychoses. In A. Tasman, J. Kay, & J.A. Lieberman (Eds.), *Psychiatry* (2nd ed.). West Sussex, England: Wiley.

Perkins, D.O., Johnson, J.L., Hamer, R.M., et al. (2006). Predictors of antipsychotic medication adherence in patients recovering from a first psychotic episode. *Schizophrenia Research, 83*(1), 53-63 (Abstract).

Tandon, R., Stuck, Z.G., Kujawa, M.J., et al. (2003). *Beyond symptoms control: Moving towards positive patient outcomes*. Paper presented at the American Psychiatric Association 55th Institute on Psychiatric Services, October 31, 2003, Boston. Retrieved January 21, 2005, from www.medscape.com/viewprogram/2835.

Tsung-Ung, W.W., Zimmer, S.V., Wojeik, J.D., et al. (2004). Treatment of schizophrenia. In A.F. Schatzberg & C.B. Nemeroff (Eds.), *The American Psychiatric Publishing textbook of psychopharmacology* (3rd ed., pp. 885-912). Washington, DC: American Psychiatric Publishing.

U.S. Department of Health and Human Services (USDHHS). (1999). *Mental health: A report of the Surgeon General*. Rockville, MD: U.S. Department of Health and Human Services, Center for Mental Health Services, National Institutes of Health.

Vidal, G. (1982). *The second American revolution and other essays (1976-1982)*. New York: Random House.

Wilkaitis, J., Mulvihill, T., & Nasrallah, H.A. (2004). In A.F. Schatzberg & C.B. Nemeroff (Eds.), *The American Psychiatric Publishing textbook of psychopharmacology* (3rd ed., pp. 437-438). Washington, DC: American Psychiatric Publishing.

CHAPTER 15

Cognitive Disorders

Elizabeth M. Varcarolis

Key Terms and Concepts

Objectives

1. Compare and contrast the clinical pictures of delirium and dementia.
2. Discuss the critical needs of a patient with delirium.
3. Summarize interventions appropriate for a patient with delirium.
4. Compare and contrast the signs and symptoms occurring in the four stages of Alzheimer's disease (AD).
5. Understand important aspects of caring for a patient with AD, including guidelines for (a) communication, (b) health maintenance, and (c) safe environment.
6. Identify at least five different types of community services and five different types of in-home services that a family might use to care for their member with AD.

evolve

For additional resources related to the content of this chapter, visit the Evolve website at http://evolve.elsevier.com/Varcarolis/essentials.

- Chapter Outline
- Chapter Review Answers
- Case Studies and Nursing Care Plans

- Nurse, Patient, and Family Resources
- Concept Map Creator

Edited by Charlotte Eliopoulos and Verna Benner Carson in the fifth edition of *Foundations of Psychiatric Mental Health Nursing*.

Cognitive processing has a direct relationship to activities of daily living. Although primarily an intellectual and perceptual process, cognition is closely integrated with an individual's emotional and spiritual values. When human beings can no longer understand facts or connect the appropriate feelings to events, they have trouble responding to the complexity of life's challenges.

There are three main **cognitive disorders:** delirium, dementia, and amnesic disorder. Cognitive disorder not otherwise specified is a category defined by the *Diagnostic and Statistical Manual of Mental Disorders (DSM-IV-TR)* that allows for the diagnosis of cognitive disorders that do not meet the criteria for delirium, dementia, or amnesic disorders (APA, 2000). Cognitive disorders not otherwise specified are presumed to be caused by a specific medical condition, a pharmacologically active agent, or possibly both.

PREVALENCE AND COMORBIDITY

Delirium "is characterized by a disturbance of consciousness and a change in cognition such as impaired attention span and disturbances of consciousness, that develop over a short period" (APA, 2000, p. 135). Delirium is always **secondary** to another condition, such as a general medical condition or substance use (drugs of abuse, a medication, or toxin exposure), or it may have multiple causes. It is a transient disorder, and if the underlying medical cause is corrected, complete recovery should occur.

Delirium, one of the most commonly encountered medical disorders in medical practice, is often overlooked or misdiagnosed. It is a significant risk for all hospitalized and older medically ill people. Delirium is present in up to 60% of nursing home residents 75 years or older at any one time, and up to 80% of people with a terminal illness develop delirium near death (APA 2000).

Dementia usually develops more slowly and is characterized by multiple cognitive deficits that include impairment in memory without impairment in consciousness. More than 80% of dementias are irreversible; those dementias that have a reversible component are **secondary** to other pathological processes (e.g., neoplasms, trauma, infections, and toxin exposure). When the underlying causes are treated, the dementia often improves. However, most dementias, such as dementias of the Alzheimer type, are related to a **primary** encephalopathy. Alzheimer's disease (AD) accounts for 60% to 80% of all dementias in the United States and is the fourth leading cause of death in adults. The average lifetime prevalence of Alzheimer's disease is about 5% by age 65, and up to 50% by age 85.

Primary dementia has no known cause or cure; thus, it is progressive and irreversible.

Amnestic disorder is characterized by loss in both short-term memory (including the inability to learn information) and long-term memory, sufficient to cause some impairment in the person's functioning. This memory impairment exists in the absence of other significant cognitive impairments. These amnestic disorders are always **secondary** to underlying causes and are classified, for example, as general medical condition, substance induced; persistent amnestic disorder; and amnestic disorder not otherwise specified.

THEORY
Alzheimer's Disease

As yet, a single cause of AD has not been identified. Most likely, several genetic and nongenetic factors—that affect each person differently—may interact to cause AD.

Age
Age seems to be the most important risk factor for AD. The number of people with the disease doubles for every 5 years beyond age 65.

Genetic Findings
Early-onset familial AD, a rare form of the disease, occurs between the ages of 30 and 60 and seems to be inherited. *Late-onset AD,* the more well-known form, occurs later in life. No obvious inheritance pattern is seen in most families (ADEAR, 2006). The only risk factor gene is a gene that makes protein, **apolipoprotein E (ApoE)**, on chromosome 19. Everyone has this gene that helps carry cholesterol in the blood and is possibly involved in neuronal repair. However, 15% of the population has a form of ApoE that increases the risk of AD (ADEAR, 2006). The ApoE gene does not by itself cause AD, so again there are many other factors involved. Likely, there are many other genes that either increase or decrease one's risk, but they are not presently known.

CULTURAL CONSIDERATIONS

AD is not affected by ethnicity, and all caregivers must learn to cope with the same kinds of behaviors (e.g., wandering, lack of sleep, incontinence, and possibly aggression). However, attitudes and perceptions of such behaviors can vary greatly among cultural groups. Strong's study (1984) found that the emotions of frustration, anger, guilt, anxiety, and conflict were closely tied to the cultural value put on the ability to maintain control.

EXAMINING THE EVIDENCE   Dementia and Reality Orientation

Last semester I was assigned to a 79-year-old woman with Alzheimer's disease. She thought that it was 1954 and that her deceased husband would soon be returning from work. She was so excited as she awaited his arrival. I didn't tell her the truth—was this wrong of me?

According to the NANDA International (2007), an appropriate nursing diagnosis for your patient would have been *Chronic confusion*. A standard and accepted intervention for disorientation is to periodically orient the patient to the environment. Related interventions for confused or delusional thoughts are (1) don't argue with the patient, and (2) focus on underlying feelings rather than the specific content of the delusion. You were in a position in which reorienting would have challenged the assertion that it was indeed 1954.

So what do the experts say? Let's take a look at the literature on reality orientation. Spector and colleagues (2000) conducted a systematic review of 43 studies and found that reorienting dementia sufferers was effective in both increasing mental acuity and on behavior. After another systematic literature review, Bates and associates (2004) concluded that reality orientation was helpful in early stages of dementia, but may lose value as mental deterioration progresses.

Surprisingly, some researchers do not support the use of reality orientation. Livingston and co-workers (2005) reviewed the literature and noted that reality orientation was ineffective compared with actively engaging patients on the ward. This group went so far as to award reality orientation with a failing grade of D.

So where does this leave you? First you need to exercise professional judgment, which includes not only weighing the evidence but also using intuition and feelings. Although, as a general rule, reality orientation may be a good intervention at best, and harmless at least, there was nothing to be gained by dashing your patient's hopes. In fact, Boccardi and Frisoni (2006) indicate that impaired memory may actually be a helpful defense against painful realities. They would consider your response to be ethically sound and directed at her well-being.

Bates, J., Boote, J., & Beverley, C. (2004). Psychosocial interventions for people with a milder dementing illness: a systematic review. *Journal of Advanced Nursing, 45,* 644-658.

Boccardi, M., & Frisoni, G.B. (2006). Cognitive rehabilitation for severe dementia: Critical observations for better use of existing knowledge. *Mechanisms of Ageing and Development, 127*(2), 166-172.

Livingston, G., Johnston, K., Katona, C., et al. (2005). Systematic review of psychological approaches to the management of neuropsychiatric symptoms of dementia. *American Journal of Psychiatry, 162,* 1996-2021.

North American Nursing Diagnosis Association International (NANDA-I). (2007). *Nursing diagnoses: Definitions and classification 2007-2008.* Philadelphia: Author.

Spector, A., Davies, S., Woods, B., & Orrell, M. (2000). Reality orientation for dementia: A systematic review of the evidence of effectiveness from randomized controlled trials. *The Gerontologist, 40,* 206-212.

The study showed that people from Native American cultures were more likely to accept their lack of control over the situation. Therefore they were far more likely to respond to their family members' situation with a sense of *loss* that life with their loved one, and life as their loved one knew it, was gone forever. This was in direct contrast to the white respondents who believed they should be able to alter or influence the situation and were more apt to feel anger, guilt, anxiety, and conflict over not being able to do so.

Health care workers who are able to assess and understand the cultural aspects of caregiving behaviors may be able to offer services and training that are more congruent with the caregiver's culture (USGPO, 1992). Health care workers have a long way to go to become more proficient in understanding the nuances of culture and how it relates to the quality of care that patients and families may ultimately accept. The issue is complicated by the fact that patients and families from a minority group may be composed of many different subcultural groups. A good example is the Hispanic population, which shares Spanish as a language; however, Hispanics comprise Mexicans, Cubans, Puerto Ricans, Salvadorans, and Nicaraguans, who all come from very distinct cultural backgrounds (USGPO, 1992).

CLINICAL PICTURE

Figure 15-1 identifies the three main cognitive disorders and gives the *DSM-IV-TR* criteria for each. This chapter addresses the broad categories of delirium and dementia because these are by far the most common conditions that nurses encounter.

Delirium

Nurses frequently encounter delirium on medical and surgical units in the general hospital setting. During certain phases of a hospital stay, confusion may be noted (e.g., after surgery or after the introduction of a new drug). The second or third hospital day may herald the onset of confusion and difficulty adjusting to an unfamiliar environment.

DSM-IV-TR CRITERIA FOR COGNITIVE DISORDERS

COGNITIVE DISORDERS

Delirium

A. Disturbance of consciousness (i.e., reduced clarity of awareness of the environment with reduced ability to focus, sustain, or shift attention).

B. A change in cognition (memory deficit, disorientation, language disturbance) or the development of a perceptual disturbance that is not better accounted for by a preexisting, established, or evolving dementia.

C. The disturbance develops over a short period of time (usually hours to days) and tends to fluctuate during the course of the day.

Due to:

1. A general medical condition
   or
2. Substance-induced (intoxication or withdrawal)
   or
3. Multiple etiologies (both 1 and 2 above)
   or
4. Not known (not otherwise specified)

Amnestic Disorder

A. The development of memory impairment as manifested by impairment in the ability to learn new information or the ability to recall previously learned information.

B. The memory disturbance causes significant impairment in social or occupational functioning and represents a significant decline from a previous level of functioning.

C. The memory disturbance does not occur exclusively during the course of a delirium or a dementia.

Dementia

A. The development of multiple cognitive deficits manifested by both:

1. **Memory impairment** (impaired ability to learn new information or to recall previously learned information).

2. One (or more) of the following cognitive disturbances:
   (a) **Aphasia** (language disturbance)
   (b) **Apraxia** (impaired ability to carry out motor activities despite intact motor function)
   (c) **Agnosia** (failure to recognize or identify objects despite intact sensory function)
   (d) Disturbance in executive functioning (i.e., planning, organizing, sequencing, abstracting)

B. The cognitive deficits in criteria A1 and A2 each cause significant impairment in social or occupational functioning and represent a significant decline from a previous level of functioning.

Figure 15-1 ▪ Diagnostic criteria for delirium, dementia, and amnestic disorder. (Adapted from American Psychiatric Association. [2000]. Diagnostic and statistical manual of mental disorders [4th ed., text rev.]. Washington, DC: Author.)

Delirium occurs more frequently in older patients. Surgery, drugs, urinary tract infections, pneumonia, cerebrovascular disease, and congestive heart failure are some of the most common causes. Delirium is also commonly seen in children with fever and in terminally ill patients.

A delayed or missed diagnosis can have serious implications because the longer a condition goes untreated, the greater the risk that the condition can cause permanent damage. Depression often masquerades as dementia, and can even co-occur with dementia; therefore a clear definition of the three can be useful during assessment. Table 15-1 offers some guidelines for distinguishing among delirium, depression, and dementia.

The essential feature of delirium is a disturbance in consciousness coupled with cognitive difficulties. Thinking, memory, attention, and perception are typically disturbed. The clinical manifestations of delirium develop over a short period (hours to days) and tend to fluctuate during the course of the day. **Sundown syndrome,** in which symptoms and problem behaviors become more pronounced in the evening, may occur in both delirium and dementia.

Because delirium increases psychological stress, supportive interventions that lower anxiety and promote calm and security can foster a sense of control. Patients with delirium may appear withdrawn, agitated, or psychotic. Also, underlying personality traits often become exaggerated. For example, a person can become more paranoid or display more disinhibition.

Box 15-1 lists common causes of delirium. Nursing interventions center on the following:

TABLE 15-1	**Comparison of Delirium, Dementia, and Depression**		
	Delirium	**Dementia**	**Depression**
Onset	Sudden, over hours to days	Slowly, over months	May have been gradual with exacerbation during crisis or stress
Cause or contributing factors	Hypoglycemia, fever, dehydration, hypotension; infection, other conditions that disrupt body's homeostasis; adverse drug reaction; head injury; change in environment (e.g., hospitalization); pain; emotional stress	Alzheimer's disease, vascular disease, human immunodeficiency virus infection, neurological disease, chronic alcoholism, head trauma	Lifelong history, losses, loneliness, crises, declining health, medical conditions
Cognition	Impaired memory, judgment, calculations, attention span; can fluctuate through the day	Impaired memory, judgment, calculations, attention span, abstract thinking; agnosia	Difficulty concentrating, forgetfulness, inattention
Level of consciousness	Altered	Not altered	Not altered
Activity level	Can be increased or reduced; restlessness, behaviors may worsen in evening (sundown syndrome); sleep-wake cycle may be reversed	Not altered; behaviors may worsen in evening (sundown syndrome)	Usually decreased; lethargy, fatigue, lack of motivation; may sleep poorly and awaken in early morning
Emotional state	Rapid swings; can be fearful, anxious, suspicious, aggressive, have hallucinations and/or delusions	Flat; delusions	Extreme sadness, apathy, irritability, anxiety, paranoid ideation
Speech and language	Rapid, inappropriate, incoherent, rambling	Incoherent, slow (sometimes due to effort to find the right word), inappropriate, rambling, repetitious	Slow, flat, low
Prognosis	Reversible with proper and timely treatment	Not reversible; progressive	Reversible with proper and timely treatment

- Performing a comprehensive nursing assessment to aid in identifying the cause
- Preventing physical harm as a result of confusion, aggression, or electrolyte and fluid imbalance
- Using supportive measures to relieve distress

Dementia

Severe memory loss is *not* a normal part of growing older. Slight forgetfulness is a common phenomenon of the aging process (age-associated memory loss), but not memory loss that interferes with one's activities of daily living. Most people who live to a very old age never experience a significant memory loss or any other symptom of dementia. Most of us know of people in their 80s and 90s who lead active lives, with the intellect intact. Margaret Mead, Pablo Picasso, Duke Ellington, Count Basie, Ansel Adams, Sonny Coles, and George Burns are all examples of people who

were still active in their careers when they died; all were older than 75 years of age (Picasso was 91; George Burns was 100). The slow, mild cognitive changes associated with aging should not impede social or occupational functioning.

Dementia, on the other hand, is marked by progressive deterioration in intellectual functioning, memory, and the ability to solve problems and learn new skills; a decline in the ability to perform activities of daily living; and a progressive deterioration of personality accompanied by impairment in judgment. A person's declining intellect often leads to emotional changes—such as mood lability, depression, and aggressive acting out—and neurological changes that produce hallucinations and delusions. There are several types of dementia, including dementia of the Alzheimer's type, vascular dementia, Lewy body disease, Pick's disease, Huntington's chorea, alcohol-related dementias (including Korsakoff's syndrome), Creutzfeldt-Jakob disease, and the

BOX 15-1

Common Causes of Delirium

Postoperative states

Drug intoxications and withdrawals
- Alcohol, anxiolytics, opioids, and central nervous system stimulants (e.g., cocaine and crack cocaine)

Infections
- Systemic: pneumonia, typhoid fever, malaria, urinary tract infection, and septicemia
- Intracranial: meningitis and encephalitis

Metabolic disorders
- Dehydration
- Hypoxia (pulmonary disease, heart disease, and anemia)
- Hypoglycemia
- Sodium, potassium, calcium, magnesium, and acid-base imbalances
- Hepatic encephalopathy or uremic encephalopathy
- Thiamine (vitamin B_1) deficiency (Wernicke's encephalopathy)
- Endocrine disorders (e.g., thyroidism or parathyroidism)
- Hypothermia or hyperthermia
- Diabetic acidosis

Drugs
- Digitalis, steroids, lithium, levodopa, anticholinergics, benzodiazepines, central nervous system depressants, tricyclic antidepressants
- Central anticholinergic syndrome as a result of using multiple drugs with anticholinergic side effects

Neurological diseases
- Seizures
- Head trauma
- Hypertensive encephalopathy

Tumor
- Primary cerebral

Psychosocial stressors
- Relocation or other sudden changes
- Sensory deprivation or overload
- Sleep deprivation
- Immobilization
- Pain

---

dementias associated with Parkinson's disease, acquired immunodeficiency syndrome (AIDS), and head trauma.

Dementias all present with common symptoms, although they may have different etiologies. Therefore care of everyone with dementia is similar. Because AD is by far the most common form of dementia, it will be used here for the prototype of caring for a patient with dementia.

Secondary Dementia

Secondary dementia occurs as a result of some other pathological process (e.g., vascular, metabolic, nutritional, or neurological). AIDS-related dementia (human immunodeficiency virus [HIV] encephalopathy) is an example of a secondary dementia. It occurs in as many as 40% of individuals with HIV. Other secondary dementias can result from viral encephalitis, pernicious anemia, folic acid deficiency, and hypothyroidism. Korsakoff's syndrome is an example of a secondary dementia and is caused by thiamine (vitamin B_1) deficiency, which may be associated with prolonged, heavy alcohol ingestion (see Chapter 16).

Alzheimer's Disease

Alzheimer's disease (AD) is a complex disease that begins to damage the brain long before the symptoms appear. Scientists believe that the disease begins with the buildup of beta amyloid protein, resulting in neuritic plaques. **Neuritic plaques** are cores of degenerated neuron material that

lie free of the cell bodies on the ground substances of the brain. The quantity of plaques has been correlated with the degree of mental deterioration.

Another abnormality found in the brains of people with Alzheimer's is **neurofibrillary tangles,** which are the damaged remains of microtubules that allow the flow of nutrients through the neurons. Theses neurofibrillary tangles form in the hippocampus, which is the part of the brain responsible for recent (short-term) memory.

Granulovascular degeneration is another active process in the disease and it results in the filling of brain cells with fluid and granular material. Increased degeneration accounts for increased loss of mental function. **Brain atrophy** is observable with wider cortical sulci and enlarged cerebral ventricles, as demonstrated by computed tomography (CT) and magnetic resonance imaging (MRI) scans. Imaging techniques reveal significant loss of cells and volume in the regions of the brain devoted to memory and higher mental functioning.

evolve

For a comprehensive case study and associated nursing care plans for a patient experiencing cognitive impairment related to Alzheimer's disease, visit the Evolve website at http://evolve. elsevier.com/Varcarolis/essentials.

Application of the Nursing Process: Delirium

ASSESSMENT

Generally the nurse suspects the presence of delirium when a patient abruptly develops a disturbance in consciousness that is manifested in reduced clarity of awareness of the environment. The person may have difficulty with orientation—first to time, then to place, and last to person. For example, a man with delirium may think that the year is 1972, that the hospital is home, and that the nurse is his wife. Orientation to person is usually intact to the extent that the person is aware of self-identity. The ability to focus, sustain, or shift attention is impaired. Questions need to be repeated because the individual's attention wanders, and the person might easily get off track and need to be refocused. Conversation is made more difficult because the person may be easily distracted by irrelevant stimuli.

Fluctuating levels of consciousness are unpredictable. Disorientation and confusion are usually markedly worse at night and during the early morning. In fact, some patients may be confused or delirious only at night and may remain lucid during the day. Some clinicians use the Mini-Mental State Examination to screen or follow the progress of an individual with delirium. Nursing assessment includes (1) cognitive and perceptual disturbances, (2) physical needs, and (3) mood and behavior.

Cognitive and Perceptual Disturbances

It may be difficult to engage patients in conversation while they are delirious because they are easily distracted, display marked attention deficits, and memory is impaired. In mild delirium, memory deficits are noted on careful questioning. In more severe delirium, memory problems usually take the form of obvious difficulty in processing and remembering recent events. For example, the person might ask when a son is coming to visit, even though the son left only an hour earlier. Perceptual disturbances are also common. Perception is the processing of information about one's internal and external environment. Various misinterpretations of reality may take the form of illusions or hallucinations.

Illusions are errors in perception of sensory stimuli. For example, a person may mistake folds in the bedclothes for white rats or the cord of a window blind for a snake. The stimulus is a real object in the environment; however, it is misinterpreted and often becomes the object of the patient's projected fear. Illusions, unlike delusions or hallucinations, can be explained and clarified for the individual.

Hallucinations are false sensory stimuli (see Chapter 14 for guidelines in dealing with hallucinations). *Visual* hallucinations are common in delirium. *Tactile* hallucinations may also be present. For example, delirious individuals may become terrified when they "see" giant spiders crawling over the bedclothes or "feel" bugs crawling on their bodies. Auditory hallucinations occur more often in other psychiatric disorders, such as schizophrenia and psychotic depression.

The delirious individual generally has an awareness that something is very wrong. For example, the delirious person may state, "My thoughts are all jumbled." When perceptual disturbances are present, the emotional response is one of fear and anxiety. Verbal and psychomotor signs of agitation should be noted.

Physical Needs

Physical Safety

A person with delirium becomes disoriented and may try to "go home." Alternatively, a person may think that he or she *is* home and may jump out of a window in an attempt to get away from "invaders." Wandering, pulling out intravenous lines and Foley catheters, and falling out of bed are common dangers that require nursing intervention.

An individual experiencing delirium has difficulty processing stimuli in the environment. Confusion magnifies the inability to recognize reality. The physical environment should be made as simple and as clear as possible. Objects such as clocks and calendars can maximize orientation to time. Eyeglasses, hearing aids, and adequate lighting without glare can maximize the person's ability to interpret more accurately what is going on in the environment. The nurse should interact with the patient whenever the patient is awake. Short periods of social interaction help reduce anxiety and misperceptions.

Biophysical Safety

Autonomic signs, such as tachycardia, sweating, flushed face, dilated pupils, and elevated blood pressure, are often present. These changes must be monitored and documented carefully and may require immediate medical attention.

Changes in the sleep-wake cycle usually are noted, and in some cases, a complete reversal of the night-day sleep-wake cycle can occur. The patient's level of consciousness may range from lethargy to stupor or from semicoma to hypervigilance. In **hypervigilance,** patients are extraordinarily alert and their eyes constantly scan the room; they may have difficulty falling asleep or may be actively disoriented and agitated throughout the night.

It is also important that the nurse assess all medications because the nurse is in a position to recognize drug reactions or potential interactions before delirium actually occurs.

Moods and Physical Behaviors

The delirious individual's behavior and mood may change dramatically within a short period. Moods may swing back and forth from fear, anger, and anxiety to euphoria, depression, and apathy. These labile moods are often accompanied by physical behaviors associated with feeling states. A person may strike out from fear or anger or may cry, call for help, curse, moan, and tear off clothing one minute and become apathetic or laugh uncontrollably the next. In short, behavior and emotions are erratic and fluctuating. Lack of concentration and disorientation complicate interventions. The following vignette illustrates the fear and confusion a patient may experience when admitted to an intensive care unit (ICU). Read the following and analyze the nurse's approach.

VIGNETTE

A 55-year-old married man, Mr. Arnold, is admitted to the ICU after having a three-vessel coronary artery bypass. Mr. Arnold's surgery took longer than usual and has necessitated his remaining on a cardiac pump for 3 hours. He arrives in the ICU without further complications. On awakening from the anesthesia, he hears the nurse exclaim, "I need to get a gas." Another nurse answers in a loud voice, "Can you take a large needle for the injection?" During this period, Mr. Arnold experiences the need to urinate and asks the nurse very calmly if he can go to the bathroom. Her reply is, "You don't need to go; you have a tube in." He again complains about his discomfort and assures the nurse that if she will let him go to the bathroom, he will be fine. The nurse informs Mr. Arnold that he cannot urinate and that he has to keep the "mask" on so that she can get the "gas" and check his "blood levels." On hearing this, Mr. Arnold begins to implore more loudly and states that he sees the bathroom sign. He assures the nurse that he will only take a minute. In reality, the sign is an exit sign.

To prove to him that a bathroom does not exist in the ICU and that the sign does not indicate a bathroom, the nurse takes off the restraints so that his head can be raised to see the sign. He abruptly breaks away from the nurse's grasp and runs toward the entrance to the ICU. He discovers a door, which is the entrance to the nurses' lounge, barricades himself in the room, and pulls out his chest tube, Foley catheter, and intravenous lines. He finds the bathroom that is connected to the lounge. Ten minutes later, the nurses and security personnel break through the barricade and escort Mr. Arnold back to bed.

When he becomes fully alert and oriented a day later, Mr. Arnold tells the nurses his perception of the previous day's events. Initially, he had thought he had been kidnapped and was being held against his will (the restraints had been tight). When the nurse yelled out about blood gas, he had thought she was going to kill him with noxious gas through his face mask (the reason he did not want to wear the face mask). All he could think about was escaping his tormentor and executioner. In this case, the nurse had not assessed the alteration in Mr. Arnold's mental status and allowed him to get out of bed. The medical jargon and loud voices had perpetuated his confusion and distortion of reality.

The nurses could have told Mr. Arnold where he was and that the nursing staff was caring for him; they could have better explained the function of his Foley catheter. What else could the nurses have done to help orient and comfort Mr. Arnold?

Assessment Guidelines

Delirium

1. Assess for fluctuating levels of consciousness, which is key in delirium.
2. Interview family or other caregivers to establish the patient's normal level of consciousness and cognition.
3. Assess for past confusional states (e.g., prior dementia diagnosis).
4. Identify other disturbances in medical status (e.g., infection, dyspnea, edema, presence of jaundice).
5. Identify any electroencephalographic, neuroimaging, or laboratory abnormalities documented in the patient's record.
6. Assess vital signs, level of consciousness, and neurological signs.
7. Assess potential for injury (is the patient safe from falls, wandering?).
8. Assess the need for comfort measures (e.g., to address pain or cold, improve positioning).
9. Monitor factors that worsen or improve symptoms.
10. Assess for availability of immediate medical interventions to help prevent irreversible brain damage.
11. Remain nonjudgmental. Confer with other staff readily when questions arise.

DIAGNOSIS

Safety needs play a substantial role in nursing care. If fever and dehydration are present, fluid and electrolyte balance will need to be managed. If the underlying cause of the patient's delirium results in fever, decreased skin turgor,

TABLE 15-2	Potential Nursing Diagnoses for the Confused Patient

Symptoms	Nursing Diagnoses
Wanders, has unsteady gait, acts out fear from hallucinations or illusions, forgets things (leaves stove on, doors open)	*Risk for injury*
Awake and disoriented during the night *(sundown syndrome),* frightened at night	*Disturbed sleep pattern* *Fear* *Acute confusion*
Too confused to take care of basic needs	*Self-care deficit (specify)* *Ineffective coping* *Functional urinary incontinence* *Imbalanced nutrition: less than body requirements* *Deficient fluid volume*
Sees frightening things that are not there *(hallucinations),* mistakes everyday objects for something sinister and frightening *(illusions),* may become paranoid and think that others are doing things to confuse him or her *(delusions)*	*Disturbed sensory perception* *Impaired environmental interpretation syndrome* *Disturbed thought processes*
Does not recognize familiar people or places, has difficulty with short- and/or long-term memory, forgetful and confused	*Impaired memory* *Impaired environmental interpretation syndrome* *Acute* or *Chronic confusion*
Has difficulty with communication, cannot find words, has difficulty in recognizing objects and/or people, incoherent	*Impaired verbal communication*
Devastated over losing place in life as known (during lucid moments), fearful and overwhelmed by what is happening to him or her	*Spiritual distress* *Hopelessness* *Situational low self-esteem* *Grieving*
Family and loved ones overburdened and overwhelmed, unable to care for patient's needs	*Disabled family coping* *Interrupted family processes* *Impaired home maintenance* *Caregiver role strain*

decreased urinary output or fluid intake, and dry skin or mucous membranes, then the nursing diagnosis of *Deficient fluid volume* is appropriate.

Any condition that alters brain activity including metabolic imbalances, infections, altered sleep, substance abuse, and medication use can be viewed as a *Risk for acute confusion.* Perceptions are disturbed during delirium and may be acted on by the patient. For example, if feeling threatened or thinking that common medical equipment is harmful, the patient may pull off an oxygen mask, pull out an intravenous or nasogastric tube, or try to flee. Hallucinations, distractibility, illusions, disorientation, agitation, restlessness, and/or misperception are major aspects of the clinical picture. When some of these symptoms are present, *Risk for injury, Fear,* or *Acute confusion* are an appropriate nursing diagnoses.

Because sleep-wake cycle may be disrupted, the patient may be less responsive during the day and may become disruptively wakeful during the night. Therefore, *Disturbed*

sleep pattern related to impaired cerebral oxygenation or disruption in consciousness is a likely diagnosis.

Sustaining communication with a delirious patient is difficult. *Impaired verbal communication* related to cerebral hypoxia or decreased cerebral blood flow, as evidenced by confusion or clouding of consciousness may be diagnosed.

Other nursing diagnoses include *Self-care deficit, Disturbed thought processes,* and *Impaired social interaction.* Table 15-2 identifies nursing diagnoses for any confused patient (delirium or dementia).

OUTCOMES IDENTIFICATION

The overall outcome is that the delirious patient will return to the premorbid level of functioning.

Although the patient can demonstrate a wide variety of needs, *Risk for injury* is always present. Appropriate outcomes are as follows:

- Patient will remain safe and free from injury while in the hospital.
- During periods of lucidity, patient will be oriented to time, place, and person with the aid of nursing interventions, such as the provision of clocks, calendars, maps, and other types of orienting information.
- Patient will remain free from falls and injury while confused with the aid of nursing safety measures throughout hospital stay.
- Patient's tubes (nasogastric [NG], intravenous [IV], O₂, etc.) will remain in place with aid of nurse, family, and/or prn medication.

Because levels of consciousness can change throughout the day, the patient needs to be checked for orientation (time, place, and person) frequently during different times of the day.

IMPLEMENTATION

Medical management of delirium involves treating the underlying organic causes. If the underlying cause of delirium is not treated, permanent brain damage may result. Judicious use of antipsychotic or antianxiety agents may also be useful in controlling behavioral symptoms.

A patient in acute delirium should never be left alone. Because most hospitals and health facilities are unable to provide one-to-one supervision of the patient, family members can be encouraged to stay with the patient. Refer to Table 15-3 for guidelines in caring for a patient with delirium.

EVALUATION

Long-term outcome criteria for a person with delirium include the following:

- Patient will remain safe.
- Patient will be oriented to time, place, and person by discharge.
- Underlying cause will be treated and ameliorated.

However, the short-term goals need constant assessment. Are the vital signs stable? Is the patient's skin turgor and urine specific gravity within normal limits?

Application of the Nursing Process: Dementia

ASSESSMENT

AD is commonly characterized by progressive deterioration of cognitive functioning. Initially, deterioration may be so subtle and insidious that others may not notice. In the early stages of the disease, the affected person may be able to

compensate for loss of memory. Some people may have superior social graces and charm that give them the ability to hide severe deficits in memory, even from experienced health care professionals. This hiding is actually a form of **denial,** which is an unconscious protective defense against the terrifying reality of losing one's place in the world. Family members may also unconsciously deny that anything is wrong as a defense against the painful awareness that a loved one is deteriorating. As time goes on, symptoms become more obvious, and other defensive maneuvers become evident.

Another defense mechanism is **confabulation,** the making up of stories or answers to maintain self-esteem when the person does not remember. For example, the nurse addresses a patient who has remained in a hospital bed all weekend:

Nurse: "Good morning, Ms. Jones. How was your weekend?"
Patient: "Wonderful. I discussed politics with the President, and he took me out to dinner."
or
Patient: "I spent the weekend with my daughter and her family." *(less grandiose)*

Confabulation is not the same as lying. When people are lying, they are aware of making up an answer; confabulation is an **unconscious** attempt to maintain self-esteem.

Perseveration (the repetition of phrases or behavior) is eventually seen and is often intensified under stress. The avoidance of answering questions is another mechanism by which the patient is able to maintain self-esteem unconsciously in the face of severe memory deficits. Therefore, (1) denial, (2) confabulation, (3) perseveration, and (4) avoidance of questions are four defensive behaviors the nurse might notice during assessment.

Cardinal symptoms observed in AD are the following (APA, 2000):

- **Amnesia or memory impairment.** Initially, the person has difficulty remembering recent events. Gradually, deterioration progresses to include both recent and remote memory.
- **Aphasia** (loss of language ability), which progresses with the disease. Initially, the person has difficulty finding the correct word, then is reduced to a few words, and finally is reduced to babbling or mutism.
- **Apraxia** (loss of purposeful movement in the absence of motor or sensory impairment). The person is unable to perform once-familiar and purposeful tasks. For example, in apraxia of gait, the person loses the ability to walk. In apraxia of dressing, the person is unable to put clothes on properly (may put arms in trousers or put a jacket on upside down).

TABLE 15-3   Interventions for a Patient with Delirium

Intervention	Rationale
1. Work with treatment team to reduce or eliminate factors causing delirium.	1. Underlying factors can lead to dementia if not reversed.
2. Monitor neurological signs on an ongoing basis.	2. Track progression or reversal of neurological disequilibrium.
3. Introduce self and call patient by name at the beginning of each contact.	3. With short-term memory impairment, person is often confused and needs frequent orienting to time, place, and person.
4. Maintain face-to-face contact.	4. If patient is easily distracted, he or she needs help to focus on one stimulus at a time.
5. Use short, simple, concrete phrases.	5. Patient may not be able to process complex information.
6. Briefly explain everything you are going to do before doing it.	6. Explanation prevents misinterpretation of action.
7. Encourage family and friends (one at a time) to take a quiet, supportive role.	7. Familiar presence lowers anxiety and increases orientation.
8. Keep room well lit.	8. Lighting provides accurate environmental stimuli to maintain and increase orientation.
9. Keep head of bed elevated.	9. Helps provide important environmental cues.
10. Provide clocks and calendars.	10. These cues help orient patient to time.
11. Encourage family members to bring in meaningful articles from home (e.g., pictures or figurines).	11. Familiar objects provide comfort and support and can aid orientation.
12. Encourage patient to wear prescribed eyeglasses or hearing aid.	12. Helps increase accurate perceptions of visual auditory stimuli.
13. Make an effort to assign the same personnel on each shift to care for patient.	13. Familiar faces minimize confusion and enhance nurse-patient relationships.
14. When hallucinations are present, clarify reality, e.g., "I know you are frightened; I do not see spiders on your sheets. I'll sit with you for a while."	14. Person feels understood and reassured while reality is validated.
15. When illusions are present, clarify reality, e.g., "This is a coat rack, not a man with a knife . . . see? You seem frightened. I'll stay with you for a while."	15. Misinterpreted objects or sounds can be clarified, once pointed out.
16. Inform patient of progress during lucid intervals.	16. Consciousness fluctuates: patient feels less anxious knowing where he or she is and who you are during lucid periods.
17. Ignore insults and name calling, and acknowledge how upset the person may be feeling. For example: **Patient:** "You incompetent jerk, get me a real nurse, someone who knows what they are doing." **Nurse:** "You are very upset. What you are going through is very difficult. I'll stay with you."	17. Terror and fear are often projected onto environment. Arguing or becoming defensive only increases patient's aggressive behaviors and defenses.
18. If patient behavior becomes physically abusive, first, set limits on behavior, e.g., "Mr. Jones, you are not to hit me or anyone else. Tell me how you feel." *or* "Mr. Jones, if you have difficulty controlling your actions, we will help you gain control." Second, check orders for use of chemical or physical restraints.	18. Clear limits need to be set to protect patient, staff, and others. Often, patient can respond to verbal commands. Chemical and physical restraints are used as a last resort, if at all.

- **Agnosia** (loss of sensory ability to recognize objects). For example, the person may lose the ability to recognize familiar sounds (auditory agnosia), such as the ring of the telephone, a car horn, or the doorbell. Loss of this ability extends to the inability to recognize familiar objects (visual or tactile agnosia), such as a glass, magazine, pencil, or toothbrush. Eventually, people are unable to recognize loved ones or even parts of their own bodies.
- **Disturbances in executive functioning** (planning, organizing, abstract thinking). The degeneration of neurons in the brain results in the wasting away of working components in the brain. These cells contain memories, receive sights and sounds, and cause hormones to secrete, produce emotions, and command muscles into motion.

Assessment for Stage of the Disease

AD is classified according to the stage of the degenerative process. The number of stages defined ranges from three to seven, depending on the source. However, four stages, as discussed subsequently, are commonly used to categorize the progressive deterioration seen in those diagnosed with AD. Table 15-4 can be used as a guide to review the four stages of AD and highlight the deficits associated with each stage.

The rate of progression varies from person to person. Some individuals in stage 1 decline quickly and may die within 3 years. Others, although their condition worsens, may still function in the community with support. Still others may remain at this level for 3 years or more. The

TABLE 15-4 Stages of Alzheimer's Disease

Stage	Hallmarks
Stage 1 (Mild) Forgetfulness	Shows short-term memory loss; loses things, forgets
	Memory aids compensate: lists, routine, organization
	Aware of the problem; concerned about lost abilities
	Depression common—worsens symptoms
	Not diagnosable at this time
Stage 2 (Moderate) Confusion	Shows progressive memory loss; short-term memory impaired; memory difficulties interfere with all abilities
	Withdrawn from social activities
	Shows declines in instrumental activities of daily living (ADL), such as money management, legal affairs, transportation, cooking, housekeeping
	Denial common; fears "losing his or her mind"
	Depression increasingly common; frightened because aware of deficits; covers up for memory loss through confabulation
	Problems intensified when stressed, fatigued, out of own environment, ill
	Commonly needs day care or in-home assistance
Stage 3 (Moderate to Severe) Ambulatory dementia	Shows ADL losses (in order): willingness and ability to bathe, grooming, choosing clothing, dressing, gait and mobility, toileting, communication, reading, and writing skills
	Shows loss of reasoning ability, safety planning, and verbal communication
	Frustration common; becomes more withdrawn and self-absorbed
	Depression resolves as awareness of losses diminishes
	Has difficulty communicating; shows increasing loss of language skills
	Shows evidence of reduced stress threshold; institutional care usually needed
Stage 4 (Late) End stage	Family recognition disappears; does not recognize self in mirror
	Nonambulatory; shows little purposeful activity; often mute; may scream spontaneously
	Forgets how to eat, swallow, chew; commonly loses weight; emaciation common
	Has problems associated with immobility (e.g., pneumonia, pressure ulcers, contractures)
	Incontinence common; seizures may develop
	Most certainly institutionalized at this point
	Return of primitive (infantile) reflexes

From Hall, G.R. (1994). Caring for people with Alzheimer's disease using the conceptual model of progressively lowered stress threshold in the clinical setting. *Nursing Clinics of North America, 29*(1), 129-141.

duration of the disease from onset of symptoms to death averages 8 to 10 years but can range from 3 to 20 years (APA, 2000).

Stage 1: Mild Alzheimer's Disease

The loss of intellectual ability is insidious. The person with mild Alzheimer's disease loses energy, drive, and initiative and has difficulty learning new things. Because personality and social behavior remain intact, others tend to minimize and underestimate the loss of the individual's abilities. The individual may still continue to work, but the extent of the dementia becomes evident in new or demanding situations. Depression may occur early in the disease but usually lessens as the disease progresses. Activities such as grocery shopping or managing finances are noticeably impaired during this phase.

VIGNETTE

Mr. Collins, a 56-year-old lineman for a telephone company, feels that he is getting old. He keeps forgetting things and writes notes to himself on scraps of paper. One day on the job, he forgets momentarily which wires to connect and connects all the wrong ones, causing mass confusion for a few hours. At home, Mr. Collins flies off the handle when his wife suggests that they invite the new neighbors for dinner. It is hard for him to admit that anything new confuses him, and he often forgets names *(aphasia)* and sometimes loses the thread of conversations. Once he even forgot his address when his car broke down on the highway. He is moody and depressed and becomes indignant when his wife finds 3 months' worth of unpaid bills stashed in his sock drawer. Mrs. Collins is bewildered, upset, and fearful that something is terribly wrong.

Stage 2: Moderate Alzheimer's Disease

Deterioration becomes evident during the moderate phase. Often the person with moderate AD cannot remember his or her address or the date. There are memory gaps in the person's history that may fluctuate from one moment to the next. Hygiene suffers, and the ability to dress appropriately is markedly affected. The person may put on clothes backward, button the buttons incorrectly, or not fasten zippers *(apraxia)*. Often, the person has to be coaxed to bathe.

Mood becomes labile, and the individual may have bursts of paranoia, anger, jealousy, and apathy. Activities such as driving are hazardous, and families are faced with the difficulty of taking away the car keys from their loved one. Care and supervision become full-time jobs for family members. Denial mercifully takes over and protects people

from the realization that they are losing control, not only of their minds but also of their lives. Along with denial, people begin to withdraw from activities and from others because they often feel overwhelmed and frustrated when they try to do things that once were easy. They may also have moments of becoming tearful and sad.

As important as it is to recognize all of the deficits of stage 2, it is helpful for caretakers to realize that the patient still retains abilities that influence care.

VIGNETTE

Mr. Collins is transferred to a less complicated work position after his inability to function is recognized. His wife drives him to work and picks him up. Mr. Collins often forgets what he is doing and stares blankly. He accuses the supervisor of spying on him. Sometimes he disappears at lunch and is unable to find his way back to work. The transfer lasts only a few months, and Mr. Collins is forced to take an early retirement. At home Mr. Collins sleeps in his clothes. He loses interest in reading and watching sports on television and often breaks into angry outbursts, seemingly over nothing. Often he becomes extremely restless and irritable and wanders around the house aimlessly.

Stage 3: Moderate to Severe Alzheimer's Disease

At the moderate to severe stage, the person is often unable to identify familiar objects or people, even a spouse *(severe agnosia)*. The person needs repeated instructions and directions to perform the simplest tasks *(advanced apraxia):* "Here is the face cloth, pick up the soap. Now, put water on the face cloth and rub the face cloth with soap." Often the individual cannot remember where the toilet is and becomes incontinent. Total care is necessary at this point, and the burden on the family can be emotionally, financially, and physically devastating. The world is very frightening to the person with AD because nothing makes sense any longer. Agitation, violence, paranoia, and delusions are commonly seen. Another problem that is frightening to family members and caregivers is wandering behavior. It is estimated that between 60% and 70% of people with AD wander and are at risk for becoming lost (ADRDA, 2004).

Institutionalization may be the most appropriate recourse at this time because the level of care is so demanding, and violent outbursts and incontinence may be burdens that the family can no longer handle. The following are some criteria that indicate the need for placement in a skilled nursing facility:

- Wandering
- Danger to self and others

- Incontinence
- Behavior affects the sleep and general health of others
- Total dependence on others for physical care

Mr. Collins is terrified. Memories come and then slip away. People come and go, but they are strangers. Someone is masquerading as his wife, and it is hard to tell what is real. Things never stay in the same place. Sometimes people hide the bathroom where he cannot find it. He in turn hides things to keep them safe, but he forgets where he hides them. Buttons and belts are confusing, and he does not know what they are doing there anyway. Sometimes he tries to walk away from the terrifying feelings and the strangers. He tries to find something he has lost long ago . . . if he could only remember what it is.

Stage 4: Late Alzheimer's Disease

Late in AD, the following symptoms may occur: **agraphia** (inability to read or write), **hyperorality** (the need to taste, chew, and put everything in one's mouth), blunting of emotions, visual agnosia (loss of ability to recognize familiar objects), and **hypermetamorphosis** (manifested by touching of everything in sight). At this stage, the ability to talk, and eventually the ability to walk, is lost. The end stage of AD is characterized by stupor and coma. Death frequently is secondary to infection or choking.

Mrs. Collins and the children keep Mr. Collins at home until his outbursts become frightening. Once, he is lost for 2 days after he somehow unlocks the front door. Finally, Mrs. Collins has her husband placed in a Veterans Administration (VA) hospital. When his wife comes to visit, Mr. Collins sometimes cries. He never talks and is always tied into his chair when she comes to see him. The staff explain to her that although Mr. Collins can still walk, he keeps getting into other people's beds and scaring them. They explain that perhaps he wants comfort and misses human touch. They encourage her visits, even though Mr. Collins does not seem to recognize her. He does respond to music. His wife brings a radio, and when she plays the country and western music he has always loved, Mr. Collins nods and claps his hands.

Mrs. Collins is torn between guilt and love, anger and despair. She is confused and depressed. She is going through the painful process of mourning the loss of the man she has loved and shared a life with for 34 years. Three months after his admission to the VA hospital, and 8 years after the incident of the crossed wires at the telephone company, Mr. Collins chokes on some food, develops pneumonia, and dies.

Diagnostic Tests for Dementia

A wide range of problems may masquerade as dementia and may be mistaken for AD. For example, depression and dementia in the older adult present with similar symptoms. It is important that nurses and other health care professionals be able to assess some of the important differences among depression, dementia, and delirium. See Table 15-1 for important differences among these three phenomena. It is important to point out that depression and dementia or depression and delirium can coexist in the same person. Therefore it is important that a complete and thorough medical exam (neurological, medical, psychiatric history, review of medications, and nutritional evaluation) be performed.

Other disorders that often mimic dementia include drug toxicity, metabolic disorders, infections, and nutritional deficiencies. A disorder that mimics dementia is sometimes referred to as a **pseudodementia.** That is, although the symptoms may suggest dementia, a careful examination may reveal another diagnosis altogether, usually depression. This reinforces the importance of performing a comprehensive assessment (including laboratory tests) when symptoms of dementia are present to identify nondementia causes.

We have no definitive test to diagnose AD and must rely on symptoms; in fact, a confirmation of the disease can only be made on autopsy. However, preliminary evidence suggests that positron emission tomography (PET) and single photon emission computed tomography (SPECT) scans can aid in the diagnosis (Rabins, 2006). Studies using MRI to measure the size of brain structures are illuminating in that those people with smaller size structure and only mild minor cognitive symptoms are often those who within 3 years will present with diagnosable AD (Rabins, 2006). Researchers have recently discovered 23 proteins in cerebrospinal fluid that may be biomarkers for AD and are optimistic that diagnosing the disease may be possible (Finehout et al., 2007).

CT, PET, and other developing scanning technologies have diagnostic capabilities because they reveal brain atrophy and rule out other conditions, such as neoplasms. The use of mental status questionnaires such as the Mini-Mental State Examination in people older than 75 is sometimes recommended to increase earlier detection (Rabins, 2006).

Assessment Guidelines

Dementia

1. Identify and treat any general medical conditions that might contribute to the dementia.

2. Evaluate potential of suicide or aggression toward others.
3. Explore how well the family is prepared for and informed about the progress of the patient's dementia (e.g., the phases and course of AD, vascular dementia, AIDS-related dementia, or dementia associated with multiple sclerosis, lupus erythematosus, or brain injury).
4. Review the medications including those from over-the-counter (OTC), herbs, complementary agents, and recreational drugs, the patient is currently taking.
5. Evaluate the patient's current level of cognitive functioning.
6. Discuss with the family members how they are coping with the patient and their main issues at this time.
7. Assess evidence of neglect or abuse.
8. Review the resources available to the family. Ask the family members to describe the help they receive from other family members, friends, and community resources. Determine if caregivers are aware of community support groups and resources.
9. Determine the appropriate safety measures needed by the patient and arrange for them to be implemented.
10. Evaluate the safety of the patient's home environment (e.g., with regard to wandering, eating inedible objects, falling, engaging in provocative behaviors toward others).
11. Identify the needs of the family for teaching and guidance (e.g., how to manage catastrophic reactions; lability of mood; aggressive behaviors; and nocturnal delirium and increased confusion and agitation at night, or sundown syndrome).

DIAGNOSIS

One of the most important areas of concern is the patient's *safety*. Many people with AD wander and may be lost for hours or days. Wandering, along with behaviors such as rummaging, may be perceived as purposeful to the patient. Wandering may result from changes in the physical environment, fear caused by hallucinations or delusions, or lack of exercise.

Seizures may occur in the later stages of this disease. Injuries from falls and accidents can occur during any stage as confusion and disorientation progress. The potential for burns exists if the patient is a smoker or is unattended when using the stove. Prescription drugs can be taken incorrectly, or bottles of noxious fluids can be mistakenly ingested, which results in a medical crisis. Therefore, *Risk for injury* is always present.

As the person's ability to recognize or name objects is decreased, *Impaired verbal communication* becomes a problem. As memory diminishes and disorientation increases, *Impaired environmental interpretation syndrome*, *Impaired memory*, and *Chronic confusion* occur.

During the course of the disease, people show personality changes, increased vulnerability, and often inappropriate behaviors. Common behaviors include hoarding, regression, and being overly demanding. Therefore nurses and family members often intervene in behaviors that signal *Ineffective coping*. Family caregivers may experience *Compromised* or even *Disabled family coping*.

Additional family issues may emerge. Perhaps some of the most crucial aspects of the patient's care are support, education, and referrals for the family. The family loses an integral part of its unit. Family members lose the love, function, support, companionship, and warmth that this person once provided. *Caregiver role strain* is always present, and planning with the family and offering community support is an integral part of appropriate care. *Anticipatory grieving* is also an important phenomenon to assess and may be an important target for intervention. Helping the family grieve can make the task ahead somewhat clearer and, at times, less painful. See Table 15-2 for potential nursing diagnoses for confused patients with dementia.

OUTCOMES IDENTIFICATION

Families who have a member with dementia are faced with an exhaustive list of issues that need addressing. Self-care needs, impaired environmental interpretation, constant confusion, ineffective individual coping, and role strain of the caregiver are just a few of the areas nurses and other health care members will need to target (Box 15-2).

PLANNING

The planning of care for a patient with dementia is geared toward the patient's immediate needs. Figure 15-2 presents the Functional Dementia Scale, which can be used by nurses and families to plan strategies for addressing immediate needs and to track progression of the dementia.

Identifying level of functioning and assessing caregivers' needs help the nurse identify appropriate community resources. Does the patient or family need the following?
- Transportation services
- Supervision and care when primary caregiver is out of the home
- Referrals to day care centers
- Information on support groups within the community
- Meals on Wheels
- Information on respite and residential services
- Telephone numbers for help lines

BOX 15-2

Suggested Outcome Criteria for Dementia*

Injury
- Patient will remain safe in the hospital or at home.
- With the aid of an identification bracelet and neighborhood or hospital alert, patient will be returned within 1 hour of wandering.
- Patient will remain free of danger during seizures.
- With the aid of interventions, patient will remain burn-free.
- With the aid of guidance and environmental manipulation, patient will not be hurt if a fall occurs.
- Patient will ingest only correct doses of prescribed medications and appropriate food and fluids.

Communication
- Patient will communicate needs.
- Patient will answer yes or no appropriately to questions.
- Patient will state needs in alternative modes when aphasic (e.g., will signal correct word on hearing it or will refer to picture or label).
- Patient will wear prescribed glasses or hearing aid each day.

Caregiver Role Strain
- Family members will have the opportunity to express "unacceptable" feelings in a supportive environment.
- Family members will have access to professional counseling.
- Family members will name two organizations within their geographical area that can offer support.
- Family members will participate in patient's plan of care, with encouragement from staff.
- Family members will state that they have outside help that allows them to take personal time for themselves each week or month.
- Family members will have the names of three resources that can help with financial burdens and legal considerations.

Impaired Environmental Interpretation: Chronic Confusion
- Patient will acknowledge the reality of an object or a sound that was misinterpreted (illusion), after it is pointed out.
- Patient will state that he or she feels safe after experiencing delusions or illusions.
- Patient will remain nonaggressive when experiencing paranoid ideation.

Self-Care Needs
- Patient will participate in self-care at optimal level.
- Patient will be able to follow step-by-step instructions for dressing, bathing, and grooming.
- Patient will put on own clothes appropriately, with aid of fastening tape (Velcro) and nursing supervision.
- Patient's skin will remain intact and free from signs of pressure.

*Not an exhaustive list.

- Home health aides
- Home health services
- The Alzheimer's Association's Safe Return program (www.alz.org)
- Additional teaching or psychopharmaceutical aids to manage distressing or harmful behaviors when appropriate

Because stress is a common occurrence when working with persons with cognitive impairments, staff need to be proactive in minimizing its effects as well as teach and provide guidelines to caregivers and loved ones. Reducing stress can be facilitated by:

- **Having a realistic understanding of the disease** so that expectations for the patient are realistic.
- **Establishing realistic outcomes** for the patient and recognizing when they are achieved. These outcomes may be as minor as *patient feeds self with spoon,* yet it must be remembered that even the smallest achievement can be a significant accomplishment for the impaired individual.
- **Maintaining good self-care.** Nurses and caregivers need to protect themselves from the negative effects of stress by obtaining adequate sleep and rest, eating a nutritious diet, exercising, engaging in relaxing activities, and addressing their own spiritual needs.

IMPLEMENTATION

The needs of a patient with dementia are complex, change over time, and can take place in a variety of settings during various stages of the disease. Care settings include the emergency department, general hospital, home settings, long-term care settings, and community.

The nurse's attitude of unconditional positive regard is the single most effective tool in caring for patients with dementia. It induces patients to cooperate with care, reduces catastrophic outbreaks, and increases family members' satisfaction with care. A warm, empathic, and nonjudgmental approach using calm, unhurried, clear communications can help allay confusion and agitation. The nurse and others

FUNCTIONAL DEMENTIA SCALE

Circle one rating for each item:
1. None or little of the time
2. Some of the time
3. Good part of the time
4. Most or all of the time

Client: _____
Observer: _____
Position or relation to patient: _____
Facility: _____
Date: _____

1	2	3	4	
1	2	3	4	1. Has difficulty in completing simple tasks on own (e.g., dressing, bathing, doing arithmetic).
1	2	3	4	2. Spends time either sitting or in apparently purposeless activity.
1	2	3	4	3. Wanders at night or needs to be restrained to prevent wandering.
1	2	3	4	4. Hears things that are not there.
1	2	3	4	5. Requires supervision or assistance in eating.
1	2	3	4	6. Loses things.
1	2	3	4	7. Appearance is disorderly if left to own devices.
1	2	3	4	8. Moans.
1	2	3	4	9. Cannot control bowel function.
1	2	3	4	10. Threatens to harm others.
1	2	3	4	11. Cannot control bladder function.
1	2	3	4	12. Needs to be watched so doesn't injure self (e.g., by careless smoking, leaving the stove on, falling).
1	2	3	4	13. Destructive of materials around him/her (e.g., breaks furniture, throws food trays, tears up magazines).
1	2	3	4	14. Shouts or yells.
1	2	3	4	15. Accuses others of doing bodily harm or stealing his or her possessions — when you are sure the accusations are not true.
	2	3	4	16. Is unaware of limitations imposed by illness.
1	2	3	4	17. Becomes confused and does not know where he or she is.
1	2	3	4	18. Has trouble remembering.
1	2	3	4	19. Has sudden changes of mood (e.g., gets upset, angered, or cries easily).
1	2	3	4	20. If left alone, wanders aimlessly during the day or needs to be restrained to prevent wandering.

Figure 15-2 ▪ Functional Dementia Scale. (From Moore, J. T., et al. [1983]. A functional dementia scale. *Journal of Family Practice, 16,* 498.)

should always introduce themselves with each encounter. Expectations should be clear and explained in simple, step-by-step instructions. To help patients maintain a sense of self-control, they should be given simple and appropriate choices in their care (e.g., "Do you want to wash your face before or after you brush your teeth?").

Because a considerable number of individuals with dementia have secondary behavioral disturbances (depression, hallucinations, delusions, agitation, insomnia, and wandering), there is an increase in the need for supervision. Many of these situations respond well to the interventions found in Tables 15-5 and 15-6. For example, a woman who is 73 years old believes that she is 23 and has babies at home would not be calmed by being told that she is 78 and has no babies. It is most helpful to reflect back to patients their feelings and to show understanding and concern for their plight (Alverez, 2002). For example, "Mrs. Green, you miss your children, and this can be a lonely place."

Intervention with family members is critical. The effects of losing a family member to dementia—that is, watching the deterioration of a person who has had an important role within the family unit and who is loved and is a vital part of his or her family's history—are devastating, exhausting, and painful. Nurses can teach families about the progression of the illness, give them guidelines for safely caring for their family member who lives at home (Tables 15-7 and 15-8), and find appropriate support for families who are grieving.

Communication Guidelines

How nurses choose to communicate with patients with dementia affects the patient's maintenance of self-esteem and ability to participate in care. People with dementia often find it difficult to express themselves. They:

- Have difficulty finding the right words.
- Use familiar words repeatedly.
- Invent new words to describe things (neologisms).
- Frequently lose their train of thought.
- Rely on nonverbal gestures.

TABLE 15-5   Interventions for Dementia: Communication

Intervention	Rationale
1. Always identify yourself and call the person by name at each meeting.	1. Patient's short term memory is impaired—requires frequent orientation to time and environment.
2. Speak slowly.	2. Patient needs time to process information.
3. Use short, simple words and phrases.	3. Patient may not be able to understand complex statements or abstract ideas.
4. Maintain face-to-face contact.	4. Verbal and nonverbal clues are maximized.
5. Be near patient when talking, one or two arm-lengths away.	5. This distance can help patient focus on speaker as well as maintain personal space.
6. Focus on one piece of information at a time.	6. Attention span of patient is poor and patient is easily distracted—helps patient focus. Too much data can be overwhelming and can increase anxiety.
7. Talk with patient about familiar and meaningful things.	7. Self-expression is promoted and reality is reinforced.
8. Encourage reminiscing about happy times in life.	8. Remembering accomplishments and shared joys helps distract patient from deficit and gives meaning to existence.
9. When patient is delusional, acknowledge patient's feelings and reinforce reality. Do not argue or refute delusions.	9. Acknowledging feelings helps patient feel understood. Pointing out realities may help patient focus on realities. Arguing can enhance adherence to false beliefs.
10. If a patient gets into an argument with another patient, stop the argument and get individuals out of each other's way. After a short while (5 minutes), explain to each patient matter of-factly why you had to intervene.	10. Escalation to physical acting-out is prevented. Patient's right to know is respected. Explaining in an adult manner helps maintain self-esteem.
11. When patient becomes verbally aggressive, acknowledge patient's feelings and shift topic to more familiar ground (e.g., "I know this is upsetting for you, because you always cared for others. Tell me about your children.")	11. Confusion and disorientation easily increase anxiety. Acknowledging feelings makes patient feel more understood and less alone. Topics patient has mastery over can remind him or her of areas of competent functioning and can increase self-esteem.
12. Have patient wear prescription eyeglasses or hearing aid.	12. Environmental awareness, orientation, and comprehension are increased, which in turn increases awareness of personal needs and the presence of others.
13. Keep patient's room well lit.	13. Environmental clues are maximized.
14. Have clocks, calendars, and personal items (e.g., family pictures or Bible) in clear view of patient while he or she is in bed.	14. These objects assist in maintaining personal identity.
15. Reinforce patient's pictures, nonverbal gestures, X's on calendars, and other methods used to anchor patient in reality.	15. When aphasia starts to hinder communication, alternate methods of communication need to be instituted.

See Table 15-5 for a variety of nursing interventions and guidelines integral for communicating with a cognitively impaired person. These interventions and guidelines also can be taught to family members.

Health Teaching and Health Promotion

Educating families who have a cognitively impaired member is one of the most important areas for nurses. Families who are caring for a member in the home need to know about strategies for communicating and structuring self-care activities (see Table 15-6).

Most important, families need to know where to get help. Help includes professional counseling and education regarding the process and the progression of the disease. Families need to know about and be referred to community-based groups that can help bear this tremendous burden (e.g., day care centers, senior citizen groups, organizations providing home visits and respite care, and family support groups). A list with definitions of some of the types of services available in the patient's community, as well as the

TABLE 15-6	Interventions for Dementia: Health Teaching and Health Promotion

Intervention	Rationale
Dressing and Bathing	
1. Always have patient perform all tasks within his or her present capacity.	1. Maintains patient's self-esteem and uses muscle groups; impedes staff burnout; minimizes further regression.
2. Always have patient wear own clothes, even if in the hospital.	2. Helps maintain patient's identity and dignity.
3. Use clothing with elastic, and substitute fastening tape (Velcro) for buttons and zippers.	3. Minimizes patient's confusion and eases independence of functioning.
4. Label clothing items with patient's name and name of item.	4. Helps identify patient if he or she wanders and gives patient additional clues when aphasia or agnosia occurs.
5. Give step-by-step instructions whenever necessary (e.g., "Take this blouse . . . Put in one arm . . . now the next arm. . . . Pull it together in the front. . . . Now . . .")	5. Patient can focus on small pieces of information more easily; allows patient to perform at optimal level.
6. Make sure that water in faucets is not too hot.	6. Judgment is lacking in patient; patient is unaware of many safety hazards.
7. If patient is resistant to performing self-care, come back later and ask again.	7. Moods may be labile, and patient may forget but often complies after short interval.
Nutrition	
1. Monitor food and fluid intake.	1. Patient may have anorexia or be too confused to eat.
2. Offer finger food that patient can take away from the dinner table.	2. Increases input throughout the day; patient may eat only small amounts at meals.
3. Weigh patient regularly (once a week).	3. Monitors fluid and nutritional status.
4. During periods of hyperorality, watch that patient does not eat nonfood items (e.g., ceramic fruit or food-shaped soaps).	4. Patient puts everything into mouth; may be unable to differentiate inedible objects made in the shape and color of food.
Bowel and Bladder Function	
1. Begin bowel and bladder program early; start with bladder control.	1. Establishing same time of day for bowel movements and toileting—in early morning, after meals and snacks, and before bedtime—can help prevent incontinence.
2. Evaluate use of disposable diapers.	2. Prevents embarrassment.
3. Label bathroom door as well as doors to other rooms.	3. Additional environmental clues can maximize independent toileting.
Sleep	
1. Because patient may awaken, be frightened, or cry out at night, keep area well lighted.	1. Reinforces orientation, minimizes possible illusions.
2. Maintain a calm atmosphere during the day.	2. Encourages a calming night's sleep.
3. Order nonbarbiturates (e.g., chloral hydrate) if necessary.	3. Barbiturates can have a paradoxical reaction, causing agitation.
4. If medications are indicated, consider neuroleptics with sedative properties, which may be the most helpful (e.g., haloperidol [Haldol]).	4. Helps clear thinking and sedates.
5. Avoid the use of restraints.	5. Can cause patient to become more terrified and fight against restraints until exhausted to a dangerous degree.

TABLE 15-7	Services for People with Dementia and their Families or Caregivers
Type of Service	**Services Provided**
Family or caregiver Some patients may live by themselves in the community; active case management is vital when this is the case.	Caregivers have a right to: • Easy access to services • Respite care • Full involvement in decision making • Assessment of the needs of the caregiver as well as those of the patient • Information and referral • Case management: coordination of community resources and follow-up
Community services	• Adult day care: provides activities, socialization, supervision • Physician services • Protective services: prevent, eliminate, and/or remedy effects of abuse or neglect • Recreational services • Transportation • Mental health services • Legal services
Home care	• Meals on Wheels • Home health aide services • Homemaker services • Hospice services • Occupational therapy • Paid companion or sitter services • Physical therapy • Skilled nursing • Personal care services: assistance in basic self-care activities • Social work services • Telephone reassurance: regular telephone calls to individuals who are isolated and homebound* • Personal emergency response systems: telephone-based systems to alert others that a person who is alone is in need of emergency assistance*

*Vital for those living alone.

names and telephone numbers of the providers of these services, should be given to the family.

The Alzheimer's Association (www.alz.org) is a national umbrella agency that provides various forms of assistance to people with the disease and their families. The Alzheimer's Association has launched Safe Return to help locate and return missing people with AD and other memory impairments. Wandering is a common behavior during the second and third stages of AD, and the Safe Return program offers peace of mind to families. Some communities are instituting small GPS systems that can be attached by a wrist- or arm-band to help locate a person with AD who wanders off for a period of time.

Information regarding housekeeping, home health aides, and companions is also available through this organization. Such outside resources can help prevent the total emotional and physical fatigue of family members. Types of resources that might be available in some communities are found in Table 15-7. When the nurse is unable to provide the relevant information, proper referrals by the social worker are needed. Information regarding advance directives, durable power of attorney, guardianship, and conservatorship should be included in the communication with the family.

Milieu Therapy

Interventions and guidelines for families in structuring a safe environment and planning appropriate activities are found in Table 15-8.

Pharmacological, Biological, and Integrative Therapies
Cognitive Impairment

There is no cure for Alzheimer's disease. However, three cholinesterase inhibitors—galantamine (Razadyne), rivastigmine (Exelon), and donepezil (Aricept)—are approved by

TABLE 15-8	Interventions for a Safe Milieu in the Home

Intervention	Rationale
Safe Environment	
1. Gradually restrict use of the car.	1. Even mild dementia increases risk of vehicular accident (APA, 2008).
2. Remove throw rugs and other objects in person's path.	2. Minimizes tripping and falling.
3. Minimize sensory stimulation.	3. Decreases sensory overload, which can increase anxiety and confusion.
4. If patient becomes verbally upset, listen briefly, give support, then change the topic.	4. Goal is to prevent escalation of anger. When attention span is short, patient can be distracted to more productive topics and activities.
5. Label all rooms and drawers. Label often-used objects (e.g., hairbrushes and toothbrushes).	5. May keep patient from wandering into other patients' rooms. Increases environmental clues to familiar objects.
6. Install safety bars in bathroom.	6. Prevents falls.
7. Supervise patient when he or she smokes.	7. Danger of burns is always present.
8. If patient has history of seizures, educate family on how to deal with seizures.	8. Seizure activity is common in advanced Alzheimer's disease.
Wandering	
1. If patient wanders during the night, put mattress on the floor.	1. Prevents falls when patient is confused.
2. Have patient wear MedicAlert bracelet that cannot be removed (with name, address, and telephone number). Provide police department with recent pictures.	2. Patient can easily be identified by police, neighbors, or hospital personnel.
3. Alert local police and neighbors about wanderer.	3. May reduce time necessary to return patient to home or hospital.
4. If patient is in hospital, have him or her wear brightly colored vest with name, unit, and phone number printed on back.	4. Makes patient easily identifiable.
5. Put complex locks on door.	5. Reduces opportunity to wander.
6. Place locks at top of door.	6. In moderate and late Alzheimer's-type dementia, ability to look up and reach upward is lost.
7. Encourage physical activity during the day.	7. Physical activity may decrease wandering at night.
8. Explore the feasibility of installing sensor devices or GPS system.	8. Sensor provides warning if patient wanders. GPS can help locate patient.
Useful Activities	
1. Provide picture magazines and children's books when patient's reading ability diminishes.	1. Allows continuation of usual activities that patient can still enjoy; provides focus.
2. Provide simple activities that allow exercise of large muscles.	2. Exercise groups, dance groups, and walking provide socialization as well as increased circulation and maintenance of muscle tone.
3. Encourage group activities that are familiar and simple to perform.	3. Activities such as group singing, dancing, reminiscing, and working with clay and paint all help to increase socialization and minimize feelings of alienation.

the U.S. Food and Drug Administration (FDA) and demonstrate positive effects not only on cognition but also on behavior and function in activities of daily living (Rabins, 2006) in mild to moderate AD disease. In July 2007, rivastigmine in the form of a transdermal patch was approved by the FDA for the treatment of mild to moderate AD. All of these medications work for a limited period until the stores of acetylcholine have been depleted. At that point, the functioning of the person with AD may fall off drastically.

Memantine (Namenda), a N-methyl-D aspartate (NMDA), is an antagonist at the NMDA-glutamatergic ion channels, thereby making more acetylcholine available. It is the first drug to target symptoms of AD during the mod-

APPLYING THE ART   A Person with Dementia

SCENARIO: I met 75-year-old Mr. Samson on our geriatric rotation. He'd recently been moved to the Memory Disorder Unit of the nursing facility. His wife of 50 years, whom he called Darlin' (her name was Darlene) had resided on the assisted living side until her sudden death from a myocardial infarction 3 weeks earlier. Mr. Samson and I regularly used the pictures in the memory wallet that his wife and the staff had put together to remind him about his life.

THERAPEUTIC GOAL: By the end of this encounter, Mr. Samson will begin to process the reality of his wife's death as evidenced by referring to her and their life together in the past tense at least part of the time.

Student-Patient Interaction	Thoughts, Communication Techniques, and Mental Health Nursing Concepts
Student: "Mr. Samson, what's wrong?" **Mr. Samson:** (crying) "My Darlin', what's wrong with my Darlin'?" *He gestures toward the sign of the memorial service to be held for "Mrs. Darlene Samson" and one other resident who had died the previous month.*	I knew from the chart that Mr. Samson had attended his wife's funeral. I should have said my name and reminded him that we'd talked a few times before, but I was worried because he was sitting in the lobby sobbing. He's crying like he just discovered "his Darlin'" died. How awful to not be able to hold on to your own life and what matters most in your memories.
Student: "Mr. Samson, I'm _____, your nursing student. You feel worried seeing your wife's name on the sign. *He nods.* Let's use your memory wallet to remember together about your Darlin'." *I wait until he makes eye contact and takes the wallet out of his hip pocket.* ***Student's feelings:*** *I am feeling a little anxious now. I hope I did okay in calling Mrs. Samson Darlin' as he does. I hope he'll remember if I show him the picture the staff put in the wallet showing Mr. Samson standing and looking at his wife in the casket. Seems unkind in some ways.*	I *introduce* myself again and use *reflection.* Diverting to the task of looking through the memory wallet provides structure to help meet *safety needs.*
Student: *Smiling encouragingly.* "Tell me about the pictures."	I know that the mental health focus needs to include helping with *reality orientation* for as long as his progressive *dementia* will allow.
Mr. Samson: *No longer crying.* "This was our house. Darlin' keeps such a great garden. I used to love her tomatoes the best. *He points to the tall plants beside the house.* ***Student's feelings:*** *He's trying so hard. I admire him. I never knew either of my grandfathers.*	He uses the present tense "keeps . . . garden," but the past tense for "was our house" and "used to love her tomatoes." He's having trouble sorting out the present from the past.
Student: "You still love tomatoes! I helped you make the tomato salad for lunch. None tastes as good as Darlin's did, I bet." ***Student's feelings:*** *I did well here by reminding him of still liking tomatoes.*	I make an *observation.* I refer to Mrs. Samson's tomatoes in the past tense to *reinforce reality.*
Mr. Samson: "Right. I wonder if Darlin' picked the tomato salad. We meet in the solarium every day." ***Student's feelings:*** *I feel frustrated that he's talking about Darlin' like she's alive. Two days ago he talked like he remembered that Mrs. Samson died 3 weeks ago.*	

Continued

APPLYING THE ART   A Person with Dementia—cont'd

Student-Patient Interaction	Thoughts, Communication Techniques, and Mental Health Nursing Concepts
Student: "Look at this next picture." *I wait as he absorbs the funeral home picture.* **Student's feelings:** *Was that too direct? I didn't know what to say when he talked about meeting her in the solarium.*	How nontherapeutic. I sound like I'm giving a command. I should have started with, "I have some sad news."
Mr. Samson: "Oh God, oh God. She died. She's gone. When did she die? How can I go on without her?" *He buries his head in his hands, sobbing.* **Student's feelings:** *He's experiencing this as though for the first time. I feel ready to cry.*	
Student: "I am with you. May I hold your hand? *He nods.* "It's so painful to say goodbye."	Touch communicates caring. I *reflect feelings* about saying goodbye. I ask permission before touching.
Mr. Samson: "We were married 50 years. She's the love of my life. Darlin' was my soul mate."	Again he mixes past and present tenses. How can he progress through the grief process when he keeps moving back to the denial stage? I can't imagine 50 years with one person. What an accomplishment.
Student: "You're really struggling with letting yourself know she died. You say, Darlin' was your soul mate. You miss her so much." **Student's feelings:** *I'll talk with the treatment team. He may need some extra support as his memory impairment grows and as he faces the memorial service.*	I use *reflection.* I also carefully *restate* to emphasize his use of the past tense. I wonder what effect the memorial service will have on him. When he comes to the point of grieving anew every time, we'll have to take out the funeral picture and emphasize feelings using *validation therapy.*
Mr. Samson: "I do, every minute of every day." *He makes eye contact as we continue talking until he's calmer and no longer crying.* **Student's feelings:** *I like him and I feel so sad about his situation.*	
Student: "Are you ready to walk together back to your room so you can get ready for reminiscence group?" *He nods.*	Giving him a choice empowers him.

erate to severe stages of the disorder. Like the cholinesterase inhibitors, the benefits of Namenda are time limited.

Targeting Behavioral Symptoms of Alzheimer's Disease

Cognitive-behavioral approaches and nursing interventions mentioned in this text are often helpful in lowering anxiety, dealing with physical agitation, and intervening with hallucinations and delusions. At times, other medications may be useful in managing behavioral symptoms of dementia, but these need to be used with extreme caution. Age alters the metabolism, absorption, and elimination of many med-

ications, and the elderly are more sensitive to these effects (APA, 2008). The rule of thumb for older patients is **"start low and go slow."**

In patients with coexisting depression, the choice of agents is usually based on the side-effect profile. SSRIs have a low side–effect profile and appear better tolerated. Bupropion (Wellbutrin) venlafaxine (Effexor), and mirtazapine (Remeron) are also good choices. Agents with anticholinergic side effects should be avoided (APA, 2008).

The use of restraints and medications to control disruptive behavior in patients with dementia is often associated with falls, worsening cognitive impairment, oversedation, and other adverse drug reactions. Physical restraints are rarely indicated. The APA (2008) suggests structural education programs for staff to help manage disruptive behaviors through behavioral interventions and or cognitive techniques in order to reduce use of both medications and restraints.

Atypical antipsychotic medications (particularly risperidone [Risperda], olanzapine [Zyprexa], and quetiapine fumarate [Seroquel]) have been used extensively for treating behavioral symptoms of AD. Some of these troubling symptoms are (1) psychoses (hallucinations and delusions), (2) severe mood swings, (3) anxiety (agitation), and (4) verbal or physical aggression (combativeness). However, current research casts into doubt the advisability of using the expensive atypical antipsychotics, none of which are approved for treating AD, for these behaviors. Schneider and colleagues (2006) found that in general whatever modest benefit this classification of medication may provide is canceled out by the side effects. The researchers recommend that atypical antipsychotics be used sparingly for the few patients who benefit from them. Anxiety, agitation, and delusional behaviors can often be tempered by timely appropriate use of nursing interventions. The updated APA guidelines (2007) for treating patients with dementia strongly suggest that non-drug treatment should be tried first. The use of antipsychotics in all settings (home, long-term care) should be limited (Busko, 2007).

EVALUATION

Outcomes need to be stated in measurable terms, be within the capability of the patient, and be evaluated frequently. As the person's condition continues to deteriorate, outcomes need to be altered to reflect the person's diminished functioning. Frequent evaluation and reformulation of outcome criteria and short-term indicators also help diminish staff and family frustration, as well as minimize the patient's anxiety by ensuring that tasks are not more complicated than the person can accomplish. The overall outcomes for treatment are to promote the patient's optimal level of functioning and to retard further regression, whenever possible. Working closely with family members and providing them with the names of available resources and support sources may help increase the quality of life for both the family and the patient.

KEY POINTS TO REMEMBER

- *Cognitive disorder* is a term that refers to disorders marked by disturbances in orientation, memory, intellect, judgment, and affect resulting from changes in the brain.
- Delirium and dementia are the cognitive disorders most frequently seen by health care workers.
- Delirium is marked by acute onset, disturbance in consciousness, and symptoms of disorientation and confusion that fluctuate by the minute, hour, or time of day.
- Delirium is always secondary to an underlying condition; therefore, it is temporary, transient, and may last from hours to days once the underlying cause is treated. If the cause is not treated, permanent damage to neurons can result.
- Dementia usually has a more insidious onset than delirium. Global deterioration of cognitive functioning (e.g., memory, judgment, ability to think abstractly, and orientation) is often progressive and irreversible, depending on the underlying cause.
- Dementia may be primary (e.g., Alzheimer's disease, vascular dementia, Pick's disease, Lewy body disease). In this case, the disease is irreversible. Or it may be secondary to other causes and when treated may be reversed.
- Alzheimer's disease accounts for up to 70% to 80% of all cases of dementia, and vascular dementia accounts for up to 20%.
- There is little known about the actual causes of AD. The incidence increases with age, and most likely several risk factor genes may interact with each other and with nongenetic factors to cause the disease.
- Signs and symptoms change according to the four stages of Alzheimer's disease: stage 1 (mild), stage 2 (moderate), stage 3 (moderate to severe), and stage 4 (late).
- The behavioral manifestations of AD include confabulation, perseveration, aphasia, apraxia, agnosia, and hyperorality.
- No known cause or cure exists for AD, although a number of drugs that increase the brain's supply of acetylcholine (a nerve communication chemical) are helpful in slowing the progress of the disease.
- People with AD have many unmet needs and present many management challenges to their families as well as to health care workers.
- Specific nursing interventions for cognitively impaired individuals can increase communication, safety, and self-care, as well as minimize confusion. The need for family teaching and support is crucial.

CRITICAL THINKING

1. Mrs. Kendel is an 82-year-old who has progressive Alzheimer's disease. She lives with her husband, who has been trying to care for her in their home. Mrs. Kendel often wears evening gowns in the morning, puts her blouse on backward, and sometimes puts her bra on backward outside her blouse. She often forgets where things are. She makes an effort to cook but often confuses frying pans and pots and sometimes has trouble turning on the stove. Once in a while, she cannot find the bathroom in time, often mistaking it for a broom closet. She becomes frightened of noises and is terrified when the telephone or doorbell rings. At times she cries because she is aware that she is losing her sense of her place in the world. She and her husband have always been close, loving companions, and he wants to keep her at home as long as possible.

A. Help Mr. Kendel by writing out a list of suggestions that he can try at home that might help facilitate (a) communication, (b) activities of daily living, and (c) maintenance of a safe home environment.
B. Identify at least seven interventions that are appropriate to this situation for each of the areas cited above.
C. Identify possible types of resources available for maintaining Mrs. Kendel in her home for as long as possible. Provide the name of one self-help group that you would urge Mr. Kendel to join.
D. Share with your clinical group the name and function of at least three community agencies in your area that could be an appropriate referral for a family in your neighborhood.

CHAPTER REVIEW

Choose the most appropriate answer.

1. A nurse assessing a patient with suspected delirium will expect to find that the patient's symptoms developed:
    1. over a period of hours to days.
    2. over a period of weeks to months.
    3. with no relationship to another condition.
    4. during middle age.
2. Of the following outcomes, which one is most appropriate for a patient with cognitive impairment related to delirium?
    1. Patient will participate fully in self-care from admission on.
    2. Patient will have stable vital signs 6 hours after admission.
    3. Patient will participate in simple activities that bring enjoyment.
    4. Patient will return to the premorbid level of functioning.
3. In caring for a patient with late Alzheimer's disease, which nursing diagnosis demands the nurse's highest priority?
    1. *Risk for injury.*

2. *Self-care deficit.*
3. *Chronic low self-esteem.*
4. *Impaired verbal communication.*

4. Nursing staff that care for cognitively impaired patients can develop burnout. Strategies to avoid the development of burnout include:
    1. setting realistic patient goals.
    2. insulating self from emotional involvement with patients.
    3. sedating patients to promote rest and minimize catastrophic episodes.
    4. encouraging the family to permit the use of restraints to promote patient safety.
5. Psychobiological agents showing promise for the treatment of cognitive impairment associated with Alzheimer's disease include:
    1. cholinesterase inhibitors.
    2. herbals, including *Ginkgo biloba*.
    3. selective serotonin reuptake inhibitors and trazodone.
    4. benzodiazepines and buspirone.

REFERENCES

Alverez, C. (2002). Anger and aggression. In E.M. Varcarolis (Ed.): Foundations of psychiatric mental health nursing: A clinical approach (4th ed.). Philadelphia: Saunders.

Alzheimer's Association. (2004). Alzheimer's Association statement on research published in *The Lancet* regarding cost effectiveness of a current Alzheimer treatment. Retrieved March 7, 2005, from www. alz.org/Media/newsreleases/2004/062404aricept.asp.

Alzheimer's Disease Education and Referral Center. (2002). *High homocysteine levels may double risk of dementia, Alzheimer's disease,*

new report suggests. Retrieved February 1, 2005, from www.nih.gov/news/pr/feb2002/nia-13.htm.

Alzheimer's Disease Education and Referral Center. (2004). *Alzheimer's disease genetics fact sheet.* Retrieved September 13, 2004, from www. alzheimers.org/pubs/genefact.html.

Alzheimer's Disease Education and Referral Center. (2006). *Causes: What causes AD?* Alzheimer's Disease Education & Referral Center. Retrieved March 21, 2007, from www.nia.nih.gov/Alzheimers/AlzheimersInformation/Causes.

Alzheimer's Disease and Related Disorders Association. (2004). *Statistics.* Retrieved March 7, 2005, from www.alz.org/Resources/FactSheets/FSAlzheimerStats.pdf.

American Psychiatric Association (APA). (2000). *Diagnostic and statistical manual of mental disorders (DSM-IV-TR)* (4th ed., text rev.). Washington, DC: Author.

American Psychiatric Association (APA). (2008). Practice guideline for the treatment of patients with Alzheimer's disease and other dementias (2nd ed.). Retrieved from www.psychiatryonline.com/popup.aspx?aID=152238.

Busko, H. (2007). APA releases updated guidelines for treating patients with dementia. Medscape Medical News. www.medscape.com/viewarticle/567497.

CenterWatch. (2001). *Drugs approved by the FDA: Drug name: Reminyl (galantamine hydrobromide).* Retrieved February 1, 2005, from www.centerwatch.com/patient/drugs/dru666.html.

Finehout, E.J., Franck, Z., Choe, L.H., et al. (2007). Cerebrospinal fluid proteomic biomarkers for Alzheimer's disease. *Annals of Neurology, 61*(2), 120-129.

Howes, M. J., Perry, N.S., & Houghton, P.J. (2003). Plants with traditional uses and activities, relevant to the management of Alzheimer's disease and other cognitive disorders. *Phytotherapy Research, 17*(1), 1-18.

Morris, J.C. (2000). *Alzheimer's disease: Unique, differentiable and treatable.* Paper presented at the 22nd Congress of the Collegium Internationale Neuro-Psycopharmacologicum, April 29-May 6, San Diego.

Prasher, V., Cumella, S., Natarajan, K., et al. (2003). Magnetic resonance imaging, Down's syndrome and Alzheimer's disease: Research and clinical implications. *Journal of Intellectual Disabilities Research, 47*(Pt 2), 90-100 (Abstract).

Rabins, P.V. (2006). *Guidelines Watch for the practice guidelines for the treatment of patients with Alzheimer's disease.* Washington, DC: American Psychiatric Association.

Ress, B. (2003). HIV disease and aging: The hidden epidemic. *Critical Care Nursing, 5,* 38-42.

Sadock, B.J., & Sadock, V.A. (2004). *Concise textbook of clinical psychiatry* (2nd ed.). Philadelphia: Lippincott Williams & Wilkins.

Schneider, L.S., Tariot, P.N., Dagerman, K.S., et al. (2006). Effectiveness of atypical antipsychotic drugs in patients with Alzheimer's disease. *New England Journal of Medicine, 355,* 1525-1538.

Shumaker, S.A., Legvalt, C., Rapp, S.R., et al. (2003). Estrogen plus progestin and the incidence of dementia and mild cognitive impairment in postmenopausal women. The Women's Health Initiative Memory Study: A randomized controlled trial. *Journal of the American Medical Association, 289*(20), 2651.

Strandberg, T.E., Pitkala, K.H., Linna Vuari, K.H., et al. (2003). Impact of viral and bacterial burden on cognitive impairment in elderly persons with cardiovascular diseases. *Stroke, 34*(9), 2126-2131.

Strong, C. (1984). Stress and caring for elderly relatives: Interpretations and coping strategies in an American Indian and white sample. *The Gerontologist, 24,* pp. 251-256.

U.S. Food and Drug Administration. (2003). *FDA News: FDA approves memantine (Namenda) for Alzheimer's disease.* Retrieved February 1, 2005, from www.fda.gov/bbs/topics/NEWS/2003/NEW00961.html.

U.S. Government Printing Office (GPO). (1992). Culture & caregiving—Confronting Alzheimer's: Help for patients and families. Retrieved December 4, 2007, from http://findarticles.com/p/articles/mi_m1000/isn363-64/ai_12519940/print.

CHAPTER 16

Addictive Disorders

Elizabeth M. Varcarolis and Kathleen Smith-DiJulio

Key Terms and Concepts

abuse, p. 329
addiction, p. 329
Al-Anon, p. 353
Alateen, p. 353
Alcoholics Anonymous (AA), p. 353
antagonistic effect, p. 338
blood alcohol level (BAL), p. 340
codependence, p. 337
dependence, p. 329

dual diagnosis, p. 338
enabling, p. 336
flashbacks, p. 337
relapse prevention, p. 349
substance-abuse intervention, p. 349
synergistic effects, p. 338
tolerance, p. 329
withdrawal, p. 337

Objectives

1. Compare and contrast substance abuse and substance dependence, as defined by *the Diagnostic and Statistical Manual of Mental Disorders (DSM-IV-TR)*.
2. Discuss the theories of substance abuse and dependence development.
3. Explain the difference between tolerance and withdrawal, and give a clinical definition of each.
4. Discuss four components of the assessment process to be used with a person who is chemically dependent.
5. Describe the difference between the behaviors of an alcoholic person and a nondrinker in relation to blood alcohol level.
6. Compare and contrast the symptoms seen in alcohol withdrawal and those seen in alcohol delirium.
7. List the appropriate steps to take if one observes an impaired co-worker.

8. Describe aspects of enabling behaviors and give examples.
9. Compare and contrast the signs and symptoms of intoxication, overdose, and withdrawal for abused substances.
10. Discuss treatment of a person who is withdrawing from alcohol delirium, including nursing care and pharmacological therapy.
11. Describe assessment strategies for people with alcohol and drug problems.
12. Discuss the meaning of synergistic and antagonistic effects of drugs in a person presenting with polydrug abuse.
13. Identify the phenomenon of relapse as it affects substance abusers during different phases of treatment, and plan steps in relapse prevention.

continued

Substance use has been around since ancient people found that chewing on the leaves of certain plants or drinking fermented fruit juice could produce feelings of well-being or altered consciousness. The degree to which substance use is accepted or condemned varies from culture to culture.

It is becoming more evident in the scientific community that drug addiction is a brain disease that evolves over a period of time and is the result of an individual's voluntarily taking drugs. Eventually, with repeated use of the drug(s), the individual develops uncontrollable and compulsive drug craving, seeking, and use that can destroy functioning, relationships with family and friends, and place in society (Leshner, 2007).

The terms *abuse* and *dependence/addiction* are particularly important to psychiatric nursing. **Abuse** is the use of a substance that falls outside of medical necessity or social acceptance resulting in adverse effects to the abuser or to others. **Dependence** or **addiction** occurs when a **tolerance** to the drug occurs and the person has to take more and more of the drug to "stay normal" or prevent withdrawal. At this point, people no longer have control over their substance use, even when it is interfering with functioning and well-being. This dependence on or addiction to a drug is progressive and can even be fatal.

It is important to keep in mind that nonchemical addictions (e.g., compulsive overeating, gambling, shopping, sex, internet) meet the criteria for dependence as well. For our purposes here, we will use an operational definition of addiction: The three Cs.

1. Behavior that is motivated by emotions ranging along the lines of **C**raving to **C**ompulsive spectrum.
2. **C**ontinued use despite adverse consequences to health, mental state, relationships, occupation, or finances).
3. Loss of **C**ontrol.

See Table 16-1 for an overview of some of the growing list of common nonchemical addictions.

PREVALENCE AND COMORBIDITY
Prevalence of Substance Abuse

Kessler and colleagues cited in their national comorbidity survey replica (2005) the lifetime prevalence for substance use disorders in the United States is 14.6%.

Alcohol

Alcohol abuse and dependence are the most common substance problems and affect more than 17.6 million Americans older than the age of 18 (8.5% of the population) (Grant et al., 2006). Over the past decade, alcohol abuse has increased from 3.3% to 4.7%, whereas alcohol dependence actually decreased from 4.4% to 3.8%. Men are more than twice as likely to both abuse alcohol and be alcohol dependent. Young adults ages 18 to 29 have the highest rate of alcohol abuse and dependence of any age-group.

Illicit Drugs

There has been a decrease in the use of marijuana, cocaine, and heroin in the United States over the past decade. However, there has been a dramatic increase in substances often referred to as **club drugs**. These substances include 3, 4-methylenedioxy-methamphetamine (MDMA; ecstasy), γ-hydroxybutyrate (GHB) (G, liquid ecstasy), flunitrazepam (Rohypnol), and methamphetamines (meth) (Gahlinger, 2004). **Marijuana** is still the most commonly abused illicit drug in the United States (DEA, 2006), but the National Institute on Drug Abuse reports that **methamphetamines** represent the fastest growing drug threat in America. Inhalants also continue to be of considerable concern, especially with those younger than 18 years of age (Magellan Health Services, 2004).

According to the National Survey on Drug Use and Health, there were approximately 3.7 million lifelong users of the **opiate** heroin in 2003 (SAMHSA, 2004). On the rise nationally is the abuse of **prescription pain medication such as oxycodone (OxyContin)**, including middle-

TABLE 16-1 **Some Nonchemical Addictions**	
Definition	**Comments**
Shopping and Spending Pattern of chronic repetitive purchasing that becomes difficult to stop and results in harmful consequences	• 6% prevalence rate • Compulsive shoppers get a "high" caused by increase of endorphins and dopamine, reinforcing the desire to spend. • May coexist in people with mood disorders, substance abuse, or eating disorders
Pathological Gambling (PG) Includes an inability to stop or control the behavior, denial, severe depression, and mood swings and results in changes in the neurochemistry of the brain	• 4% to 6% of gamblers become pathological or problem gamblers. • PG and major depression often co-occur. • Presence of gambling opportunities can double the prevalence of PG and problem gamblers. • Youth (11-18 years old) show a 4% to 7% prevalence rate of problem gambling.
Internet • Compulsive Internet use provides a high, and the person needs that high to feel normal. • The Internet becomes the predominant priority in a person's life and negatively affects relationships, work or school, marriages, finances, etc. • A large subgroup participates in sexual encounters resulting in divorces, separations, and problems at home.	• About 5% to 10% of Internet users are compulsive users. • More than 50% of people "addicted" to the Internet suffer from other addictions (drugs, sex, alcohol, and smoking). • Types of Internet addictions include cyber porn, sexual encounters, online gaming, auctions, excessive e-mailing.
Sexual Addiction The pursuit of persistent and escalating patterns of sexual behavior despite negative consequences to self and others	• 18 to 24 million Americans are addicted to sex. • Sexual addictions include compulsive masturbation, anonymous sex with multiple partners, multiple affairs outside a committed relationship, computer sex, and more. • Sexual compulsivity often co-occurs with other addictive behaviors.

and hihg-school youth (NIDA, 2007e). The abuse of prescription pain medication (opiates and narcotics) alone accounts for a total of 2.5 million abusers, the majority of whom are adult females (Magellan Health Services, 2004). Fortunately, treatment for opiate dependence can be highly effective (APA, 2006). The misuse of other prescription drugs, such as amphetamines and benzodiazepines, is also increasing on a national level and often results in dangerous addictions requiring withdrawal precautions during hospitalization.

Anabolic Steroids

The abuse of **anabolic steroids**, synthetic substances related to male hormones (e.g., testosterone) is no longer associated with body builders and professional athletes but has become widespread in American society. Initially in the 1950s and 1960s, some athletes used these drugs to build muscles and boost athletic performance. Today the use of anabolic steroids has become more prevalent and may rank between 1% and 6% among athletes (Volkow, 2006). Unfortunately, steroid abuse has spread to include school-age children, models, business professionals, and others.

There has been an increase of steroid use among 12th graders from 2000 to 2005. The Centers for Disease Control and Prevention (CDC) reported that their survey revealed nearly 5% of all high school students reported lifetime use of steroids (NIDA, 2005). The actual preva-

EXAMINING THE EVIDENCE   Alcoholism: Disease or Bad Behavior?

From reading this chapter, nurses might think that they should urge people who have problems with alcohol to stop drinking, and if they relapse, they should work to regain abstinence. This is puzzling because it seems like drinking is a behavior and not a typical illness.

Without a doubt, the dominant model for alcoholism and its treatment is the disease model. This model identifies alcoholism as a disease that is predominantly genetically mediated. In this model alcoholism is treated with psychosocial and pharmacological interventions accompanied by complete abstinence. The American Psychiatric Association has identified alcoholism as a *DSM-IV-TR* Axis I disorder; most treatment clinics operate under this model, and Alcoholics Anonymous is based on this concept.

What's the evidence to support alcoholism as a disease? We know that risk for alcohol abuse is greater (three or four times) among close relatives (Schuckit, 2000), but perhaps culture and family lifestyle affect excessive alcohol intake (consider the Amish culture, in which alcohol abuse is a fraction of the general population). For a definitive answer, researchers would find a gene or gene combination present in every person who abused alcohol and not present in nonabusers, but so far this isn't the case. Most researchers agree that genetics account for only 40% to 60% of inheritability for alcoholism (Heath et al., 1997; McGue, 1997; Schuckit, 2000).

Opponents of the disease model cite its destructiveness saying that it frees the afflicted from taking responsibility for their actions and guilt. The alcohol abuser may feel like a helpless victim of a predetermined genetic fate, although at least one study reports that this is not the case (Gamm et al., 2004). Further, those who believe alcoholism is a behavioral choice claim that the *DSM-IV* classification was primarily developed as a means to get reimbursement from insurance companies. They contend that alcoholics can learn new behaviors and to eventually drink in moderation and point out that half of all smokers in the United States have quit smoking without support groups or treatment (Peele, 2003). In fact, according to the National Quality Forum (2007), "cessation or *reduction* of substance abuse" is a target outcome of evidence-based care. On the other hand, the APA (2006) states that the evidence to date suggests that substance-dependent individuals who sustain sobriety have the best long-term outcomes. One determining factor for healthcare providers to consider for recommending either controlled drinking or abstinence is the severity of the drinking problem. Often abstinence is recommended to those with more severe drinking problems and controlled drinking for those with lower severity drinking problems (Cox et al., 2004).

The disease-versus-choice controversy rages on and people passionately embrace their positions. But treatment for alcohol abuse can go forward while we await definitive answers. Considering the untold loss and tragic consequences of alcohol abuse, this is a good thing. Awareness of alcohol abuse, reducing it, and cessation—especially for those with the most serious problems—are all desirable goals.

American Psychiatric Association (APA). (2006). *Practice guidelines for the treatment of patients with substance use disorders* (2nd ed.). Retrieved November 4, 2006, from www.psychiatryonline.com/content.aspx?aID=141079.

Cox, W.M., Rosenberg, H., Hodgins, C.H.A., et al. (2004). United Kingdom and United States health care providers' recommendations of abstinence versus controlled drinking. *Alcohol and Alcoholism 39*(2), 130-134.

Gamm, J.L., Nussbaum, R.L., & Biesecker, B.B. (2004). Genetics and alcoholism among at-risk relatives I: Perceptions of cause, risk, and control. *American Journal of Medical Genetics Part A,128*(2), 144-150.

Heath, A.C., Bucholz, K.K., Madden, P.A.F., et al. (1997). Genetic and environmental contributions to alcohol dependence risk in a national twin sample: Consistency of findings in women and men. *Psychological Medicine, 27*, 1381-1396.

McGue, M. (1997). A behavioral-genetic perspective on children of alcoholics. *Alcohol, Health, and Research World, 21*, 210-217.

National Quality Forum. (2007). *National voluntary consensus standards for the treatment of substance abuse conditions: Evidence-based treatment practices.* Washington, DC: Author.

Peele, S. (2003). Addiction: Choice or disease. *Psychiatric Times, 20*(2), 11-12.

Schuckit, M.A. (2000). Genetics of the risk for alcoholism. *American Journal of Addictions, 9*,103-112.

lence of steroid abuse in the United States is extremely difficult to ascertain because most studies that measure drug abuse do not include steroids.

Nicotine

Nicotine is highly addictive. It alters mood, appetite, and alertness in ways users find pleasant and beneficial (GDCADA, 2006a). There are about 46 million individuals in the United States who smoke cigarettes, and tobacco is responsible for about 430,000 preventable U.S. deaths annually (GDCADA, 2006b).

Psychiatric Comorbidity

It is estimated that at least 50% of people with a serious mental illness have a substance use disorder as well. For example, data from the Epidemiologic Catchment Area Study found that 55% of patients with schizophrenia and 62% of patients with bipolar disorder had a comorbid substance use disorder (Minkoff, 2003). Other psychiatric disorders that may be seen concurrently in people addicted to substances include acute and chronic cognitive impairment disorders, attention deficit disorder, borderline and antisocial personality disorders, anxiety disorders, and depression. Substance abuse contributes to emotional problems in young and old alike. Eating disorders and compulsive behaviors (e.g., gambling) are also associated with substance use.

Suicide is a high risk among individuals who abuse alcohol or drugs. The rate of suicide is three to four times higher in substance abusers than in the general population, with a lifetime mortality rate of 15% in this group (APA, 2000b). Substance abuse increases the risk of suicide among children, adolescents, adults, and older adults. Refer to Chapters 8 through 15 as well as Chapter 20 for more information on the relationship between substance abuse and the rates of suicide among various clinical disorders.

People with comorbid mental illness or dual diagnosis often experience more severe and chronic medical, social, and emotional problems. Because these individuals have two or more disorders, they are vulnerable to both substance abuse relapse and worsening of the psychiatric disorder. In addition, substance abuse relapse often leads to psychiatric decompensations, and worsening of psychiatric problems often leads to substance abuse relapse.

Medical Comorbidity

Although marijuana is the most common illicit drug of abuse, alcohol abuse is the most prevalent of the substance abuse disorders. Therefore *alcohol*-related medical problems are the comorbidities most commonly seen in medical settings. The risk of health problems related to alcohol abuse is almost endless. Alcohol can affect all organ systems, in particular the central nervous system (Wernicke's encephalopathy and Korsakoff's psychosis) and the gastrointestinal system (esophagitis, gastritis, pancreatitis, alcoholic hepatitis, and cirrhosis of the liver).

Cardiovascular risks are also significant. Alcohol can raise the levels of triglycerides in the blood. Excessive alcohol intake results in stroke, cardiomyopathy, cardiac dysrhythmia, and sudden cardiac death (AHA, 2007). Also commonly associated with long-term alcohol use or abuse are tuberculosis, all types of accidents, suicide, and homicide.

Cocaine abusers may experience extreme weight loss and malnutrition, myocardial infarction, and stroke. Methamphetamine abusers experience, among other things, hypo-

thermia, seizures, brain damage, kidney damage, stroke, and death. Abuse of anabolic steroids can include liver and heart disease, stroke, and increased aggression. One of the most dangerous side effects, however, is depression that can occur during withdrawal. When not treated, the depression can lead to suicide weeks after the drug has been discontinued (NIDA, 2005).

Nicotine in the form of tobacco can cause chronic lung disease, coronary heart disease, and stroke, as well as cancer of the lungs, larynx, esophagus, mouth, and bladder (GDCADA, 2006b). About 50% of nonsmoking Americans are exposed to secondhand smoke. A comprehensive scientific report concluded that there is no risk-free level of exposure to secondhand smoke. Secondhand smoke is responsible for heart disease and lung cancer in nonsmoking adults and is extremely harmful to infants and children (USDHHS, 2006).

Most effects of *steroid abuse* are reversible if the person stops taking the drug. Some effects can be serious and permanent. For example, liver cancer, heart attack, and elevated cholesterol levels among adolescents may stop bone growth (NIDA, 2006a) and cause violent mood swings.

The route of drug administration influences medical complications as well affecting a person's addictive potential. **Intravenous drug users** have a higher incidence of infections and sclerosing of veins. **Intranasal users** may have sinusitis and a perforated nasal septum. **Smoking a substance** increases the likelihood of respiratory problems. Both smoked and injected drugs enter the brain within seconds, producing a powerful rush of pleasure lasting a short period of time, necessitating taking more of the drug more often to recapture the high (NIDA, 2007a). Refer to Table 16-2 for a look at physical complications associated with various classes of drugs and their routes of administration.

THEORY

Addiction is characterized by (1) loss of control of substance consumption, (2) substance use despite associated problems, and (3) tendency to relapse. The reason one person becomes addicted and another does not seems to relate to physical, developmental, psychosocial, and environmental factors, as well as genetic predisposition (Lingford-Hughes et al., 2003; Sinha et al., 2001). The difficulty in determining cause and effect is that the diagnosis of addiction generally occurs many years after the onset of use. Various factors are involved over the course of those years.

Scientific research has confirmed that addiction is a disease that affects both brain and behavior. There are biological and environmental factors, and genetic variations

TABLE 16-2   Physical Complications Related to Drug Abuse

Route	Physical Complications
Narcotics (e.g., Heroin), Phencyclidine Piperidine (PCP), Cocaine or Crack, Methamphetamine	
Intravenous*	Human immunodeficiency virus (HIV)
	Acquired immunodeficiency syndrome (AIDS)
	Hepatitis
	Bacterial endocarditis
	Renal failure
	Cardiac arrest
	Coma
	Seizures
	Respiratory arrest
	Dermatitis
	Pulmonary emboli
	Tetanus
	Abscesses—osteomyelitis
	Septicemia
Cocaine, Methamphetamine	
Intravenous, intranasal, smoking	Perforation of nasal septum (when taken intranasally)
	Respiratory paralysis
	Cardiovascular collapse
	Hyperpyrexia
	Intracerebral hemorrhage
Caffeine	
Ingestion	Gastroesophageal reflux
	Peptic ulcer
	Increased intraocular pressure in unregulated glaucoma
	Tachycardia
	Increased plasma glucose and lipid levels
PCP	
Ingestion	Respiratory arrest
Marijuana	
Smoking, ingestion	Impaired lung structure
	Chromosomal mutation—increased incidence of birth defects
	Micronucleic white blood cells—increased risk of disease as a result of decreased resistance to infection
	Stroke
	Possible long-term effects on short-term memory
Nicotine	
Smoking, chewing	Heavy chronic use associated with:
	Emphysema
	Cancer of the larynx and esophagus
	Lung cancer
	Peripheral vascular diseases
	Cancer of the mouth
	Cardiovascular disease
	Hypertension

*The complications listed can result from any drug taken intravenously.

Continued

TABLE 16-2	Physical Complications Related to Drug Abuse—cont'd
Route	**Physical Complications**
Heroin	
Intravenous*, smoking	Constipation
	Dermatitis
	Malnutrition
	Hypoglycemia
	Dental caries
	Amenorrhea
Inhalants	
Sniffing, snorting, bagging (inhalation of fumes from a plastic bag), huffing (placing an inhalant-soaked rag in the mouth)	Respiratory arrest
	Tachycardia
	Dysrhythmias
	Nervous system damage

*The complications listed can result from any drug taken intravenously.

that contribute to this disease, and research in this area is ongoing (NIDA, 2007b). Biological, psychological, and sociocultural theories are examined here briefly.

Biological Theories

Genetic factors are believed to account for between 40% and 60% of a personal vulnerability to addiction (NIDA, 2007a). A Norwegian study of 1400 pairs of twins supported previous findings that genetic factors are an important risk factor for psychoactive drug use (Kendler et al., 2006). Alcoholism is three to four times more likely to occur in children of alcoholic parents than in children of nonalcoholic parents (APA, 2000a).

It has been demonstrated more recently that alcohol and drugs of abuse have specific effects on selected neurotransmitter systems. Dopamine is a neurotransmitter that plays a major role in addiction, but the concepts that apply to dopamine can apply to other neurotransmitters as well.

Dopamine is the brain chemical present in regions of the brain that regulates motivation, emotion, cognition or learning, and the ability to experience pleasure and pain.

All drugs of abuse (e.g. nicotine, cocaine, marijuana, methamphetamine) directly or indirectly affect the limbic (reward) system. The reward system is made up of the ventral tegmental area (VTA), nucleus accumbens, and part of the cerebral cortex. The first time an individual uses a drug of abuse, neurons in the reward pathway release dopamine into specific areas of the brain. The neurons in the

reward pathway communicate through electrical signals that are passed on to the next neuron across a small gap called a synapse. Dopamine is then released into the synapse and crosses to the next neuron and binds to that neuron's dopamine receptor (NIDA, 2007a,b). It is this binding that produces the initial unnaturally intense feelings of pleasure.

As a result of this flood of neurotransmitters (dopamine in this case), the neurons try to regulate the level of dopamine in the brain by either reducing the number of dopamine receptors, or make less dopamine. Eventually, dopamine's ability to stimulate the reward center becomes very low, and the individual uses more and more of the drug to get the dopamine levels up to normal or higher, and the vicious cycle of taking more and more of the drug to even feel "normal" begins the cycle of tolerance to the drug and eventual dependence or addiction. Other nerve cells release γ-aminobutyric acid (GABA), which is an inhibitory neurotransmitter that helps moderate neuronal activity and works to help the receptor nerve from becoming overstimulated (NIDA, 2007a,b).

Opioid drugs act on opioid receptors. Alcohol and other central nervous system (CNS) depressants act on GABA receptors. This finding helps explain the addictive and cross-tolerance effects that occur when the use of alcohol is combined with use of barbiturates and benzodiazepines. Cocaine and amphetamines act on the dopamine and serotonin systems, producing the intense rush and resulting intense lows, reinforcing compulsive use.

Psychological Theories

Although no known addictive personality type exists, associated psychodynamic factors have been identified such as lack of tolerance for frustration and pain, impulsiveness, lack of success in life, lack of affectionate and meaningful relationships, low self-esteem, lack of self-regard, and strong propensity for risk-taking. Polysubstance abusers (two or more drugs) are more likely to report an unstable childhood and self-medicate than are those who abuse alcohol alone. Multiple studies link personality disorders (e.g., antisocial, borderline, and narcissistic) and substance abuse.

There is no single cause of substance abuse. Multiple factors contribute to substance use, abuse, and addiction in any individual. For example, a child of an alcoholic parent may have a biochemical deficiency predisposing him or her to alcoholism and may grow up with low self-esteem in a society that has no rituals governing alcohol use.

CULTURAL CONSIDERATIONS

There does seem to be some interesting differences among cultural groups. For example, in Asian cultures, the prevalence rate for alcohol abuse is believed to be relatively low. This is partly because of a deficiency in about 50% of the population of aldehyde dehydrogenase, the chemical that breaks down alcohol acetaldehyde. As the level of alcohol acetaldehyde increases in the blood, a severe flush and palpitations may occur (APA, 2000a). This reaction is thought to effectively keeps many Asians from drinking. In contrast, in Native Americans and Alaska Natives, the prevalence rate for alcohol dependence or abuse is quite high: 70% compared with 11% to 32% for their white, African American, and Japanese American counterparts (USDHHS, 1999).

Women in general are diagnosed with substance use at lower rates than men (SAMHSA, 2006). However, girls and young women get hooked faster and suffer the consequences sooner than boys and young men (CASA, 2003). Addicted women are viewed much more negatively than addicted men in many cultural groups. This negative attitude may lead to avoidance of the diagnosis and thus to a lack of treatment services.

Special Populations

Pregnant Women and Their Partners

Alcohol use during pregnancy can have negative physical, mental, and behavioral consequences. If a pregnant woman takes a drink, the unborn child takes the same drink. Alcohol is extremely neurotoxic and interferes with the fetus's ability to get enough oxygen and nourishment for normal cell development in the brain as well as other organs. The most extreme examples of the effect of alcohol on fetal development are fetal alcohol syndrome (FAS) or the lesser of the two syndromes, fetal alcohol spectrum disorders (FASD).

There are three basic criteria in that need to be present in order to make the diagnosis of FAS: (1) mental retardation, (2) delayed growth and development, and (3) distinctive facial abnormalities. FAS and FASD are lifelong conditions that result in permanent physical disabilities (e.g., hearing, eyesight, facial abnormalities, organ deformities, heart and kidney defects), mental disabilities (e.g., mental retardation, learning disabilities, memory impairment, CNS handicaps), and behavioral problems (e.g., hyperactivity, poor impulse control, irritability, criminal behavior) (CDC, 2006).

Women who smoke cigarettes prenatally are twice as likely to deliver low-birth-weight babies. There is also an increased risk of congenital abnormalities and respiratory problems. Recent research indicates that exposure to prenatal tobacco can affect the neurological system of the newborn (e.g., significant CNS changes and gastrointestinal and visual effects) (Williams, 2004). These infants also required more handling to keep them quiet and alert (NIDA, 2004). Teenage children of mothers who smoked during pregnancy are found to perform more poorly on tasks requiring auditory memory and of general intelligence than do children who were not exposed to cigarette smoke prenatally (NIDA, 2004).

Secondhand smoke exposure is known to be a cause of sudden infant death syndrome (SIDS), respiratory problems, ear infections, and asthma attacks in infants and children (USDHHS, 2006a).

Mothers who take opiates during pregnancy are more likely to experience intrauterine fetal deaths and are at a higher risk for infant death. Infants born to opiate-dependent mothers exhibit withdrawal symptoms.

Chemically Impaired Nurses and Health Care Workers

Impairment of a health care professional is the inability or impending inability to practice according to accepted standards as a result of substance use, abuse, or dependency (Baldisseri, 2007). Generally, health care workers are more apt to have higher rates of abuse with benzodiazepines and opiates.

Nurses have a 32% to 50% higher rate of chemical dependency than the general population. Estimates of the proportion of practicing nurses who are chemically dependent range from 10% to 20%. Helping the chemically impaired nurse is difficult but not impossible. The choices for action are varied, and *the only choice that is clearly wrong is to do nothing.* Without intervention or treatment, the problems associated with the chemical dependency escalate, and the potential for patient harm increases, as well as the health and well-being of the health care worker.

Often, the impaired nurse volunteers to work additional shifts to be nearer to the source of the drug. The nurse may leave the unit frequently or spend a lot of time in the bathroom. When the impaired nurse is on duty, more patients may complain that their pain is unrelieved by their narcotic analgesic or that they are unable to sleep, despite receiving sedative medications. Increases in inaccurate drug counts and vial breakage may occur.

If indicators of impaired practice are observed, they must be reported to the nurse manager. Intervention is the responsibility of the nurse manager and other nursing administrators. **The nurse manager's emphasis is on patient safety first; everything else, including work performance is secondary.** However, clear documentation by co-workers (specific dates, times, events, consequences) is crucial. Once the nurse manager has been informed, the legal and ethical responsibilities for in-house reporting have been met. If the impaired nurse remains in the situation and no action is taken by the nurse manager, then the information must be taken to the next level in the chain of command. These measures can prevent harm to patients under the impaired nurse's care and can save a colleague's professional career or even life.

Reporting an impaired colleague is not easy, even though it is our responsibility. Often he or she has high levels of denial and is not receptive of interventions. By the same token, the colleague of an impaired nurse may not see what is going on. In order *not* to see what is going on, nurses may deny or rationalize, thus **enabling** the impaired nurse to potentially endanger lives while becoming sicker and more isolated (Box 16-1 can be used as a check to discern enabling behaviors).

Referral to a treatment program should always be an option. Programs for chemically dependent nurses have been developed in some states in response to a policy statement issued by the American Nurses Association. Some state boards of nursing allow impaired nurses to avoid disciplinary action if they seek treatment. The aim of these programs is to protect patients and to keep the nurse in active practice (perhaps with limitations) or return to practice after suspension and professional help. Nurses who continue to show signs of impaired practice should not be returned to direct patient care.

Many programs have been created for helping not only nurses with substance abuse problems but also all health care providers who develop abuse and dependency. The National Association of Social Workers, the American Psychological Association, International Nurses Anonymous,

---

BOX 16-1

Have I Enabled?

Have I:

Excused or ignored behaviors in a peer that may be suggestive of impairment and justified those behaviors as "just having a bad day" or "stress"?

Never told the supervisor about behaviors possibly indicative of impairment that I observed because I was afraid of being wrong and did not want anyone to get angry at me?

Accepted responsibility for my colleague's unfinished work and at times attempted to counsel and solve his or her problem?

Believed that nurses do not use drugs or alcohol to the point of practice impairment and that substance use can be stopped at any time unless the person is morally weak?

Liked to use drugs or alcohol myself to relax or enjoy with friends? I do not want anyone to look at me. In fact, I have used a few discontinued drugs from work myself. Doesn't everyone?

Exonerated a peer's irresponsible actions by covering for attendance or tardiness? Have I cosigned wastes I have not truly witnessed or corrected the narcotic count to account for a discrepancy?

Defended a colleague when it was suggested there may be a problem with impairment?

From Smith, L., Taylor, B.B., & Hughes, T.L. (1998). Effective peer response to impaired nursing practice. *Nursing Clinics of North America, 33*(1), 105-118.

Nurses in Recovery, and American Counseling Association have developed programs to treat impaired social workers, psychologists, nurses, and counselors (Baldisseri, 2007).

CLINICAL PICTURE

The diagnostic scheme in the *DSM-IV-TR* (APA, 2000a) focuses on the behavioral aspects and the pathological patterns of substance use, emphasizing the physical symptoms of tolerance and withdrawal. An overview of *DSM-IV-TR* diagnostic criteria for substance abuse and dependence is provided in Figure 16-1.

evolve

For a comprehensive case study and associated nursing care plan for a patient experiencing alcohol dependence, visit the Evolve website at http:// evolve.elsevier.com/Varcarolis/essentials.

DSM-IV-TR CRITERIA FOR SUBSTANCE ABUSE AND DEPENDENCE

SUBSTANCE ABUSE AND DEPENDENCE

Substance Abuse

Maladaptive pattern of substance use leading to clinically significant impairment or distress, manifested by one or more of the following within a 12-month period:

1. Inability to fulfill major role obligations at work, school, and home

2. Participation in physically hazardous situations while impaired (driving a car, operating a machine, exacerbating existing problem [e.g., ulcer])

3. Recurrent legal or interpersonal problems

4. Continued use despite recurrent social and interpersonal problems

Substance Dependence

Maladaptive pattern of substance use leading to clinically significant impairment or distress, manifested by three or more of the following within a 12-month period:

1. Presence of tolerance to the drug

2. Presence of withdrawal syndrome

3. Substance is taken in larger amounts/for longer period than intended

4. Unsuccessful or persistent desire to cut down or control use

5. Increased time spent in getting, taking, and recovering from the substance; may withdraw from family or friends

6. Reduction or absence of important social, occupational, or recreational activities

7. Substance used despite knowledge of recurrent physical or psychological problems or that problems were caused or exacerbated by one substance

Figure 16-1 ■ Diagnostic criteria for substance abuse and dependence. (Adapted from American Psychiatric Association. [2000]. *Diagnostic and statistical manual of mental disorders* [4th ed., text rev.]. Washington, DC: Author.)

Tolerance and Withdrawal

The diagnosis of substance dependence involves the concepts of tolerance and withdrawal. **Tolerance** is a need for higher and higher doses to achieve the desired effect. **Withdrawal** occurs after a long period of continued use, so that stopping or reducing use results in specific physical and psychological signs and symptoms. Because alcohol is still the most common drug of abuse in the United States and poses the greatest withdrawal danger, *DSM-IV-TR* diagnostic criteria for alcohol intoxication, withdrawal, and delirium are highlighted in Figure 16-2. Information on signs and symptoms of intoxication and withdrawal from other substances of abuse is given later in this chapter.

Flashbacks

Flashbacks are transitory recurrences of perceptual disturbance caused by a person's earlier hallucinogenic drug use

when he or she is in a drug-free state (APA, 2000a). Visual distortions, time expansion, loss of ego boundaries, and intense emotions are reported. Often flashbacks are mild and perhaps pleasant, but at other times, individuals experience repeated recurrences of frightening images or thoughts. Flashbacks are common in individuals who are suffering from posttraumatic stress disorder (PTSD) as well.

Codependence

Codependence is a cluster of behaviors originally identified through research involving the families of alcoholic patients. Living with a substance-abusing or alcoholic individual is a source of stress and requires family system adjustments. People who are codependent often exhibit over-responsible behavior—doing for others what others could just as well do for themselves. They have a constellation of maladaptive thoughts, feelings, behaviors, and attitudes that effectively prevent them from living full and satisfying lives. Symp-

DSM-IV-TR CRITERIA FOR ALCOHOL-RELATED DISORDERS

ALCOHOL-RELATED DISORDERS

Alcohol Intoxication	Alcohol Withdrawal	Substance-Induced Delirium
1. Recent ingestion 2. Clinically significant, maladaptive behavior or psychological changes (sexual, aggressive, mood, and judgment) 3. At least one of the following: • Slurred speech • Incoordination • Unsteady gait • Nystagmus • Impairment in attention or memory • Stupor or coma 4. Symptoms not due to another medical/mental condition	1. Cessation (reduction) of alcohol use that has been heavy or prolonged 2. Two (or more) of the following: • Nausea or vomiting • Anxiety • Transient visual, tactile, or auditory hallucinations or illusions • Autonomic hyperactivity (e.g., sweating, increased pulse over 100 beats/min) • Psychomotor agitation • Insomnia • Grand mal seizures • Increased hand tremor	1. Impaired consciousness (reduced awareness of environment) 2. Changes in cognition (memory impairment, disorientation, language impairment, visual or tactile hallucinations, illusions) 3. Develops over short period of time — hours to days — and fluctuates over a day 4. Evidence of substance use (history, physical, laboratory findings) and symptoms developed during withdrawal

Figure 16-2 ■ Diagnostic criteria for alcohol-related disorders. (Adapted from American Psychiatric Association. [2000]. *Diagnostic and statistical manual of mental disorders* [4th ed., text rev.]. Washington, DC: Author.)

tomatic of codependence is valuing oneself by what one does, what one looks like, and what one has, rather than by who one is (Box 16-2).

Synergistic Effects

When some drugs are taken together, the effect of either or both of the drugs is intensified or prolonged. For example, combinations of alcohol plus a benzodiazepine, alcohol plus an opiate, and alcohol plus a barbiturate produce **synergistic effects**. All these drugs are CNS depressants. Taking two of these drugs together results in far greater CNS depression than the simple sum of the effects of each drug. Many unintentional deaths have resulted from lethal drug combinations.

Antagonistic Effects

Many people combine drugs to weaken or inhibit the effect of one of the drugs (i.e., for **antagonistic effect**). For example, cocaine is often mixed with heroin (speedball). The heroin (CNS depressant) is meant to soften the intense letdown of withdrawal from cocaine (CNS stimulant).

Naloxone (Narcan), an opiate antagonist, is often given to people who have overdosed on an opiate (usually heroin) to reverse respiratory and CNS depression. Because the duration of action of naloxone may be less than that of the narcotic that was taken, further monitoring and possible additional doses of naloxone may be needed.

Application of the Nursing Process
ASSESSMENT

Assessment of chemical impairment is becoming more complex because of the increase in the simultaneous use of many substances **(polydrug abuse)**, as well as the coexistence of psychiatric disease (**dual diagnosis**) and comorbid physical illnesses, including human immunodeficiency virus (HIV) infection, acquired immunodeficiency syndrome (AIDS), dementia, and encephalopathy.

Sensitivity to multicultural and racial issues is important in interpreting symptoms, making diagnoses, providing clinical care, and designing prevention strategies. Refer to Box 16-3 for areas to be covered in overall assessment for patients who use substances.

BOX 16-2

Over-responsible (Codependent) Behaviors

Codependent individuals find themselves:

- Attempting to control someone else's drug use.
- Spending inordinate time thinking about the addicted person.
- Finding excuses for the person's substance abuse.
- Covering up the person's drinking or drug taking or lying.
- Feeling responsible for the person's drinking or drug use.
- Feeling guilty for the addicted person's behavior.
- Avoiding family and social events because of concerns or shame about the addicted member's behavior.
- Making threats regarding the consequences of the alcoholic's or drug abuser's behavior and failing to follow through.
- Eliciting promises for change.
- Feeling like they are "walking on eggshells" on a routine basis to avoid causing problems, especially in relation to alcohol or drug use.
- Allowing moods to be influenced by those of the addicted person.
- Searching for, hiding, and destroying the abuser's drug or alcohol supply.
- Assuming the alcoholic's or substance abuser's duties and responsibilities.
- Feeling forced to increase control over the family's finances.
- Often bailing the addicted person out of financial or legal problems.

BOX 16-3

Overall Assessment Guide for Substance Use

History of Patient's Substance Use

1. What are the date of first use, number of substances being taken, pattern of use, amount, frequency, periods of sobriety, time last taken?
2. Was patient treated previously for substance abuse? What was the outcome?
3. Is there a history of blackouts, delirium, or seizures?
4. Is there a history of withdrawal symptoms, overdoses, and complications from past substance use?
5. Is there a family history of drug or alcohol problems?

Medical History

1. Does the patient have any coexisting physical conditions (e.g., HIV infection)?
2. What medications does the patient presently take?
3. What is the patient's current medical status? Mental status?

Psychiatric History

1. Is there a history of comorbid psychiatric problems (dual diagnosis)? Depression? Personality disorder? Conduct disorder? Schizophrenia?
2. Has the patient undergone treatment for a specific disorder? What medications were given and what was the outcome?
3. Is there a history of abuse (physical, sexual)? Family violence?

4. Is there a history of suicide? Violence toward others?
5. Is the patient having suicidal thoughts?

Psychosocial Issues

1. Does the patient have a poor work record related to substance use?
2. How has the patient's substance use affected his or her relationships with others?
   - Family
   - Friends
   - Professional relationships
   - Community involvement
3. How has the substance use affected the patient's ability to meet usual role expectations (e.g., parent, spouse, friend, employee)?
4. Is there a police or criminal record or legal problems related to substance use (e.g., vehicle accidents, driving while intoxicated, physical violence)?
5. Whom does the patient identify as his or her support system? Whom does the patient trust? Who cares for the patient? Who will help the patient if the patient asks for help?
6. Does the patient use coping styles that contribute to the maintenance of his or her drug or alcohol lifestyle?

Initial Interview Guidelines

Current alcohol or other drug problems can be detected by asking two questions that are easily integrated into a clinical interview (Brown et al., 2001). These two questions are:

1. In the past year, have you ever drunk or used drugs more than you meant to?
2. Have you felt you wanted or needed to cut down on your drinking or drug use in the past year?

From those two initial questions, the nurse can then pinpoint specific drugs depending on the particular clinical situation. The nurse should ask questions in a matter-of-fact, nonjudgmental fashion. Specific details include name(s) of drug(s) used, route, quantity, time of last use, and usual pattern of use. The CAGE-AID assessment is a commonly used tool in screening alcohol and substance abuse (Box 16-4).

Responses that serve as red flags indicating the need for further assessment are rationalizations ("You'd smoke dope, too, if . . ."); automatic responses, as if the question were predicted; and slow, prolonged responses, as if the person were being careful about what to say. If the person is not able to provide a drug history, the nurse should assess for indications of substance abuse, such as dilated or constricted pupils, abnormal vital signs, needle marks, tremors, and alcohol on the breath. The nurse should also obtain history information from family and friends. Clothing should be checked for drug paraphernalia, such as used syringes, crack vials, white powder, razor blades, bent spoons, and pipes.

Further Initial Assessment

There is a consistent and significant association between alcohol and drug use and injury (Miller et al., 2001). Intracranial hematomas, subdural hematomas, and other conditions can go unnoticed if symptoms of acute alcohol intoxication and withdrawal are not distinguished from the symptoms of a brain injury. Therefore neurological signs (pupil size, equality, and reaction to light) should be assessed, especially in comatose patients suspected of having traumatic injuries. In addition, questions about alcohol or drug use should be asked as part of the assessment of any trauma. A urine **toxicology screen** or **blood alcohol level (BAL)** can be useful for assessment purposes.

Assessment strategies must include collection of data pertaining to both substance dependence and psychiatric impairment. Individuals with previously established psychiatric impairment may be experiencing substance abuse or dependence if they exhibit increasing frequency of symptoms, exacerbation without obvious reason, chronic noncompliance with treatment regimens, and self-medication or use of a substance in response to symptomatology secondary to psychiatric impairment or social stressors (Compton et al., 2003). Substance abuse can go undetected in those who are depressed, suicidal, or anxious unless a thorough history is taken. Similarly, the understanding and treatment of substance-dependent people are enhanced by inquiries about symptoms of depression and anxiety.

Once specific data are obtained, it is helpful to know if the person is abusing a substance or is actively dependent on the substance (see Figure 16-1 for guidance in making this distinction).

BOX 16-4

CAGE-AID Screening Tool

C—Have you ever felt you ought to **C**ut down on your drinking (or drug use)?

A—Have people **A**nnoyed you by criticizing your drinking (drug use)?

G—Have you ever felt bad or **G**uilty about your drinking (drug use)?

E—Have you ever had a drink (used drugs) first thing in the morning (**E**ye-opener) to steady your nerves or get rid of a hangover?

AID—**A**dapted to **I**nclude **D**rugs. One positive answer indicates a possible problem; two positive answers indicate a probable problem.

From Ewing, J.A. (1984). Detecting alcoholism: The CAGE questionnaire. *Journal of the American Medical Association, 252,* 1905-1907.

Psychological Changes

Certain psychological characteristics are associated with substance abuse, including denial, depression, anxiety, dependency, hopelessness, low self-esteem, and various psychiatric disorders. It is often difficult to determine which comes first, psychological changes or substance abuse. Some people self-medicate in an attempt to cope with psychiatric symptoms. For these people, symptoms of psychological difficulty remain, even after months of sobriety.

Substance-abusing people are threatened on many levels in their interactions with nurses. First, they are concerned about being rejected. They are acutely aware that not all nurses are equally willing to care for addicted people, and in fact, many patients have experienced instances of rejection in past encounters with nursing personnel. Second, substance abusers may be anxious about recovering because to do so they must give up the substance they think they need to survive. Third, addicts are concerned about failure in recovery. Addiction is a chronic relapsing condition. In fact, relapse is one of the criteria for diagnosing addiction. Most addicts have tried recovery at least once before and have experienced relapse. As a result, many become discouraged about their chances of ever succeeding.

These concerns can threaten the addict's sense of security and sense of self, increasing anxiety levels. To protect against these feelings, the addict establishes a **predictable defensive style.** The elements of this style include various defense mechanisms (denial, projection, rationalization), as well as characteristic thought processes (all-or-none thinking, selective attention) and behaviors (conflict minimization and avoidance, passivity, and manipulation). Refer to Chapter 8 for more discussion on defense mechanisms. The substance abuser is not able to give up these maladaptive coping styles until more positive and functional skills are learned.

Signs of Intoxication and Withdrawal
Central Nervous System Depressants

CNS depressant drugs include alcohol, benzodiazepines, and barbiturates. Symptoms of intoxication, overdose, and withdrawal, along with possible treatments, are presented in Table 16-3.

Withdrawal reactions to alcohol and other CNS depressants are associated with severe morbidity and mortality, unlike withdrawal from other drugs. The syndrome for alcohol withdrawal is the same as that for the entire class of CNS depressant drugs. Alcohol is used here as the prototype. The time intervals are delayed when other CNS depressants are the main drugs of choice or are used in combination with alcohol. In addition, as patients age, their symptoms of withdrawal continue for longer periods and are more severe than in younger patients.

TABLE 16-3 Central Nervous System Depressants

Drugs	Intoxication Effects	Overdose Effects	Possible Overdose Treatments	Withdrawal Effects	Possible Withdrawal Treatments
Barbiturates Benzodiazepines Chloral hydrate Glutethimide Meprobamate Alcohol (ETOH)	*Physical:* Slurred speech Incoordination Unsteady gait Drowsiness Decreased blood pressure *Psychological-perceptual:* Disinhibition of sexual or aggressive drives Impaired judgment Impaired social or occupational function Impaired attention or memory Irritability	Cardiovascular or respiratory depression or arrest (mostly with barbiturates) Coma Shock Convulsions Death	*If awake:* Keep awake. Induce vomiting. Give activated charcoal to aid absorption of drug. Every 15 minutes check vital signs (VS). *Coma:* Clear airway; insert endotracheal tube. Give intravenous (IV) fluids. Perform gastric lavage with activated charcoal. Check VS frequently for shock and cardiac arrest after patient is stable. Initiate seizure precautions Possibly perform hemodialysis or peritoneal dialysis. Administer flumazenil (Romazicon) IV.	*Cessation of prolonged heavy use:* Nausea and vomiting Tachycardia Diaphoresis Anxiety or irritability Tremors in hands, fingers, eyelids Marked insomnia Grand mal seizures *After 5 to 15 years of heavy use:* Delirium	Perform carefully titrated detoxification with similar drug. *Note:* Abrupt withdrawal can lead to death.

Multiple drug and alcohol dependencies can result in simultaneous withdrawal syndromes that present a bizarre clinical picture and may pose problems for safe withdrawal. Family and friends may help provide important information that can assist in care planning. The *DSM-IV-TR* identifies two alcohol withdrawal syndromes: (1) alcohol withdrawal and (2) the more severe alcohol withdrawal delirium (see Figure 16-2).

Alcohol Withdrawal

The early signs of withdrawal develop within a few hours after cessation or reduction of alcohol (ethanol) intake; they peak after 24 to 48 hours and then rapidly and dramatically disappear, unless the withdrawal progresses to alcohol withdrawal delirium. The person may appear hyperalert, manifest jerky movements and irritability, startle easily, and experience subjective distress often described as "shaking inside." Grand mal seizures may appear 7 to 48 hours after cessation of alcohol intake, particularly in people with a history of seizures. Careful assessment followed by appropriate medical and nursing interventions can prevent the more serious withdrawal reaction of delirium.

A nurse's kind, warm, supportive manner can allay anxiety and provide a sense of security. Consistent and frequent orientation to time and place may be necessary. Encouraging the family or close friends (one at a time) to stay with the patient in quiet surroundings can help increase orientation and minimize confusion and anxiety.

Illusions are usually terrifying for the patient. Illusions are misinterpretations of objects in the environment, usually of a threatening nature. For example, a person may think that spots on the wallpaper are blood-sucking ants. However, illusions can be clarified; this reduces the patient's terror: "See, they are not ants, they are just part of the wallpaper pattern." If a person experiencing withdrawal is argumentative, hostile, or demanding, it is often because of deep-seated anxiety and feelings of guilt and shame. The nurse can make relief and hope possible by demonstrating an accepting attitude and showing strong support for efforts at recovery.

Alcohol Withdrawal Delirium

Alcohol withdrawal delirium is considered a medical emergency and can result in death even if treated (Webb et al., 2000). Death is usually a result of sepsis, myocardial infarction, fat embolism, peripheral vascular collapse, electrolyte imbalance, aspiration pneumonia, or suicide. The state of delirium usually peaks 2 to 3 days (48 to 72 hours) after cessation or reduction of intake (although it can occur later) and lasts 2 to 3 days.

In addition to anxiety, insomnia, anorexia, and delirium, features include the following:

- Autonomic hyperactivity (e.g., tachycardia, diaphoresis, elevated blood pressure)
- Severe disturbance in sensorium (e.g., disorientation, clouding of consciousness)
- Perceptual disturbances (e.g., visual or tactile hallucinations)
- Fluctuating levels of consciousness (e.g., ranging from hyperexcitability to lethargy)
- Delusions (paranoid), agitated behaviors, and fever (100° to 103° F).

Immediate medical attention is warranted in alcohol withdrawal delirium (see Pharmacological, Biological, and Integrative Therapies for a full discussion of medical treatments).

Alcohol is the only drug for which objective measures of intoxication exist. The relationship between BAL and behavior in a nontolerant individual is shown in Table 16-4. Knowledge of the BAL assists the nurse in determining the level of intoxication and the level of tolerance, and in ascertaining whether the person accurately reported recent drinking during the nursing history. These factors are also assessed by means of behavioral cues. As tolerance develops,

TABLE 16-4	**Relationship Between Blood Alcohol Level and Effects in a Nontolerant Drinker**	
Blood Alcohol Level	**Blood Alcohol Accumulation**	**Effects**
0.05 mg%	1-2 drinks	Changes in mood and behavior; impaired judgment
0.10 mg%	5-6 drinks	**Legal level of intoxication in most states.** Clumsiness in voluntary motor activity
0.20 mg%	10-12 drinks	Depressed function of entire motor area of the brain, causing staggering and ataxia; emotional lability
0.30 mg%	15-18 drinks	Confusion, stupor
0.40 mg%	20-24 drinks	Coma
0.50 mg%	25-30 drinks	Death caused by respiratory depression

a discrepancy is seen between BAL and expected behavior. A person with tolerance to alcohol may have a high BAL but minimal signs of impairment, as indicated in the following vignette.

VIGNETTE

Clarence comes to the emergency department with a BAL of 0.41 mg%. He is stuporous, ataxic, and has slurred speech. The fact that he is still alive indicates a high tolerance for alcohol. A nursing history conducted as the patient sobers reveals an extensive drinking history. When the blood alcohol level is this high, assessing for withdrawal symptoms is important.

The nursing history, physical examination, and laboratory tests are used to gather data about drug-related physical problems. The extent of impairment depends on individual susceptibility as well as the amount of drug used and the route of administration. Each class of drugs has its own physiological signs and symptoms of intoxication, which are summarized in the tables for each substance class.

Central Nervous System Stimulants

Table 16-5 outlines the physical and psychological effects of intoxication from abuse of amphetamines and other psychostimulants, possible life-threatening results of over-

TABLE 16-5   Central Nervous System Stimulants

Drugs	Intoxication Effects	Overdose Effects	Possible Overdose Treatments	Withdrawal Effects	Possible Withdrawal Treatments
Cocaine, crack (*short acting*) *Note:* High obtained in: snorted, 3 minutes; injected, 30 seconds; smoked (crack), 4-6 seconds Average high lasts 15-30 minutes for cocaine; 5-7 minutes for crack	*Physical:* Tachycardia Dilated pupils Elevated blood pressure Nausea and vomiting Insomnia *Psychological-perceptual:* Assaultiveness Grandiosity Impaired judgment Impaired social and occupational functioning Euphoria	Respiratory distress Ataxia Hyperpyrexia Convulsions Coma Stroke Myocardial infarction Death	Antipsychotics Medical and nursing management for: Hyperpyrexia (ambient cooling) Convulsions (diazepam) Respiratory distress Cardiovascular shock Acidification of urine (ammonium chloride for amphetamine)	Fatigue Depression Agitation Apathy Anxiety Sleepiness Disorientation Lethargy Craving	Antidepressants (desipramine) Dopamine agonist Bromocriptine
Amphetamines (*long acting*) Dextroamphetamine Methamphetamine Ice (synthesized for street use)	Increased energy Increased wakefulness, increased respirations, increased hyperthermia, and euphoria *Severe effects:* State resembling paranoid schizophrenia Paranoia with delusions Psychosis Visual, auditory, and tactile hallucinations Severe to panic levels of anxiety Potential for violence **Note: Paranoia and ideas of reference may persist for months afterward**	Same as above	Same as above	Same as above	Same as above

dose, and emergency measures for both overdose and withdrawal. All stimulants accelerate the normal functioning of the body and affect the CNS. Common signs of stimulant abuse include dilation of the pupils, dryness of the nasal cavity, and excessive motor activity.

When a person who has ingested a stimulant experiences chest pain, has an irregular pulse, or has a history of heart trouble, the person should be taken to an emergency department immediately.

Cocaine and Crack

Cocaine is a naturally occurring stimulant extracted from the leaf of the coca bush. Crack is a cheap, widely available alkalinized form of cocaine. When crack is smoked, it takes effect in 4 to 6 seconds, producing a fleeting high (5 to 7 minutes) followed by a period of deep depression that reinforces addictive behavior patterns and guarantees continued use of the drug. Cocaine is classified as a schedule II substance—"high abuse potential with some recognized medical use."

Cocaine exerts two main effects on the body: anesthetic and stimulant. As an anesthetic it blocks the conduction of electrical impulses within the nerve cells that are involved in sensory transmission, primarily pain transmission. It also acts as a stimulant for both sexual arousal and violent behavior. Cocaine produces an imbalance of neurotransmitters (dopamine and norepinephrine) that may be responsible for many of the physical withdrawal symptoms reported by heavy chronic cocaine users: depression, paranoia, lethargy, anxiety, insomnia, nausea and vomiting, and sweating and chills—all signs of the body's struggling to regain its normal chemical balance.

Methamphetamine

Methamphetamine is a highly addictive stimulant related to amphetamines, but has a longer lasting and more toxic effect on the CNS. Methamphetamines have neurotoxic (brain damaging) effects, destroying brain cells that contain dopamine and serotonin. Over time, as a result of reduced levels of dopamine, Parkinson-like symptoms can develop. Prolonged use can also include cracked teeth, skin infections, strokes, lung disease, kidney or liver damage, birth defects, and death (CESAR, 2005).

Nicotine

Nicotine is highly addictive and used worldwide. At least 20% of the U.S. population meets the criteria for nicotine dependence. A high proportion of psychiatric outpatients are nicotine dependent, which makes them even more susceptible to the medical sequelae of cigarette smoking. High among the list are lung cancer, emphysema, and cardiovascular disease.

Nicotine can act as a stimulant, depressant, or tranquilizer. Nicotine can also be chewed (in smokeless tobacco), which adds mouth cancer to the list of dangers. Wellbutrin (Zyban) and nicotine replacement therapy are successful treatments for many individuals during smoking cessation.

Opiates

The opiate drug class includes opium, morphine, heroin, codeine, fentanyl and its analogues, methadone, and meperidine. Use of heroin by American teenagers is increasing as it becomes cheaper and more potent (Hopfer et al., 2002). Novices are starting with nasal administration. Table 16-6 lists signs and symptoms of opiate intoxication, overdose, and withdrawal, as well as possible treatments.

Marijuana

Marijuana *(Cannabis sativa)* is an Indian hemp plant in which **tetrahydrocannabinol (THC)** is the active ingredient. Research has established that marijuana is addictive, and heavy use impairs the ability of young people to concentrate, learn and retain information (Brown University, 2008). THC has mixed depressant and hallucinogenic properties. Marijuana, the leaves of the cannabis plant, is generally smoked, but it can be ingested. It is the most widely used illicit drug in the United States. Desired effects include euphoria, detachment, and relaxation. Other effects include talkativeness, slowed perception of time, inappropriate hilarity, heightened sensitivity to external stimuli, and anxiety or paranoia. Overdose and withdrawal (other than craving) rarely occur.

In 2001, the Supreme Court ruled that marijuana has no medical value as determined by Congress, and the decision was upheld in 2001 by the Court of Appeals.

Hallucinogens

See Table 16-7 for signs and symptoms of hallucinogen intoxication and overdose.

Lysergic Acid Diethylamide (LSD) and LSD-Like Drugs

LSD (also known as "acid"), **mescaline** (peyote), and **psilocybin** (magic mushroom) are hallucinogens. Mescaline and the mushroom *Psilocybe mexicana* (from which psilocybin is isolated) have been used for centuries in religious rites by Native Americans living in the southwestern United States and northern Mexico. The hallucinogenic experience produced by LSD is called a trip.

Phencyclidine Piperidine (PCP)

PCP is also known as angel dust, horse tranquilizer, and peace pill. When it is taken orally the onset of symptoms occurs about 1 hour after ingestion. When the drug is taken

TABLE 16-6	Opiates				
Drugs	**Intoxication Effects**	**Overdose Effects**	**Possible Overdose Treatments**	**Withdrawal Effects**	**Possible Withdrawal Treatments**
Opium (paregoric)	*Physical:*	Possible dilation	Narcotic antagonist	Yawning	Methadone tapering
Heroin	Constricted pupils	of pupils as a	(e.g., naloxone	Insomnia	Clonidine-naltrexone
Meperidine	Decreased respiration	result of anoxia	[Narcan]) to	Irritability	detoxification
(Demerol)	Drowsiness	Respiratory	quickly reverse	Runny nose	Buprenorphine
Morphine	Decreased blood	depression or	central nervous	(rhinorrhea)	substitution
Codeine	pressure	arrest	system depression	Panic	
Methadone	Slurred speech	Cardiac arrest		Diaphoresis	
(Dolophine)	Psychomotor	and death		Cramps	
Hydromorphone	retardation	Coma		Nausea and	
(Dilaudid)	*Psychological-perceptual:*	Shock		vomiting	
Fentanyl	Initial euphoria	Convulsions		Muscle aches	
(Sublimaze)	followed by	Death		("bone pain")	
Fentanyl analogues	dysphoria and			Chills	
	impairment of			Fever	
	attention, judgment,			Lacrimation	
	and memory			Diarrhea	

Note: An opiate is a derivative or synthetic that affects the central nervous system and the autonomic nervous system. Medically it is used primarily as an analgesic (pain killer). Consistent use causes tolerance and distressing withdrawal symptoms.

intravenously, sniffed, or smoked, the onset of symptoms may occur within 5 minutes. The signs and symptoms of PCP intoxication range from acute anxiety to acute psychosis. The drug produces a generalized anesthesia that lessens the sensations of touch and pain and makes staff interventions difficult. Chronic use of PCP can result in long-term effects such as dulled thinking, lethargy, loss of impulse control, poor memory, and depression.

Suicidal risk is always assessed, especially in cases of toxicity or coma. If the patient awakens and appears to be suicidal, the nurse should determine whether previous suicide attempts have occurred. Information regarding suicide history of family members is also elicited. Additional history may be obtained through family as well as a review of medical records. Refer to Chapter 20 for more information on suicide assessment.

Inhalants
About 19% of adolescents in the U.S. say that they have sniffed inhalants—usually volatile solvents such as spray paint, glue, cigarette lighter fluid, and propellant gases used in aerosols—at least once in their lives (Espeland, 2000). Types of inhalants, signs of intoxication, and side effects are given in Table 16-8. Inhalant use may be an early marker of substance abuse and should be the focus of increased preventive efforts and early diagnosis and treatment.

Rave and Techno Drugs, "Club Drugs," Date Rape Drugs
Raves or techno dances are all-night dance parties attended by large numbers of youth, sometimes in excess of 20,000. Raves are known for their electric music and the liberal use of techno drugs such as ecstasy. **Ecstasy** (also called MDMA, Adam, yaba, and XTC), is a prototype of a class of substituted amphetamines that also includes MDA (methylenedioxy-amphetamine, or "love") and MDE (3,4-methylenedioxy-ethylamphetamine, or "Eve"). These recreational drugs produce subjective effects resembling those of stimulants and hallucinogens.

After MDMA is taken, subjective side effects include euphoria, increased energy, increased self-confidence, increased sociability, and a feeling of closeness to people. Because of their psychostimulant and psychedelic effects, ecstasy and the other drugs listed are increasingly abused, especially within the rave subculture.

Adverse effects such as hyperthermia, heart failure, and kidney failure have occurred. Deaths from acute dehydration have been reported (Leshner, 2000). Morgan (2000) states that there is growing evidence that chronic heavy recreational use of ecstasy is associated with sleep disorders, depressed mood, persistent elevation of anxiety level, impulsiveness, and hostility as well as selective impairment of episodic memory and weakening of memory and attention.

TABLE 16-7	Hallucinogens		
Drugs	**Intoxication Effects**	**Overdose Effects**	**Possible Overdose Treatments**
Lysergic acid diethylamide (LSD) Mescaline (peyote) Psilocybin	*Physical:* Pupil dilation Tachycardia Diaphoresis Palpitations Tremors Incoordination Elevated temperature, pulse, respiration *Psychological-perceptual:* Fear of going crazy Paranoid ideas Marked anxiety, depression Synesthesia (e.g., colors are heard; sounds are seen) Depersonalization Hallucinations, although sensorium is clear Grandiosity (e.g., thinking one can fly)	Psychosis Brain damage Death	Keep patient in room with low stimuli—minimal light, sound, activity. Have one person stay with patient; reassure patient, "talk down" patient. Speak slowly and clearly in low voice. Give diazepam or chloral hydrate for extreme anxiety or tension.
Phencyclidine piperidine (PCP)	*Physical:* Vertical or horizontal nystagmus Increased blood pressure, pulse, and temperature Ataxia Muscle rigidity Seizures Blank stare Chronic jerking Agitated, repetitive movements Belligerence, assaultiveness, impulsiveness Impaired judgment, impaired social and occupational functioning *Severe effects:* Hallucinations, paranoia Bizarre behavior (e.g., barking like a dog, grimacing, repetitive chanting speech) Regressive behavior **Violent, bizarre behaviors** Very labile behaviors	Psychosis Possible hypertensive crisis or cardiovascular accident Respiratory arrest Hyperthermia Seizures	*If alert:* *Caution:* Gastric lavage can lead to laryngeal spasms or aspiration. Acidify urine (cranberry juice, ascorbic acid); in acute stage, ammonium chloride acidifies urine to help excrete drug from body— may continue for 10-14 days. Put in room with minimal stimuli. Do not attempt to talk down! Speak slowly, clearly, and in a low voice. Administer diazepam. Haloperidol may be used for severe behavioral disturbance (*not* a phenothiazine). *Institute medical intervention for:* Hyperthermia High blood pressure Respiratory distress Hypertension

Note: A hallucinogen produces *abnormal mental phenomena* in the cognitive and perceptual spheres; for example, distortion in space and time, hallucinations, delusions (paranoid or grandiose), and synesthesia may occur.

TABLE 16-8	Inhalants		
Drug	**Intoxication Effects**	**Overdose Effects**	**Treatment**
Solvents (paint thinners, glues, gasoline) Gases (butane, propane, nitrous oxide)	Similar to alcohol: Slurred speech, lack of inhibitions, drunkenness, violent behavior, etc.	Liver and brain damage, heart failure, respiratory arrest, suffocation, coma, death	Support affected systems.
Nitrates (isoamyl, isobutyl)		Capable of interfering with oxygen supply to vital organs by knocking out oxygen carrying ability to red blood cells; associated with fatal cardiac rhythm	Neurological symptoms may respond to vitamin B_{12} and folate.

Data from National Institute on Drug Abuse. (1998). *Research report series: Inhalant use* (NIH Publication No. 94-3818). Washington, DC: U.S. Department of Health and Human Services.

The drugs most frequently used to facilitate a sexual assault (rape) are flunitrazepam (Rohypnol or "roofies"), which is a fast-acting benzodiazepine, and γ-hydroxybutyric acid (GHB) and its congeners (Schwartz et al., 2000). They are odorless, tasteless, and colorless, mix easily with drinks, and can leave a person unconscious in a matter of minutes. Perpetrators use these drugs because they rapidly produce disinhibition and relaxation of voluntary muscles; they also cause the victim to have lasting anterograde amnesia. Alcohol potentiates their effects. See Chapter 19 for more on these drugs.

Assessment Guidelines

Chemically Impaired Patients

1. Assess for a severe or major withdrawal syndrome.
2. Assess for an overdose to a drug or alcohol that warrants immediate medical attention.
3. Assess the patient for suicidal thoughts or other self-destructive behaviors.
4. Evaluate the patient for any physical complications related to drug abuse.
5. Explore the patient's interests in doing something about his or her drug or alcohol problem.
6. Assess the patient and family for knowledge of community resources for alcohol and drug treatment.

DIAGNOSIS

Nursing diagnoses for patients with psychoactive substance use disorders are many and varied because of the large range of physical and psychological effects of drug abuse or dependence on the user and his or her family. Comorbid psychiatric problems also must be addressed. Potential nursing diagnoses for people with substance use disorders are listed in Table 16-9.

OUTCOMES IDENTIFICATION

When planning care for patients with substance use problems, the patient's cultural background and values need to be factored in to the plan of care. Examples might include:

- Remaining free from injury while withdrawing from substance
- Attending programs for treatment and maintenance of sobriety (e.g., Alcoholics Anonymous [AA], Cocaine Anonymous [CA], Narcotics Anonymous [NA], or group therapy, cognitive-behavioral therapy or other)
- Attending a relapse prevention program during active course of treatment
- Verbalizing cues or situations that pose increased risk of drug use
- Having a stable group of drug-free friends and socializes with them at least three times a week (by *date*)
- Demonstrating (1, 2, or 3) new skills in dealing with troubling feelings (anger, loneliness, cravings, anxiety)

PLANNING

Planning care requires attention to the patient's social status, income, ethnic background, gender, age, substance use history, and current condition. It is safest to propose abstinence as a treatment goal for all addicts. Abstinence is strongly related to good work adjustment, positive health status, comfortable interpersonal relationships, and general social stability. Planning must also address the patient's major psychological, social, and medical problems as well as the substance-using behavior. Involvement of appropriate family members is essential.

TABLE 16-9 · Potential Nursing Diagnoses for Substance Abuse

Signs and Symptoms	Nursing Diagnoses
Vomiting, diarrhea, poor nutritional and fluid intake	*Imbalanced nutrition: less than body requirements* *Deficient fluid volume*
Audiovisual hallucinations, impaired judgment, memory deficits, cognitive impairments related to substance intoxication or withdrawal (deficits in problem solving, ability to attend to tasks and grasp ideas)	*Disturbed thought processes* *Disturbed sensory perception* *Acute* or *Chronic confusion*
Changes in sleep-wake cycle, interference with stage 4 sleep, inability to sleep or long periods of sleeping related to effects of or withdrawal from substance	*Disturbed sleep pattern*
Lack of self-care (hygiene, grooming), failure to care for basic health needs	*Ineffective health maintenance* *Self-care deficit* *Nonadherence to health care regimen*
Feelings of hopelessness, inability to change, feelings of worthlessness, feeling that life has no meaning or future	*Hopelessness* *Spiritual distress* *Situational low self-esteem* *Chronic low self-esteem* *Risk for self-directed violence* *Risk for suicide*
Family crises and family pain, ineffective parenting, emotional neglect of others, increased incidence of physical and sexual abuse of others, increased self-hate projected to others	*Interrupted family processes* *Impaired parenting* *Risk for other-directed violence*
Excessive substance abuse affecting all areas of a person's life: loss of friends, poor job performance, increased illness rates, proneness to accidents and overdoses	*Ineffective coping* *Impaired verbal communication* *Social isolation* *Risk for loneliness* *Anxiety* *Risk for suicide*
Increased health problems related to substance used and route of use, as well as overdose	*Activity intolerance* *Ineffective airway clearance* *Ineffective breathing pattern* *Impaired oral mucous membrane* *Risk for infection* *Decreased cardiac output* *Sexual dysfunction* *Risk for impaired liver function*
Total preoccupation with and majority of time consumed by taking and withdrawing from drug	*Delayed growth and development* *Ineffective coping* *Impaired social interaction* *Dysfunctional family processes: substance dependence*

Unfortunately, a person's social status and social relations often deteriorate as a result of addiction. Job demotion or loss of job, with resultant reduced or nonexistent income, may occur. Meeting basic needs for food, shelter, and clothing is thereby hampered. Marriage and other close relationships deteriorate and fail, and the person is often left alone and isolated. The lack of interpersonal and social supports is a complicating factor in treatment planning for the addict.

IMPLEMENTATION

The aim of treatment is self-responsibility, not compliance. A major challenge is improving treatment effectiveness by matching subtypes of patients to specific types of treatment. Although addicts share some characteristics and dynamics, significant differences exist within the addict population with regard to physiological, psychological, and sociocultural processes. These differences influence the recovery process either positively or negatively.

Often the choice of inpatient or outpatient care depends on cost and the availability of insurance coverage. Outpatient programs work best for employed substance abusers who have an involved social support system. People who have no support and structure in their day often do better in inpatient programs when these programs are available.

In addition, neuropsychological deficits have been associated with long-term alcohol abuse as well as other substances (e.g., methamphetamines). Impairment has been found in abstract reasoning ability, ability to use feedback in learning new concepts, attention and concentration spans, cognitive flexibility, and subtle memory functions. These deficits undoubtedly have an impact on the process of treatment.

At all levels of practice, the nurse can play an important role in the intervention process by recognizing the signs of substance abuse in both the patient and the family and by being familiar with the resources available to help with the problem.

Communication Guidelines

Communication strategies are designed to address behaviors that almost all substance abusers have in common, including dysfunctional anger, manipulation, impulsiveness, and grandiosity. The nurse's ability to develop a warm, accepting relationship with an addicted patient can help the patient feel safe enough to start looking at problems with some degree of openness and honesty. It is important to communicate in culturally appropriate ways.

A useful tool for helping the resistant addict develop a willingness to engage in treatment is known as **substance-abuse intervention**. The concept behind this approach is that addiction is a progressive illness and rarely goes into remission without outside help. Significant others arrange for a meeting with the addict to point out current problems and to offer treatment alternatives. The steps or elements are outlined in Box 16-5 and can be applied not only to alcohol but also other substances.

Health Teaching and Health Promotion
Relapse Prevention

Relapses are common during a person's recovery and they are in all chronic medical illnesses, such as diabetes, hypertension, asthma which also have both physiological and behavioral components (NIDA, 2007d). The goal of **relapse prevention** is to help the person learn from these situations so that periods of sobriety can be lengthened over time and so that lapses and relapses are not viewed as total failure. Relapse can result in a renewed and refined effort toward change.

BOX 16-5
Steps in Substance Abuse Intervention for the Resistant Addict

1. All the people concerned about and affected by the person's substance abuse are gathered together to present their case. The intervention must be rehearsed before it is actually carried out, usually with the support and guidance of a counselor.
2. Specific evidence related to the substance abuse is presented by each person, and it is written down so that each person does not have to rely on memory in a tense situation.
3. Timing must be right:
   • There must be current evidence available.
   • The intervention must take place after a crisis is precipitated by substance use and *not* when the person is under the influence of the substance or in severe withdrawal.
4. The intervention requires privacy. It is held in a place where no interruptions can occur.

5. The use of defenses is anticipated. No reaction is made to them.
6. Genuine, but firm, concern is demonstrated.
7. Substance abuse is understood as a disease.
8. Treatment alternatives are presented.
9. Responses to possible outcomes are prepared. The goal is to get the affected person into treatment. If the substance abusing person agrees to accept treatment, then he or she is taken immediately to a detoxification unit, where arrangements have been made previously. If the person refuses, then family members state that his or her decision must force them to make decisions of their own because they are no longer willing to live with the addicted person's behavior.

Adapted from Johnson, V.E. (1986). *Intervention: How to help someone who doesn't want help.* Minneapolis: Johnson Institute.

APPLYING THE ART   A Person with Chemical Dependency

SCENARIO: During our previous two one-to-ones, 34-year-old Kristen had repeatedly insisted she would "quit using and take my med." Now Kristen, a single mom, had just learned that her own mother had gained legal custody of Kristen's three preschool-aged children related to charges of child neglect. Prior to each of her two psychiatric hospitalizations in the past year, Kristen had chosen heroin over taking her psychotropic medication, and that decision then impaired taking care of her children.

THERAPEUTIC GOAL: By the end of this interaction, Kristen will show progress towards taking responsibility for acting-out behavior and acknowledge that choosing heroin when feeling out of control compounds her losses.

Student-Patient Interaction	Thoughts, Communication Techniques, and Mental Health Nursing Concepts
Kristen: *Glances my way and motions "come on" as she rapidly paces the hallway.* **Student's feelings:** *I'm surprised Kristen did not even stop to greet me.*	
Student: "Kristen, I'm having trouble keeping up with you. You seem really upset." **Student's feelings:** *Addiction makes me angry. Kristen shows such promise, then abandons everything when heroin calls. I know that some people at school see nothing wrong with "recreational" use of drugs. I look around the addictions unit and see pain everywhere.*	I had learned in report about Kristen losing custody of her children. Initially she had cried out but her tears quickly turned to angry pacing. I *offer self* by walking with Kristen, then *reflect* feelings.
Kristen: "Yes, I'm upset. My so-called mother stole my kids! I never injured my kids. I just asked my 5-year-old whether he wanted new shoes or wanted Mommy to feel better. It's not my fault. So my mother gets upset and bought the shoes. She thinks she can buy their love."	Kristen uses *projection*, blaming her mother for the loss of her children. I remember that clients with addiction use *"stinking-thinking,"* which includes *denial* ("I'd never hurt my kids"), *rationalization* ("It wasn't me who chose heroin over shoes"), and *projection*.
Student: "Kristen, I'm concerned with what is happening with you, but I'm having trouble keeping up. Could you walk a little slower, so I can hear you clearly?" **Student's feelings:** *I really am concerned with her welfare even though I feel frustrated that she totally denies her addiction.*	I think Kristen may be *ambivalent*, not sure if she can tolerate me or anyone.
Kristen: *Kicks over a chair, whirls and grabs my forearm, pulling me toward her.* "Get up here then if you care so much!" **Student's feelings:** *Okay. I am okay. I need to mindfully breathe and stay calm and in charge of me. I must admit though I don't like my arm being grabbed.*	She's escalating. I see staff on their way to help. Anxiety is communicated interpersonally. I need to talk her down.
Student: "Kristen, stop." *Louder voice, then quieter.* "You're hurting my arm." *Quietly concerned, trying to make eye contact.*	I *set limits* and *give information.*
Kristen: *Meets my eyes and loosens her grip. Sarcastically:* "Here comes the cavalry!" *Three staff approach, but wait as I speak.* **Student's feelings:** *I feel kind of honored that the staff trusts that I am doing well enough to wait to see if they're needed.*	Though Kristen uses sarcasm, she nonetheless responds to the staff's arrival by loosening her grip on my arm.

APPLYING THE ART   A Person with Chemical Dependency—cont'd

Student-Patient Interaction	Thoughts, Communication Techniques, and Mental Health Nursing Concepts
Student: "Kristen, I trust that you and I can get through this." *Pausing.* "Thank you for loosening your grip." *Concerned look.* "I know you're upset. Please let go." *She does.* "Thank you Kristen." *Staff step back carefully watching as Kristen slowly walks to the chair. Kristen uprights the chair she kicked over, then we both sit down.* **Student's feelings:** *I made it through this with no one hurt. I feel more confident but I'm also really relieved that the staff responded so quickly. I know the staff was ready to intervene if needed.*	I *offer self* and use *reflection.* I treat Kristen with respect as well as model socially appropriate interactions by saying please and thanks to Kristen for letting go of my arm.
Kristen: "I don't know what got into me. I never meant to hurt you."	She not only let go of me, she also fixed the chair.
Student: *I make eye contact.* "It's frightening to be grabbed. I'm okay now. How about you?"	I assess and also let Kristen know my feelings. Her choices affect others. I nonjudgmentally accept Kristen, but not the hurtful behavior.
Kristen: *Nods.* "I'm sorry. Sometimes I feel so out of control." **Student's feelings:** *Kristen tries to make things right by apologizing and fixing the chair.*	
Student: "You kicked the chair and grabbed my arm but you were also able to say 'sorry.' "	I name the observed *acting-out behavior* but also give *support* by saying, "You were able to. . . ."
Kristen: "I meant the 'sorry.' I always mean it. Then the pressure builds and . . ." *Points to the needle tracks on her arms.*	She uses heroin as a dysfunctional way to cope with anxiety. Then the heroin compounds her problems.
Student: "So when you feel out of control, maybe even overwhelmed, you turn to heroin? *Kristen nods.* And then. . . ." **Student's feelings:** *I can identify with feeling overwhelmed. I am so thankful I have other ways to cope and people who care about me.*	
Kristen: "I am gone. No more Kristen. I forget all the hassles. Then it all crashes down. I lose everything. I've screwed up everything again." **Student's feelings:** *Some days I think how far I still have to go to be a nurse. Then I think of Kristen's long, long road to reach a drug-free life.*	In choosing heroin she also chooses "no more Kristen." The drug erodes her self-esteem and even her sense of self.
Student: "Everything?"	I use *restatement,* encouraging her to go on.
Kristen: "Myself, my kids." *Starts to cry.*	Kristen shows *partial insight* but so far, avoids attending *Narcotics Anonymous.*

Continued

APPLYING THE ART   A Person with Chemical Dependency—cont'd

Student-Patient Interaction	Thoughts, Communication Techniques, and Mental Health Nursing Concepts
Student: *I lean forward, waiting quietly.* **Student's feelings:** *I want to fill the silences, but I contain my anxiety.*	I use *attending behavior.*
Kristen: "I miss them so much! They deserve better than me. I need to go lie down." *She begins to turn away.* **Student's feelings:** *Kristen feels exhausted by all of the emotions she's experienced.*	Kristen uses *withdrawal* by physically retreating to her room.
Student: "Okay, I'll check with you after lunch." **Student's feelings:** *I need to debrief in a clinical conference. I'm feeling exhausted too.*	I *give information* and accept Kristen's decision to leave in order to give her control and build trust.
Kristen: *Nods, walking toward her room.*	

VIGNETTE

Bill, 20 years old and single, is brought to the emergency department in a coma. He is accompanied by his mother, with whom Bill lives in a small apartment. Bill had been in his room at home. When his mother was not able to rouse him, she dialed 911 for an ambulance. A syringe and some white powder were found next to Bill. His breathing is labored, and pupils are constricted. Vital signs are taken; his blood pressure is 60/40 mm Hg, and his pulse is 132 beats per minute. Bill's situation is determined to be life threatening.

Bill's mother is extremely distressed, but she is able to report to the staff that Bill has a substance abuse problem and had been taking heroin for 6 months before entering a methadone maintenance program. It is decided at this point to administer a narcotic antagonist, and naloxone is given intramuscularly. After this, Bill's breathing improves, and he responds to verbal stimuli. His mother later tells staff that Bill has been in the methadone maintenance program for the past year but has not attended the program or received his methadone for the past week. At their urging, she calls the program, which arranges to send an outreach worker, Mr. Rodriguez, to talk to her and Bill. An appointment is made with Mr. Rodriguez for the following Monday. Mr. Rodriguez knows that Bill's future ultimately rests with Bill and talks to him regarding how he perceives his situation, where he wants to go, and what he thinks he needs to get there.

After talking to Bill and reviewing Bill's history, the health care team decides that a self-help, abstinence-oriented recovery program might be the most helpful treatment. Bill has not been taking drugs a long time, he has a job, and he appears motivated. Naltrexone (Trexan) will be given in conjunction with relapse prevention training, and Bill will regularly attend Narcotics Anonymous meetings.

General strategies for relapse prevention are cognitive and behavioral: recognizing and learning how to avoid or cope with threats to recovery; changing lifestyle; learning how to participate fully in society without drugs; and securing help from other people, or social support. Box 16-6 identifies relapse prevention strategies.

Awareness of Dual-Diagnosis Principles

The nurse needs to be aware of clinical practice guidelines that have been developed through research involving the dual-diagnosis population. The following six principles are applicable in inpatient and outpatient settings (Minkoff, 2003):

1. Expect a patient to have a dual diagnosis—it is not the exception.
2. Treatment success is increased when providers are empathic and hopeful, and work as a team.
3. Addiction programs and mental health programs both need a dual focus, which requires appropriate training for staff.
4. The substance use disorder and the psychiatric disorder are considered primary and need simultaneous treatment.
5. Recovery occurs in stages, and treatment should be matched to the patient's needs and level of motivation and engagement.
6. Outcomes must be individualized to support progress in small steps over a long period.

BOX 16-6
Relapse Prevention Strategies

Basics
1. Keep the program simple at first; 40% to 50% of patients who abuse substances have mild to moderate cognitive problems while actively using.
2. Review instructions with health team members.
3. Use a notebook and write down important information and telephone numbers.

Skills
Take advantage of cognitive-behavioral therapy to increase your coping skills. Identify which important life skills are needed:
1. Which situations do you have difficulty handling?
2. Which situations are you managing more effectively?
3. For which situations would you like to develop more skills to act more effectively?

Relapse Prevention Groups
Become a member of a relapse prevention group. These groups work on:
1. Rehearsing stressful situations using a variety of techniques.
2. Finding ways to deal with current problems or ones that are likely to arise as you become drug free.
3. Providing role models to help you make necessary life changes.

Enhancement of Personal Insight
Therapy—group, individual, or family—can help you gain insight and control over a variety of psychological concerns, for example:
1. What drives your addictions?
2. What constitutes a healthy supportive relationship?
3. How can you increase your sense of self and self-worth?
4. What does your addictive substance give you that you think you need and cannot find otherwise?

Adapted from Zerbe, K.J. (1999). *Women's mental health in primary care* (pp. 94-95). Philadelphia: Saunders.

Psychotherapy and Therapeutic Modalities

Nurses with advanced training may be involved in psychotherapy with substance-using patients. Psychotherapy assists patients in identifying and using alternative coping mechanisms to reduce reliance on substances. Eventually, psychotherapy can assist recovering addicts to become increasingly comfortable with sobriety. Evidence-based practice and data indicate that cognitive-behavioral therapies, psychodynamic and interpersonal therapies, group therapy, and family therapy are effective for selected substance use disorders (APA, 2000b, 2006).

Many critical issues arise during the first 6 months of sobriety. These include the following:
- Physical changes take place as the body adapts to functioning without substances.
- Numerous signals occur in the patient's internal and external world that previously were cues to drinking and drug use. Different responses to these cues need to be learned.
- Emotional responses (feelings that were formerly diluted by substance use) are now experienced full strength. Because they are so unfamiliar, they can produce anxiety.
- Responses of family and co-workers to the patient's new behavior must be addressed. Sobriety disrupts a system, and everyone in that system needs to adjust to the change.
- New coping skills must be developed to prevent relapse and ensure prolonged sobriety.

Psychotherapy needs to be directive, open and honest, and caring. The therapeutic process involves teaching the patient to identify the physical and emotional changes that are occurring in the here and now. The nurse therapist can then assist in the problem-solving process. Confidentiality must be maintained throughout therapy *except* when this conflicts with requirements for mandatory reporting in certain circumstances (e.g., child abuse, danger to self or others).

Self-Help Groups for Patient and Family
Counseling and support should be encouraged for all families with a drug-dependent member. **Al-Anon** and **Alateen** are self-help groups that offer support and guidance for adults and teenagers, respectively, in families with a chemically dependent member. Other such organizations include Adult Children of Alcoholics (ACA), Pills Anonymous (PA), and Narcotics Anonymous (NA), to name but a few.

Self-help groups assist family members in dealing with many common issues. Their work is based on a combination of educational and operational principles centered on acceptance of the disease model of addiction, including pragmatic methods for avoiding enabling behaviors.

Twelve-Step Programs
The most effective treatment modality for all addictions has been the twelve-step program. **Alcoholics Anonymous**

(AA) is the prototype for all the 12-step programs that were subsequently developed for many types of addiction. These programs offer the behavioral, cognitive, and dynamic structure needed in recovery. Three basic concepts are fundamental to all 12-step programs:

1. Individuals with addictive disorders are powerless over their addiction, and their lives are unmanageable.
2. Although individuals with addictive disorders are not responsible for their disease, they are responsible for their recovery.
3. Individuals can no longer blame people, places, and things for their addiction; they must face their problems and their feelings.

Using the 12 steps is often referred to as "working the steps" and helps a person refrain from addictive behaviors as well as fostering individual change and growth. In addition to AA, other 12-step programs include PA, NA, CA, and Valium Anonymous.

Residential Programs

Residential treatment programs are best suited for individuals who have a long history of antisocial behavior. The goal of treatment is to effect a change in lifestyle, including abstinence, development of social skills, and elimination of antisocial behavior. Follow-up studies suggest that patients who stay in such programs 90 days or longer exhibit a significant decrease in illicit drug use and recorded arrests and an increase in legitimate employment. Length of stay increases when treatment is family focused (McComish et al., 2000).

Intensive Outpatient Programs

Most treatments for substance-abusing patients take place in the community. The steps addicted people follow in an intensive outpatient program include a variety of psychotherapeutic and pharmacological interventions along with behavioral monitoring. Intensive outpatient treatment programs are becoming more popular because they are viewed as flexible, diverse, cost effective, and responsive to the specific needs of the individual. Reduction in program length can significantly increase the number of patients completing a program without affecting clinical effectiveness (Bamford et al., 2003).

Outpatient Drug-Free Programs and Employee-Assistance Programs

Outpatient drug-free programs are better suited to the polydrug-abusing or alcoholic patient than to the patient who is heavily addicted to heroin. These centers may offer vocational education and placement, counseling, and individual or group psychotherapy. Employee assistance programs have been developed to provide the delivery of mental health services in occupational settings. Many hospitals and corporations offer their employees counseling and support as an alternative to job termination when the employee's work performance is negatively affected by his or her impairment.

Pharmacological, Biological, and Integrative Therapies
Alcohol Withdrawal Treatment

The treatment of withdrawal symptoms has two major goals (APA, 2006):

1. Help the person achieve detoxification as safely and comfortably as possible.
2. Enhance the person's motivation for abstinence and recovery.

Not all people who stop drinking require management of withdrawal. This decision depends on the length of time and the amount the patient has been drinking, history of withdrawal complications, and overall health status. Medication should not be given until the symptoms of withdrawal are seen. Drugs that are useful in treating alcohol withdrawal delirium are listed in Table 16-10. For an overview of pharmacotherapy for substance use disorders, see Table 16-11.

EVALUATION

Favorable treatment outcome is judged by increased lengths of time in abstinence, decreased denial, acceptable occupational functioning, improved family relationships, and ultimately, ability to relate normally and comfortably to other human beings. The ability to use existing supports and skills learned in treatment is important for ongoing recovery. For example, recovery is actively viable if, in response to cues to use the substance, the patient calls his or her sponsor or other recovering persons; increases attendance at 12-step meetings, aftercare, or other group meetings; or writes feelings in a log and considers alternative action. Continuous monitoring and evaluation increase the chances for prolonged recovery.

TABLE 16-10 Treatment of Alcohol Withdrawal Delirium

Drug	Dosage	Purpose
Sedatives		
*Benzodiazepines**		
Chlordiazepoxide (Librium)	25-100 mg PO q4h tapered to zero over 3-7 days	Provides *safe* withdrawal, and has anticonvulsant effects; chlordiazepoxide and diazepam are cross-addicting
Diazepam (Valium)	5-10 mg PO q2-4h in tapering doses	Has anticonvulsant qualities
Oxazepam (Serax)	30-90 mg PO qid and 45 mg at bedtime and tapered to zero over 5-7 days	Not metabolized in the liver
Lorazepam (Ativan)	1-2 mg qid, then tapered	Not metabolized in the liver
Seizure Control		
Carbamazepine (Tegretol), or valproate (Depacote)		Reduces the requirement (dose) of a benzodiazepine; not effective when used alone
Magnesium sulfate	1 g IM q6h for 2 days	Increases effectiveness of vitamin B_1 and helps reduce post-withdrawal seizures
Thiamine (vitamin B_1)	100 mg PO daily for 3 days	Given intramuscularly or intravenously before glucose loading to prevent Wernicke's encephalopathy
Alleviation of Autonomic Nervous System		
β-blockers (propranolol) or	10 mg q6h	May help reduce ANS hyperactivity (e.g., tremor, tachycardia, elevated blood pressure, diaphoresis
α-blockers (clonidine)	0.5 mg bid or tid	
Folic acid	1 mg PO daily	Most effective in short time
Multivitamins	1 daily	Malabsorption due to heavy long-term alcohol abuse causes deficiencies in many vitamins

Data from Mack, A.H., Franklin, J.E., & Francis, J.F. (2003). Substance use disorders. In R.E. Hales & S.C. Yudofsky (Eds.), *Textbook of clinical psychiatry*, Washington, DC: American Psychiatric Publishing; American Psychiatric Association. (2006). *Guidelines: Treatment of patients with substance use disorders.* Retrieved November 4, 2006, from www.psych,org/psych_pract/treatg/pg/prac.
*Benzodiazepines should be discontinued once detoxification is complete.
bid, Twice daily; *IM*, intramuscular; *PO*, by mouth; *qid*, four times a day; *tid*, three times a day; *ANS,* autonomic nervous system.

TABLE 16-11 Pharmacotherapy for Substance Use Disorders

Indications	Prescribing	Advantages	Risks
Disulfiram (Antabuse)			
Helps prevent relapse of alcohol abuse. Ingested in combination with alcohol, it will cause nausea, vomiting, headache, and flushing.	**Induction:** 250-500 mg daily for 2 weeks **Maintenance:** 250 mg daily. Range is 125-500 mg daily **Labs:** liver function tests (LFT)s initially, then at 10-14 days, every 6 months thereafter	Useful in patients who have maintained sobriety but who have a history of relapse, current motivation, and a witnessed ingestion.	Metallic aftertaste; dermatitis; severe reaction or death could result from alcohol ingestion.

TABLE 16-11 Pharmacotherapy for Substance Use Disorders—cont'd

Indications	Prescribing	Advantages	Risks
Naltrexone (Revia)			
Helps with alcohol cravings, possibly by reducing the reinforcing effects of alcohol. Also used to block the effects of opiates.	**Induction for opiate dependence:** Be sure patient is opioid-free for 7-10 days; confirm by urine drug screen (UDS). Start 25 mg. If no withdrawal reaction, increase by another 25 mg. Continue at 50 mg daily.	Very useful in the acute recovery phase of alcohol dependence (first 12 weeks).	Nausea, abdominal pain; constipation; dizziness; headache; anxiety; fatigue
Vivitrol (naltrexone for extended-release, injectable suspension)			
Vivitrol is used for alcohol abuse only (should not be used if patient has opioid dependence).	**Induction for alcohol dependence:** Start at 50 mg daily. Continue at 50 mg daily. *Vivitrol (injection in buttocks)*—be sure patient is alcohol-free for at least a week: 380 mg/vial. **Labs:** UDS, LFTs prior to 6 months thereafter.	Vivitrol may be easier for patients recovering from alcohol dependency to use consistently.	Vivitrol should not be used by a patient who is also using opioids, such as heroin.
Acamprosate (Campral)			
Helps with alcohol cravings, possibly by reducing intensity of prolonged withdrawal syndrome. Benefit emerges after 30 to 90 days.	**Induction:** Begin two, 333-mg tablets, tid. Patients with renal impairment may need dosage reduction. **Maintenance:** 666 mg tid. **Labs:** blood urea nitrogen (BUN), creatine, creatinine clearance.	Reasonably safe in patients with mild to moderate hepatic impairment (excreted via the kidneys). Need to have been abstinent at least 7 or more days.	Diarrhea and increased libido
Buprenorphine hydrochloride (Subutex); Buprenorphine hydrochloride and Naloxone hydrochloride (Suboxone)			
Treatment for outpatient detoxification and maintenance by specially trained and registered physicians.	**Induction:** Begin 8 mg SL on day 1, 16 mg day 2. **Maintenance:** Continue 16 mg SL daily thereafter. Range is 4-24 mg daily. **Labs:** UDS at induction, and monthly thereafter. LFTs on induction, every 6 months thereafter.	Buprenorphine can prevent symptoms of withdrawal in patients addicted to opiates; an alternative maintenance treatment to methadone.	Dizziness; nausea; respiratory depression

Modified from Magellan Health Services. *Magellan substance use disorders tip sheet.* Retrieved July 14, 2007, from www.magellanprovider.com/MHS/ MGL/providing_care/clinical_guidelines/clin_prac_guidelines/sa_tipsheet.pdf. Information derived from National Institute on Alcohol Abuse and Alcoholism (NIAAA): (2005). *Helping patients who drink too much: A clinician's guide* (Updated edition). Available at http://pubs.niaaa.nih.gov/ publications/Practitioner/CliniciansGuide2005/guide.pdf.
bid, Twice daily, *PO*, by mouth; *SL*, sublingual (under the tongue); *tid*, three times daily.

KEY POINTS TO REMEMBER

- Substance use and dependence occur on a continuum, and addiction develops over a period of time.
- The tendency to abuse a substance can be influenced by a combination of genetic, biological, and environmental factors.
- Assessment of patients with substance use disorders needs to be comprehensive, aimed at identifying common medical and psychiatric comorbidities.
- Patients with a dual diagnosis have more severe symptoms, experience more crises, and require longer treatment for successful outcomes.
- The effects of a person's substance use or addiction affects everybody: family, friends, co-workers, and others and may lead them to adopt codependent behaviors to cope and minimize what is going on with the abuser.

- Relapse is an expected complication in the recovery of addictions, and treatment includes a significant focus on teaching relapse prevention.
- Successful treatment modalities include a dual-diagnosis approach, relapse prevention, self-help groups, psychotherapy, and psychopharmacotherapy.
- Nurses need to be aware of their own feelings about substance use so that they can provide empathy and hope to patients.
- Nurses themselves are at higher risk for substance use disorders and should be vigilant for signs of impairment in colleagues to ensure patient safety and referral to treatment for the chemically dependent nurse.

CRITICAL THINKING

1. Write a paragraph describing your possible reactions to a drug-dependent patient to whom you are assigned.
    A. Would your response be different depending on the substance, for example, alcohol versus heroin, or marijuana versus cocaine? Give reasons for your answers.
    B. Would your response be different if the substance-dependent person were a professional colleague? How?
2. Rosetta Seymour is a 15-year-old teenager who has started using heroin nasally.
    A. Briefly discuss the trend in heroin use among teenagers.
    B. When Ms. Seymour asks you why she needs to take more and more to get "high," how would you explain to her the concept of tolerance?
    C. If she had just taken heroin, what would you find on assessment of physical and behavioral-psychological signs and symptoms?

    D. If she came into the emergency department with an overdose of heroin, what would be the emergency care? What might be effective long-term care?
3. Tony Garmond is a 45-year-old mechanic. He has a 20-year history of heavy drinking and he says he wants to quit but needs help.
    A. Role-play with a classmate an initial assessment. Identify the kinds of information you would need to have in order to plan holistic care.
    B. Mr. Garmond tried stopping by himself but is in the emergency department with delirium tremens. What are the dangers for Mr. Garmond? What are the appropriate medical interventions?
    C. What are some possible treatment alternatives for Mr. Garmond when he is safely detoxified? How would you explain to him the usefulness and function of AA? What are some additional treatment options that might be useful to Mr. Garmond? What are available as referrals for Mr. Garmond in your community?

CHAPTER REVIEW

Choose the most appropriate answer.

1. When intervening with a patient who is intoxicated from alcohol, it is useful for a nurse to first:
    1. let the patient sober up.
    2. decide immediately on care goals.
    3. ask which drugs other than alcohol the patient has recently used.
    4. gain compliance by sharing personal drinking habits with the patient.

2. A principle of counseling intervention that should be observed by a nurse caring for a chemically dependent patient is to:
    1. develop a warm, accepting relationship.
    2. communicate that clinicians expect relapses to occur.
    3. recognize that recovery is considered complete and absolute.
    4. refrain from conveying hopeful empathy in order to promote resilience.

CHAPTER REVIEW—cont'd

3. As a nurse evaluates a patient's progress, which treatment outcome would indicate a poor general prognosis for long-term recovery from substance abuse? Patient demonstrates:
   1. improved self-esteem.
   2. enhanced coping abilities.
   3. improved relationships with others.
   4. expectations for only occasional drug use in the future.
4. Which statement relates most specifically to nursing assessment for a patient who is experiencing the effects of CNS stimulant abuse?
   1. Symptoms of intoxication include dilated pupils, dry nasal cavity, and excessive motor activity.

2. Medical management focuses on removing the drugs from the body.
3. Withdrawal is simple and rarely complicated.
4. Postwithdrawal symptoms include fatigue and depression.

5. Severe morbidity and mortality are associated with withdrawal from which of the following combinations?
   1. Alcohol and CNS depressants
   2. CNS stimulants and hallucinogens
   3. Narcotic antagonists and caffeine
   4. Opiates and inhalants

REFERENCES

American Heart Association (AHA). (2007). Alcohol, wine and cardiovascular disease. Retrieved July 23, 2007, from www.americanheart.org/presenter.jhtml?identifier=4422.

American Psychiatric Association (APA). (2000a). *Diagnostic and statistical manual of mental disorders (DSM-IV-TR)* (4th ed., text rev.). Washington, DC: Author.

American Psychiatric Association (APA). (2000b). *Practice guidelines for the treatment of psychiatric disorders: Compendium 2000.* Washington, DC: Author.

American Psychiatric Association (APA). (2006). *Practice guidelines for the treatment of patients with substance use disorders* (2nd ed.). Retrieved November 4, 2006, from www.psychiatryonline.com/content.aspx?aID=141079.

Baldisseri, M.R. (2007). Impaired healthcare professional. *Critical Care Medicine, 35*(2), 106-116.

Bamford, Z., Booth, P.G., McGuire, P.G., et al. (2003). Treatment outcome following day care for alcohol dependency: The effects of reducing program length. *Health and Social Care in the Community, 11*(5), 440-445.

Brown, R.L., Leonard, T., Saunders, L.A., et al. (2001). A two-item conjoint screen for alcohol and other drug problems. *Journal of the American Board of Family Practice, 14*(2), 95-106.

Brown University Health Education (2008). Marijuana. http://www.brown.edu/student_services/health_services/health-education/atod/marijuana. Retrieved April 2, 2008.

Centers for Disease Control and Prevention (2006). Fetal Alcohol Spectrum Disorders. Retrieved July 30, 2007, from www.cdc.gov/ncbddd/fas/fasask.htm.

CESAR (Center for Substance Abuse Research). (2005). *Methamphetamine.* Retrieved November 4, 2006, from www.cesar.umd.edu/cesar/drugs/meth.asp.

Compton, W.M., Cottler, L.B., Jacobs, J.L., et al. (2003). The role of psychiatric disorders in predicting drug dependence treatment outcomes. *American Journal of Psychiatry, 160*(5), 890-895.

Espeland, K.E. (2000). Inhalant abuse. *Lippincott's primary care practice, 4,* 336.

Gahlinger, P.M. (2004). Club drugs: MDMA, gamma hydroxybutyrate (GHB), Rohypnol, and ketamine. *American Family Physician, 69*(1).

GDCADA (Greater Dallas Council on Alcohol and Drug Abuse). (2006a). Steroids. Retrieved July 23, 2007, from www.gdcada.org/statistics/steroids.htm.

GDCADA (Greater Dallas Council on Alcohol and Drug Abuse). (2006b).Tobacco/smoking. Retrieved July 23, 2007, from www.gdcada.org/statistics/tobacco.htm.

Grant, B.F., Dawson, D.A., Stinson, F.S., et al. (2006). The 12-month prevalence and trends in DSM-IV alcohol abuse and dependence. *Alcohol Research and Health, 29*(2), 131-142.

Hopfer, C.J., Khuri, E., Crowley, T.J., et al. (2002). Adolescent heroin use: A review of the descriptive and treatment literature. *Journal of Substance Abuse Treatment, 23*(3), 231-237.

Kendler, K.S., Aggen, S.H., Tambs, K., et al. (2006). Illicit psychoactive substance use, abuse and dependence in a population-based sample of Norwegian twins. *Psychological Medicine, 36*(7), 955-962.

Kessler, R.C., Berglund, P., Demler, O., et al. (2005). Lifetime prevalence and age-of-onset distributions of DSM-1V disorders in the national comorbidity survey replica. *Archives of General Psychiatry, 62* (6), 593-602

Leshner, A.I. (2000). A club drug alert. *NIDA notes, 14*(6), 3-4.

Leshner, A.I. (2007). *Addiction is a brain disease. Issues in science and technology.* University of Texas at Dallas.

Lingford-Hughes, A.R., Davies S.J., McIver S., et al. (2003). Addiction. *British Medical Bulletin, 65*(4), 209-222.

Magellan Health Services (2005). *Marijuana's impact on teen's health, education, and welfare.* Retrieved November 4, 2006, from www.magellanassit.com/mem/library/default.asp?topicid=2&8&categoryid=d&articleid=51.

McComish, J.F., Greenberg, R., Ager, J., et al. (2000). Survival analysis of three treatment modalities in a residential substance abuse program for women and children. *Outcomes Management for Nursing Practice, 4*(2), 71.

Miller, T.R., Lestina, D.C., & Smith, G.S. (2001). Injury risk among medically identified alcohol and drug abusers. *Alcoholism: Clinical and Experimental Research, 25*(1), 54-59.

Minkoff, K. (2003). Dual diagnoses. In A. Tasman, J. Kay, & J.A. Lieberman (Eds.), *Psychiatry* (2nd ed., vol. 2, pp. 2333-2341). West Sussex, England: Wiley.

Morgan, M.J. (2000). Ecstasy (MDMA): A review of possible persistent effects. *Psychopharmacology (Berlin), 152*(3), 230-241.

National Center on Addiction and Substance Abuse at Columbia University (CASA). (2003). *The formative years: Pathways to substance abuse among girls and young women ages 8-22.* Retrieved from http://www.casacolumbia.org/Absolutenm/articlefiles/151006.pdf.

National Institute of Health (NIDA). (2004). The neurobehavioral legacy of prenatal tobacco exposure. Retrieved July 25, 2007, from www.nida.nida.nih./gov/nide_notes./nnvol18N67legacy.htm/.

National Institute on Drug Abuse (NIDA). (2005). *NIDA web site addresses consequences of steroid abuse.* Retrieved from http://drugabuse.gov/NIDA_notes/NNvol20N2/tearoff.html.

National Institute on Drug Abuse (NIDA). (2006). *Research report series—Anabolic steroid abuse.* Retrieved July 23, 2007, from www.drugabuse.gov/ResearchReports/Steroids/anabolicsteroids2.html.

National Institute on Drug Abuse (NIDA). (2007a). *Brain & addiction.* Retrieved July 25, 2007, from www.teens.drugabuse.gov/facts/facts_brain1.asp.

National Institute on Drug Abuse (NIDA). (2007b). *Drugs and the brain.* Retrieved July 25, 2007, from www.nida.nih.gov/scienceofaddiction/brain.html.

National Institute on Drug Abuse (NIDA). (2007c). *Drug abuse and addiction.* Retrieved July 25, 2007, from www.nida.nih.gov/scienceofaddiction/addiction.html.

National Institute on Drug Abuse (NIDA). (2007d). *NIDA infofacts: High school and youth trends.* Retrieved July 24, 2007, from www.drugabuse.gov/infofacts/HSYouthtrends.html.

National Institute on Drug Abuse (NIDA). (2007). *The science of drug abuse and addiction.* Retrieved July 23, 2007, from www.nida.nih.gov/scienceofaddiction/treatment.html.

Sinha, R., Drummond, D.C., & Orford, J. (2001). How does stress increase risk of drug abuse and relapse? *Psychopharmacology (Berlin), 158*(4), 343-359.

Substance Abuse and Mental Health Services Administration (SAMHSA). (2004). Results from the *2003 National Survey of Drug Use Health: National Findings.* (Office of Applied Studies, NSDUH serious H-25, DHHS publication No. SMA 04 3964) Rockville, MD.

Substance Abuse and Mental Health Services Administration (SAMHSA). (2006). Results from the *2005 National Survey of Drug Use Health: National Findings,* September.

U.S. Department of Health and Human Services. (1999). *Mental health: Culture, race and ethnicity. A supplement to mental health: A report of the Surgeon General.* Retrieved February 6, 2004, from www.mentalhealth.org/cre/default.asp.

U.S. Department of Health and Human Services (USDHHS). (2006). *New Surgeon General's report focuses on the effects of second-hand smoke.* Retrieved June 10, 2007, from www.hhs.gov/news/press/2006pres/20060627.html.

U.S. Drug Enforcement Administration (DEA). (2006). *Marijuana.* Retrieved June 10, 2007, from www.usdoj.gov/dea/concern/marijuana.html.

Volkow, N.D. (2006). *Steroid abuse is a high-risk route to the finish line.* Retrieved July 23, 2007, from www.drugabuse.gov/NIDA_notes/NNvol21N1/DirRepVol21N1.html.

Webb, J.M., Carlton, E.F., & Geehan, D.M. (2000). Delirium in the intensive care unit: Are we helping the patient? *Critical Care Nursing Quarterly, 22*(4), 47-60.

Williams, J.S. (2004). The neurobehavioral legacy of prenatal tobacco exposure. Retrieved July 25, 2007, from www.nida.nih.gov/NIDA_notes/NNvol18N6/Legacy.html.

Communicating with and Planning Care for Patients Experiencing Psychiatric Emergencies

CHAPTER 17

Crisis and Disaster

Elizabeth M. Varcarolis

Key Terms and Concepts

Objectives

1. Differentiate among the three types of crises.
2. Discuss aspects of crises that have relevance for nurses involved in crisis intervention.
3. Compare and contrast the differences among primary, secondary, and tertiary intervention, including appropriate intervention strategies.
4. Describe the initial needs of people in a disaster situation (adventitious crisis).
5. Explain the need for triage during a disaster.
6. Summarize the areas to assess during a crisis, giving examples of the kinds of questions for each area.
7. Give an overview of critical incident stress debriefing (CISD) including its purpose and process.

evolve

For additional resources related to the content of this chapter, visit the Evolve site at http://evolve.elsevier.com/Varcarolis/essentials.

- Chapter Outline
- Chapter Review Answers
- Case Sutdy and Nursing Care Plans

- Nurse, Patient, and Family Resources
- Concept Map Creator

Edited by Carolyn M. Scott in the fifth edition of
Foundations of Psychiatric Mental Health Nursing

The U.S. Department of Homeland Security raises the terror alert to "high" and warns American citizens to be watchful for any suspicious behavior. A child is killed in a drive-by shooting—the bullet intended for a neighborhood drug dealer. A husband announces to his wife of 30 years that he no longer loves her and wants a divorce. Tornadoes grind through Oklahoma and Kansas, leaving massive damage, flooding, deaths, injuries, homelessness, and the devastation of an entire town. A young nursing student discovers she is pregnant, and the father of the baby abandons her. What do these situations have in common? Each of these situations could be the precipitant of a crisis—an event that leaves individuals, families, or whole communities struggling to cope.

Nurses work with people in crisis all of the time: in the emergency department (ED); on medical, surgical, psychiatric, obstetric, and pediatric units; with family and friends; and in their own lives. Nurses need to constantly monitor personal feelings and thoughts when dealing with people in crisis and be aware when they need self-help. Self-monitoring and taking care of personal needs is especially important with mass casualties and natural disasters. Nurses may respond with anxiety to a patient's situation or anxiety level and try to repress such feelings to maintain personal comfort.

When nurses are unaware of personal feelings and reactions, they may unconsciously prevent the expression of the painful feelings in the patient that are precipitating the nurse's own discomfort. Thus closing off feelings in the patient can render the nurse ineffective. There may be times when the nurse, perhaps for personal reasons, feels he or she cannot deal effectively with a patient's situation. The nurse might ask a colleague to work with a particular patient. This will give the nurse a chance to work through some uncomfortable or painful personal issues.

It is crucial in beginning crisis intervention that supervision be available as an integral part of the training process. The supervisor should be an experienced professional, such as a nurse counselor or a nursing supervisor. Nurses new to crisis intervention often face common problems that must be dealt with before they become comfortable and competent in the role of crisis counselor. For example, nurses set unrealistic goals and become frustrated or have difficulty dealing with some issues, such as suicide. A number of schools of nursing now offer master's degrees in disaster nursing.

Even seasoned nurses and other health care workers working in disaster situations can become overwhelmed by witnessing catastrophic loss of human life (as in acts of terrorism, plane crashes, school shootings) or mass destruction of people's homes and belongings (as in floods, fires, tornadoes) that leave many families bereft of a sense of stability, well-being, and shelter. Disaster nurses need supportive ties and access to debriefing. Debriefing is an important step for staff in coming to terms with overwhelming violent or otherwise disastrous situations once they are over. It helps staff place the crisis in perspective and begin healing themselves. Debriefing is discussed in more detail later in the chapter.

Everyone experiences crises. The experience itself is not pathological but rather represents a struggle for equilibrium and adjustment when problems seem unsolvable. A crisis presents both a danger to personality organization and a potential opportunity for personality growth. The outcome depends on how the individual, family, or community perceives and deals with the crisis and what outside supports are available at the time the crisis occurs.

Crises are acute, time-limited occurrences experienced as overwhelming emotional reactions to:
- A stressful situational event
- A developmental event
- A societal event
- A cultural event
- The perception of an event

Crisis intervention is what nurses and other health professionals do to assist those in crisis to cope. Interventions are broad, creative, and flexible.

PREVALENCE AND COMORBIDITY

Many factors may limit a person's ability to problem solve or cope with stressful life events or situations. Some of these factors include the presence of other stressful life events, mental illness, substance abuse, history of poor coping skills, diminished cognitive abilities, preexisting physical health problems, limited social support network, and developmental or physical challenges.

THEORY

An early crisis theorist, **Erich Lindemann,** conducted a classic study in the 1940s on the grief reactions of close relatives of victims who died in the Coconut Grove nightclub fire in Boston. This study formed the foundation of crisis theory and clinical intervention. Lindemann was convinced that even though acute grief is a normal reaction to a distressing situation, preventive interventions could eliminate or decrease serious personality disorganization and devastating psychological consequences from the sustained effects of severe anxiety. He believed that the same interventions that were helpful in bereavement would prove just as helpful in dealing with other types of stressful events and

EXAMINING THE EVIDENCE   First Responders and PTSD

My aunt lives near New Orleans. She is a nurse and was one of the people who helped in the rescue efforts after Hurricane Katrina. For about a month after the disaster she was a different person; she was anxious, irritable, and barely slept. What was going on with her?

It sounds like your aunt might have been suffering from symptoms of posttraumatic stress disorder (PTSD) caused by being a "first responder." A first responder is a person who is directly involved in a traumatic event by being among the first at the scene. Natural and man-made disasters and terrorist attacks are all types of traumatic incidents that can affect first responders such as police, firefighters, and emergency health care professionals (including nurses). It's hard to imagine the helplessness and horror that accompanies witnessing such events. Additionally, as a resident of New Orleans your aunt suffered a dual trauma; she was dealing not only with the stress of being a first responder to family and friends, but also the stresses of rebuilding her own life (Jordan, 2007).

Recently, American researchers have had the unfortunate opportunity to study PTSD responses in some depth and have arrived at varying conclusions as to the extent of the problem. One week after the attacks on the World Trade Center, researchers surveyed a random sample of Americans and concluded that 44% showed significant signs of stress (McNally et al., 2003). Based on statistics gathered after the Oklahoma City bombing in 1995, it was believed that about 35% of those directly exposed to the events of September 11, 2001, would develop PTSD (Yehuda, 2002). New York City braced itself for the outpouring of people who would need disaster debriefing and put together an impressive program for counseling

people involved in this disaster. However, of the 2.5 million people they expected to treat, only about 25% actually sought help (Gittrich, 2003).

Even though first responders may not be directly involved with the catastrophe, research supports that they are affected, although again the question of "to what degree?" should be raised. Robbers and Jenkins (2005) report that after the attacks on the Pentagon, 36% of police officers at an Arlington, Virginia, police station met the diagnostic criteria for PTSD. However, according to North and associates (2002), of 176 male firefighters who had rescued and aided in recovery efforts at the Oklahoma City bombing site, only 13% had disaster-related PTSD, as opposed to 23% of 88 males who were immediately involved in the bombing. Battles (2007) explored the prevalence of PTSD signs and symptoms in emergency department nurses working in New Orleans during Hurricane Katrina found that 20% had symptoms consistent with PTSD.

Although researchers don't agree on the rates of PTSD in first responders, most agree that it exists. These disaster responses are typically believed to be diagnosable mental disorders, but some researchers classify them as normal and expectable stress responses to horrific situations (Wakefield & Spitzer, 2002). One of the most important recommendations to come out of the tremendous number of research studies since the Oklahoma bombing, 9/11, and Hurricane Katrina is extremely important to first responders: being intellectually and psychologically prepared for disasters are protective factors that may help first responders in the future (North et al., 2002). Outcomes of studies of first responders who have undergone extensive disaster-preparedness education based on inevitable future disasters will bear out the wisdom of this recommendation.

(See Chapter 8 for more on posttraumatic stress disorder.)

Battles, E.D., (2007). An exploration of posttraumatic stress disorder in emergency nurses following hurricane Katrina. *Journal of Emergency Nursing, 33*(4), 314-318.

Gittrich, G. (2003). $90 million in Project Liberty mental health funds remains unspent. *New York Daily News,* May 27, p. 1.

Jordan, K. (2007). A case study: Factors to consider when doing 1:1 crisis counseling with local first responders with dual trauma after Hurricane Katrina. *Brief Treatment Crisis Intervention, 7*(2), 91-101.

McNally, R.J., Bryant, R.A., & Ehlers, A. (2003). Does early psychological intervention promote recovery from post-traumatic stress? *Psychology, 4*(2), 45-79.

North, C.S., Tivis, L., McMillen, J.C., et al. (2002). Psychiatric disorders in rescue workers after the Oklahoma City bombing. *American Journal of Psychiatry, 159*, 857-859.

Robbers, M.L.P., & Jenkins, J.M. (2005). Symptomatology of posttraumatic stress disorder among first responders to the Pentagon on 9/11: A preliminary analysis of Arlington county police first responders. *Police Practice and Research, 6*(3), 235-249.

Wakefield, J.C., & Spitzer, R.L. (2002). Lowered estimates—But of what? *Archives of General Psychiatry, 59*, 129-130.

Yehuda, R., (2002). Post-traumatic stress disorder. *The New England Journal of Medicine, 346*(2), 108-114.

A special thanks to Renee Pennington, RN, University of Akron graduate student, for her research assistance.

proposed a crisis intervention model as a major element of preventive psychiatry in the community.

In the early 1960s, **Gerald Caplan** (1964) further elaborated crisis theory and outlined crisis intervention strategies. Since that time, our understanding of crisis and effective

intervention has continued to be refined and enhanced by numerous contemporary clinicians and theorists (Behrman & Reid, 2002; Roberts, 2000).

In 1961, a report of the Joint Commission on Mental Illness and Mental Health addressed the need for commu-

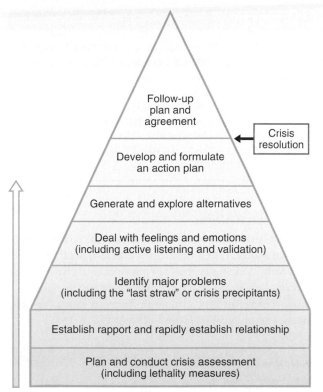

Figure 17-1 ■ Roberts' seven-stage model of crisis intervention. (From Roberts, A.R. [Ed.]. [2005]. *Crisis intervention handbook* [3rd ed.]. New York: Oxford University Press.)

nity mental health centers throughout the country. This report stimulated the establishment of crisis services, which are now an important part of mental health programs in hospitals and communities.

Donna Aguilera and **Janice Mesnick** (1970) provided a framework for nurses for crisis assessment and intervention, which has grown in scope and practice. Aguilera (1998) continues to set a standard in the practice of crisis assessment and intervention.

Roberts's seven-stage model of crisis intervention (2000) is a more contemporary model useful in helping individuals who have suffered from an acute situational crisis as well as people who are diagnosed with acute stress disorder (Figure 17-1).

The devastating effects of the 9/11 World Trade Center terrorist attack and the distressing lack of response to hurricane Katrina emphasized the need for crisis assessment and intervention by community mental health providers throughout the country to deal with all types of crises and the people who had been traumatized—victims, families, rescue workers, and observers (Everly, 2000; Howard & Goelitz, 2004; Lowry & Lating, 2002). Crisis theory defines

---

Foundation for Crisis Intervention

• A crisis is self-limiting and is usually resolved within 4 to 6 weeks.
• The resolution of a crisis results in achievement of one of three different functional levels. The person will emerge at:
  • A *higher* level of functioning.
  • The *same* level of functioning.
  • A *lower* level of functioning.
• The goal of crisis intervention is to return the individual to the precrisis level of functioning.
• The form of resolution of the crisis depends on the actions of the individual and the intervention of others.
• During a crisis people are often more open to outside intervention than they are at times of stable functioning. With intervention a person can learn different adaptive means of problem solving to correct inadequate solutions.
• A person in a crisis situation is assumed to be mentally healthy and to have functioned well in the past but is presently in a state of disequilibrium.
• Crisis intervention deals with the person's present problem and resolution of the immediate crisis only. Dealing with material not directly related to the crisis can take place at a later time. Crisis intervention deals with the "here and now."
• A nurse must be willing to take an active, even directive, role in intervention; this is in direct contrast to what occurs in conventional therapeutic intervention, which stresses a more passive and nondirective role for the practitioner.
• Early intervention probably increases the chances for a good prognosis.
• A patient is encouraged to set realistic goals and plan an intervention with the nurse that is focused on the current situation.

---

specific aspects of crisis basic to crisis intervention (Box 17-1).

The ways of assessing crisis described in the following sections are derived from established crisis theory and constitute a sound knowledge base for the application of the nursing process to treatment of a patient in crisis. An understanding of three areas of crisis theory enables application of the nursing process: (1) types of crisis, (2) phases of crisis, and (3) aspects of crisis that have relevance for nurses.

CLINICAL PICTURE
Types of Crises

There are three basic types of crises: (1) maturational, (2) situational, and (3) adventitious (disasters). It is possible to experience two types of crisis situations simultaneously. For example, a 51-year-old woman may be going through a midlife crisis (maturational) when her husband dies suddenly of cancer (situational). The presence of more than one crisis further taxes the individual's coping skills. People who have preexisting mental health problems are vulnerable and prone to crisis. Psychiatric emergencies are covered in the following four chapters.

Maturational Crisis

A process of maturation occurs throughout life. Erik Erikson (1902–1994) identified eight stages of growth and development in which specific maturational tasks must be mastered. The path (stages) to adulthood is stressful and at times can be overwhelming. Erikson declared that each of these stages constitutes a crisis in personal growth and development. Each developmental stage can thus be referred to as a **maturational crisis**.

When a person arrives at a new stage, formerly used coping styles are no longer appropriate, and new coping mechanisms have yet to be developed. For a time, the person is without effective defenses. This often leads to increased anxiety, which may manifest as variations in the person's normal behavior. Marriage, the birth of a child, and retirement are examples of maturational crises.

Alcohol and drug addiction can interrupt an individual's progression through the maturational stages. This phenomenon is too often seen among teenagers. When the addictive behavior is controlled (by the late teens), the young person's growth and development will resume at the point at which it was interrupted. A young person whose addiction is arrested at 19 years of age may have the social and problem-solving skills of a 14-year-old. Often these teenagers do not receive or accept treatment, and their adult coping skills are diminished or absent.

Successful resolution of these maturational tasks leads to development of basic human qualities. Erikson believed that the way these crises are resolved at one stage affects the ability to pass through subsequent stages because each crisis provides the starting point for moving to the next stage. If a person lacks support systems and adequate role models, successful resolution may be difficult or may not occur. Unresolved problems in the past and inadequate coping mechanisms can adversely affect what is learned in each developmental stage.

When a person is experiencing severe difficulty during a maturational crisis, professional intervention may be indicated.

> ### VIGNETTE
>
> Loretta, 41 years old, gets married for the first time to her high school sweetheart. Although he was previously married with children, the couple planned to have a child early in their marriage. When Loretta finds that she is unable to conceive because of early menopause, she becomes distraught. She is severely anxious, experiences extreme feelings of guilt, is unable to sleep, and consequently no longer is able to function as a manager of a small software company. Her concerned husband takes her to the community health center.

Situational Crisis

A **situational crisis** arises from an external rather than an internal source. Often the crisis is unanticipated. Examples of external situations that can precipitate a crisis include loss of a job, death of a loved one, unwanted pregnancy, a move, change of job, change in financial status, divorce, and severe physical or mental illness.

> ### VIGNETTE
>
> Don, 56 years old, has held a middle management position in his company for 25 years. When his company downsized, letting many of the middle managers go, Don was devastated. He has been looking for another job for 9 months, but so far has no prospects. His family's health care is about to expire. His perception of himself as a competent family provider is shattered and his self-esteem has plummeted. He has been drinking heavily, staying up late, and sleeping late into the morning. He has closed himself off from family and friends.

Some refer to these events as "critical life problems" because they are encountered by most people during the course of their lives. Whether these events precipitate a crisis depends on such factors as the degree of support available from caring friends and family members, a person's general emotional and physical status, social supports in the community, and a person's ability to understand and cope with the meaning of the stressful event.

As in all crises or potential crisis situations, the stressful event involves a loss or change that threatens a person's self-concept and self-esteem. To varying degrees, successful resolution of a crisis depends on resolution of the grief associated with the loss.

Adventitious Crisis

An **adventitious crisis**, or **crisis of disaster**, is not a part of everyday life; it is unplanned and accidental. Adventitious crises may result from (1) a natural disaster (e.g., flood, fire, earthquake), (2) a national disaster (e.g., acts of terrorism, war, riots, airplane crashes), or (3) a crime of violence (e.g., rape, assault, murder in the workplace or school, bombing in crowded areas, spousal or child abuse). Every disaster is a unique challenge.

Disasters, whether natural or human caused, result in excessive morbidity and mortality along with extensive damage to property, roadways, and electrical lines, limiting a region's ability to respond. These disasters can leave local governmental operations, medical systems, and local first responders overwhelmed and exhausted.

Even today, thousands of people are still trying to recover from the never to be forgotten 2005 Atlantic hurricane Katrina in New Orleans, Louisiana. Although the media frenzy has long abated, people are still trying to put their lives together, get homes built, and recover from the long-term effects of trauma. This points out the dire need for better planning in vulnerable areas and clearer lines of communication among community, state, and federal disaster agencies in order to be effective in mitigating morbidity and mortality.

From 1990 to 2000, 460 major disasters were declared, higher than any other decade on record (Cox & Briggs, 2004). Since the turn of the century, we have all lived through some of the most shattering disasters in recent memory. No one in America can ever forget the infamous day in 2001 now known as 9/11. In December 2004, the world watched in horror the TV footage of the Indonesian tsunami disaster. And school shootings (e.g., Virginia Tech, Columbine) continue to dot the headlines leaving families, communities, and our youth changed forever.

Efficient response to disaster requires a **triage** team and ability to distribute casualties to the most appropriate facility or holding ground for proper care. The underlying principle of triage is to separate out those who need rapid medical care from those with more minor injuries, thus reducing the urgent burden on medical facilities and organizations and making the most efficient use of available resources. Triage helps responders do the greatest good for the greatest number of casualties.

During a disaster often the first needs are rescue efforts, evacuation plans and execution, food and shelter, medical attention, and physical safety. Since 2000, the Department of Homeland Security oversees a variety of agencies that focus on the safety and security of people in disasters in the United States. Providing medical disaster relief is under the jurisdiction of the National Disaster Medical System (NDMS). There are, however, nongovernmental agencies as well who take volunteer nurses and doctors to various parts of the United States and the world to help disaster victims, including the International Medical Corps (IMC). This group sends medical personnel to places such as Indonesia during the catastrophic tsunami disaster, Darfur, etc.

After immediate needs are met, people need help in reconstructing and normalizing their lives. People need housing, food, jobs, and availability of posttrauma counseling.

Common phenomena experienced following a disaster are *cognitive* (e.g., memory impairment, difficulty making decisions or problem solving, recurring or intrusive images), *behavioral* (e.g., withdrawal, relapse in chemically dependent people, under- or overeating or sleeping), or *emotional* (e.g., flood of emotions like anxiety, fear, anger, numbness, helplessness). Common sequelae of crisis, particularly a disaster are posttrauma, posttraumatic stress disorder, and depression. **The need for psychological first aid (crisis intervention) and debriefing after any crisis situation for all age-groups (children, adolescents, adults, and older adults) cannot be overstressed.** *Critical incident stress debriefing* is discussed later in this chapter.

Disaster nursing, stemming from critical care nursing, is a new frontier, and from the preceding information, one can see the great need for nurses in this area.

evolve

For a comprehensive case study and associated nursing care plans for patients and staff experiencing crises, visit the Evolve website at http://evolve.elsevier.com/Varcarolis/essentials.

Phases of Crisis

Caplan (1964) identified four distinct **phases of crisis**.

- Phase 1: A person confronted by a conflict or problem that threatens the self-concept responds with increased feelings of anxiety. The increase in anxiety stimulates the use of problem-solving techniques and defense mechanisms in an effort to solve the problem and lower anxiety.
- Phase 2: If the usual defensive response fails, and if the threat persists, anxiety continues to rise and produce feelings of extreme discomfort. Individual functioning becomes disorganized. Trial-and-error attempts at solving the problem and restoring a normal balance begin.
- Phase 3: If the trial-and-error attempts fail, anxiety can escalate to severe and panic levels, and the person mobilizes automatic relief behaviors, such as withdrawal and flight. Some form of resolution (e.g., compromising needs or redefining the situation to reach an acceptable solution) may be made in this stage.
- Phase 4: If the problem is not solved and new coping skills are ineffective, anxiety can overwhelm the person and lead to serious personality disorganization, depression, confusion, violence against others, or suicidal behavior (Greenstone & Leviton, 2002; Jordan, 2003; Lowry & Lating, 2002).

Application of the Nursing Process

ASSESSMENT

A person's equilibrium may be adversely affected by one or more of the following: (1) an unrealistic perception of the precipitating event, (2) inadequate situational supports, and (3) inadequate coping mechanisms (Aguilera, 1998). It is crucial to assess these factors when a crisis situation is evaluated because data gained from the assessment are used as guides for both the nurse and the patient in setting realistic and meaningful goals as well as in planning possible solutions to the problem situation.

After determining whether there is a need for external controls because of suicidal or homicidal ideation or gestures, the nurse assesses three main areas: (1) the patient's perception of the precipitating event, (2) the patient's situational supports, and (3) the patient's personal coping skills.

Assessing the Patient's Perception of the Precipitating Event

Whether an event is a crisis is based on the perspective and strengths of the patient. Whereas having a doctor's appointment canceled would seem to be a trivial annoyance to most people, for someone who is vulnerable from severe schizophrenia, the change could bring on a crisis and lead to disorganization. Therefore it is important to see the event through the eyes of the patient. The nurse's initial task is to assess the individual or family's perception of the problem. The more clearly the problem can be defined, the better the chance that an effective solution will be found. Sample questions that may facilitate the assessment include the following:

- Has anything particularly upsetting happened to you within the past few days or weeks?
- What was happening in your life before you started to feel this way?
- What leads you to seek help now?
- Describe how you are feeling right now.
- How does this situation affect your life?
- How do you see this event as affecting your future?
- What would need to be done to resolve this situation?

VIGNETTE

Laura, a 15-year-old, is brought to the emergency department (ED) after slashing her wrists. She was found by her mother, who returned home early from a date. Her mother called the police, and they rushed Laura to the hospital. After Laura is seen by the medical personnel, she is taken to the psychiatric nurse working in the ED. The nurse speaks calmly, introduces herself, and tells Laura she would like to spend some time with her. The nurse states, "It looks as if things are pretty overwhelming. Is that how you are feeling?" The nurse makes the observation that things must be very bad if Laura wants to kill herself. Laura sits slumped in a chair, her head hanging down, with tears in her eyes.

Assessing Laura's Perception of the Precipitating Event

Nurse: "Laura, tell me what has happened."

Laura: "I can't . . . I can't go home. No one cares. No one believes me. I can't go through it again."

Nurse: "Tell me what you can't go through again, Laura."

Laura starts to cry, shaking with sobs. The nurse sits quietly for a while, offers her some tissues, and then speaks.

Nurse: "Tell me what is so terrible. Let's look at it together."

After a while, Laura starts telling the nurse that when she was 9 years old, her mother had a boyfriend. When the mother would go to work, the boyfriend would touch her and eventually forced her to have sex, threatening to kill her if she told anyone. When she was 11, the boyfriend moved out. Two weeks ago Laura's mother told her that the old boyfriend was coming back to live with them. When Laura told her mother what had happened years ago, her mother called her a liar and said if it was a choice between Laura and the boyfriend, she would choose the boyfriend.

Assessing the Patient's Situational Supports

The patient's support systems are assessed to determine the resources available. Does the stressful event involve important people in the support system? Is the patient isolated from others, or are there family and friends who can provide the vital support? Family and friends may be called on to aid the individual by offering material or emotional support (e.g., lending money, offering services, being available to give affection and understanding). If these resources are not available, the nurse or counselor acts as a temporary support system while relationships with individuals or groups in the community are established. The following are some sample questions to ask:

- With whom do you live?
- To whom do you talk when you feel overwhelmed?
- Whom can you trust?
- Who is available to help you?
- Where do you go to worship (or talk to God)? Where do you go to school or to other community-based activities?
- During difficult times in the past, who did you want most to help you?
- Who is the most helpful?

VIGNETTE

Assessing Laura's Situational Supports

Nurse: "Laura, who can you go to? Do you have any other family?"

Laura: "No, my dad left when I was little, and we are pretty much alone. My mom never allowed me to play with other kids."

Nurse: "Do you have anyone you can talk to?"

Laura: "No, I really don't have any friends. The other kids think I am stuck up. My mom always had something for me to do in the house."

Nurse: "What about teachers or a minister or rabbi?"

Laura: "My teachers are nice, but I can't tell them things like this. Besides, they wouldn't believe me either."

Assessing the Patient's Personal Coping Skills

In crisis situations it is important to evaluate the person's level of anxiety. Common coping mechanisms may be overeating, drinking, smoking, withdrawing, seeking out someone to talk to, yelling, fighting, or engaging in other physical activity (Behrman & Reid, 2002). The potential for suicide or homicide must be assessed. If the patient is suicidal, homicidal, or unable to take care of personal needs, hospitalization should be considered (Aguilera, 1998). Some sample questions to ask are the following:

- Have you thought of killing yourself or someone else? If yes, have you thought of how you would do this?
- What do you usually do to feel better?
- Did you try it this time? If so, what was different?
- What helped you through difficult times in the past?
- What do you think might happen now?

VIGNETTE

The nurse learns that Laura does very well in school. Laura explains that when she studies, she can forget her problems and get lost in other worlds. Getting good grades also has another reward: it is the only time her mother says anything nice about her.

Assessing Laura's Personal Coping Skills

Nurse: "What do you think would help your situation?"

Laura: "I don't want to die. I just don't know where to turn."

The nurse tells Laura that she wants to work with her to find a solution, and that she is concerned for Laura's safety and well-being.

Assessment Guidelines

Crisis

1. Identify whether the patient's response to the crisis warrants psychiatric treatment or hospitalization to minimize decompensation (suicidal behavior, psychotic thinking, and violent behavior).
2. Identify whether the patient is able to identify the *precipitating event.*
3. Assess the patient's understanding of his or her present *situational supports.*
4. Identify the patient's usual *coping skills* and determine what coping mechanisms may help the present situation.
5. Determine whether there are certain religious or cultural beliefs that need to be considered in assessing and intervening in this person's crisis.
6. Assess whether this situation is one in which the patient needs primary intervention (education, environmental manipulation, or new coping skills), secondary intervention (crisis intervention), or tertiary intervention (rehabilitation).

DIAGNOSIS

A person in crisis may exhibit various behaviors that indicate a number of problems. See Table 17-1 for some signs and symptoms of people in crisis that may be used as a guide for identifying potential nursing diagnoses.

For the example in the preceding vignette, the assessment of Laura's (1) perception of the precipitating event, (2) situational supports, and (3) personal coping skills provides the nurse enough data to formulate two diagnoses and to work with Laura in setting goals and planning interventions.

VIGNETTE

Nursing Diagnoses for Laura

The nurse formulates the following nursing diagnoses for Laura:

- *Anxiety (moderate/severe)* related to fear of renewed sexual abuse and lack of protection as evidenced by ineffectual problem solving and feelings of impending doom
- *Compromised family coping* related to inadequate understanding by her mother's inability to listen to daughter's fears

TABLE 17-1	Potential Nursing Diagnoses for Crisis Intervention
Signs and Symptoms	**Nursing Diagnoses**
Overwhelmed, depressed, states that has nothing in life worthwhile, self-hate and feelings of being ineffectual are assessed	*Risk for self-directed violence* *Chronic low self-esteem* *Spiritual distress* *Hopelessness* *Powerlessness*
Confused, highly anxious, incoherent, crying or sobbing, shows extreme emotional pain	*Anxiety (moderate, severe, panic)* *Acute confusion* *Disturbed thought processes* *Sleep deprivation*
Has difficulty with interpersonal relationships, isolated, has few or no social supports	*Social isolation* *Risk for loneliness* *Impaired social interaction*
Unable to function at work, school, or home at previous level, has difficulty concentrating or completing simple tasks	*Ineffective coping* *Interrupted family processes* *Caregiver role strain*
Has experienced traumatic, emotionally overwhelming event or loss; unable to work through overwhelming loss or event	*Risk for post-trauma syndrome* *Rape-trauma syndrome* *Dysfunctional grieving* *Chronic sorrow*

OUTCOMES IDENTIFICATION

The planning of realistic patient outcomes is done together with the patient or family. Realistic outcomes are made to fit within the person's cultural and personal values. The nurse will document the outcomes as measurable goals that are realistic and include a time estimate (ANA, 2007). Without the patient's involvement, the outcome criteria (goals at the end of 4 to 8 weeks) may be irrelevant or unacceptable solutions to that person's crisis.

For example, a nurse new to crisis intervention who suggests that a woman leave her husband because he beats her may be surprised to find that the woman has different thoughts on what she wants as a solution. Thus outcomes are always established with the patient, and they have to be congruent with the patient's needs, values, and (in some instances) cultural expectations. The nurse evaluates the outcome for safety as well as other factors and works on contingency plans when necessary.

VIGNETTE

A social worker is called. Laura, the nurse, and the social worker meet together. All agree that Laura should not return to her mother's home if the boyfriend returns. The nurse then meets with Laura and her mother; however, her mother continues to berate Laura for lying. She says she doesn't care what Laura says. She has her own life to live and if Laura doesn't like it, she can move out.

The nurse and Laura set four goals together:
1. Laura will return to her precrisis state within 2 to 6 weeks.
2. Laura and staff will find a safe environment for her before the boyfriend moves back.
3. Laura, with the support of staff, will have at least two outside supports available within 24 hours.
4. Laura will receive continued evaluation and support until the immediate crisis is over (6 to 8 weeks).

PLANNING

Nurses are called on to plan and intervene through a variety of crisis intervention modalities, such as disaster nursing, mobile crisis units, group work, health education and crisis prevention, victim outreach programs, and telephone hotlines.

The nurse may be involved in planning and intervention for an individual (e.g., cases of physical abuse), for a group (e.g., students after a classmate's suicide event or shooting), or for a community (e.g., disaster nursing after tornadoes, shootings, and airplane crashes).

The following questions are answered (Aguilera, 1998):

- How much has this crisis affected the person's life? Can the patient still go to work? Attend school? Care for family members?
- How is the state of disequilibrium affecting significant people in the patient's life (wife, husband, children, other family members, boss, boyfriend, girlfriend)?

Data from the answers to these two questions will guide the nurse in determining what kinds of immediate action to take.

IMPLEMENTATION

Crisis intervention is considered to be a function of the basic level nurse and has two basic initial goals:

1. **Patient safety.** External controls may be applied for protection of the person in crisis if the person is suicidal or homicidal.
2. **Anxiety reduction.** Anxiety reduction techniques are used so that inner resources can be mobilized.

During the initial interview, the person in crisis first needs to gain a feeling of safety. Solutions to the crisis may be offered, so that the patient is aware of other options. Feelings of support and hope will temporarily diminish anxiety. The nurse needs to play an active role by indicating that help is available. The availability of help is conveyed by the competent use of crisis intervention skills and genuine interest and support. It is not conveyed by the use of false reassurances and platitudes, such as "Everything will be all right." Crisis intervention requires a creative and flexible approach through the use of traditional and nontraditional therapeutic methods. The nurse may act as educator, adviser, and model, always keeping in mind that it is the patient who solves the problem, not the nurse. The following are important assumptions when working with a patient in crisis:

- The person is in charge of his or her own life.
- The person is able to make decisions.
- The crisis counseling relationship is one between partners.

The nurse helps the patient refocus to gain new perspectives on the situation. The nurse supports the patient during the process of finding constructive ways to solve or cope with the problem. It is important for the nurse to be mindful of how difficult it is for the patient to change his or her behavior. See Table 17-2 for crisis interventions and corresponding rationales.

TABLE 17-2   Interventions for Patients in Crisis

Intervention	Rationale
1. Assess for any suicidal or homicidal thoughts or plans.	1. Safety is always the first consideration.
2. Take initial steps to make patient feel safe and to lower anxiety.	2. When a person feels safe and anxiety decreases, the individual is able to problem-solve solutions with the nurse.
3. Listen carefully (e.g., make eye contact, give frequent feedback to make sure you understand, summarize what patient says at the end).	3. When a person believes that someone is really listening, this can translate into the belief that someone cares about the person's situation and that help may be available. This offers hope.
4. Crisis intervention calls for directive and creative approaches. Initially the nurse may make phone calls (arrange babysitters, schedule a visiting nurse, find shelter, contact a social worker).	4. Initially a person may be so confused and frightened that performing usual tasks is not possible at that moment.
5. Assess patient's support systems. Rally existing supports (with patient's permission) if patient is overwhelmed.	5. People are often overwhelmed and nurses often need to take an active role.
6. Identify needed social supports (with patient's input) and mobilize the most needed first.	6. Patient's needs for shelter, help with care for children or elders, medical workup, emergency medical attention, hospitalization, food, safe housing, and self-help group are determined.
7. Identify needed coping skills (problem solving, relaxation, assertiveness, job training, newborn care, self-esteem raising).	7. Increasing coping skills and learning new ones can help with current crisis and help minimize future crises.
8. Plan with patient interventions acceptable to both counselor and patient.	8. Patient's sense of control, self-esteem, and compliance with plan are increased.
9. Plan regular follow-up to assess patient's progress (e.g., phone calls, clinic visits, home visits as appropriate).	9. Plan is evaluated to see what works and what doesn't work.

Levels of Nursing Care

There are three levels of nursing care in crisis intervention. These three levels are (1) primary, (2) secondary, and (3) tertiary. Psychotherapeutic nursing interventions in crisis are directed toward these three levels of care.

Primary

Primary care promotes mental health and reduces mental illness to decrease the incidence of crisis. On this level, the nurse can:

- Work with an individual to recognize potential problems by evaluating the stressful life events the person is experiencing.
- Teach individual specific coping skills, such as decision making, problem solving, assertiveness skills, meditation, and relaxation skills, to handle stressful events.
- Assist an individual in evaluating the timing or reduction of life changes to decrease the negative effects of stress as much as possible. This may involve working with a patient to plan environmental changes, make important interpersonal decisions, and rethink changes in occupational roles.

Secondary

Secondary care establishes intervention during an acute crisis to *prevent* prolonged anxiety from diminishing personal effectiveness and personality organization. The nurse's primary focus is to ensure the safety of the patient. After safety issues are dealt with, the nurse works with the patient to assess the patient's problem, support systems, and coping styles. Desired goals are explored and interventions planned. Secondary care lessens the time a person is mentally disabled during a crisis. Secondary-level care occurs in hospital units, emergency departments, clinics, or mental health centers, usually during daytime hours.

Tertiary

Tertiary care provides support for those who have experienced a severe crisis and are now recovering from a disabling mental state. Social and community facilities that offer tertiary intervention include rehabilitation centers, sheltered workshops, day hospitals, and outpatient clinics. Primary goals are to *facilitate optimal levels of functioning and prevent further emotional disruptions*. People with severe and persistent mental problems are often extremely susceptible to crisis, and community facilities provide the structured environment that can help prevent problem situations. See Chapter 24 for an extensive discussion on community supports for people with severe and persistent mental problems.

Critical Incident Stress Debriefing

Critical incident stress debriefing (CISD) is an example of a tertiary intervention directed toward a group that has experienced a crisis (Everly et al., 2000). CISD consists of a seven-phase group meeting that offers individuals the opportunity to share their thoughts and feelings in a safe and controlled environment. CISD is used to debrief staff on an inpatient unit following the suicide of a patient (see Chapter 20); to debrief staff following incidents of patient violence; to debrief crisis hotline volunteers; to debrief schoolchildren and school personnel after shootings have occurred in a school; and to debrief rescue and health care workers who have responded to a natural disaster or a terrorist attack such as that on the World Trade Center (Hammond & Brooks, 2001).

The phases of CISD are the following (Everly et al., 2000):

- *Introductory phase*—The purpose of the meeting is explained; an overview of the debriefing process is provided; participants are motivated; confidentiality is assured; guidelines are explained; team members are identified; and questions are answered.
- *Fact phase*—Participants are assisted in discussing the facts of the incident; participants are asked to introduce themselves and tell how they were involved in the incident and what happened from their perspective.
- *Thought phase*—All participants are asked to discuss their first thoughts of the incident.
- *Reaction phase*—Participants engage in freewheeling discussion and talk about the worst thing about the incident—what they would like to forget and what was most painful.
- *Symptom phase*—Participants describe cognitive, physical, emotional, or behavioral experiences that they had at the scene of the incident and describe any symptoms they felt following the initial experience.
- *Teaching phase*—The normality of the symptoms that have been expressed is acknowledged and affirmed; anticipatory guidance is offered regarding future symptoms that may be experienced by participants; the group is involved in stress management techniques.

APPLYING THE ART   A Person Needing Crisis Intervention

SCENARIO: I met 38-year-old Richard when he brought his son Lamar to the community health free-clinic for his allergy shot. Richard asked if I had time to talk during Lamar's post-injection waiting period. Lamar played with other children as Richard first described his gratitude that his son was able to get allergy injections despite Richard's lack of health insurance. He went on to recount his mixed feelings about his wife being 2 months pregnant. He saw no way to care for his expanding family on his minimum wage income.

THERAPEUTIC GOAL: By the end of this interaction, Richard will acknowledge controlled breathing as one method of limiting a panic attack and make the decision to enter psychotherapy.

Student-Patient Interaction	Thoughts, Communication Techniques, and Mental Health Nursing Concepts
Richard: *After several silent moments.* "You're a nursing student right? May I ask you a question?"	
Student: "Go on." *Nodding.* **Student's feelings:** *When I get anxious, I must remind myself that I don't have to know everything. My instructor is nearby.*	I wonder where this is going and if I'll know the answer to his question. I give a *general lead* encouraging Richard to continue.
Richard: "How long can a person's heart pound really hard and fast before it gives out?" *At my immediately alert expression, Richard added,* "It's not happening now." **Student's feelings:** *I have to become more aware of what I show non-verbally. Hopefully, I just looked alert and not panicked.*	Belatedly, I use my assessment skills. Richard is not hyperventilating; his breaths are even and slow. His face is not flushed. He does not talk or look like he's experiencing pain nor vertigo.
Student: "You are trying to understand some symptoms you've been having?" *He nods.* "Tell me more." **Student's feelings:** *Our distribution of health care dollars falls short for the Richards of the world. I feel sadness then anger. I worry about all my debt from school, but in comparison, the pressure Richard must feel seems overwhelming.*	I *clarify* then ask an *indirect question.* I wonder if he has ever had a full cardiac work-up. Probably not, because he doesn't have health insurance.
Richard: "A few weeks ago, out of the blue my heart starts pounding for at least 15 minutes. It always feels like my heart will pound right out of my chest!"	Richard sounds like he may be in a crisis. I will need to assess the crisis balancing factors: his perception of the events, his coping mechanisms, and situational supports.
Student: "That would be so frightening. You said 'it always feels,' so these 'heart pounding' times continue?" **Student's feelings:** *I would worry too if my heart started pounding for no reason I could figure out.*	I use restatement and ask a direct question. I know that physiologically such palpitations alone from a healthy heart muscle aren't life threatening.
Richard: "Yes, my chest pounds and I start breathing fast. It feels like any minute now, I'm going to die." **Student's feelings:** *I feel empathy for Richard. The wife's pregnancy likely set Richard up for crisis but something within the last 24–48 hours acted as a precipitating event. In other words, I wonder what made today the day that Richard recognized he needed help? What in the last 48 hours makes this overwhelming?*	If there is nothing physically wrong with Richard's heart, and his symptoms are from anxiety, then the biochemical changes from moderate-severe levels of anxiety should abate in a few minutes. However, if Richard re-fuels the flight-or-fight response with catastrophic thinking like, 'I'll die!" his anxiety can grow into a full fledged panic attack.
Student: "How do you get yourself through all of this?"	I ask an *open question.* I also imply that Richard has been able to *cope* (the second balancing factor), despite his fears.

Continued

APPLYING THE ART   A Person Needing Crisis Intervention—cont'd

Student-Patient Interaction	Thoughts, Communication Techniques, and Mental Health Nursing Concepts
Richard: "The first few times I rushed to the ER, but after the second or third time they checked out my heart; they said there was nothing wrong with my heart. That made me feel stupid. The doctor said I was panicking. Like I'm a nut case." *Shakes his head.* "Maybe I am." **Student's feelings:** *Satisfied that there is no physical heart problem, I feel frustrated that there is such a stigma about mental illness, unlike physical illnesses.*	Richard uses *projection* when he says the ER staff made him feel stupid. Maybe he wonders that about himself. Richard re-encounters *autonomy vs. shame and doubt* with the palpitations beyond his control, he feels shame when he says words like "stupid" and "nut case."
Student: "Sounds like you're upset at how you were treated but maybe you're also worried something is really wrong with your heart or your head or both." **Student's feelings:** *Maybe I went too far with that "really wrong" part. Sometimes it's hard to know when to allow the patient space or when to try for insight.*	I again *attempt to translate into feelings,* which communicates empathy.
Richard: *Impatiently brushing away tears.* "What if this panic thing hits me at work? What happens to my family?" **Student's feelings:** *I admire how Richard cares so much for his family. I feel that way about my family, too. Sometimes, I feel guilty about all the time and money it takes for me to get through nursing school. Sometimes the demands of school take so much away from my family. I need to mindfully breathe. Right now my focus needs to be on Richard.*	He was able to let himself know how overwhelmed he feels, even though he quickly gets rid of the tears. In crisis intervention work, *perception* of oneself rests at the core of the patient's *perception* of the *crisis event.*
Student: "Right now you feel as though facing the problem means you will not be able to work." *He nods.* "I wonder if it's possible that knowing more about panic disorder could, on the other hand, bring a way to regain some control in your life."	I *validate* then ask an *indirect question.* I remember that the fear of having a panic attack out in public or for Richard, at work, adds to the sense of loss of control and can even contribute to agoraphobia.
Richard: *Takes a deep breath, then begins hyperventilating with a scared look on his face.* **Student's feelings:** *I am breathing faster too, feeling anxious.*	Richard is starting to have a panic attack!
Student: "Calm down! Please calm down." *Richard starts breathing even faster.* **Student's feelings:** *What's wrong with me! When someone tells me to calm down it usually makes me angry instead. It's like one more pressure on me when I'm already having trouble. I need to offer self to work with Richard first. I need to be in charge of my actions and reactions. I will stay calm and use my listening skills to talk Richard through this. Where, oh where is my teacher?*	I gave premature advice. In essence I said, "You calm down," like a parent would say. If Richard were able to, he would have already found a way to *cope* with my non-therapeutic advice. I know that anxiety is communicated interpersonally. I need to think this through.

APPLYING THE ART   A Person Needing Crisis Intervention—cont'd

Student-Patient Interaction	Thoughts, Communication Techniques, and Mental Health Nursing Concepts
Student: "Richard, could you breathe with me?" *He makes fleeting eye contact.* "Now slowly exhale all the air as I count." *I slow my pace.* "One . . . two . . . three . . . four . . . Now breathe in slowly . . . one . . . two . . . three . . . Again fully and slowly exhale: one . . . two . . . three . . . and four. Now slowly inhale counting one . . . two . . . three . . . Again, exhale, always one count longer. You have the rhythm now. Keep breathing and counting as I lightly put my fingers on your pulse." **Student's feelings:** *Richard seems to be responding. I'm relieved. I will have a lot to talk about in post-conference.*	From studying about panic disorder I learned the benefits of *controlled breathing* during an attack. Counting distracts the patient from automatic catastrophic thoughts while exhaling for one count longer than the inhale combats the tendency to hyperventilate. *Asking* Richard to breathe with me and *role modeling* how to do so works a lot better than commanding him to "calm down." By breathing together, I *offer self.*
Richard: *After 4 minutes of breathing and counting.* "I can't believe it. I'm getting to be okay." **Student's feelings:** *I'm amazed that what I did actually helped Richard. It's really true that mental health nursing comes in handy anywhere and everywhere.*	Richard's pulse rate gradually changes from 180 down to 85. I watch and breathe with him, only counting aloud as needed to remind him to breathe slowly.
Student: "You were able to breathe and count and thus take some control over the panic episode."	I give *support* by saying "you were able to . . ."
Richard: "I don't understand. Why did that work?"	
Student: "The rapid breathing and scary thoughts that worsen the heart palpitations cannot happen when you exhale completely and keep on slowly counting each breath."	I *teach* about how mindfully controlling the breathing inhibits hyperventilation and distracts Richard away from automatic dysfunctional thoughts like, "I'm going to die."
Richard: *Sighs.* "I still don't get why this panic thing is happening, but at least now I feel some hope." **Student's feelings:** *Richard feels hope and that combats powerlessness. I feel hopeful for him. It almost always helps me to talk someone I trust about painful things in my own life. Finding someone to talk to would help Richard with the third balancing factor: situational support.*	An advanced-practice nurse psychotherapist could help Richard learn more about the physiology of panic as well as ways to manage stress. He'd also most likely keep a record of his *dysfunctional thoughts* and learn how to do *health self-talk* instead.
Student: "I'm guessing the panic episodes might be your body's way of letting you know you might need to take some time for you." *Nodding, Richard sighs.* "Would you be ready to talk with someone who could help?"	I do some *teaching* as I suggest a *plan of action.* With help, Richard may look deeper at the onset of his panic symptoms. They started right around the time of learning that he was going to be a father again.
Richard: *Nods.* "If I could get good at that breathing thing, I could manage the panic even if it happens at work." **Student's feelings:** *I really hope Richard will find therapy that he can afford. I care about what happens to him.*	Something at work in the last 48 hours may have been the trigger for Richard to ask for my help today.
Student: *My instructor rounds the corner.* "Let's ask about a referral."	I *offer self* by saying, "let's *together* ask . . ." The minimum crisis intervention goal targets Richard to return to the pre-crisis state with no panic attacks. The maximum goal aims for growth.
Richard: "Thank you."	

- *Reentry phase*—Participants review old material discussed; introduce new topics they want to discuss; ask questions; and discuss how they would like to bring closure to the debriefing. Debriefing team members answer questions, inform, and reassure; provide handouts and other written material; provide information on referral sources for additional help; and summarize the debriefing experience with encouragement, support, and appreciation.

VIGNETTE

The nurse performs secondary crisis intervention and meets with Laura twice weekly during the next 4 weeks. Laura is motivated to work with the social worker and the nurse to find another place to live. The nurse suggests several times that Laura start to see a counselor in the outpatient clinic after the crisis is over so that she can talk about some of her pain. Laura is not interested, and says she will talk to the school counselor if she needs to talk. Three weeks after the attempted suicide, foster placement is found for Laura. The couple seems interested in Laura, and Laura appears happy about the attention she is receiving.

EVALUATION

The evaluation for a person in crisis is usually performed 4 to 8 weeks after the initial interview, although it can be done earlier (e.g., by the end of the visit the anxiety level will decrease from severe to moderate). If the intervention has been successful, the person's level of anxiety and ability to function should be at precrisis levels. Appropriate questions to ask during evaluation are as follows:

- Is the patient safe?
- Has the patient developed more adaptive ways to cope with stress and anxiety?
- Does the patient have a stronger existing support system?
- Has the patient maintained an optimum level of functioning?
- Has the patient returned to the precrisis level of functioning?

Often a person chooses to follow up on additional areas of concern and is referred to other agencies for more long-term work. Crisis intervention often serves to prepare a person for further treatment.

VIGNETTE

After 6 weeks Laura and the nurse decide that the crisis is over. Laura remains aloof and distant. The nurse evaluates Laura as being in a moderate amount of emotional pain, but Laura feels she is doing well and is beginning to feel more secure and accepted. The nurse's assessment indicates that Laura has other serious issues (e.g., the issue of her earlier sexual assaults), and the nurse strongly suggests that she could benefit from further counseling. The decision, however, is up to Laura, who says she is satisfied with the way things are and again states that if she has any problems she will talk to her school counselor.

KEY POINTS TO REMEMBER

- A crisis is not a pathological state but a struggle for emotional balance.
- Crises offer opportunities for emotional growth but can also lead to personality disorganization.
- There are three types of crisis: maturational, situational, and adventitious.
- Crises are usually resolved within 4 to 6 weeks.
- Crisis intervention therapy is short term, from 1 to 6 weeks, and focuses on the present problem only.
- Resolution of a crisis takes three forms: a person emerges at a higher level, at the precrisis level, or at a lower level of functioning.
- Social support and intervention can promote successful resolution.
- Crisis therapists take an active and directive approach with the patient in crisis.
- The patient is an active participant in setting goals and planning possible solutions.

- Crisis intervention is usually aimed at the mentally healthy person who generally is functioning well but is temporarily overwhelmed and unable to function.
- The crisis model can be adapted to meet the needs of people in crisis who have long-term and persistent mental problems.
- The steps in crisis intervention are consistent with the steps of the nursing process.
- Specific qualities in the nurse that can facilitate effective intervention are a caring attitude, flexibility in planning care, an ability to listen, and an active approach.
- The basic goals of crisis intervention are to reduce the individual's anxiety level and to support the effort to return to the person's precrisis level of functioning.
- During a disaster triage helps make the most efficient use of available resources.
- Critical incident stress debriefing is a group approach that helps groups of people who have been exposed to a crisis situation.

CRITICAL THINKING

1. List the three important areas of crisis assessment once safety concerns have been identified. Give examples of two questions in each area that need to be answered before planning can take place.

2. Barbara is 21 years old and a junior in nursing school. She tells her nursing instructor that her father (age 45 years) has just lost his job. Her father has been drinking heavily for years, and Barbara is having difficulty coping. Because of her father's alcoholism and the increased stress in her family, Barbara wants to leave school. Her mother has multiple sclerosis and thinks Barbara should quit school to take care of her.

    A. How many different types of crisis are going on in this family? Discuss the crises from the viewpoint of each family member.

    B. If this family came for crisis counseling, what areas would you assess and what kinds of questions would you ask to evaluate each member's needs and the needs of the family as a unit (perception of events, coping styles, social supports)?

    C. Formulate some tentative goals you might set in conjunction with the family.

    D. Identify by name appropriate referral agencies in your area that would be helpful if members of this family were willing to expand their use of outside resources and stabilize the situation.

    E. How would you set up follow-up visits for this family? Would you see the family members together, alone, or in a combination during the crisis period (4 to 6 weeks)? How would you decide whether follow-up counseling was indicated?

CHAPTER REVIEW

Choose the most appropriate answer.

1. Which statement about crisis theory provides a basis for nursing intervention?
    1. A crisis is an acute, time-limited phenomenon experienced as an overwhelming emotional reaction to a problem perceived as unsolvable.
    2. A person in crisis usually has had adjustment problems and has coped inadequately in his or her usual life situations.
    3. Crisis is precipitated by an event that enhances the person's self-concept and self-esteem.
    4. Nursing intervention in crisis situations rarely has the effect of ameliorating the crisis.

2. Ms. T., a single mother of four, comes to the crisis center 24 hours after an apartment fire in which all the family's household goods and clothing were lost. Ms. T. has no family in the area. Her efforts to mobilize assistance have been disorganized, and she is still without shelter. She is distraught and confused. The nurse assesses the situation as:
    1. a maturational crisis.
    2. a situational crisis.
    3. an adventitious crisis.
    4. evidence of an inadequate personality.

3. As the nurse responds to the patient in question 2, the intervention that takes priority is to:
    1. reduce anxiety.
    2. arrange long-term shelter.
    3. contact out-of-area family.
    4. hospitalize and place on suicide precautions.

4. For a nurse working in crisis intervention, which belief would be least helpful?
    1. A person in crisis is incapable of making decisions.
    2. The crisis counseling relationship is one between partners.
    3. Crisis counseling helps the patient refocus to gain new perspectives on the situation.
    4. Anxiety reduction techniques are used so the patient's inner resources can be accessed.

5. Which of the following is not a function of critical incident stress debriefing (CISD)? To debrief:
    1. staff after incidents of patient violence.
    2. a hotline volunteer after a patient's suicide.
    3. a patient after transplant surgery.
    4. search and rescue workers after a natural disaster.

REFERENCES

Aguilera, D.C. (1998). *Crisis intervention: Theory and methodology* (8th ed.). St. Louis: Mosby.

Aguilera, D.C., & Mesnick, J. (1970). *Crisis intervention: Theory and methodology.* St. Louis: Mosby.

American Nurses Association (ANA), American Psychiatric Nurses Association, & International Society of Psychiatric–Mental Health Nurses. (2007). *Psychiatric–mental health nursing: Scope and standards of practice.* Washington, DC: Nursesbooks.org.

Behrman, G., & Reid, W.J. (2002). Post-trauma intervention: Basic tasks. *Brief Treatment and Crisis Intervention, 2,* 39-48.

Caplan, G. (1964). *Symptoms of preventive psychiatry.* New York: Basic Books.

Cox, E., & Briggs, S. (2004). Disaster nursing: New frontiers for critical care. *Critical Care Nurse, 24,* 6-24.

Everly, G.S., Jr. (2000). Crisis management briefings (CMB): Large group crisis intervention in response to terrorism, disasters and violence. *International Journal of Emergency Mental Health, 2,* 53-57.

Everly, G.S., Jr., Lating, J.M., & Mitchell, J.T. (2000). Innovations in group crisis intervention: Critical incident debriefing (CISD) and critical incident stress management (CISM). In A.R. Roberts (Ed.), *Crisis interventions handbook: Assessment, treatment, and research* (2nd ed., pp. 77-100). New York: Oxford University Press.

Greenstone, J.L., & Leviton, S.C. (2002). *Elements of crisis intervention: Crises and how to respond to them* (2nd ed.). Pacific Grove, CA: Brooks/Cole.

Hammond, J., & Brooks, J. (2001). The world trade center attack. Helping the helpers: The role of critical incident stress management. *Critical Care, 5*(6), 315-317.

Holmes, T.H., & Rahe, R.H. (1967). The social readjustment rating scale. *Journal of Psychosomatic Research, 11*(2), 213-218.

Howard, J.M., & Goelitz, A. (2004). Psychoeducation as a response to community disaster. *Brief Treatment and Crisis Intervention, 4,* 1-10.

Jordan, K. (2003). A trauma and recovery model for victims and their families after a catastrophic school shooting: Focusing on behavioral, cognitive, and psychological effects and needs. *Brief Treatment and Crisis Intervention, 3,* 397-411.

Lowry, J.L., & Lating, J.M. (2002). Reflections on the response to mass terrorist attacks: An elaboration on Everly and Mitchell's 10 commandments. *Brief Treatment and Crisis Intervention, 2,* 95-104.

Roberts, A.R. (Ed.). (2000). *Crisis intervention handbook: Assessment, treatment, and research* (2nd ed., pp. 77-100). New York: Oxford University Press.

CHAPTER 18

Child, Partner, and Elder Abuse

Elizabeth M. Varcarolis

Key Terms and Concepts

Adult Protective Services (APS), p. 394
child abuse, p. 381
Child Protective Services, p. 389
cycle of violence, p. 387
elder abuse, p. 390
emotional abuse, p. 380

intimate partner violence (IPV), p. 385
perpetrators, p. 381
physical abuse, p. 380
safety plan, p. 390
victims, p. 381

Objectives

1. Differentiate among the three types of family abuse and give two physical and behavioral indicators for each.
2. Identify interview guidelines for assessing child abuse or intimate partner violence (IPV).
3. Compare and contrast at least five characteristics of an abusive parent or caretaker with that of an abusive partner or older adult.
4. Compare and contrast the forensic data gathered for a child with that of the forensic data gathered for an abused partner. Describe the procedures.
5. Delineate the factors that make an older adult more vulnerable to abuse.
6. Explain what Adult Protective Services (APS) can provide to an abused older adult.
7. Relate the procedure and contact number in your state for reporting suspected child and elder abuse.
8. Identify at lcast two referrals in your community for a victim of IPV to find safety and group or individual therapeutic support.

evolve

For additional resources related to the content of this chapter, visit the Evolve website at http://evolve.elsevier.com/Varcarolis/essentials.

- Chapter Outline
- Chapter Review Answers
- Case Study and Nursing Care Plans

- Nurse, Patient, and Family Resources
- Concept Map Creator

Physical and psychological trauma causes long-lasting and devastating damage to people's lives, their children's lives, and lives of generations to come. Violence has moved from the home to schools, the workplace, neighborhoods, the road, and the air and touches every corner of community life. Family violence and abuse is prevalent among all ethnic, socioeconomic, age, and social groups (Bartol et al., 2004). Besides family abuse, abuse by trusted authority figures is part of the picture of violence in our society. Spiritual abuse (pastors, priests, faith healers) and caregiver abuse (physicians, dentists, babysitters) are examples of violence that can be devastating and cause lifelong trauma.

The nurse is often the first point of contact for people experiencing family violence and is in the ideal position to contribute to prevention, detection, and effective intervention. All forms of interpersonal abuse can be devastating. Abuse can take the form of emotional, physical, or sexual abuse and neglect. **Emotional abuse** kills the spirit and the ability to succeed later in life, feel deeply, or make emotional contact with others.

Physical abuse includes emotional abuse in addition to the potential for long-term physical deformity, internal damage, and acute painful tissue damage, bone damage, and, in some cases, death. The consequences of being sexually abused may never be resolved if treatment is unavailable, and can cause behavioral and emotional difficulties throughout a person's life.

Sensitivity is required on the part of the nurse who suspects family violence. A person who feels judged or accused of wrongdoing is most likely to become defensive, and any attempts at changing coping strategies in the family will be thwarted. It is better for the nurse to ask about ways of solving disagreements or methods of disciplining children, rather than use the word *abuse* or *violence*, which appear judgmental and are therefore threatening to the family.

Some findings that should alert the nurse to the possibility of family violence are listed in Box 18-1.

THEORY

Most theories of intrafamily violence are related to psychology, sociology, or culture. According to DeKeseredy and Perry (2006), most conventional explanations of intrafamily violence remain partial and incomplete. These authors assert that most theories of violence are one-dimensional and separately emphasize different yet related phenomena. They advocate for a theory of violence that provides a comprehensive explanation that incorporates an integration of interpersonal, institutional, and structural violence. Domestic violence is extremely complex. There is no single theory that explains intrafamily violence, but rather it is

---

BOX 18-1

Indicators for Family Violence

- Recurrent emergency department (ED) visits for injuries attributed to being "accident prone"
- Presenting problems reflecting signs of high anxiety and chronic stress:
  - Hyperventilation
  - Panic attacks
  - Gastrointestinal disturbances
  - Hypertension
  - Physical injuries
- Depression
- Stress related conditions:
  - Insomnia
  - Violent nightmares
  - Anxiety
  - Extreme fatigue
- Eczema
- Loss of hair

---

most likely an interaction of societal, cultural, and psychological factors.

Social Learning Theory

Learning theory or **intergenerational violence theory** of family violence relies on role modeling, identification, and human interaction (Sadock & Sadock, 2007). Learning theory proposes that a child who witnesses abuse or is abused in the family of origin learns that violence is an acceptable reaction to stress, and internalizes the violent behavior as a behavioral norm. If the violent acting out behaviors are condoned in the family or social milieu, then the person is rewarded with a sense of power and control over others. Intergenerational abuse is considered a contributing factor in some cases of intimate partner violence (IPV), elder abuse (adults who were abused as children retaliate against their parents in later life), and child abuse.

Societal and Cultural Factors

According to Walker (1979), some correlates that exist when family abuse is high include the following:
- Poverty or unemployment
- Communities with inadequate resources
- Overcrowding
- Social isolation of families

The "frustration-aggression" hypothesis (Dollard et al., 1939) proposes that when frustration is high in response to the societal situations mentioned in the preceding text, frustration leads to aggression. Although these factors do correlate with family violence, they do not "cause" family violence. Not all frustrated individuals respond to frustration with violence. Some people respond to high levels of frustration with despair, depression, and resignation or attempt to change the situation (Sadock & Sadock, 2007).

The "patriarchal theory" (often referred to as feminist theory), which is advanced by social and behavioral scientists, holds the view that male dominance in our political and economic structure exists to enforce the differential status of men and woman. In many subcultures, women are viewed as property of or "belonging to" men, are subservient, and are kept relatively powerless. Research indicates that domestic violence does have its roots in societies where the role of the women is subordinate to men both in their public and private lives (MAHR, 2006). The United Nations Declaration on the Elimination of Violence Against Women (1994) states:

Recognizing that violence against women is a manifestation of historically unequal power relations between men and women, which have led to domination of the discrimination against women by men and to the prevention of the full advancement of women, and that violence against women is one of the crucial social mechanisms by which women are forced into a subordinate position compared to men.

Psychological Factors

Psychological theories focus on the abuser having personality traits that "cause" abusiveness. The abuser has no control over his or her violence and, as such, is not at fault. For example, the perpetrators of violence have no control because they have a mental illness, or they are addicted to drugs and alcohol. It is now known that many abusers, as well as their victims, are considered "normal" after psychological testing. By the same token, most people who have a mental disorder do not demonstrate violent behavior.

The use of legal and illegal drugs (e.g., prescription, over-the-counter, or illicit drugs; alcohol; or solvents) may coexist with family violence, but not everyone who abuses substances is involved in family violence and vice versa (NCFV, 2005). However, when the two do coexist, it is a matter of real concern. Both family violence and substance abuse problems usually require outside assistance, and both need to be addressed together. Unfortunately often when an abuser stops abusing a substance, family violence does not stop (NCFV, 2005).

Some abusers argue that they are physically unable to control their anger and aggression. This "loss of control" is not supported by their behavior, however. Perpetrators of family violence will most likely choose not to hit their bosses or a policeman, no matter how frustrated or angry they become. Abusers often plan where (in the home), when (no one is around), and how (leave no visible marks) when they inflict violence (MAHR, 2006). See Chapter 21 for neurobiological factors related to violence and interventions for angry and aggressive patients.

Other psychological factors include some of the following traits: low self-esteem, poor problem-solving skills, history of impulsive behavior, hypersensitivity (sees self as victim), and self-centered (lacks compassion for others) (Sadock & Sadock, 2007). People with aggressive traits are usually immature (although some are able to put up a mature façade to the outside world).

evolve

For a comprehensive case study and associated nursing care plans for a family experiencing violence, visit the Evolve website at http://evolve. elsevier.com/Varcarolis/essentials.

CHILD ABUSE

Child abuse takes place when a child is harmed by someone else physically, psychologically, sexually, or by acts of neglect. Each state is responsible for providing its own definition of child abuse. These definitions must meet the minimum standards set by the federal government through the Child Abuse and Prevention Act (CAPA):

Any recent act or failure to act on the part of a parent or caregiver, which results in death, serious physical harm, sexual abuse or exploitation, or act of failure to act which presents an immediate risk of serious harm.

Generally, most states recognize four different types of abuse: physical, emotional, sexual, and neglect. Table 18-1 provides definitions of different types of child abuse, some physical indicators, and some behavioral indicators.

The actual occurrence rates of child abuse are grossly underreported. Parents appear to account for 78.9% of child abuse (USDHHS: Childrens Bureau, 2006). Siblings can also be perpetrators of emotional, physical, and sexual abuse. Statistics concerning this common, yet unrecognized abuse are even less available. Among children confirmed by child protective agencies as being maltreated, 61% experienced neglect, 19% were physically abused, 10% were sexually abused, and 5% were emotionally or psychologically abused (USDHHS, 2005). However, more than one type of abuse can co-occur, and emotional abuse is always part of the picture.

TABLE 18-1   Types of Child Abuse and Physical and Behavioral Indicators

Type of Abuse	Physical Indications	Behavioral Indications
Physical Abuse Occurs when a caretaker allows or inflicts intentional physical injury that causes a substantial risk to the child's well-being and health.	Bruises/wounds in differing stages of healing Unexplained burns, bruises, welts, broken bones, internal injuries, bite marks, etc. Bald patches on scalp Subdural hematoma (child younger than 2) Retinal hemorrhage	Excessive fear of parents or constant effort to please Wary of adult contact Posttrauma syndrome, e.g., nightmares Obvious attempts to hide bruises or injuries Withdrawn, depressed or aggressive disruptive behavior Regressive behavior
Neglect Failure to provide for the child's basic needs.	*Physical neglect:* Malnourished Underweight, poor growth pattern Inadequately supervised Poor hygiene Unattended physical problems Inappropriate dress *Educational neglect:* School problems or failure Not enrolled in mandatory school for age of child	Soiled clothing, poor hygiene Begging, stealing food Emaciated or have distended belly Extended stay at school (early arrival–late departure) Psychosomatic complaints Delinquency Alcohol or drug abuse Abandonment Chronic truancy Special educational needs not being attended
Sexual Abuse Sexual abuse perpetrated on nonfamily member. Some types include: • Exhibitionism • Touching or manipulating the child's sexual organs • Oral, anal, or vaginal sex • Having child touch perpetrator • Masturbation in front of or with the child	Difficulty in walking or sitting Vulvovaginitis Urinary tract infections Torn, stained, or bloody underclothing Bruises or bleeding in external genitalia, vaginal or anal areas Venereal disease, especially in preteens In boys, pain on urination or penile swelling or discharge Foreign matter in rectum, vagina, or urethra	Mistrust of adults Abnormal or distorted view of sex. Bizarre, sophisticated or unusual sexual behavior or knowledge Phobias: fear of the dark, men, strangers, leaving the house Delinquent or running away. Self-injury or suicidal thoughts or behaviors Mental disorders may develop (e.g., posttraumatic stress disorder, depression, multiple personality disorder, eating disorders, conduct disorders, anxiety disorder)
Emotional or Psychological Abuse Behaviors that convey to the child that he or she is worthless, flawed, unloved, or unwanted: • Constant criticism • Insults • Harsh demands • Threats and yelling • Ignoring the child • Denying child opportunities to receive positive reinforcement	Speech disorders Lag in physical development	Difficulty in learning and living up to potential Lack of self-confidence Inappropriate adult-like behavior or infantile behavior Dramatic behavior changes, e.g., aggressiveness, compulsive seeking affection or approval

Children younger than 4 years of age are at greatest risk of severe injury or death. In 2003, children younger than 4 years accounted for 70% of child maltreatment fatalities, with infants younger than 1 year accounting for 44% of deaths (USDHHS, 2005).

A growing problem in industrialized countries—where financial resources have increased and family size has decreased—is overindulgence of children, which is considered an abuse of neglect. While overindulgence is the farthest issue from a health care worker's mind during an assessment, it is a serious problem that results in social impairment, emotional stunting (particularly empathy), and physical problems caused by inactivity and obesity.

Application of the Nursing Process
ASSESSMENT
Child

Often the abused child is excessively fearful of a parent or caregiver. The child may appear disheveled and neglected and have a history of absenteeism. Guidelines for interviewing the child suspected of being abused are presented in Box 18-2.

Reassure children that they will not be punished or hurt and that they did not do anything wrong. Children should not feel pressured to talk about any topics they are unwilling or unable to discuss. The experience should be non-threatening and supportive and not resemble a trial or inquisition. Preschoolers may be better able to express their experiences through playing out the incident with dolls or drawings. Open-ended questions are best. Possible questions include the following:
- How did this happen to you?
- Who takes care of you?
- What do you do after school?
- Who are your friends?
- What happens when you do something wrong?

Parent or Caregiver

Abusing parents vary by degrees of intelligence, education, and come from all socioeconomic backgrounds and religious affiliations. Specific characteristics are often found either singly or in combination among parents who abuse their children (Box 18-3). Guidelines for interviewing a parent or caregiver suspected of abusing a child are presented in Box 18-4.

Questions that are open ended and require a descriptive response can be less threatening and elicit more relevant

---

BOX 18-2
Interview Guidelines for Assessment of a Child

Do
- Conduct the interview in private.
- Sit next to the child, not across the table or desk.
- Tell the child that the interview is confidential.
- Use language the child understands.
- Ask the child to clarify words that you do not understand.
- Tell the child if any action will be required.

Do Not
- Allow the child to feel "in trouble" or "at fault."
- Suggest answers to the child.
- Probe or press for answers the child is not willing to give.
- Display shock or disapproval of parent, child, or situation.
- Force the child to remove clothing.
- Conduct the interview with a group of interviewers.

BOX 18-3
Characteristics of Abusive Parents

- A history of violence, neglect, or emotional deprivation as a child
- Low self-esteem, feelings of worthlessness, depression
- Poor coping skills
- Social isolation (may be suspicious of others)
- Few or no friends, little or no involvement in social or community activities
- Involved in a crisis situation—unemployment, divorce, financial difficulties
- Rigid, unrealistic expectations of child's behavior
- Frequently uses harsh punishment
- History of severe mental illness, such as schizophrenia
- Violent temper outbursts
- Looks to child for satisfaction of needs for love, support, and reassurance
- Projects blame onto the child for his or her "troubles"
- Lack of effective parenting skills
- Inability to seek help from others
- Perceives the child as bad or evil
- History of drug or alcohol abuse
- Feels little or no control over life
- Low tolerance for frustration
- Poor impulse control

BOX 18-4

Interview Guidelines for Assessment of a Parent or Caregiver

Do
- Conduct the interview in private.
- Be direct, honest, and professional.
- Be understanding.
- Be attentive.
- Inform the person if you must make a referral to Child Protective Services and explain the process.

Do Not
- Try to "prove" accusations or demands.
- Display horror, anger, or disapproval of parents or situation.
- Place blame on or make judgments about the parent(s) or child.

information than questions that can be answered yes or no. For example:
- What arrangements do you make when you have to leave your child alone?
- How do you punish your child?
- When your infant cries for a long time, how do you get him or her to stop?
- What does the child do to make you cry?
- Do you get time for yourself?
- How are things between you and your partner?

DIAGNOSIS AND OUTCOMES IDENTIFICATION

The most immediate concern is to ensure the child's safety and well-being. Therefore safety, injury, and *Risk for injury* are primary. Other nursing diagnoses might include *Disabled family coping*, *Post-trauma syndrome*, *Anxiety*, *Fear*, *Impaired parenting*, *Acute pain*, *Delayed growth and development*, and *Imbalanced nutrition: less than body requirement*.

The following is a list of short-term goals for the child experiencing abuse, the outcome of which should be "physical abuse, sexual abuse, or neglect has ceased."
1. Receive medical care for injuries within an hour.
2. Notify proper state authorities to ensure continued safety for child after abuse is suspected.
3. Be safe until adequate home and family assessment can be made.

IMPLEMENTATION

When child abuse is suspected, nurses are *legally* responsible for reporting to the appropriate child protective agency designated by each state (as are social workers, medical and mental health professionals, teachers, and childcare providers). Each state mandates that a report must be filed when "suspected" abuse or neglect is encountered. Some states require all people to report suspected child abuse. Reports remain confidential. (For more on reporting child abuse and neglect go to www.childwelfare.gov.)

The emergency department (ED) is usually where first contact is made with the abused child and family. Table 18-2 includes a list of nursing interventions to be used with the abused child and his or her family and rationales for the interventions.

The physician or nurse practitioner caring for an abused child should bring in help from a variety of sources to ensure the long-term safety of the child. For example, social workers, home health agencies, financial counselors, local mental health facilities, alcohol and drug treatment centers, and parenting centers.

Follow-up Care

There have been long-standing questions over whether treatment for abuse and neglect of children is valuable. A comprehensive analysis of interventions for child maltreatment (Skowron & Reinemann, 2005) found that "On average, individuals involved in a counseling or therapeutic program were better off than 71 percent of those who did not experience treatment in terms of various psychological, cognitive and behavioral outcomes (e.g. anxiety, depression, aggressiveness, etc.)."

Primary Prevention

Many factors exist in cases of child abuse. An estimated 40% of confirmed cases of child abuse are related to substance abuse (Shore, 1997). Additional related factors are single parenthood, teen parents, or parents with mental retardation or disorders; a vulnerable child (unwanted pregnancy, low-birth-weight baby; or a child that is difficult to care for because of physical or mental handicap, hyperactivity, colic, etc.). Mothers who were abused as children or are abused by their partner are more likely to abuse their child.

Societal risk factors also play an important role. Poverty is thought to be the most frequently and persistently noted risk factor for child abuse. Other societal risk factors according to Bethea (1999) are "inaccessible and unaffordable health care, fragmented social services, and lack of support from extended families and community."

TABLE 18-2   Interventions for the Abused Child and the Child's Family

Intervention	Rationale
1. Adopt a nonthreatening, nonjudgmental relationship with parents.	1. If parents feel judged or blamed or become defensive, they may take the child and either seek help elsewhere or seek no help at all.
2. Understand that children do not want to betray their parents.	2. Even in an intolerable situation, the parents are the only security the child knows.
3. Provide (or have physician provide) a complete physical assessment of the child.	3. To provide competent care and to substantiate reporting to child welfare agency, if required.
4. Use of dolls might help child tell how "accident" happened.	4. Child might not know how to articulate what happened or might be afraid of punishment. Dolls can be an easier way for child to act out what happened.
Forensic Issues	
1. **Be aware of your agency's and state's policy in reporting child abuse.** Contact supervisor or social worker to implement appropriate reporting.	1. Health care workers are mandated to report any cases of suspected or actual child abuse.
2. Ensure that proper procedures are followed, and evidence collected.	2. If child is temporarily taken to a safe environment, appropriate evidence helps protect the child's welfare.
3. Keep accurate and detailed records of incident: • Verbatim statements of who caused the injury and when it occurred • A body map to indicate size, color, shape, areas, and types of injuries with explanation • Physical evidence, when possible, of sexual abuse • Use of photos can be helpful. Check hospital policy.	3. Accurate records could help ensure child's safety and court presentation.
4. Forensic examination of the sexually assaulted child should be conducted according to specific protocols: • Provided by law enforcement agencies • Follow state guidelines (www.childwelfare.gov)	4. Proper collection, handling, and storage of forensic specimens are crucial to court presentation.

Adapted from Varcarolis (2006). *Manual of psychiatric nursing care plans: Diagnoses, clinical tools, and psychopharmacology* (3rd ed.). Saunders: St. Louis.

BOX 18-5

Common Features of a Successful Child Abuse Protection Program

• Strengthen and establish links with family and community support systems.
• Create opportunities for parents to feel empowered to act on their own behalf.
• Enhance coordination and integration of services needed by families.
  • Parenting skills
  • Coping skills
• Anger management
• Normal child development
• Parent support group
• Provide settings where parents and children can gather, interact, support, and learn from each other.
• Enhance community awareness of the importance of healthy parenting practices.
• Provide emergency support for parents 24 hours a day.

Adapted from Bethea, L. (1999). Primary prevention of child abuse. *American Family Physician, 59*(15).

Early diagnosis of actual or potential child abuse and intervention correlates with a more positive prognosis. Box 18-5 on p. 385 identifies common features of a successful child abuse prevention program.

INTIMATE PARTNER VIOLENCE

Intimate partner violence (IPV) is defined as current or former emotional, psychological, physical, or sexual abuse between current or former partners of an intimate relationship, regardless of gender or marital status (Goodman, 2006).

Although the majority of the victims of reported domestic violence are women, and domestic violence is the number one cause of ED visits by women, an estimated 25% to 33% of domestic violence cases involve women abusing men and abuse among homosexual couples (Halpern et al., 2004). Because it is accepted that woman are more likely to be the assaulted partner, this discussion will use the female pronoun to denote the battered person. For the same reason, the male pronoun will be used when speaking of the violent partner, with the understanding that males are also the victim of IPV.

Although the exact numbers of abused domestic partners are not known, some estimate that up to 37% of all women experience battering, and that of those that are battered, 60% are battered during pregnancy (AADA, 2004). Equally disturbing is that physical violence is estimated to occur in 20% to 35% of dating relationships. Even high school– and college-age dating couples have engaged in an estimated 20% to 52% of reported physical abuse (AADA, 2004).

It has well been established that the abused as well as those who become the violent domestic partner can come from any race and religious, economic, or educational background. Either can be of any age, married, single, divorced, or never married.

An abusive relationship is all about instilling fear and wanting to have power and control in the relationship. Anger is one way that the abuser tries to gain authority. He may also turn to physical violence (kicking, punching, grabbing, slapping, or strangulation), sexual violence (forcing sexual intercourse or performing sexual acts against the victim's will), or psychological violence (threats of death or death of a child, use of weapons) (Women's Health, 2006).

IPV has severe, long-reaching effects. Children who reside in homes where IPV occurs are vulnerable to feelings of responsibility, guilt, emotional distress, behavioral regression, somatic complaints, posttrauma disorder, alcohol or drug abuse, and more. Children who live in an atmosphere of IPV are 30% to 60% likely to be abused as well (Goodman, 2006).

Unfortunately children from violent homes are more likely to model the actions they see around them in their own lives and carry the legacy of a violent home forward.

CHARACTERISTICS OF INTIMATE PARTNER VIOLENCE

The Battered Partner

Women do not ask to be beaten, nor do they enjoy being battered. The battered partner lives in terror of the next beating. Women do not usually initiate the violence, but when they are aggressive toward their violent mate, it is usually in self-defense. Approximately 93% of women who killed their mates had been battered by them (AADA, 2004).

The abused woman is often the subject of extreme and irrational jealousy, isolation, and verbal as well as physical abuse. Feelings of powerlessness and low self-esteem are common. After constant belittlement, insults, and degradation, the abused becomes so psychologically destroyed that she begins to believe that what the abuser says is true. Because of the physical or sexual abuse and threats, the abused lives in a world of terror and fear for her life and the lives of her children. These families are usually isolated, and they have few if any friends or outside influences. The violence and pain that exist inside the home remain secret. Table 18-3 lists characteristics of the abused woman and violent partner.

The Batterer

Violence is a learned behavior used by a person to control others. Frequently violent partners were brought up in a home where they themselves were beaten or where they witnessed parental beatings. A batterer has a low sense of self, poor impulse control, and limited tolerance for frustration, and senses a lack of control in his life. Abusing someone less powerful or more vulnerable helps the violent partner feel more in control, powerful, and masculine (if male). Men who batter have no guilt and lack concern over their aggressiveness. Batterers may appear well adjusted from the outside, but usually have only superficial relationships with others. They are extremely possessive, pathologically jealous, believe in male supremacy in relationships, and often have a drug or alcohol problem, which is not a cause of the abuse but often an excuse for the abuse.

Cycle of Violence

Abuse toward a person in a partner relationship is not merely an exchange of blows, but rather a process that increases in

TABLE 18-3	Behavioral Characteristics of Intimate Partner Violence
Characteristics of Violent Partner	**Characteristics of Battered Partner**
Denial and Blame: Denies that abuse occurs, shifts responsibility to abuse to partner	Comes to believe that if they do or say "the right thing," the abuse will stop. If they don't do anything "wrong" abuse won't happen.
Emotional Abuse: Belittles, criticizes, insults, uses name calling, undermines	Becomes psychologically devastated and begins to believe partner's words
Control Through Isolation: Limits family or friends, controls activities and social events, tracks time or mileage on car, activities, stalks at work, takes to and from work or school, may demand permission to leave house	Gradually loses sight of personal boundaries for self, children; becomes unable to assess blame without validation from a supportive network
Control Through Intimidation: Uses behaviors to instill fear such as through vile threats, breaks things, destroys property, abuses pets, displays weapons, threatens children, and threatens homicide or suicide, increasing physical, sexual, or psychological abuse	Results in constant fear and terror that becomes cumulative and oppressive; contemplates suicide, completes suicide, contemplates homicide, occasionally completes suicide in self-defense
Control Through Economic Abuse: Controls money, makes account for all money spent; if partner works, calls excessively, forces partner to miss work. Refuses to share money.	Economic and emotional and economic dependency may result in depression, high risk for secret drug or alcohol abuse. If works, frequently loses job from partner stalking and harassing
Control Through Power: Makes all decisions, defines role in the relationship, treats spouse like a servant, and takes charge of the home and social life.	Continues to lose sense of self, becomes unsure of who she is, defines self in terms of partner, children, job, others, lacks self power

intensity and escalates over time without valid provocation. The abusive relationship may start subtly. It may start by the abuser being critical of the way the partner dresses, disciplines the kids, cares for the home. Or the abuser becomes unreasonably jealous, possessive, and watchful of the partner's activities. No matter how it begins, the process is always slowly progressive. The abuse becomes more frequent, intense, and life threatening over time. In Walker's classic study of 400 women in violent families (1979), the **cycle of violence** was first operationally defined. The theory consists of three phases: (1) tension-building phase, (2) acute battering phase, and (3) honeymoon phase. Figure 18-1 shows behaviors that characterize the steps in the cycle.

The cycle of violence is a continuing cycle that is hard to break without help. It is important to recognize, however, that the cycle does not apply to many cases of IPV. However, many women report that their partner never repents, nor is the violence cyclical, but is a constant presence in their lives.

Why Abused Partners Stay

There are many reasons women stay in violent domestic situations. Perhaps one of the *strongest* motives for staying is fear that the attacks will become even more violent, or she or her children could be killed if found by the batterer once they leave. This is a very real concern, and women are

at a high risk of further violence or even death when they threaten to leave or if they are later found by their abuser. Other reasons many women cannot leave are that:
- They have no other means of financial support.
- They have no support system after living in isolation for long periods.
- They are afraid to be alone or think they cannot survive without the partner.
- They experience depression or loss of psychological energy necessary to leave.
- Their self-esteem is low, and they believe that the batterer is powerful and omniscient.

Some women may also believe that they:
- Deserve the beatings because they did something "wrong."
- Can control the beatings by not doing anything to upset their partners.
- Need to stay for the sake of the children.
- Are still positively reinforced by the honeymoon phase of the battering cycle.

Application of the Nursing Process
ASSESSMENT

Women are most often seen in the ED, but they may be seen in a physician's office or clinic. There is wide agree-

EXAMINING THE EVIDENCE   Helping the Abuser, Protecting the Abused

Coming from a home where my father communicated by throwing things, hitting, shoving, and shouting, I found this chapter to be extremely interesting. Our house was like growing up in a war zone. I remember Dad grabbing Mom by the arms and nearly pushing her down the steps to the basement. I always wondered if he and Mom could have gotten help. Is there any treatment available for men who abuse their spouses?

In a word, yes, there is treatment available. The next question is, how effective is the treatment? It wasn't until the past two decades of the 21st century that the United States began to take a close look at family violence. Before then, domestic issues were largely considered private and something best left behind closed doors (Rosenfeld, 1992). Now we deal with spousal abuse from a criminal perspective, in which the perpetrator may be jailed, and from a rehabilitation perspective, in which the perpetrator receives treatment to, it is hoped, eradicate the violent behavior.

Some groups of abusers may be more or less responsive to treatment. Berns and colleagues (1999) classify abusers as Type I and Type II. Type I constitutes 20% of all batterers. Chillingly, they have heart rates that become lower as they become more aggressive. This group frequently meets criteria for anti-social personality disorder and are considered more dangerous, belligerent, contemptuous, and more likely to use lethal weapons. Type II refers to the remaining 80% of all batterers; they have increased heart rates as they become more aggressive

and are characterized by being slower to anger. According to Berns and colleagues, whereas Type II spouse abusers may derive some benefits from treatment, Type I batterers derive almost no value.

Overall, positive outcomes from interventions are not supported by research. In a systematic review of the current literature (a meta-analysis), Babcock and associates (2004) examined 22 studies. They concluded that treatment methods do little to reduce the rate at which batterers will reoffend (recidivism). Feder and Wilson (2005) reviewed the literature to determine the effectiveness of court-ordered treatment. They, too, expressed doubt at the efficacy of treatment for batterers.

The spouses of volatile partners live with fear, anxiety, hopelessness, and incredibly low self-esteem. Randall and Smith (2007) studied abused wives' responses to their partners attending a batterers' intervention program. They found that engagement in treatment offered abused wives a source of hope, yet noted that this hope is not supported by the literature.

Currently our best bet in reducing the problem of spousal abuse is to strengthen the legal system in the form of sanctions and in developing alternative sanctions to improve treatment compliance. At the same time, these treatments should be tested for effectiveness and developed (Babcock, Green, & Robie, 2004). Researchers, clinicians, and policymakers are deeply concerned about people whose lives are disrupted as yours was by this horrible problem and are continuing to devote time and financial resources to improve the care we have to offer.

Babcock, J.C., Green, C.E., & Robie, E. (2004). Does batterers' treatment work? A meta-analytic review of domestic violence treatment. *Clinical Psychology Review, 23*, 1023-1053.

Berns, S.B., Jacobson, N.S., & Gottman, J.M. (1999). Demand/withdraw interaction patterns between different types of batterers and their spouses. *Journal of Marital and Family Therapy*, 25(3), 337-348.

Feder, L., & Wilson, D.B. (2005). A meta-analytic review of court-mandated batterer intervention programs: Can courts affect abusers' behavior? *Journal of Experimental Criminology, 1*, 239-262.

Randall, M.E., & Smith, E.J. (2007). Batterer intervention program: The victim's hope in ending the abuse and maintaining the relationship. *Issues in Mental Health Nursing, 28*, 1045-1063.

Rosenfeld, B.D. (1992). Court ordered treatment of spouse abuse. *Clinical Psychology Review, 12*, 205-226.

ment that improved health care response to victims of domestic violence is needed. Many hospitals and health care systems across the country are designing and implementing screening and intervention programs to help meet this need (AHRQ, 2002).

If an injury that brings a woman to the ED does not match the explanation, or if the patient minimizes the abuse, IPV might be suspected. If IPV is suspected, a complete physical history needs to be done, including x-rays and a neurological examination. Because rape may be part of the abusive scenario, this should be evaluated as well, especially if the woman is pregnant, exposed to sexually

transmitted diseases (STDs), or has any signs of infection or trauma.

Signs of abuse may include burns, bruises, scars, and other wounds in various stages of healing, particularly around the head and neck. Physical examination includes assessing for signs of internal injuries such as concussions, perforated eardrums, abdominal injuries, eye injuries, and strangulation marks on the neck. Broken or fractured bones such as arms, pelvis, ribs, clavicle, legs, and jaw are other signs of abuse. An examination might reveal burns from cigarettes, acids, scalding liquids, or appliances.

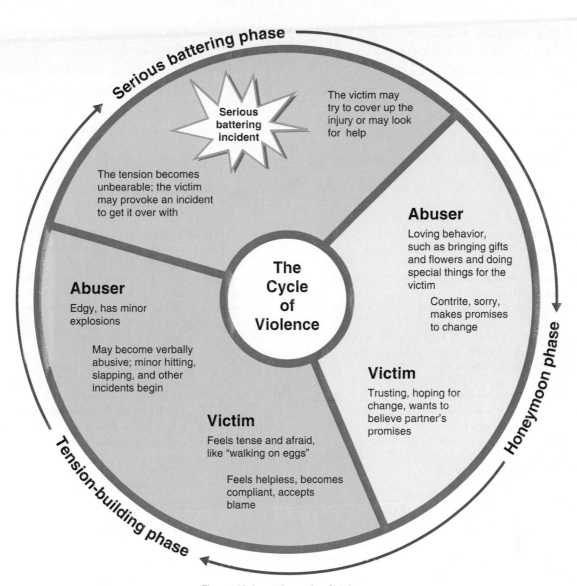

Serious battering phase

Serious battering incident

The victim may try to cover up the injury or may look for help

The tension becomes unbearable; the victim may provoke an incident to get it over with

Abuser
Loving behavior, such as bringing gifts and flowers and doing special things for the victim

Contrite, sorry, makes promises to change

The Cycle of Violence

Abuser
Edgy, has minor explosions

May become verbally abusive; minor hitting, slapping, and other incidents begin

Victim
Trusting, hoping for change, wants to believe partner's promises

Honeymoon phase

Victim
Feels tense and afraid, like "walking on eggs"

Feels helpless, becomes compliant, accepts blame

Tension-building phase

Figure 18-1 ■ The cycle of violence.

Always there are psychological and emotional scars. The woman might present with signs of high anxiety and stress and complain of insomnia, chest pain, back pain, dizziness, stomach upset, trouble eating, severe headache, and so on. Signs of posttraumatic stress disorder (PTSD) are often present and should be part of an assessment. A brief history may reveal a series of falls, "accidents," and recent department visits. A woman with any indication of IPV should always be seen alone, without her partner present.

Three questions are often sufficient to reveal current or prior IPV (Feldhaus et al., 1997):

1. Have you been hit, kicked, punched, or otherwise hurt by someone within the past year? If so, by whom?

2. Do you feel safe in your current relationship?

3. Is there a partner from a previous relationship who is making you feel unsafe now?

Always ask if the children are also being hit or hurt in any way, and if suspected or confirmed, **Child Protective Services** need to become involved.

An assessment of the patient's support systems, suicide potential, and coping responses (learned helplessness, substance abuse) should be included. Once the history of abuse has been ascertained, carefully document verbal statements as well as physical findings as outlined in the forensic part of interventions. Ask the woman if she would allow photos to be taken.

TABLE 18-4   Interventions for Intimate Partner Violence: Emergency Department

Intervention	Rationale
1. Ensure that medical attention is provided to patient. Ask permission to take photos.	1. If patient wants to file charges, photos boost victim's confidence to press charges now or in the future.
2. Set up interview in private and ensure confidentiality.	2. Patient might be terrified of retribution and further attacks from partner if she tells.
3. Assess in a nonthreatening manner information concerning: • Sexual abuse • Chemical abuse • Thoughts of suicide or homicide.	3. These are all vital issues in determining appropriate interventions: • Increases risk for posttrauma • Many victims self-medicate. • May seem the only way out of an intolerable, catastrophic situation.
4. Encourage patient to talk about the battering incident without interruptions.	4. When patients share their stories, attentive listening is essential.
5. Ask how patient is faring with the children in the home.	5. In homes in which the mother is abused, children also tend to be abused.
6. Assess if patients have a safe place to go when violence is escalating. If no, include a list of shelters or safe houses with other written information.	6. When abused patients are ready to go, they will need to go quickly.

Forensic Issues

Intervention	Rationale
1. Identify if patient is interested in pressing charges. If yes, give verbal and written information on: • Local attorneys who handle spouse abuse cases • Legal clinics • Battered women's advocates	1. Often spouse or partner is afraid of retaliation, but when ready to seek legal advice, an appropriate list of lawyers well trained in this area is needed.
2. Know the requirement in your state about reporting suspected spouse abuse.	2. Many states have or are developing laws or guidelines for protecting battered women.
3. Discuss with patient an escape plan during escalation of anxiety before actual violence erupts (see Box 18-2).	3. Write out plan and include shelter and referral numbers. This can prevent further abuse to children and patient.
4. Throughout work with battered spouses emphasize that the beatings are not their fault.	4. When self-esteem is eroded, people often buy into the myth that they deserved the beatings because they did something "wrong," and if they had not done X, then it would not have happened.
5. Encourage patient to reach out to family and friends whom they might have been avoiding.	5. Old friends and relatives can make helpful allies and validate that patient does not deserve to be beaten.
6. Know the psychotherapists in the community who have experience working with battered spouses or partners.	6. Psychotherapy with victims of trauma requires special skills on the part of even an experienced therapist.
7. If patient is not ready to take action at this time, provide a list of community resources: a. Hotlines b. Shelters c. Battered women's groups d. Battered women's advocates e. Social services f. Medical assistance or Aid to Families with Dependent Children (AFDC)	7. It can take time for patients to make decisions to change their life situation. People need appropriate information.

Adapted from Varcarolis (2006). *Manual of psychiatric nursing care plans: Diagnoses, clinical tools, and psychopharmacology* (3rd ed.). Saunders: St. Louis.

APPLYING THE ART   A Person Experiencing Partner Violence

SCENARIO: I met 28-year-old Maddie in the emergency department where she had been seen 3 weeks before for a dislocated shoulder, which she attributed to falling down the basement steps while carrying a basket of laundry. This time she described cramping in this, her second month of pregnancy. Her left eye showed bruising, partially masked by heavy makeup. I introduced myself and my role as Maddie rested in an exam room waiting for the nurse-midwife.

THERAPEUTIC GOAL: By the conclusion of this interaction, Maddie will verbalize the intent to access her support system, decreasing her isolation.

Student-Patient Interaction	Thoughts, Communication Techniques, and Mental Health Nursing Concepts
Maddie: "I feel better now. The cramps barely hurt. I don't need that exam. I need to get home. I'm fine really." ***Student's feelings:*** *Falling down the steps plus a bruised face and now cramping, I feel deeply concerned, and I wonder if there's a connection.*	She uses *denial* that she does not need the exam, and that she's "fine really."
Student: "You say you feel better, but still you're cramping." *She shrugs her shoulders.* "You're anxious to leave, almost as though you're fearful." *She wrings her hands, looking downward.* ***Student's feelings:*** *I'm worried for her. I need to work up the courage to ask her about abuse.*	I use *restatement* then *attempt to translate into feelings.* She's moving into *moderate anxiety.* She's still able to focus her thoughts.
Maddie: "It's not worth it."	
Student: "Not worth it. The exam?" ***Student's feelings:*** *I feel concerned that she actually may see herself as "not worth it."*	I *restated* then asked a *direct question* to *clarify.* Maybe I should have stopped after "not worth it" to keep her options for answering open. Physical abuse is always emotionally damaging, too.
Maddie: *Glancing at me.* "I just need to get home before 5:30." ***Student's feelings:*** *I hope she will open up to me. I must take charge of my feelings. There's stigma attached to abuse, almost like it's the victim's fault. I want her to know whatever happens, she's okay by me.*	I need to focus on building her comfort level with me.
Student: "Maddie, I appreciate how difficult this must be. I am concerned about you." *I learn toward her and make eye contact.*	*Attempting to translate into feelings* facilitates empathy. My *nonverbals* and words need to be *congruent* and show *nonjudgmental acceptance.*
Maddie: *Silent. Bites her lip.*	
Student: "Could you share with me what happens at 5:30?"	Using the word "could" in my *question* gives her a choice, which empowers her.
Maddie: "He gets home. He can't know about the baby." *She starts to cry.* ***Student's feelings:*** *I feel sad at all she has to worry about.*	She must feel overwhelmed.
Student: "The 'he' is your husband?" *She nods.* "You seem afraid of him." *She opens her mouth then closes it again.* "I sense you've been hurt by him before."	I clarify the indefinite pronoun "he" and *attempt to translate into feelings.*

Continued

APPLYING THE ART   A Person Experiencing Partner Violence—cont'd

Student-Patient Interaction	Thoughts, Communication Techniques, and Mental Health Nursing Concepts
Maddie: "Before, after, and during! I used to be better at reading Steve's moods but I've been so worried about my baby. He punched my stomach when I didn't cook his eggs right this morning. He punched my stomach!" *Begins to tear up.* "Maybe he suspects." **Student's feelings:** *I just realized why I'm feeling so anxious. When I was young, I remember a neighbor and her kids that my family sheltered one night. She cringed describing the beating, but she also went back to her husband the very next morning.*	Like many *battered women*, Maddie describes how she anticipates her husband's needs. She may show *codependent behavior* by needing to be needed.
Student: "Maybe he suspects?" **Student's feelings:** *I'm hoping she shares some of her burden with me.*	*Restatement says,* "go on." Sharing her pain with me decreases its intensity.
Maddie: "That I'm pregnant. He's always accusing me of running around, but I swear I never did! I never would. I love him." *Sobs.* "He's wonderful on his good days."	
Student: "He's wonderful on the good days, but not so wonderful on the bad days."	I *verbalize the implied* opposite pole, e.g., "good days" implies bad days, too. My *acceptance* gives her permission to talk more about the painful parts.
Maddie: *Nods.* "The bad days happen more often. One day he's going to kill me." *Winces with another cramp.* "I'll never forgive him or myself if I lose my baby."	I'm remembering that people in chronically abusive relationships suffer *depression* and *anxiety.* Over time *posttraumatic stress disorder* can emerge.
Student: "You feel in danger for you life and now, for your baby's life, too." **Student's feelings:** *Should I focus on her danger first or her not feeling able to forgive herself? She's carrying so much. What kind of man beats his wife? How can she think him wonderful, at all?*	I *summarize* her deepest fears. Any part that's "wonderful" undoubtedly occurs during the *honeymoon phase* of the *abuse cycle.*
Maddie: *Closes her eyes. Silent for 3 minutes.* **Student's feelings:** *It's tough for me to wait quietly. I want her to leave him but this is her life, not mine. I'll mindfully breathe to keep myself calm, yet focused. My instructor will be making rounds soon. I feel a need to debrief.*	I need to think this through. I don't want to add to the stigma by judging her. I remember about *learned helplessness,* when battering chips away at *self-esteem,* initiative, and hope.
Maddie: "You're still here." *Smiles and makes eye contact.*	
Student: "Yes, Maddie, I'm guessing you're thinking deeply about your options. Is there anyone who can help you through this?" **Student's feelings:** *I so much want to tell her to leave him but then I'm just one more person telling her what to do.*	She's *ambivalent.* She wrestles with the pain of leaving as compared to the pain of staying. Maybe she'll accept some information or at least the number for the women's shelter.
Maddie: "I think it's time I told my parents. I know they suspect something. I've lied and lied. I feel so ashamed."	

APPLYING THE ART   A Person Experiencing Partner Violence—cont'd

Student-Patient Interaction	Thoughts, Communication Techniques, and Mental Health Nursing Concepts
Student: "Sounds to me that, like other battered women, you made tough choices that enabled you to survive." *I look at Maddie and offer my hand.* **Student's feelings:** *I'm taking a risk in calling her a battered woman if she's not ready.*	I *give information* as I *offer self* by reaching for her hand.
Maddie: *Holds my hand, looking up as the nurse-midwife comes in.*	
Maddie: *Nods.* "I don't know what I'm going to do yet, but I'm going to call my mom." **Student's feelings:** *She recognizes her loneliness. I feel so proud of her courage.*	*Isolation* from supports fits the victimizer's agenda of ensuring dependency on the abuser alone.
Student: "You're making the decision to tell her about the abuse."	My statement acts like an *indirect question.*
Maddie: "Yes, I've been so lonely. Yes." **Student's feelings:** *Maddie really may take this step. I feel hopeful.*	

DIAGNOSIS AND OUTCOMES IDENTIFICATION

IPV is a situational crisis that threatens a woman's physical and psychological health, as well as her life and possibly the lives of her children. Therefore, *Risk for violence, Risk for injury, Acute/Chronic pain, Risk for trauma,* and *Risk for self-directed or other-directed violence* are all nursing diagnoses that might need immediate focus. Others that need to be considered include *Social isolation, Disturbed sleep pattern, Powerlessness, Disturbed personal identity, Risk for post-trauma syndrome,* and *Disabled family coping.*

Unfortunately women who are treated in the ED may admit to IPV but seldom come for treatment. Nurses often have strong reactions when children or women are violently treated. However, in the case of partner abuse, it is up to the abused partner to make the decision to stay in the battering situation or to leave. It is most helpful for the woman if the nurse can accept the woman's decision in a nonjudgmental way and support the woman in her decision.

Therefore the obvious outcome for health care personnel would be to see the woman opt for a safe environment for herself and her children in the form safe houses, a caring relative, or a friend. Because that is not usually the woman's decision, the nurse can provide the woman with referrals

BOX 18-6

Basic Intimate Partner Violence Safety Plan

- Move to a room with more than one exit, avoiding rooms with potential weapons (e.g., kitchen knives).
- Know the quickest route out of your home.
- Know the quickest route out of your workplace. Find out what resources they have to protect employees.
- Pack a bag with essential clothes, valuables, and documents for you and each of your children. Keep it hidden but make it easy to grab quickly.
- Tell your neighbors about your abuse and ask them to call the police when they hear a disturbance.
- Have a code word to use with your kids, family, and friends when you need help.
- Have a safe place selected in case you ever have to leave.
- Use your instincts.
- You have the right to protect yourself and your kids.

Goodman, P.E. (2006). The relationship between intimate partner violence and other forms of family and societal violence. *Emergency Medical Clinics of North America, 21,* 889-903.

(numbers for safe houses, hotlines, and support groups, legal counseling in verbal and written forms) as well as a **safety plan.** Box 18-6 contains an example of a basic IPV safety plan.

IMPLEMENTATION

Table 18-4 on p. 390 lists several interventions and their rationales related to the initial ED visit. It is important that the battered partner begins to understand that:

- No one deserves to be beaten.
- She cannot make anyone hurt her.
- It is not her fault.

ELDER ABUSE

Elder abuse is a serious and rapidly growing problem with an estimated one out of every 20 older Americans being abused each year (Elder Abuse Unit, 2005). The World Health Organization (2002) states that elder abuse is "a violation of human rights and a significant cause of injury, illness, lost productivity, isolation and despair." There are three common categories of elder abuse: domestic, institutional, and self-neglect. The four common kinds of elder abuse are physical or sexual, psychological, financial abuse or exploitation, and neglect (Box 18-7).

As a public policy issue, elder abuse has a long and convoluted history first emerging in the 1970s as "granny abuse." Unfortunately even today elder abuse has not received major attention at the national level (Quinn & Zielke, 2005). The extent of the incidence and prevalence of elder abuse in the United States is unknown. The 2004 Survey of State Adult Protective Services reported a 19.7% increase in the combined total of reported cases of elder and vulnerable adult abuse and neglect and a 15.6% increase in substantiated cases from 2000 to 2004 (Wood, 2006). Unfortunately it is estimated that up to four out of five cases are never reported (ICN, 2005).

All 50 states have some form of elder abuse prevention laws and have set up reporting systems. It is the **Adult Protective Services (APS)** of each state that receives and investigates reports of suspected elder abuse. To be eligible for APS help in most states, an older adult has to be deemed unable to care for himself or herself. This leaves many older adults who are mentally and physically healthy unprotected in a situation in which they are physically or financially being exploited by family members. The result is that the definitions of elder abuse and the APS programs differ from state to state, resulting in a "patchwork of laws, definitions, and services throughout the country" (Quinn & Zielke, 2005, p. 451). These widely differing definitions and terminologies makes it impossible to know the actual extent of the problem or to conduct sound research. Gorbien (2005) states that fortunately there have been some recent movements at the national level to standardize the approach to the study of elder mistreatment.

CHARACTERISTICS OF ELDER ABUSE

The Abused Elder

The percentage of older adults (defined as 60 years or older) is growing in the United States as people are living longer. Seniors can be especially vulnerable to abuse as well as to other crimes. Age-related syndromes often result in frailty and functional decline, making an older adult even more at risk for abuse, neglect, and self-neglect. This frailty and decline also puts older adults at greater risk for sexual abuse that, when reported, is often disbelieved. Elder abuse is most often diagnosed in older adults who have depression, alcohol or drug abuse, dementia, psychosis, loss of executive function, or other psychiatric illness, which compounds an older adult's vulnerability.

People older than 80 years of age are two to three times more likely to suffer abuse and neglect than their proportion of the older population, and victims of elder abuse are three times more likely to die than older adults who are not mistreated (Quinn & Zielke, 2005). Older women are more likely than men to suffer from abuse or neglect, and the majority of victims are white.

BOX 18-7

Five Kinds of Elder Abuse

1. **Physical abuse:** The infliction of physical pain or injury (e.g., slapping, bruising, sexually molesting, restraining) (approx. 20%).
2. **Psychological abuse:** The infliction of mental anguish (e.g., humiliating, intimidating, threatening) (approx. 20%).
3. **Financial abuse or exploitation:** The misuse of someone's property and resources by another person (approx. 20%).
4. **Neglect:** Failure to fulfill a caretaking obligation to provide goods and services (e.g., abandonment, denial of food or health-related services) (approx. 40%). This category may also include self-neglect.
5. **Sexual abuse:** Nonconsensual (either by refusal or incapacity to refuse) sexual contact (% unknown).

From International Council of Nurses. *Elder abuse.* www.icn.ch/matters_elder.htm.

The Abuser

Early studies on elder abuse focused on the caretaker's stress and burden as a causative factor in elder abuse. More recent research indicates that the characteristics of the abuser more closely resemble those characteristics of the abuser in partner abuse (IPV) (Quinn & Zielke, 2005). Although institutional abuse of older adults is a troubling phenomenon, it is believed that among known perpetrators of abuse and neglect, the perpetrator was a family member in about 90% of the cases, with two thirds being adult children or spouses (DHHS, 2007).

Application of the Nursing Process

ASSESSMENT

Physicians, nurses, and other health care professionals are often the only outside contact an older adult may have. In most states, health care workers (nurses, nurses' aides, and physicians) are mandated to report elder abuse and neglect to APS. However, it is likely that only a very small fraction of reportable cases get referred to APS.

Victims of violence have twice as many physician and clinic visits as those not subjected to abuse. Because victims of abuse or neglect are most likely to be abused by family members, the abused is often afraid to speak out. There may be threats against disclosure, the abused may experience deep shame, or the abused may want to protect a loved one. It is important, therefore, that family and friends speak out. Health care workers should make careful evaluation when older adults visit health care facilities, especially on a frequent basis.

The signs of abuse are very similar to those of the victim in child or IPV. Some additional red flags include the following:

- Fear of being alone with caregiver
- Obvious malnutrition
- Bedsores or skin lesions
- Begging for food
- In need of medical or dental care
- Left unattended for long periods
- Reports of abuse or neglect
- Passive, withdrawn, or emotionless behavior
- Concern over finances
- Valuables missing

When patients are referred by friends, family, police, social services, or others in situations in which the patient cannot leave the home, house calls are necessary. House calls allow the clinician to make an assessment of how the older adult functions in his or her own environment, and

often self-neglect, abuse, or financial exploitation is easier to detect (Dyer et al., 2005).

DIAGNOSIS AND OUTCOMES IDENTIFICATION

Nursing diagnoses for abused older adults are much the same as with other cases of abuse. *Risk for injury, Acute or Chronic pain, Fear, Anxiety, Risk for self-directed*, and *Risk for other-directed violence* have been discussed. However, two areas that particularly apply to an abused older adult are neglect and financial exploitation. Nursing diagnoses that may be appropriate include *Impaired home maintenance, Self-care deficit, Caregiver role strain, Adult failure to thrive*, and *Powerlessness*.

Successful long-term outcomes include the following:
1. Physical, emotional, sexual abuse has ceased.
2. Neglect or financial exploitation has ceased.
3. Plans are in place to maintain safety.

Most hospitals and community centers have protocols that offer guidelines for nurses and other health care workers for suspected elder abuse. Immediate physical safety is always the first concern. Each state has its own protocols, but they all provide guidance to health care workers in case of suspected elder abuse. However, not all the needs of a particular older adult may be met through the protocols. Once abuse is suspected, referral to APS is appropriate.

There are a number of services APS can offer to address issues of patient neglect, abuse, and other mistreatment. These services are voluntary, and the patient has the right to accept or decline them. According to Dyer and colleagues, APS interventions include the following:

- Arranging for housing services (e.g., emergency housing, repairs, modification for disabilities)
- Obtaining medical services
- Addressing personal needs (e.g., food delivery, food stamps, caretaker services)
- Providing service coordination (case manager, referrals to appropriate service groups)
- Serving as patient advocate
- Implementing legal interventions

IMPLEMENTATION

Interventions include providing medical services, legal intervention, and involving social services. Table 18-5 includes interventions for suspected elder abuse.

TABLE 18-5	Interventions for Suspected Elder Abuse

Intervention	Rationale
1. Check your state for laws regarding elder abuse.	1. All states have adopted laws to help protect elders and support their needs for safety.
2. Involve Adult Protective Services (APS) if abuse is suspected.	2. APS can offer many sources to help guard the safety and well-being of abused elders.
3. Meet with other family members and others to identify stressors and problem areas.	3. Other family members might not be aware of the strain the abuser is under or the lack of safety to the abused family member.
4. If there are no other family members, notify other community agencies that might help abuser and elder stabilize situation, for example: • Support group for elder • Support group for abuser • Meals on Wheels • Day care for seniors • Respite services • Visiting nurse services	4. Minimizes family stress and isolation, and increases safety.
5. Encourage abuser's use of counseling.	5. Increases coping skills and social supports.
6. Suggest that family members meet together on a regular basis for problem solving and support.	6. Encourages family to learn and solve problems together.

EVALUATION

Failures in interventions with abusive families often are related to personal deficits but to deficits in the social, economic, and political systems in which we all live. A very real problem is that of social exclusion "by which multidimensionally disadvantaged individuals are prohibited from obtaining formal helping services" (Hilbert & Krishnan, 2000). Nurses can direct interventions to the social environment and can question, among other things, the acceptance of corporal punishment as a technique for guiding behavior in children, the unequal burden of caregiving responsibilities placed on women, the low priority given to education and preparation for parenthood, and the belief that one has little social value if one is older.

Evaluation of interventions (IPV, child, elder) can be based on whether the survivor acknowledges the violence, is willing to accept intervention, or is removed from the violent situation. With more long-term interventions, evaluation should be made by all members of the health care team on an ongoing basis. Because violence is a symptom of a family in distress, diagnosis, interventions, and evaluation should ideally be carried out by a multidisciplinary team that includes a physician, a nurse, a social worker, an attorney, and perhaps a psychiatrist. Follow-up is crucial in helping decrease the frequency of family violence.

KEY POINTS TO REMEMBER

- Physical and emotional trauma cause long-lasting and devastating damage to people's lives, and is often passed down to future generations.
- The actual incidence of child or partner and elder abuse is unknown, but current statistics most likely represent the tip of the iceberg.
- All states have mandatory guidelines for reporting child abuse and elder abuse. Individuals involved in IPV can be given guidelines for reporting and legal help, but reporting is their decision to make.

- Guidelines for "what to do" and "what not to do" when interviewing a child suspected of abuse are included.
- Characteristics of the parent or caregiver who abuse their child are outlined.
- Characteristics of a violent partner and caregiver to abused elder are discussed.
- Abuse never just goes away; it usually escalates over time and in intensity, and for victims of IPV the cycle of violence is a classic phenomenon.

KEY POINTS TO REMEMBER—cont'd

- Forensic examination of a child and for abusive partners (IPV) is outlined, and the responsibility of the nurse, clinician, or physician is described.
- Nursing diagnoses and long-term outcomes are similar in all abuse cases, although each individual has unique needs.

- Guidelines for nursing interventions for child, partner, and elder abuse in each section of this chapter have been outlined.

CRITICAL THINKING

1. Six-year-old Sammy is rushed to the ED by a neighbor who found him wandering in the street in only a dirty undershirt, seemingly dazed. He is covered in what appears to be cigarette burns, is cachectic, and has bruises on his wrists and ankles. He appears fearful, confused, and does not respond to questioning except to say, "I hurt. I don't feel good."
    A. What is your first priority?
    B. Write documentation following forensic nursing guidelines (draw a map and describe physical behaviors and verbatim comments).

C. What else could you do to document his injuries?
D. What other evidence might you and the health team gather?
E. Role-play with a classmate what you would say when reporting Sammy's situation to Child Protective Services.

CHAPTER REVIEW

Choose the most appropriate answer.

1. When nurses provide health teaching about how to recognize behaviors and situations that might trigger violence in families, they are engaging in:
    1. primary prevention.
    2. secondary prevention.
    3. tertiary prevention.
    4. nonintervention.
2. When treating a woman who has been trapped in an abusive marriage for many years, which statement would a nurse expect not to hear?
    1. "If I'm patient, he'll change."
    2. "I deserve to be beaten."
    3. "I'll stay for the sake of the children."
    4. "No adult has the right to control or harm another."
3. When making assessments the nurse should bear in mind that a common characteristic of an abusing parent is:
    1. being female.
    2. having poor coping skills.
    3. having realistic expectations of child behavior.

4. abstaining from use of chemical substances of abuse.
4. During a nursing assessment, which of the following is a "red flag" for suspecting that a patient has been a victim of physical violence?
    1. Patient's explanation does not match the injury.
    2. Patient has no history of stress-related physical problems.
    3. Patient mentions having a concerned, supportive spouse.
    4. Patient is anxious but open and direct in explaining the complaint or injury.
5. Which of the following nursing diagnoses is most appropriate for the Jones family? The husband is disabled, unable to work, drinks episodically, and abuses his two preschool-age children when drinking. The wife works outside the home.
    1. *Powerlessness*
    2. *Caregiver role strain*
    3. *Low self-esteem*
    4. *Disabled family coping*

REFERENCES

Agency for Healthcare Research and Quality (AHRQ). (2002). *Evaluating domestic violence programs.* Retrieved February 3, 2007, from www.AHRQ.gov/research/domesticviol.
Asians Against Domestic Abuse (AADA). (2004). *National statistics.* Retrieved January 28, 2007, from www.aadainc.org/Statistics.htm.

Barak, G. (2003). *Violence and nonviolence: Pathways to understanding.* Thousand Oaks, CA: Sage.
Bartol, C.R., Bartol, A.M., and Bartol, A. (2004). *Criminal behavior: A psychosocial approach.* Upper Saddle River, N.J.: Prentice Hall.

Bethea, L. (1999). Primary prevention of child abuse. *American Family Physician*, *59*(6).

Department of Health and Human Services (DHHS). (2007). Administration on Aging Fact sheet: Elder abuse and prevention: Elder abuse is a serious problem. Retrieved April 8, 2008 from http://www.aoa.gov/press/fact/alpha/fact_elder_abuse.asp.

Dollard, J., Doob, L., Miller, N., et al. (1939). *Frustration and aggression*. New Haven, CT: Yale University Press.

Dyer, C.B., Heisler, C.J., Hill, C.A., & Kim, L.C. (2005). Community approaches to elder abuse. *Clinics in Geriatric Medicine*, *21*(2), 429-447.

Elder Abuse Unit. (2005). Division of Criminal Justice: Office of the Chief State's Attorney, Rocky Hill, CT. Retrieved January 25, 2007, from www.ct.gov/csao/cwp/view.asp?a=1798&q=285768.

Feldhaus, K.M., Koziol-McLain, J., Amsbury, H.L., et al. Accuracy of 3 brief screening questions for detecting partner violence in the emergency department (1997). *Journal of the American Medical Association*, *277*, 1357-1361.

General Assembly United Nations (1994). Declaration of the elimination of violence against women (resolution 48/104). Retrieved February 3, 2007, http://daccessdds.un.org/doc/UNDOC/GEN/N94/095/05/PDF/N9409505.pdf.

Goodman, P.E. (2006). The relationship between intimate partner violence and other forms of family and societal violence. *Emergency Medicine Clinics of North America*, *24*(4), 889-903.

Gorbien, M.J. (2005). Elder abuse and neglect. *Clinics in Geriatric Medicine*, *21*(2), 279-292.

Halpern, C.T., Young, M.L., Waller, M.W., et al. (2004). Prevalence of partner violence in same-sex romantic and sexual relationships in a national sample of adolescents. *Journal of Adolescent Health*, *35*(2), 124-131.

Hilbert, J.C., & Krishnan, S.P. (2000). Addressing barriers to community care of battered women in rural environments: Creating a policy of social inclusion. *Journal of Health Social Policy*, *12*(1), 41-52.

International Council of Nurses Fact Sheet. *Elder abuse*. Retrieved February 10, 2007, from www.icn.ch/matters_elder.htm.

Mayo Clinic Staff (2006). *Domestic violence toward women: Recognize the patterns and seek help*. Retrieved February 1, 2007, from www.mayoclinic.com/health/domestic-violence/wO00044.

Minnesota Advocates for Human Rights (MAHR): *Stop violence against women: Evolution of theories of violence*. (2006). Retrieved August 14, 2007, from www.stopvaw.org/Evolution_of_Theories_of_Violence.html.

National Clearinghouse on Family Violence (NCFV). (2005). *Fact sheet on family violence and substance abuse*. Retrieved August 13, 2007, from http://phac-aspc.gc.ca/ncfv-cnivf/familyviolence/html/fvsubstance_e.html.

Quinn, K., & Zielke, H. (2005). Elder abuse, neglect, and exploitation: Policy issues. *Clinics in Geriatric Medicine*, *21*(2), 449-457.

Sadock, B.J., & Sadock, V.A. (2007). *Kaplan & Sadock's synopsis of psychiatry: Behavioral sciences/clinical psychiatry* (10th ed.). Philadelphia: Lippincott Williams & Wilkins.

Shore, R. (1997). *Rethinking the brain: New insights into early development*. New York: Families and Work Institute.

Skowron, E.A., & Reineman, D.H.S. (2005). Psychological interventions for child maltreatment. *Psychotherapy: Theory Research, Practice, and Training*, *42*, 52-71.

U.S. Department of Health and Human Services (USDHHS). (2005). Administration on Children Youth, and Families (ACF). *Child maltreatment 2003*. Washington, DC: Government printing office. Retrieved April 5, 2007, from www.acf.hhs.gov/programs/cb/pubs/cm03/index.htm.

U.S. Department of Health and Human Services (USDHHS). (2006). Administration on Children, Youth, and Families (ACF). *Child multreatment 2004*. Washington, DC: Government Printing Office. Retrieved February 10, 2007.

Walker, L. (1979). *The battered woman*. New York: Harper & Row.

Wood, E.F. (2006) *The availability and utility of interdisciplinary data on elder abuse: A white paper for the national center on elder abuse*. American Bar Association Commission on Law and Aging for the National Center on Elder Abuse, Washington D.C., April 2006.

World Health Organization (2002). ACTVCAGING. A policy statement. Geneva, Switzerland.

CHAPTER 19

Sexual Assault

Elizabeth M. Varcarolis

Key Terms and Concepts

acquaintance rape, p. 400
date rape, p. 400
date rape drug, p. 403
forensic evidence, p. 400
institutional protocol, p. 402

marital rape, p. 400
rape kits, p. 402
rape-trauma syndrome, p. 403

Objectives

1. Identify vulnerabilities that might be risk factors for sexual assault.
2. Summarize the characteristics of a perpetrator of sexual assault.
3. Summarize the types of data collected in the forensic component of the assessment that may be used as criminal evidence in court.
4. State the guidelines for emergency treatment of a woman who has been sexually assaulted according to the Centers for Disease Control and Prevention and the American College of Obstetrics and Gynecology.
5. Relate the symptoms of posttraumatic stress disorder to rape-trauma syndrome.
6. Discuss the kinds of community supports that can be offered to the assaulted patient.
7. Identify the most important aspects of care for a sexually abused patient. Be specific.

evolve

For additional resources related to the content of this chapter, visit the Evolve website at http://evolve.elsevier.com/Varcarolis/essentials.

- Chapter Outline
- Chapter Review Answers
- Case Study

- Nursing Care Plan
- Nurse, Patient, and Family Resources
- Concept Map Creator

Sexual assault is an act of violence not sex, and most often results in devastating severe and long-term trauma. It is often committed in context of unequal power in order to demonstrate dominance and control. Legal definitions of rape vary by state, but in general sexual assault includes the use of force or any nonconsensual contact involving the breasts, genitals, or anus with or without penetration. Sexual assault is an umbrella term encompassing the crimes of rape, **date rape**, **acquaintance rape**, **marital rape**, within partner relationships (intimate partner violence [IPV]), molestation or incest, and sexual assault of older adults (Blackwood, 2005). Rape is a legal term rather than a medical diagnosis. Rape should be considered a criminal act with wide-ranging medical, psychological, legal, and social sequelae (Viguera & Mian, 2004).

Presently, there is no mandated reporting for crimes of sexual assault unless it involves abuse of a minor or an elder. It is up to the survivors of the assault to make the decision to report the crime. It is up to health care workers to offer support, information on obtaining legal counsel, and—with the patient's permission—securing **forensic evidence** (evidence that can be used in court) for future prosecution.

PREVALENCE AND COMORBIDITY

Sexual assault is usually committed by men against women, but it can be committed by women against men or between people of the same gender. The majority of perpetrators are male; however, women also sexually assault men. Women can force men to have sex, particularly if the male is younger and more vulnerable, and often through blackmail. Women also sexually assault other women, although the statistics are difficult to ascertain.

According to the National Crime Survivorization Survey (2003), 1 in every 10 rape survivors are male. Gay men are victims of sexual assault slightly more often than heterosexual men, especially if they are the target of hate crimes. However, heterosexual men are raped in very large numbers. The vast majority of men who are sexually assaulted are assaulted by men who consider themselves heterosexual (which is in keeping with the understanding that rape is a crime of violence and control) (Starman, 2006). Although a great percentage of male rapes take place in prisons, male rape also happens in the military, colleges, universities, work, or in the home.

Sexual assault is one of the most underreported crimes. The available data greatly underestimate the true magnitude of this crime. Findings from the National Violence Against Women Survey 2005 (NVAWS) found that only one in five adult women reported rapes to the police (Tjaden & Thoennes, 2006). Because male sexual assault survivors do not generally seek medical or legal help, the incidence of male rape is unknown (Viguera & Mian, 2004). One of the reasons for massive underreporting of sexual assault to the police is thought to be because of fear of retaliation. This fear is best understood when we realize that 73% of sexual assaults are committed by a nonstranger (38% by a friend, 28% intimates, and 7% another relative) (National Crime and Victim Survey 2005). Other reasons include the survivor's embarrassment, shame, and feelings of discomfort and mistrust toward the official(s) to whom the assault is reported.

In intimate partner violence (IPV), sexual abuse may be part of the picture. It has been reported that more than 50% of gay men and lesbians reported at least one incidence of coercion by a same-sex partner. Gay and lesbian sexual survivors may not come forward for fear of facing homophobia and prejudice as well as making their personal lives more public (DC Rape Crisis Center, Washington, DC).

People who are raped suffer severe, deep, and emotional scars that may stay with them the rest of their lives. Beyond the physical trauma such as risk of sexually transmitted disease (STD), human immunodeficiency virus (HIV), or pregnancy, psychological sequelae often develop. Common long-term psychological traumas include depression, suicide, anxiety, difficulties with daily functioning, low self-esteem, eating disorders, self-destructive behaviors, and substance abuse disorders. Although the risk exists for both male and female rape survivors, male rape survivors are more likely to commit suicide and contact acquired immunodeficiency disease syndrome (AIDS) through anal tears than are women (Starman, 2006). Timely and age-appropriate interventions can greatly help mitigate the devastating psychological sequelae.

evolve

For a comprehensive case study and a nursing care plan for a patient who has been a victim of rape, visit the Evolve website at http://evolve.elsevier.com/Varcarolis/essentials.

CULTURAL CONSIDERATIONS

Cultural and societal factors play a part in forming attitudes, for example, cultural and societal norms that maintain women's inferiority and support male superiority and sexual entitlement. In such groups, often weak laws and policies related to gender equity, and high tolerance for crimes of violence coexist. Some college fraternities reflect needed societal context that could encourage violence toward

EXAMINING THE EVIDENCE   Counteracting the Oldest Date Rape Drug

I'm working with a 19-year-old female college student on the psychiatric unit who is terribly depressed. She went on a date with an older guy, who encouraged her to drink. Although the details of what happened that evening are a blur, she does remember kissing, then telling him she wouldn't go any further, and being raped. She feels guilty for letting this happen and terrified that it could happen again.

Your patient experienced acquaintance rape, a disturbingly common and underreported college and university problem, one made far worse by alcohol. In fact, alcohol may be the most common "date-rape" drug. Researchers in Ireland report that alleged sexual assault victims had blood alcohol levels exceeding the drunk driving limit by three times and that not a trace of the classic drink-spiking drugs—Rohypnol, GHB, or ketamine—was found in victims in the study (University of Ulster, 2007).

According to Abbey (2002) nearly half of all sexual assaults involve alcohol consumption on the part of the victim, the perpetrator, or both. There is little doubt that drinking places potential victims at increased risk, especially with people who they don't know well (Davis et al., 2004). From the standpoint of the victim, alcohol can impair a person's ability to perceive danger and resist effectively. From the standpoint of the perpetrator, alcohol may lead to a misperception that the other is interested in sexual advances and increases the likelihood of

aggressive behavior (Abbey et al., 2001). Is drunkenness an excuse for committing rape? In one study, college-age perpetrators didn't view themselves as real criminals, but rather blamed alcohol for their behavior (Abbey, 1991).

Nasta and associates (2005) indicate that once an assault occurs victims are either unaware of reporting mechanisms or are reluctant to do so, and found that only 4% report the incident to university safety services. Colleges and universities are beginning to offer assault prevention programs and are reporting a decrease in victimization for most students (Rotherman & Silverman, 2007). One of the simplest, most effective, and empowering prevention methods is learning self-defense (Sochting et al., 2004). Researchers have also examined a complementary strategy; a prevention/education program aimed at males that promotes empathy; one particularly effective empathy-producing method is accomplished by describing male-on-male rape (Foubert & Newberry, 2006).

In a culture that ostensibly supports the rights of women, your patient was a victim of a too-common and unacceptable crime. This crime may have even opened old scars. She will benefit from listening, acceptance, education, and possibly considering pressing charges. Carefully interviewing her to assess whether she has experienced other trauma may be a first step to deal with possible stress-related disorders such as anxiety or even posttraumatic stress disorder.

Abbey, A. (1991). Acquaintance rape and alcohol consumption on college campuses. *Journal of American College Health, 39*(1).

Abbey, A. (2002). Alcohol-related sexual assault: A common problem among college students. *Journal of Studies on Alcohol*, (Suppl)*14*, 118-128.

Abbey, A., Zawacki, T., Buck, P.O., et al. (2001). Alcohol and sexual assault. *Alcohol Health and Research World, 25*(1).

Davis, K.C., George, W.H., & Norris, J. (2004) Women's responses to unwanted sexual advances: The role of alcohol and inhibition conflict. *Psychology of Women Quarterly, 28*, 3330-3343.

Foubert, J.D., & Newberry, J.T. (2006). Effects of two versions of an empathy-based rape prevention program on fraternity men's survivor empathy, attitudes, and behavioral intent to commit rape or sexual assault. *Journal of College Student Development, 47*(2), 133-148.

Nasta, A., Shah, B., Brahmanandam, S., et al. (2005). Sexual victimization: Incidence, knowledge, and resource use among a population of college women. *Journal of Pediatric Adolescent Gynecology, 18*(2), 91-96.

Rotherman, E., & Silverman, J. (2007). The effect of a college sexual assault prevention program on first-year students' victimization rates. *Journal of American College Health, 55*(5), 283-290.

Sochting, I., Fairbrother, N., & Koch, W.J. (2004). Sexual assault of women: Prevention efforts and risk factors. *Violence Against Women, 10*(1), 73-93.

University of Ulster. (2007). *Alcohol is most common "date rape" drug.* Retrieved December 18, 2007, from www.sciencedaily.com/releases/2007/10/071020113144.htm.

women, and sexual assault on campus appears to be increasing. The military is another societal group in which sexual assaults of women resulting from gender inequality along with norms that support masculine dominance have become a concern, and changes within military policy have been made. In order to affect substantial change, there needs to be strong enforceable laws in place and recognition that rape is a punishable crime and the perpetrator will be punished.

THEORY
The Person Vulnerable to Sexual Assault

Sexual assault occurs within all age-groups, genders, cultures, and socioeconomic backgrounds, but some groups appear more vulnerable, and some situations are more conducive to sexual assault. For example, a 2000 study by Fisher and associates concluded that between one in four and one in six women experienced completed or attempted rape during their college years. Other vulnerability factors associated with sexual assault include the following:

- **Gender:** 78% of rapes are of women, 22% men.
- **Age:** More than half of all rapes of women (54%) occur before age 12. For men, 48% of rapes occur before age 12 and 75% before age 18. Hopper (2007) estimates that one in six boys is sexually abused before the age of 16.
- **Older adults:** Domestic violence against older adults includes physical and sexual abuse most often by adult children, most often the sons (Quinn & Zielke 2005).
- When an older adult is cognitively or functionally impaired, the likelihood of being sexually assaulted increases (Blackwood, 2005).
- **History of sexual violence:** Tjaden and Thoennes (2000) found that women who are raped before the age of 18 are twice as likely to be raped as adults.
- **Drug and alcohol use:** Use of alcohol or drugs by the perpetrator, the victim, or both is related to increased rates of victimization.
- **High-risk sexual behaviors:** High-risk sexual behavior is a vulnerability that is often a consequence of childhood sexual abuse.
- **Poverty:** Poverty can make women and children more vulnerable and place them in more dangerous situations. Poor women may be at risk when they need to support themselves or their children and trade sex for food, clothing, money, or other necessary items.
- **Ethnicity or Culture:** American Indian and Alaskan Native women are more likely (34%) to report being raped than African American women (19%), white women (18%), or Hispanic women (15%) (Tjaden & Thoennes, 2000).

The Perpetrator of Sexual Assault

The causes of violence toward women are multifaceted and involve biological, psychological, and social factors.

Biological Factors

From a *biological* perspective, neurophysiological factors may be a risk factor in violent behavior. Alterations in the functioning of neurotransmitters, such as serotonin, dopamine, norepinepthrine, acetylcholine, and γ-aminobutyric acid, may interfere with cognition and behavior (Chapter 21).

Psychosocial Factors

From a *psychosocial* standpoint, studies have found a high incidence of psychopathology and personality disorders among sexual offenders. Antisocial personality, in which people are viewed as objects, is one of the most prevalent. The act involves a need for control, power, degradation, and dominance over others rather than sexual satisfaction. It is thought that some sexual offenders have difficulty finding willing sexual partners and resort to coercion or rape.

Many characteristics of a perpetrator of sexual assault are the same as the perpetrator in child abuse, IPV, and elder abuse (Chapter 18). Not surprisingly, most perpetrators of sexual abuse report being sexually assaulted as children. Some other characteristics include:

- Impulsive and antisocial tendencies
- Association with sexually aggressive and delinquent peers
- Preference for impersonal sex
- Hostility toward women
- Childhood history of sexual and physical abuse, or witness of family violence as a child
- Membership in a gang

Application of the Nursing Process
ASSESSMENT

When an individual who has been sexually assaulted seeks treatment, he or she is most likely seen in the emergency department (ED). People who have been sexually assaulted often go to the ED to find emotional support, help in regaining a sense of control, and reassurance regarding their safety (Viguera & Mian, 2004). A sexual assault survivor who arrives at the ED should not be left alone. The staff should provide privacy, and the victim should be a priority in triage.

The nature of sexual assault carries with it complex implications, and the individual requires medical care, collection of specimens for use as forensic evidence, and psychological support. Often the physical examination and the collection of evidence are performed by a gynecologist or an ED attending. However, sexual assault nurse examiner (SANE) programs are established in many parts of the country; in these programs, certified nurses provide forensic evidence collection and expertise (Viguera & Mian, 2004). Most hospitals have an **institutional protocol** for evidence collection and use **"rape kits."** Correct preservation of body fluids and swabs is essential because DNA (deoxyribonucleic acid; genetic mapping) can help identify the rapist.

The individual has the right to refuse legal and medical examination. Therefore *consent forms must be signed* in order to take photographs, perform a pelvic examination, and carry out whatever other procedures might be needed to collect evidence and provide treatment. The victim needs to know that all documentation is confidential, and that no one can access the information without permission, unless the case goes to court.

Viguera and Mian (2004) caution against the use of pejorative language when documenting the history, findings, and verbatim statements. For example:

- Instead of alleged, use *reported*
- Instead of refused, use *declined*
- Instead of intercourse, use *penetration*
- Instead of in no acute distress, *describe the behavior*

After the immediate medical issues of the patient have been taken care of, it is important to perform as many elements of the *forensic examinations* the individual allows. Once the evidence is collected, it is imperative that providers maintain a "chain of custody" until it is turned over to the authorities.

Assessment Guidelines

Sexual Assault

1. Assess and document the circumstances of the event, including presence of threats (force, trauma, weapons, resistance, sexual acts), where it took place, and circumstances surrounding the assault. *Document in patient's own words* when possible.
2. Gather data that may be used as criminal evidence in court using the institution's protocol.
3. After consent forms have been signed, forensic evidence (debris) should be obtained from clothing, fingernail scrapings, head, hair, and pubic hair; smears for sperm and/or acid phosphatase should be taken from any orifice involved. Permission for any photographs taken during the assessment also needs to be obtained. Numbers 3, 4, 5, 6, 7, and 8 are all considered forensic evidence and can be used in court at a later date.
4. Assess for evidence of any physical trauma (e.g., bites, stab wounds, contusions, gunshot or stab wounds). Use drawings and photos.
5. Perform pelvic exam to identify vaginal and cervical trauma (anal exam for males). Culture for STDs.
6. Perform psychological assessment noting reactions to the rape event (e.g., crying, fearfulness, agitation, preoccupation). Describe all behavior in writing.
7. Perform a mental status examination.
8. Determine drug use by either assailant or survivor. Assess situation for potential involvement of **"date rape drug"** if it occurred in a large gathering (e.g., college campus, bar, etc.). If not too much time has passed, a urine sample might be useful. Emphasize to individuals that even if they were drinking, they are *not* at fault for being assaulted. (See Table 19-1 for drugs associated with sexual assault.)

9. Identify the survivor's support system (family and friends), and ask for permission to involve them. Explain possible delayed reactions that might occur.

DIAGNOSIS

Rape-Trauma Syndrome

The nursing diagnosis *Rape-trauma syndrome* is a variant of posttraumatic stress disorder (PTSD) and is common sequela of psychological trauma. Left untreated, psychologically traumatic events can have devastating effects. Nearly 70% of people who have been sexually assaulted develop PTSD (Blackwood, 2005). PTSD, depression, panic disorder, suicidal ideation and attempts, and substance abuse are high among survivors of sexual assault.

There are two phases of **rape-trauma syndrome**. The acute phase begins immediately after the crisis, followed by the long-term phase, which may occur as long as 2 weeks after the rape and may last years if untreated. *Rape-trauma syndrome: compound reaction* is also a likely diagnosis and includes both the acute phase of disorganization and the long-term recovery phase. Unfortunately, some people with PTSD (as a result of rape or other trauma) never fully resolve or recover from devastating traumatic events.

The Acute Phase

Typical reactions to crisis often reflect cognitive, affective, and behavioral disruptions. The most common responses are shock, numbness, and disbelief. A person may appear self-contained and calm. At other times, cognitive function may be impaired, and the person may have difficulty making decisions, solving problems, or concentrating. Or the person may cry, become hysterical, be restless, or even smile.

The Long-Term Phase

It is important to let victims know what to expect during this phase so they will be prepared. It is also important to understand that all assault survivors will deal with the event in their own manner. Common symptoms of PTSD related to sexual assault include the following (RAINN 2006a):

- **Re-Experiencing the Trauma:** Recurrent nightmares about the rape, flashbacks, or uninvited, intrusive thoughts day or night
- **Social Withdrawal:** Called "psychic numbing" and involves not experiencing feelings of any kind
- **Avoidance Behaviors and Actions:** Avoidance of all places and activities, as well as thoughts or feelings, that could recall events about the rape
- **Increased Psychological Arousal Characteristics:** Exaggerated startle response, hypervigilance, sleep disorders, or difficulty concentrating

TABLE 19-1	**Drugs Associated with Sexual Assault**	
Mechanism of Action	**Effect**	**Additional Information**
GHB (γ-hydroxybutyric acid) (liquid ecstasy, salty water, scoop)		
Central nervous system depressant	Onset is within 5 to 20 minutes; duration is dose related and is from 1 to 2 hours. Produces euphoria, amnesia, hypotonia, and depressed respiration. Can also cause seizures, unconsciousness, nausea, and vomiting, coma and death.	Causes respiratory depression, coma, and death. GHB leaves the body in 12 hours. Used to treat narcolepsy.
Rohypnol (flunitrazepam) ("forget" drug; also roofies, club drug, roachies, and rophies)		
Potent benzodiazepine; 10 times stronger than diazepam	Impact is within 10 to 30 minutes and lasts 2 to 12 hours; becomes more potent when combined with alcohol; causes dizziness, amnesia, lack of motor coordination, confusion, nausea and vomiting, respiratory depression, and blackout episodes lasting 8 to 24 hours.	Not legal in the United States. Detected in urine for up to 72 hours
Ketamine (special K, K, vitamin K, bump, kitkat, purple, super C)		
Anesthetic frequently used in veterinary practice; also a hallucinogenic substance related to PCP (phencyclidine)	Onset is rapid, 20 minutes orally; duration is only 30 to 60 minutes; amnesia effects may last longer; usually administered as a powder that is snorted, smoked, injected, or dissolved in drinks. Causes dissociative reaction with a dreamlike state leading to deep amnesia and analgesia and complete compliance of the survivor. Later, survivor may be confused, paranoid, delirious, combative, with drooling and hallucinations.	

Adapted from Lynch, J.S. (2003). *Date rape and drug-assisted rape: Clinical implications.* Paper presented at the National Association of Nurse Practitioners in Women's Health 6th Annual Conference, October 15-18, 2003, Savannah, GA.

* **Fears and phobias:** Fear of being alone, fear of sexual encounters, fear of the indoors or outdoors, etc.

OUTCOMES IDENTIFICATION

Short-Term Goals

The patient will:

* Have a short-term plan for handling immediate situational needs before leaving the ED.
* Have a written list of common physical, social, and emotional reactions that may follow a sexual assault before leaving the ED.
* State the results of the physical examination completed in the ED.
* Have written access to information on obtaining competent legal counsel and community supports (individual or group) before leaving the ED.
* Have a follow-up appointment with a rape counselor or crisis counselor.
* Have support from family and friends.

Long-Term Goals

The hoped for outcome is that the person eventually will be able to:

* Return to precrisis level of functioning without any residual symptoms.
* Experience hopefulness and confidence in going ahead with life plans.

IMPLEMENTATION

Follow the sexual assault protocol provided in your ED procedure manual. The nurse should approach the person who has been sexually assaulted in a nonjudgmental and empathic manner. Patients need to hear and understand that the rape is *not their* fault, and confidentiality should be stressed repeatedly. It is important to help survivors and their significant others separate the issues of vulnerability from blame. Although individuals may have made choices that made them more vulnerable to assault, they are **not** to

APPLYING THE ART   A Person Experiencing Sexual Assault

SCENARIO: A neighbor brought 40-year-old Margaret to the ED following her report of a sexual assault by a 20-something male who gained access to Margaret's home by claiming the need to make a phone call because of car trouble. The ED staff bustled about caring for many acute patients. My student status enabled me to provide continuity of care so Margaret never needed to be left alone despite the coming and going of staff. I established the contact, struggling to hear Margaret, who spoke in a whisper.

THERAPEUTIC GOAL: By the close of this interaction, Margaret will allow herself to acknowledge her survival and to express her concerns.

Student-Patient Interaction	Thoughts, Communication Techniques, and Mental Health Nursing Concepts
Margaret: *Voice tense.* "I don't want to be alone. Not now. Not ever." **Student's feelings**: *I would be afraid to be alone, too, if someone attacked me in my own home. But why did she trust a stranger? I struggle with countertransference. I have to be alert to not blame the victim as a way to distance myself; if I make this Margaret's fault, then rape cannot happen to me.*	Margaret started our interaction with a whisper, which makes me think she may be reacting with the *controlled style* in this *acute phase of the rape-trauma syndrome*. Yet, her tense assertion of not wanting to be alone may indicate the *expressed style*.
Student: "I am staying right here with you. You've been through a terrible ordeal."	I *offer self* and *attempt to translate into feelings*.
Margaret: "I feel so ashamed."	Earlier Margaret asked for water and I had to say no until all the evidence is collected. I'm staying alert and especially careful to follow the rape-crisis protocol for this ED for Margaret's sake and for any legal ramifications.
Student: "What happened was not your fault. You don't have anything to be ashamed of." **Student's feelings:** *Without thinking, I immediately reassured Margaret that she has no reason to be ashamed. Even as I speak the words, I notice Margaret pulling away. I wonder now, if I wasn't really reassuring myself.*	Reassurance seems supportive but actually discounts the patient's feelings. Margaret feels more alone now.
Margaret: "You don't understand. No one does." *Looking downward.*	
Student: "You're right. I don't understand what you went through. Margaret, I care about what happened you and I want to understand." **Student's feelings:** *I do care about Margaret.*	I offer self and give control to Margaret, acknowledging that only she knows her experience.
Margaret: "I don't know how I will ever tell my husband." *Eyes swell with tears, which she angrily brushes away, then proceeds to rub her temples.*	
Student: "You feel worried about his reaction."	I *attempt to translate into feelings* by saying "worried." I assess Margaret's *anxiety* to be at least *moderate*. *Physical signs* arise at the *severe level* and Margaret is now rubbing her temples, as though she has a headache. Though she didn't report a headache at the intake assessment, Margaret's stress and anxiety may be stimulating additional physiological responses.

Continued

APPLYING THE ART   A Person Experiencing Sexual Assault—cont'd

Student-Patient Interaction	Thoughts, Communication Techniques, and Mental Health Nursing Concepts
Margaret: "Why would he even want to be with me—damaged goods."	
Student: "You feel damaged, unlovable." ***Student's feelings:*** *I feel sad that she has the added burden of dealing with the reactions of loved ones who might not be supportive.*	I use *restatement* and *attempt to translate into feelings*.
Margaret: "Unlovable." *Eyes again fill with tears. Margaret presses her fists against her eyelids.*	
Student: "Margaret, it's okay to cry." *Margaret shakes her head.*	I give permission to lend *support* and *acceptance*.
Student: "I wonder what it would mean to you to cry."	I ask an *indirect question* to assess underlying dynamics.
Margaret: *Breathing deeply to suppress tears.* "That I am a weak woman, so weak I couldn't stop that monster." ***Student's feelings:*** It's kind of scary. This could be me at another time.	She uses the word "monster." It must have been such a horrible violation of her personhood.
Student: "You had the strength to stay alive. You did what you had to do to survive. Your instincts acted properly to keep you alive."	I give *support* affirming that Margaret was, in fact, able to stay alive. She survived the assault.
Margaret: "I am alive. Damaged, but alive." *Eyes water.*	
Student: "You look close to tears." *She nods.* "It's okay to grieve, to let your feelings out."	I *make an observation*. Sharing the pain and allowing the *grief* decrease the intensity of the pain.
Margaret: *Sobs, accepts a tissue and holds on to my hand.* ***Student's feelings:*** *I feel Margaret's trust that she reaches for my hand.*	Just then the rape-crisis counselor and sexual assault nurse examiner arrive.

blame for the rape. See Table 19-2 for a list of interventions to be used for the victim of sexual assault.

Pharmacological, Biological, and Integrative Therapies
Emergency Department

Treatment of the survivor should address physical injuries, pregnancy prophylaxis, and sexually transmitted diseases. Common examples of physical injuries may be abrasions or contusions. More serious injuries might include broken bones, knife wounds, and injuries around the eyes, nose, and abdomen. The most common injuries are to the face, head, neck, and extremities.

According to the 2005 National Crime Victimization Study, 5% of rapes resulted in pregnancy for a one-time unprotected sexual assault (RAINN, 2006). The American College of Obstetricians and Gynecologists recommends offering emergency contraception to all women who have been assaulted or are at risk of pregnancy (ACOG, 2004). Even if a woman chooses not to take the medication for personal reasons, treatment should be available.

The Centers for Disease Control and Prevention (CDC) recommend prophylactic STD treatment for the most

TABLE 19-2   Interventions for Sexual Assault

Intervention	Rationale
1. Have someone stay with the patient (friend, neighbor, or staff member) while he or she is waiting to be treated in the ED.	1. People in high levels of anxiety need someone with them until anxiety level is down to moderate. **Never leave the patient alone.**
2. **Very important:** Approach patient in a nonjudgmental manner.	2. Nurses' attitudes can have an important therapeutic effect. Displays of shock, horror, disgust, or disbelief can increase anxiety and shame.
3. **Confidentiality is crucial.**	3. The patient's situation is not to be discussed with anyone other than medical personnel involved unless patient gives consent.
4. Explain to the patient the signs and symptoms that many people experience during the long-term phase, for example: a. Nightmares b. Phobias c. Anxiety, depression d. Insomnia e. Somatic symptoms	4. Many individuals think they are going crazy as time goes on and are not aware that this is a process that many people in their situation have experienced.
5. Listen and let the patient talk. **Do not** press the patient to talk.	5. When people feel understood, they feel more in control of their situation.
6. Stress that the patient did the right thing to save his or her life.	6. Rape survivors might feel guilt or shame. Reinforcing that they did what they had to do to stay alive can reduce guilt and maintain self-esteem.
7. **Do not** use judgmental language (Viguera & Mian, 2004): • Reported *not* alleged • Declined *not* refused • Penetration *not* intercourse • Instead of reporting "no acute distress," describe the behavior.	7. Pejorative terms often reflect old myths and a lack of knowledge and understanding regarding the rape victim's experience and need for immediate intervention. Words like "alleged," "refused," and "intercourse" all minimize the devastation of the event.

Forensic Examination and Issues

1. Assess the signs and symptoms of physical trauma.	1. Most common injuries are to face, head, neck, extremities.
2. **Explain and get permission from patient to take photos and specimens.**	2. Patient's consent is needed to collect and document evidence which may be later used in court.
3. Make a body map to identify size, color, and location of injuries. Ask permission to take photos.	3. Accurate records and photos can be used as legal evidence for the future.
4. Carefully explain all procedures before doing them (e.g., "We would like to do a vaginal [rectal] examination and do a swab. Have you had a vaginal [rectal] examination before?").	4. The individual is experiencing high levels of anxiety. Matter-of-factly explaining what you plan to do and why you are doing it can help reduce fear and anxiety.
5. Explain the forensic specimens you plan to collect; inform patient that they can be used for identification and prosecution of the rapist, for example: • Debris in hair and pubic hair • Skin from underneath nails • Semen samples • Blood	5. Collecting body fluids and swabs is essential (DNA) for identifying the rapist.
6. Encourage patient to consider treatment and evaluation for sexually transmitted diseases before leaving the ED.	6. Many survivors are lost to follow-up after being seen in the ED or crisis center and will not otherwise get protection.

Continued

TABLE 19-2	Interventions for Sexual Assault—cont'd

Intervention	Rationale
7. Offer prophylaxis to pregnancy.	7. Approximately 5% of women who are raped become pregnant.
8. All data must be carefully documented: • Verbatim statements • Detailed observations of physical trauma • Detailed observation of emotional status • Results from the physical examination • All lab tests should be noted	8. Accurate and detailed documentation is crucial legal evidence.
9. Arrange for support follow-up: • Rape counselor • Support group • Group therapy • Individual therapy • Crisis counseling	9. Many individuals carry with them constant emotional trauma. Depression and suicidal ideation are frequent sequelae of rape. The sooner the intervention, the less complicated the recovery may be.

common sexually transmitted diseases (chlamydia, gonorrhea, trichomoniasis, and bacterial vaginosis [BV]). The guidelines also recommend a collection of serum for immediate evaluation for HIV, hepatitis B (if not immunized), and syphilis. Any survivor with abrasions should be immunized for tetanus if 5 years have elapsed since the last immunization.

Pharmacology

Short-term treatment with a benzodiazepine may help ameliorate acute anxiety and agitation that follows a trauma. Antidepressants (selective serotonin reuptake inhibitors [SSRIs]) may be helpful for symptoms of PTSD such as hyperarousal, agitation, insomnia, and in the treatment of depression and panic attacks.

Psychotherapy

Crisis counseling should be available to any person who has been sexually assaulted. Information on support groups, therapists, and attorneys who work with sexual assault survivors should be provided before the person leaves the ED. Caring for survivors is not completed in a single visit. Their emotional state and other psychological needs should be assessed within 24 to 48 hours by phone after being treated.

Follow-up Care

Follow-up visits should occur at least 2, 4, and 6 weeks after the initial visit to the ED. At each visit the survivor should be assessed for psychological progress, the presence of a sexually transmitted disease, pregnancy, and need for legal counsel.

Community-Based Supports

Group therapy or support groups can be beneficial for survivors. Sharing experiences with others who are going through the devastating physical and emotional aftermath of rape can be healing and break through feelings of isolation, shame, and guilt.

Therapy for Rapists

Changing in thinking and behavior needs to be undertaken in order to effect change. Unfortunately, most rapists do not acknowledge the need for change. No single method or program of treatment has been found to be totally effective.

EVALUATION

Most patients will be able to eventually resume their previous lives after supportive services and crisis counseling. If survivors are relatively free of signs of PTSD and their lifestyles are close to their lifestyles before the rape, the recovery is successful. Too often, without counseling of some kind, various sequelae of the assault may remain for years or a lifetime.

KEY POINTS TO REMEMBER

- Sexual assault is an act of violence and a criminal offense that often results in severe long-term psychiatric trauma.
- Contact with the sexual assault patient usually takes place in the ED. Nurses with special training assess the patient, collect data, and provide information and referrals (therapists, legal counsel, support groups) for patients before they leave the ED.
- Permission is necessary for collecting forensic data, performing a pelvic examination, and taking photographs. Confidentiality is stressed.
- Forensic examination is conducted, and evidence is collected. The patient should be given medications against STDs, evaluated for pregnancy, offered prophylaxis, and tested for HIV and syphilis. If abrasions are noted, a tetanus shot may be indicated.

- Careful documentation of findings (diagrams and photos), observations of emotional status, and description of the events surrounding the assault are documented using verbatim statement.
- Assessment for "date rape" drugs should be included if description of the event indicates that possibility. In such a case, a urine sample may be obtained.
- Everything is explained to individual patient before it is done to prepare him or her and to help allay anxiety.
- Before leaving the ED, sexually assaulted individuals are told what kinds of reactions are commonly experienced by sexually traumatized survivors following a crisis.
- Follow-up counseling, support groups, and resources to effective legal attorneys who specialize in sexual assault should always be given before discharge from the ED.

CRITICAL THINKING

1. Sally M. is brought by a friend to the ED. She is dazed, and the friend explains that a few friends went to a bar and met some guy Sally had met at a party on campus. He bought them all drinks. Sally said that after a few drinks she felt funny and doesn't remember much except that she woke up outside the back of the bar with her underclothes off and a number of reddened marks and abrasions on her breasts and arms. She felt pain and burning in her pelvic region. Her friends found her semiconscious and brought her to the ED. Sally appears confused and alternates between crying uncontrollably and staring into space. She repeatedly says she wants to wash up and change clothes, but her friend wanted her to come into the ED as soon as possible.
    A. Chart the signs and symptoms of Sally's physical and emotional trauma using the guidelines outlined in the chapter.

    B. Once Sally agrees to photos and pelvic examination, how would you describe to her the procedures that will be performed during the forensic and pelvic examination?
    C. Why might you ask her for a urine specimen at this time?
    D. She is afraid and does not want her parents or anyone on campus to know what happened. What would you say to her?
    E. Describe the emergency medical treatment that should be offered to all sexually assaulted individuals.
    F. Knowing that the sequelae of rape can be devastating and take years or longer to resolve, what kinds of supports and referrals should Sally be given before she leaves the ED?

CHAPTER REVIEW

Choose the most appropriate answer.
1. Rape-trauma syndrome is most similar to:
    1. posttraumatic stress disorder.
    2. dissociative identity disorder.
    3. unresolved grief reaction.
    4. developmental crisis.
2. In the medical record of a survivor of rape, which of the following types of data are inappropriate to document?
    1. Observations of the patient's physical trauma using a body map
    2. Assessment of signs and symptoms of emotional trauma
    3. Verbatim statements made by the patient
    4. Details of the patient's sexual history

3. When an ED nurse is providing care to a rape survivor, which two of the following are important elements of care?
    1. Providing nonjudgmental care
    2. Conveying disgust that this would happen
    3. Aligning with her sense of blaming herself
    4. Assuring confidentiality
4. Which of the following observations, if found in the medical record of a sexual assault survivor, would indicate that "reorganization" after a rape crisis was not yet complete? The patient is:
    1. free from somatic reactions.
    2. generally positive about self.
    3. calm and relaxed during interactions.
    4. experiencing frequent nightmares.

REFERENCES

Abbey, A. (1991). Acquaintance rape and alcohol consumption on college campuses. *Journal of American College Health, 39*(1).

American College of Obstetrics and Gynecology (ACOG). (2004). Acute care of sexual assault victims. Retrieved July 30, 2007, from www.acog.org/departments/dept_notice.cfm?recno=17&bulletin=1625.

Blackwood, C.L. (2005). Sexual assault. *Clinics in Family Practice, 7*(1).

Centers for Disease Control and Prevention (CDC). (2007). *Sexual violence fact sheet.* National Center for Injury Prevention and Control. Retrieved February 8, 2007, from www.cdc.gov/ncipc/pub-res/images/SV%20Factsheet.pdf.

DC Rape Crisis Center. Retrieved February 10, 2007, from www.dcrcc.org/same-sex.htm.

Fisher, B.S., Cullen, F.T., & Turner, M.G. (2000). *The sexual victimization of college women.* Retrieved February 12, 2007, from www.ncjrs.gov/txtfiles1/nij/182369.txt.

Hopper, J. (2007). *Sexual abuse of males: Prevalence, possible lasting effects and resources.* Retrieved February 12, 2007, from www.jimhopper.com/male-ab.

National Crime Victimization Survey. (2005). *Crime and Victims Statistics,* Retrieved February 8, 2007, from www.ojp.usdoj.gov/bjs/cvict.htm.

National Crime and Victim Survey (2003). Retrieved February 8, 2007, from www.ojp.usdoj.gov/bjs/pub/pdf/cv03.pdf.

Quinn, K., Zielke, H. (2005). Elder abuse, neglect, and exploitation: policy issues. *Clinics in Geriatric Medicine, 21*(2).

Rape Abuse and Incest National Network (RAINN). (2006b). *Pregnancies resulting from rape.* Retrieved February 8, 2007, from rainn.org/get-information/statistics/sexual-assault-victims.

Starman, U.K. (2006). Myths about male rape, the rape of men. Abused empowered survive thrive. Retrieved July 27, 2007, from www.aest.org.uk/survivors/male/myths_about_male_rape.htm.

Tjaden, P., & Thoennes, N. (2000). *Full report of the prevalence, incidence, and consequences of violence against women: findings from the national violence against women survey.* Washington: National Institute of Justice. Report NCJ 183781.

Tjaden P., & Thoennes, N. (2006). *Extent, nature, and consequences of rape survivorization: Findings from the national violence against women survey.* Washington: National Institute of Justice. Report NCJ 2103346.

Viguera, A.C., & Mian, P. (2004.) The patient who has been sexually assaulted. In T.A. Stern, J.B. Herman, & P.L Salvin (Eds.), *Massachusetts General Hospital guide to primary care psychiatry* (2nd ed.). New York: McGraw-Hill.

CHAPTER 20

Suicidal Thoughts and Behaviors

Elizabeth M. Varcarolis

Key Terms and Concepts

physician-assisted suicide (PAS), p. 412
postvention, p. 417
suicidal ideation, p. 412

suicide, p. 412
suicide attempt, p. 412

Objectives

1. Understand the pros and the cons of the "right to die" issue.
2. Explain the role of culture and socioeconomic status as they relate to suicidal risk.
3. Using the SAD PERSONS scale, discuss in detail the 10 risk factors to consider when assessing for suicide.
4. Understand the overt, covert, and behavioral clues in a person who may be contemplating suicide.
5. Compare the interventions during the crisis period to those after the crisis period.

evolve

For additional resources related to the content of this chapter, visit the Evolve site at http://evolve.elsevier.com/Varcarolis/essentials.

- Chapter Outline
- Chapter Review Answers
- Case Study and Nursing Care Plan

- Nurse, Patient, and Family Resources
- Concept Map Creator

Suicide or **completed suicide** is the act of intentionally ending one's own life and opting for nonexistence. The act of purposeful self-destruction by taking one's own life arouses intense and complex emotions in others. **Suicide attempt** includes all willful, self-inflicted, life-threatening attempts that have not led to death. **Suicidal ideation** means a person is thinking about self-harm. *Always* take a person very seriously if he or she mentions some form of suicidal ideation. *Always* ask, "Are you thinking of harming [killing] yourself?" Listen very carefully to what the person does and does not say. Appropriate nursing interventions are outlined later in this chapter.

Suicide can be understood from a variety of different perspectives: religious, philosophical, sociological, psychological, and biological. The meaning of suicide has traditionally reflected the religious beliefs of a culture. For example, in cultures derived from the Judeo-Christian background, life is considered a gift, and to take away one's life is a sin. Cultures that derived from Catholic teachings (South America, Spain, Italy, Ireland) often have lower rates of suicide (Carroll-Ghosh et al., 2003). By the same token, people who practice the Japanese Shinto religion believe in reincarnation. Therefore death may be seen an honorable solution to life problems (Range et al., 1999).

The more recent growth of the secular philosophy—the foundation of which is respect for an individual's will and basic human rights—has influenced the perception of suicide in our society. This philosophy has lead to a movement that supports the right of mentally competent adults to humanely end their own suffering (Caroll-Ghosh et al., 2003). The natural extension of this perspective is the practice of **physician-assisted suicide (PAS)** for the terminally ill, which operates under very strict guidelines (Emanuel et al., 2000). The patient must have:

- Absence of neuromedical or psychiatric conditions that impair capacity to reason and process information.
- Understanding of the consequence of his or her decisions based on a realistic view of his or her situation.
- Strong desire to end his or her suffering from a terminal condition.

At present, only a few jurisdictions legally sanction PAS, including Australia's Northern Territory, Canada, Colombia, the Netherlands, and the U.S state of Oregon. The "right to die" issue is vastly controversial and complex.

PREVALENCE AND COMORBIDITY

Suicide is the 11th leading cause of death in the United States (CDC, 2004) and is the third leading cause of death for adolescents and young adults. Among older adults, suicide rates increase alarmingly with age. Epidemiological surveys have demonstrated that the vast majority of completed suicides are in individuals with diagnosable psychiatric conditions, most prominently that of **depression** and **alcohol or substance abuse.**

The risk of suicide in people with a major depressive disorder (MDD) is about 20 times that of the general population. Patients who have schizophrenia, dementia, bipolar disorder, anxiety disorder (especially panic disorder and PTSD), personality disorders (borderline, paranoid, and antisocial), and other psychiatric disorders all have a higher rates of suicide than people in the general population.

Physical illnesses may also play a role in increasing suicide risk. For example, people with AIDS, cancer, chronic renal failure with hemodialysis, head injury, multiple sclerosis, and Parkinson's disease are at an increased risk for suicide. Intentional death, either physician-assisted or self-inflicted, may be a means of escaping from intolerable pain and extreme limitations imposed by illness. Therefore nurses might encounter suicidal individuals in outpatient settings, intensive care units, nursing homes, or medical-surgical units, during home visits, or even among one's own circle of family and friends.

It is important for nurses to know that some medications can contribute to symptoms of depression, thus raising an individual's risk for suicide. Some medications commonly associated with depression are antihypertensives, benzodiazepines, calcium channel blockers, corticosteroids, hormonal medications, and medications to treat pain.

THEORY

Sigmund Freud (1856-1939) developed some of the first psychological theories of suicide in the early 1900s. Freud described suicide as a murderous attack on an ambivalently loved, internalized significant person, often referred to as murder in the 180th degree. Building on Freud's theory, **Karl Menninger** (1893-1990) suggested that all suicides experience three interrelated emotions: revenge, depression, and guilt.

Edwin Shneidman (b.1918) proposed that victims of suicide suffer unbearable psychological pain, a sense of isolation, and the perception that death is the only solution to their situation. In essence, an individual feels that "there is no way out." Shneidman identified self-destructive behaviors (e.g., compulsive use of drugs, hyperobesity, gambling, self-harmful sexual behaviors, and medical noncompliance) as **sub-intentioned suicide.**

Herbert Hendin, medical director of the American Foundation of Suicide Prevention, states that Shneidman was the first person in the United States to call public attention to the problem of suicide. Hendin goes on to say that, "however, the biggest advances in the field of suicide prevention in the last 15 years have been in the field of biology and the pharmacology of depression and suicide; it borders on malpractice for a doctor not to prescribe medication for seriously depressed individuals" (Curwen, 2004).

Risk Factors for Suicide

Many risk factors may be involved, but there is no single theory that explains suicide. There are, however, some commonalities. People who attempt or complete suicide are often poor problem solvers, have troubled emotional lives (depression, anger, anxiety, guilt, boredom), have a low threshold for emotional pain, are often impulsive, and might engage in extreme solutions sooner than non— suicide-prone individuals. Please note that a person may experience one or more risk factors and not be suicidal. However, acute risk is associated with anxiety, insomnia, and substance abuse. See Figure 1-1 on page 6 for a clinical algorithm for the suspicion of suicide risk.

Biological

Suicide seems to cluster in some families; therefore family history is pertinent. A striking example is the novelist Ernest Hemingway's family in which five members in four generations committed suicide (a number of Hemingway's family members suffered from mental illness or substance abuse) (Sadock and Sadock, 2007).Twin studies have shown that monozygotic twins pairs (identical twins) have significantly greater concordance rates for suicide as well as attempted suicide than dizygotic twin pairs (fraternal twins) (Roy et al., 1991).

A recent study of 21,168 suicides spanning a 17-year period in Denmark demonstrated the suicide mortality of first-degree relatives of suicide victims was about 3.5 times greater than first-degree relatives of live controls that matched for age, sex, and date of suicide (Qin, 2003). This could be the result of inherited markers for depression, learned problem-solving behavior within the family, or a genetic factor associated with suicide, such as inherited low cerebrospinal fluid (CSF) levels of 5-hydroxyindole acetic acid (5-HIAA). 5-HIAA is a metabolite of the neurotransmitter serotonin (5-HT). Scientists now believe that there is an association between suicidal behavior and the molecular genetics of the neurotransmitter serotonin. Low levels of serotonin metabolite 5-HIAA in the cerebral spinal fluid are associated with suicidal and aggressive behavior (Qin, 2003).

Cultural and Societal

Societal factors that may increase the potential for suicide include loss, lack of social supports, negative life events, and severe life stress. Therefore suicide potential is apt to be higher among individuals facing these circumstances, including those who are impoverished; recently divorced, separated, or bereaved; childless, homeless; those who live alone; have few to no supports; and are grappling with recent negative life events. Suicide also seems to be higher among the unemployed. Epidemiological studies have shown a relationship between suicide or suicidal behaviors and socioeconomic disadvantage, such as unemployment, particularly among the young and those who have experienced a recent loss of employment as opposed to chronic unemployment (AISRAP, 2003; Carroll-Ghosh et al., 2003).

Psychological

People who are psychotic are at a high risk for suicide, especially those who experience command hallucinations telling them to kill themselves or delusions that they must die. There is a trio of psychological-emotional factors often present when people become suicidal: hopelessness, helplessness, and feelings of worthlessness. Hopelessness refers to lack of purpose in life, helplessness refers to lack of social supports, and worthlessness refers to low self-esteem or lack of love for self. In other words, people may contemplate suicide when they feel trapped and there is "no way out." Often this type of thinking is precipitated or intensified by a negative and overwhelming event.

Suicide risk factors include: (NIMH, 2006; Silverman, 2005)

- Presence of a plan
- Previous suicide attempt
- History of mental disorder particularly depression, alcohol or drug abuse
- Impulsive or aggressive tendencies
- Adverse life events, recent or expected loss
- Feelings of hopelessness or isolation
- Family history of mental or substance abuse disorder
- Family history of suicide, or prior suicide attempt
- Family violence, including physical or sexual abuse
- Incarceration
- Exposure to suicidal behavior of others, including family, peers, in the news or fiction
- Chronic physical illness, particularly if associated with chronic pain

Age
Adolescents and Young Adults
Suicide is the third leading cause of death for 14- to 24-year-olds after accidents and homicides. American Indian

and Alaska Native male adolescents have the highest suicide rate (NAHIC, 2006). The strongest risk factors for youth are substance abuse, aggression, disruptive behaviors, depression, and social isolation. Other factors related to youth suicide are:

- Frequent episodes of running away
- Frequent expressions of rage
- Family loss or instability
- Frequent problems with parents
- Withdrawal from family and friends

- Expression of suicidal thoughts or talk of death or the afterlife when sad or bored
- Difficulty dealing with sexual orientation
- Unplanned pregnancy

Older Adults

People 65 and older have the highest suicide rate of any group in the country. Most older adults who commit suicide have visited their primary care physician in the month before the suicide, sometimes that very day. Recog-

---

EXAMINING THE EVIDENCE   Antidepressants and Suicide Risk in Children

I heard on the news that giving antidepressants to children increases their risk of suicide. I'm doing a rotation on a child psychiatric unit and most of the kids there are on antidepressants. Should they be taking these drugs?

Clinicians have long known that there may be an increased risk of suicide in early antidepressant treatment. One study identifies the risk of suicide as being four times higher in the 9 days after initial treatment than in the subsequent 80 days (Simon et al., 2006). The reason for this risk may be a result of activating the energy of previously apathetic people, but we don't know why selective serotonin reuptake inhibitors (SSRIs) may bring about agitation and unusual behavior in some children and adolescents.

In October 2003, the U.S. Food and Drug Administration (FDA) issued a public health advisory about the risk of suicidal thinking and behavior in pediatric patients taking SSRIs. By 2004, the FDA ordered all pharmaceutical companies to add a serious warning, or a black box, to all antidepressant advertising. This black box said:

> Antidepressants increase the risk of suicidal thinking and behavior in children and adolescents with major depressive disorder and other psychiatric disorders.

This warning was spurred on by testimony from grieving parents whose children committed suicide while taking antidepressants. This resulted in an extensive review by the FDA of the literature and clinical trials of antidepressants and children.

Findings from the review revealed that among the more than 2000 children taking SSRIs there were no completed suicides, yet about 4% of these children experienced suicidal thinking or behavior (even attempted suicide), a rate twice that of children taking placebos.

The warning resulted in alarmed parents refusing to allow their children to take antidepressants and in practitioners becoming far more conservative in prescribing SSRIs to pre-adults. In fact, research indicates that between 2003 and 2005 pediatric prescriptions for SSRIs fell by more than 50%, the diagnosis of depression decreased, and between 2003 and 2004 suicide among teens increased by a record 18% (Libby et al., 2007).

Critics of the black box warning call for its lifting, saying that it has done more harm than good and that the few children who are adversely affected by SSRIs pale in comparison to the hundreds of children whose lives are saved. The director of the National Institute of Mental Health (2007), Thomas Insel, agrees, "Although we cannot ignore the possibility that antidepressants may exacerbate suicidal thoughts and actions in some children, it would be worse to let these children go untreated."

Bridge and associates (2007) conducted further research on suicidality in children and concluded that the FDA may have underestimated the benefits and overestimated the risks. They recommend the continued use of SSRIs in children, but emphasize the need to assess how well the child is doing (if not responding favorably to the drug, there's no point in continuing it) and careful monitoring for behavioral changes.

Bridge, J.A., Birmaher, B., and Brent, D.A. (2007). Benefits and harms of pediatric antidepressant medications. *Journal of the American Medical Association, 298*(6): 627.

U.S. Food and Drug Administration. (2004). *Public health advisory.* Retrieved from www.fda.gov/cder/drug/antidepressants/default.htm.

Gibbons, R.D., Hur, K., Bhaumik, D.K., & Mann, J.J. (2006). The relationship between antidepressant prescription rates and rate of early adolescent suicide. *American Journal of Psychiatry, 163,* 1898-1904.

Libby, A.M., Brent, D.A, Morrato, E.H., et al. (2007). Decline in treatment of pediatric depression after FDA advisory on risk of suicidality with SSRIs. *American Journal of Psychiatry, 164,* 884-891.

National Institute of Mental Health. (2007). *Science update.* Retrieved from www.nimh.nih.gov/science-news/2007/benefits-of-antidepressants-may-outweigh-risks-for-kids.shtml.

Simon, G.E., Savarino, J., Operskalski, B., & Wang, P.S. (2006). Suicide risk during antidepressant treatment. *American Journal of Psychiatry, 163,* 41-47.

A special thanks to Carly Albert-Kiber, graduate student at the University of Akron, for her research assistance.

nition and treatment of depression in the medical setting are promising ways to prevent suicide in older adults. Risk factors include social isolation, solitary living arrangements, widowhood, lack of financial resources, poor health, and feelings of hopelessness.

Gender

Although women seek help for depression at a rate of five to one and *attempt* suicide three times more often than men, men are at significantly more risk for *completing* suicide (CDC, 2004). In fact, men are four times as likely to commit suicide as women (NIMH, 2006). When race and ethnicity are considered, white men have the highest rates. One factor that contributes to this gender difference is that men tend to use the most lethal methods: firearms, knives, hanging, and drowning. Also men tend to lack strong networks of social support and are reluctant to get help because of greater societal stigma for depression in men.

CULTURAL CONSIDERATIONS

Generally, in the United States, European Americans have twice the suicide rate of minority groups (Hispanic Americans, African Americans, and Asian Americans) (APA, 2003). The exception is Native Americans, among whom the suicide rate is equal to that of European Americans. Among African Americans, men commit suicide more often than women, and the peak rate occurs in adolescence and young adulthood. Protective factors for this group as a whole include religion and the role of the extended family, both of which provide a strong social support system. Among Hispanic Americans, the Roman Catholic religion (in which suicide is a sin) and the importance given to the extended family decrease the risk for suicide. Among Asian Americans, suicide rates are noted to increase with age. Beliefs that reduce suicide include adherence to religions that tend to emphasize interdependence between the individual and society (i.e., self destruction is seen as disrespectful to the group or selfish).

Application of the Nursing Process

ASSESSMENT

There are a number of tools one can use to ascertain risk factors when assessing for potential suicidal behaviors. An acronym that can facilitate the health care worker's recall when in the midst of crisis situations is the SAD PERSONS scale (Patterson et al., 1983) (Box 20-1). This scale is commonly used in emergency rooms to evaluate need for referrals to mental health sources (Mitchell & Dennis, 2006).

BOX 20-1

SAD PERSONS Scale

S	Sex	1 if male
A	Age	1 if 15-24, 25-40 years, or 65+ years
D	Depression	1 if present
P	Previous attempts	1 if present
E	Etho (alcohol) or drug use	1 if present
R	Rational thinking loss	1 if psychotic for any reason
S	Social supports lacking	1 if lacking, especially if recent loss
O	Organized plan	1 if plan with lethal method
N	No spouse	1 if divorced, widowed, separated, or single male
S	Sickness	1 if severe or chronic

Guidelines for Action

Points	Clinical Action
0-2	Send home with follow-up
3-4	Closely follow up; consider hospitalization
5-6	Strongly consider hospitalization
7-10	Hospitalize or commit

Data from Patterson, W.M., Dohn, H.H., Bird, J., et al. (1983). Evaluation of suicidal patients: The SAD PERSONS scale. *Psychosomatics 24,* 343-349.

Verbal Clues

Always take a suicide threat seriously. Whether a person makes 1 or 1000 threats, take the threat seriously. Assessing verbal clues includes:

Overt statements
- "I can't take it anymore."
- "Life isn't worth living anymore."
- "I wish I were dead."
- "Everyone would be better off if I died."

Covert statements
- "It's okay now. Everything will be fine."
- "Things will never work out."
- "I won't be a problem much longer."
- "Nothing feels good to me anymore, and probably never will."
- "How can I give my body to medical science?"

Behavioral Clues

Sudden behavioral changes may be noticed, for example:
- Giving away prized possessions
- Writing farewell notes
- Making out a will

- Putting personal affairs in order
- Global insomnia
- Exhibiting a sudden and unexpected improvement in mood after being depressed or withdrawn
- Neglecting personal hygiene

Lethality of Plan

The evaluation of a plan is extremely important in determining the degree of suicide risk. The main elements in assessment should include:
- How detailed is the plan?
- How lethal is the proposed method?
  - Guns, hanging, carbon monoxide, staging a car crash are extremely lethal.
  - Slashing wrists, inhaling natural gas, ingesting pills are lower-risk methods.
- Availability of means. Does the person have a gun? Access to a tall building? Availability is a crucial factor when carrying out a plan.

Assessment Guidelines

Suicide Risk

1. If a person appears depressed, displays any verbal or behavioral clues, or for any reason you feel concern, **always ask "Are you thinking of harming or killing yourself?"**
2. Assess precipitating event. "Is there something difficult you are facing?"
3. Assess risk factors *as well as* protective factors.
4. Assess history of suicide (in family, friends, etc.), degree of hopelessness and helplessness, and lethality of plan.
5. If there is a history of suicide attempt, assess:
   - **Intent:** Is there a high probability of being discovered?
   - **Lethality:** Was the method used highly lethal or less lethal?
   - **Injury:** Did the patient suffer physical harm (e.g., was the patient admitted to an intensive care unit)?
6. Determine whether the patient's age, medical condition, or psychiatric diagnosis put the patient at higher risk.
7. Red flags include:
   - The patient suddenly goes from sad or depressed to happy and peaceful. Often a decision to commit suicide gives a feeling of relief and calm.
   - The patient gives away treasured possessions
8. If the patient is to be managed on an outpatient basis, also assess:
   - Social supports.
   - Significant others' knowledge of the signs of potential suicidal ideation (e.g., increasing withdrawal, preoccupation, silence, and remorse).

- Knowledge of community resources that the patient and family could use for support during the crisis.

evolve

For a comprehensive case study and associated nursing care plan for a suicidal patient, visit the Evolve website at http://evolve.elsevier.com/Varcarolis/essentials.

DIAGNOSIS

Risk for suicide is the most immediately important nursing diagnosis, and self-restraint from suicide is the hoped-for outcome. Other nursing diagnoses include *Ineffective coping*, *Hopelessness*, *Social isolation*, *Spiritual distress*, *Chronic low self-esteem*, *Disturbed thought processes*, among others.

OUTCOMES IDENTIFICATION AND PLANNING

Interventions during the crisis attempt to accomplish optimizing events and environmental factors to help minimize further self-destructive acts. Outcomes for working with suicidal patients are to help explore alternatives, problem solve, increase coping skills, minimize feelings of isolation and loneliness, and find treatment for co-occurring mental health issues (e.g., depression, substance abuse) would be the thrust of the work with the patient on a long-term basis.

IMPLEMENTATION

Unfortunately, there seems to be a lack of evidence that supports any particular approach to suicide prevention. Although restriction of access to means, treatment of depression, assisting with problem solving and other therapies, and prescription of psychotropic medications may be effective, none of these interventions have been systematically investigated (International Suicide Rates, 2003).

Some factors are thought to support a person's resilience and act as protective factors. According to Silverman (2005), they include the following:
- Family and community support
- Effective and appropriate clinical care for mental, physical, and substance abuse disorders
- Restricted access to highly lethal methods of suicide
- Cultural and religious beliefs that discourage suicide and support self-preservation instincts
- Acquisition of learned skills for problem solving, conflict resolution, and nonviolent management of disputes

TABLE 20-1	Interventions During the Crisis Period
Intervention	**Rationale**
Forensic Issues	
1. **Follow institutional protocol** for suicide regarding creating a safe environment (taking away potential weapons—belts, sharp objects; checking what visitors bring in, etc.)	1. Provide safe environment during time patient is actively suicidal and impulsive; self-destructive acts are perceived as the only way out of an intolerable situation.
2. Keep accurate and thorough records of patient's behavior—both verbal and physical—as well as all nursing and physician actions.	2. These might become court documents. If patient's needs or requests are not documented, they do not exist in a court of law.
3. Put on either *suicide precaution* (one-on-one monitoring at arm's length away) or *suicide observation* (15-minute visual check of mood, behavior, and verbatim statements), depending on level of suicide potential.	3. Protection and preservation of the patient's life at all costs during crisis is part of medical and nursing staff responsibility. **Follow institutional protocol.**
4. Keep accurate and timely records and document patient's activity—usually every 15 minutes—including what patient is doing, with whom, etc. **Follow institutional protocols.**	4. Accurate documentation is vital. The chart is a legal document regarding patient's "ongoing status," interventions taken, and by whom.
5. If accepted at your institution, construct a *no-suicide contract* with the suicidal patient. Use clear, simple language. When contract is up, it is renegotiated.	5. The no-suicide contract helps patients know what to do when they begin to feel overwhelmed by pain (e.g., "I will speak to my nurse/counselor/support group/family member when I first begin to think of harming myself").
6. Encourage patients to talk about their feelings and problem-solve alternatives.	6. Talking about feelings and looking at alternatives can minimize suicidal acting-out.

See Table 20-1 for interventions *during* the crisis period and Table 20-2 for interventions *after* the crisis period.

Communication Guidelines

Nurses and other health care providers use communication skills and counseling techniques as one of their most important tools. Communication and counseling skills used by the nurse working with a suicidal person are practiced (1) in the community, (2) in the hospital, and (3) on telephone hotlines. During suicidal crisis, the following information should be conveyed to the patient in all settings:

- The crisis is temporary
- Unbearable pain can be survived
- Help is available
- You are not alone

Psychotherapy

See Table 20-3 for interventions to be used during follow-up psychotherapy.

Postvention

Intervention for family and friends ("survivors") of a person who has committed suicide—**postvention**—should be ini-

tiated within 24 to 72 hours after the death. Natural feelings of denial and avoidance predominate during the first 24 hours (Thompson, 1996). Mourning the death of a loved one who has committed suicide is painful at all times. Family and friends are often faced with the process of mourning without the normal social supports—unfortunately, neighbors, acquaintances, and even family and friends are often confused and may blame the family for the death. Families with members who have committed suicide are often stigmatized and isolated.

Survivors often feel that they are "going crazy" and need to be told that these feelings are normal. Survivors also need outlets for the undercurrent of anger against the deceased, who is responsible for the trauma, confusion, and pain inflicted on them. Unfortunately, few friends or family members of a person who has committed suicide seek counseling. Pronounced feelings of anger and guilt are common reactions.

People exposed to traumatic events such as suicide or sudden loss often manifest the following posttraumatic stress reactions: irritability, sleep disturbance, anxiety, startle reaction, nausea, headache, difficulty concentrating, confusion, fear, guilt, withdrawal, anger, and reactive depression. The particular pattern of the emotional reaction and type of response differ with each survivor depending on the relationship of the deceased, circumstances surrounding the death, and coping mechanisms of the survivors. The

TABLE 20-2   Interventions After the Crisis Period

Intervention	Rationale
1. Arrange for patient to stay with family or friends. If no one is available and the person is highly suicidal, hospitalization must be considered.	1. Relieve isolation and provide safety and comfort.
2. Weapons and pills are removed by friends, relatives, or the nurse.	2. To help ensure safety.
3. Encourage patients to talk freely about feelings (anger, disappointments) and help plan alternative ways of handling anger and frustration.	3. Gives patients alternative ways of dealing with overwhelming emotions and gaining a sense of control over their lives.
4. Encourage patient to avoid decisions during the time of crisis until alternatives can be considered.	4. During crisis situations, people are unable to think clearly or evaluate their options.
5. Contact family members, arrange for individual or family crisis counseling.	5. Reestablishes social ties and mobilizes family support to deal with precipitating event(s) or overwhelming situation.
6. Activate links to social supports in the community, e.g., self-help groups	6. Diminished sense of isolation, and provides contact with individuals who care about the suicidal person.
7. If anxiety is extremely high, or patient has not slept in days, an antianxiety or antidepressant might be prescribed. **Only a 1- to 3-day supply of medication should be given. Family member or significant other should monitor pills for safety.**	7. Relief of anxiety and restoration of sleep loss can help the patient think more clearly and might help restore some sense of well-being. Use of SSRIs is felt to be safe for a depressed adult. **Fluoxetine is the only FDA-approved antidepressant for treatment in children** (Barclay & Vega, 2006).

TABLE 20-3   Interventions for Follow-up Psychotherapy

Intervention	Rationale
1. Identify situations that trigger suicidal thoughts (define the precipitating event).	1. Identify targets for learning more adaptive coping skills.
2. Assess patient's strengths and positive coping skills (talking to others, creative outlets, social activities, problem-solving abilities).	2. Use to build on and draw from when planning alternatives to self-defeating behaviors.
3. Assess patient's coping behaviors that are not effective and that result in negative emotional sequelae: drinking, angry outbursts, withdrawal, denial, and procrastination.	3. Identify areas to target for teaching and planning strategies for supplanting more effective and self-enhancing behaviors.
4. Encourage patients to look into their negative thinking, and reframe negative thinking into neutral objective thinking.	4. Cognitive reframing helps people look at situations in ways that allow for alternative approaches.
5. Point out unrealistic and perfectionistic thinking.	5. Constructive interpretations of events and behavior open up more realistic and satisfying options for the future.
6. Spend time discussing patient's dreams and wishes for the future. Identify short-term goals that can be set for the future.	6. Renewing realistic dreams and hopes can give promise to the future and meaning to life.
7. Identify things that have given meaning and joy to life in the past. Discuss how these things can be reincorporated into the present lifestyle (e.g., religious or spiritual beliefs, group activities, creative endeavors).	7. Reawakens in patient abilities and experiences that tapped areas of strength and creativity. Creative activities give people intrinsic pleasure and joy, and a great deal of life satisfaction.

APPLYING THE ART   A Person with Suicidal Behaviors

SCENARIO: I met 55-year-old Raymond on the adult unit following a suicide attempt and surgical repair of a gunshot wound where he had damaged the right side of his neck, face, and part of his ear, but missed every vital vessel and somehow lived. He had shown improvement by participating more actively in group and had progressed from one-to-one observation (no farther than an arm's length away), to close constant observation within continuous visual range. I was meeting with him for a third time.

THERAPEUTIC GOAL: By the conclusion of this encounter, Raymond will feel comfortable enough with me to reveal his suicide attempt.

Student-Patient Interaction	Thoughts, Communication Techniques, and Mental Health Nursing Concepts
Student: "Raymond, I'm here after lunch as agreed."	I *offer self.* Being back when I said I would be builds trust.
Raymond: *Avoids eye contact.* "You can stay if you want. I don't feel like talking much." *Glances up briefly then stares at the floor.* **Student's feelings:** *While reserved, earlier Raymond's voice had more animation. He also made eye contact. Did I do something wrong to impair the relationship?*	While I need to *evaluate* my *nursing practice*, Raymond's behavior change most likely came from his *mood disorder.* *Depression* influences his perception of just about everything.
Student: "I'll stay here with you." I lean toward him with a concerned expression. **Student's feelings:** *I have the hardest time waiting. I keep wanting to fill the silence. I sit on the left because Raymond has hearing loss on the right from the gunshot wound.*	I offer *self* with words and with attending behavior. My silence shows nonjudgmental acceptance.
Raymond: Silent for 4 minutes. "My wife wants a divorce." **Student's feelings:** *Divorce. Another loss. I am beginning to pick up his feelings of hopelessness.*	Does this increase his suicide risk further? Such a lethal method . . . to shoot yourself. I remember that sometimes when a suicide fails the patient sees self once again as a failure.
Student: "How devastating. How hurtful." **Student's feelings:** *Sometimes when I use reflection, I worry that it sounds fake. Maybe because I'm still having to think about how to ask things. Even if I'm wrong about his feelings, I hope he senses that I care, because I do.*	Reflection communicates empathy because I have to really connect to be able to discern his probable feeling.
Raymond: *Nods.* "She said she can't take it anymore."	
Student: "You say she can't take it anymore?"	*Restatement* helps him elaborate.
Raymond: "My depression. Doing this." Touches the dressing on his ear, carefully shakes his head side to side, then stares downward. **Student's feelings:** *I wonder what his marriage was like before this. When I have trouble with the people I love I often feel bad about myself too.*	*Suicide* acts as a two-edged sword, hurting the survivors as well as the patient. I remember reading that suicide also acts as an *attempt* to *communicate*, but what?
Student: "You shake your head, like you feel regret."	I *make an observation* and use *reflection.*

Continued

APPLYING THE ART   A Person with Suicidal Behaviors—cont'd

Student-Patient Interaction	Thoughts, Communication Techniques, and Mental Health Nursing Concepts
Raymond: "About so many things. At my age I should be able to readily name my accomplishments but all I see are my failures. I can't believe she had an affair. Then I look at how I've screwed up and no wonder. I can't even kill myself right." **Student's feelings:** *Where do I start? His despair makes me feel down, too.*	At the root of all this rests low self-esteem paired with depression. Was his suicide attempt a way to punish his wife as well as himself for being as he says "a screw-up"? His age puts him into *generativity vs. stagnation*. To feel he has no accomplishments sounds like stagnation rather than meeting the generativity task.
Student: "You're having trouble finding any reason to choose to live." **Student's feelings:** *I should have checked the chart to see if he has attempted suicide before.*	The 3-month period after an attempt remains high risk for another suicide attempt. I need to actively assess his suicide potential.
Raymond: "Some days more than others." **Student's feelings:** *I'm feeling worried that he may attempt again.*	He feels *ambivalent*. I double-check that the staff member assigned to the close constant observation is indeed watching him.
Student: "So, sometimes you are able to find something in you worth saving." **Student's feelings:** *I feel hopeful that he lets himself experience "some days" when he finds a reason to choose life. I need to help him get the feelings out, both the despair and the hope.*	I give *support*. Using the words, "you are able to" reinforces his *self-esteem*.
Raymond: "I guess so, but not today. Not with divorce papers in my hand." **Student's feelings:** *He sounds unsure. It's painful to struggle with depression. I know what depression feels like.*	In report this morning, the nurse indicated that Raymond's antidepressant and therapies may be starting to help. I remember that as *depression lifts*, the patient may experience the energy needed to carry through the *suicide plan*.
Student: "Today you're feeling pretty hopeless." *He nods.* "So hopeless you're thinking about suicide again?" **Student's feelings:** *My anxiety skyrockets. Okay. I am right here in the chair next to him. He and I are both safe right now. I can do this.*	His *suicide risk* suddenly increased with the impact of the divorce papers. He doesn't have a weapon but he could rip out his stitches. I stay alert and watch his hands.
Raymond: *Nods.*	
Student: "Do you have a plan right now?" **Student's feelings:** *My heart rate is increasing but I'm keeping my voice calm.*	I ask a *direct question* to *assess suicide risk*. I need to tell staff as soon as I can. He needs to be on a one-to-one with staff only an arm's length away.
Raymond: "It'd be easier at home." **Student's feelings:** *He's given a lot of thought to this. I'm doing okay with connecting with Raymond.*	Raymond continues to talk and that's so much healthier than hurting himself.
Student: "So you've thought of suicide while in the hospital, too."	The *current risk* takes precedence over thoughts of suicide at home. I *validate* with him.
Raymond: *Looks down.* **Student's feelings:** *Is Raymond avoiding eye contact? I don't want to lose the connection.*	He uses *avoidance*. What is he hiding?
Student: "Raymond, I care about you. Have you done or are you planning to do something to yourself right now?"	I assess suicidality with a *direct question*. Communicating caring gives support. A *caring relationship* deters suicide.

APPLYING THE ART   A Person with Suicidal Behaviors—cont'd

Student-Patient Interaction	Thoughts, Communication Techniques, and Mental Health Nursing Concepts
Raymond: *Mumbles.*	
Student: *Moving closer.* "Raymond, I need your help with this. Please. Did you do something?" ***Student's feelings:*** *Part of me prays he will answer me!*	
Raymond: "I saved up all my pills and took them all."	
Student: "When? What? How many?" ***Student's feelings:*** *I feel frantic. Okay, self, mindfully breathe.*	Too many *questions* at once. I'll overload him. I need help now.
Student: *I stop asking questions. I call and motion to staff. The nurse comes over to assess and begin emergency intervention with Raymond.* ***Student's feelings:*** *I feel relieved to get help.*	The whole *treatment team* on the psych unit works together. *Confidentiality* always includes the explanation that danger to self or others always gets reported.
Student: *As Raymond is transported off the unit, I walk alongside and I hold out my hand.* "Raymond, you were able to tell me about overdosing. That's a beginning of caring about yourself." ***Student's feelings:*** *By holding out my hand, I nonverbally ask permission to touch.*	My words and nonverbals give *support.*
Raymond: *Squeezes my hand.* ***Student's feelings:*** *I needed to know that he knows that I care.*	

BOX 20-2

Guidelines for Survivors of Suicide

- Know you can survive. You may not think so, but you can.
- Know you may feel overwhelmed by the intensity of your feelings, but all your feelings are normal.
- Anger, guilt, confusion, and forgetfulness are common responses. You are not crazy; you are in mourning.
- Having suicidal thoughts is common. It does not mean that you will act on these thoughts.
- Find a good listener with whom to share. Call someone if you need to talk.
- Don't be afraid to cry. Tears are healing.
- Give yourself time to heal.
- Remember, the choice was not yours. No one is the sole influence in another's life.

- Give yourself permission to get help.
- Be aware of the pain of your family and friends.
- Steer clear of people who tell you what or how to feel.
- Know that there are support groups that can be helpful. If you can't find one, ask a professional to help start one.
- Call on your personal faith to help you through.
- It is common to experience physical reactions to your grief, such as headaches, loss of appetite, inability to sleep.
- Wear out all of your questions, anger, guilt, or other feelings until you can let them go. Letting go doesn't mean forgetting.
- Know that you will never be the same again, but you can survive and go beyond just surviving.

Modified from Dunne, E., McIntosh, J., & Dunne-Maxim, K. (1987). *Suicide and its aftermath: Understanding and counseling the survivors.* New York: Norton.

ultimate contribution of suicide or sudden loss intervention in survivor groups is to create an appropriate and meaningful opportunity to respond to suicide or sudden death. To reduce the trauma associated with the sudden loss, post-traumatic loss debriefing can help initiate an adaptive grief process and prevent self-defeating behaviors.

Self-help groups are extremely beneficial for survivors of a suicidal family member or friend. Many people join self-help groups, even if the suicide took place 25 to 30 years before. Self-help groups for the survivors of a family member or friend who committed suicide are similar to all other self-help groups. Essentially these groups are run by people who have lost someone through suicide.

Box 20-2 gives some guidelines for coping with a suicide loss. Also, the American Foundation for Suicide Prevention can provide helpful information (www.afsp.org).

KEY POINTS TO REMEMBER

- People who attempt or complete suicide often share many risk factors, but people who have experienced the same risk factors are not always suicidal.
- Psychosis, substance abuse, poor problem solving, impulsivity, and low threshold for pain put people at high risk for suicide when overwhelmed.
- Adolescents, older adults, white males, and Native Americans have the highest rates of *completed* suicide. Some cultures play a protective role.
- Always try to identify the precipitating event for clues to areas of intervention.
- Assessment should include verbal clues, behavioral clues, and lethality of the plan as evaluation of the risk factors.

- The SAD PERSONS scale gives a quick overview of major risk factors.
- If suicidal risk is assessed, always ask point blank, "Are you thinking of killing yourself?"
- During the crisis period when a person is acutely suicidal, specific interventions can prove helpful (in or out of the hospital) and many save lives (see Table 20-1).
- After the crisis period is over, other interventions can prove helpful in increasing coping skills, problem solving, and minimizing isolation and loneliness (see Table 20-2).
- Intervention for family and friends of a person who has completed suicide is called postvention. Postvention can help lessen the guilt, anger, grief, pain, and myriad emotions that can stay with survivors for years.

CRITICAL THINKING

1. Sam Tee is a 66-year-old whose wife recently died of leukemia. His only son moved to California 2 years ago with his two daughters. Sam had been caring for his wife for 3 years before her death and has become withdrawn and despondent since her death. He does admit to having a gun in the house for protection. He is now in the ED after a "fender bender" and is getting two stitches on his ear. You ask Mr. Tee if he has thought about harming himself, and he says, "Well, there is always a last resort, isn't there?"

A. How many risk factors does Sam have?
B. Do you think he needs hospitalization? Explain the rationale behind your answer.
C. What are Sam's needs? What kinds of referrals do you think would help him over this crisis?
D. What do you think about the "fender bender"?
E. Name at least three groups in your community to which you could refer Sam.

CHAPTER REVIEW

Choose the most appropriate answer.
1. Charles Brown, age 52, lost his wife in an automobile accident 4 months ago. Since then, he has been severely depressed, withdrawn from contacts with family and friends, and taken to drinking to "numb the pain." On the SAD PERSONS assessment scale, how many points does Mr. Brown have?
  1. Three
  2. Four
  3. Five
  4. Six

2. Which of the following is an example of primary intervention in suicide?
  1. Working with the family of a recent suicide victim.
  2. Placing a hospitalized patient on suicide precautions.
  3. Keeping the caller to a crisis hotline on the phone and working out alternatives to suicide for a patient.
  4. Providing a seminar for older adults that focuses on coping with loneliness and physical changes.

CHAPTER REVIEW—cont'd

3. Miss B. has a concrete plan to commit suicide by hanging. She refuses to make a no-suicide contract because she believes there is no hope for a better life now that her fiancé has left her and God has abandoned her. She believes the breakup with her fiancé was because he found out "how worthless I am." Which of Miss B.'s nursing diagnoses is of highest priority?
   1. *Hopelessness*
   2. *Spiritual distress*
   3. *Low self-esteem*
   4. *Risk for suicide*

4. Which of the following groups is known to have the highest suicide rate?
   1. Asian Americans
   2. African Americans
   3. Native Americans
   4. Hispanic Americans

REFERENCES

American Psychiatric Association (2003) Practice guidelines for the assessment and treatment of patients with suicidal behaviors. *American Journal of Psychiatry, 160* (Suppl 11), 1-60.

Australian Institute for Suicide Research and Prevention (AISRAP) (2003). *International suicide rates: Recent trends and implications for Australia.* Retrieved July 12, 2007, from www.health.gov.au/internet/wcms/publishing.nsf/content/1D2B4E895BCD429ECA2572290027094D/$File/intcov.pdf.

Barclay, L., & Vega, C. (2006) *Antidepressants linked with attempted suicide risk in certain patients.* Retrieved January 18, 2007, from www.medscape.com/viewarticle/548961.

Carroll-Ghosh, T., Victor, B.S., & Bourgeois, J.A. (2003). Suicide. In R.E. Hales & S.C. Yudofsky (Eds.), *Textbook of clinical psychiatry* (4th ed.). Washington, DC: American Psychiatric Publishing Co.

Centers for Disease Control and Prevention, National Center for Injury Prevention and Control (producer). (2004). *Web based injury statistics query and reporting system* [Online]. Retrieved January 11, 2007. from www.cdc.gov/ncipc/wisqars/default.htm.

Curwen, T. (2004). *His work is still full of life.* Retrieved July 13, 2007, from www.cartercenter.org/news/documents/doc1755.html.

Emanuel, E.J., Fairclough, D.L., & Emanuel, L.L. (200). Attitudes and desires related to euthanasia and physician-assisted suicide among terminally ill patients and their caregivers. *JAMA, 284,* 2460-2468.

Law and Psychiatric Institution, North Shore, Long Island, Jewish Health System. *Suicide fact sheet.* Retrieved January 1, 2007, from www.northshorelij.com/body.cfm?id=741.

Mitchell, A.J., & Dennis, M. (2006). Self-harm and attempted suicide in adults: 10 practical questions and answers for emergency room staff. *Emergency Medicine Journal, 23,* 251-155.

National Adolescent Health Information Center (NAHIC). (2006). *Suicide: Adolescents & young adults: 2006 fact sheet.* Retrieved July 23, 2007, from http://nahic.ucsf.edu/downloads/Suicide.pdf.

National Institute of Mental Health (HIMH). (2006). *Suicide in the U.S.: Statistics and prevention.* Retrieved January 11, 2007, from www.nimh.nih.gov/health/publications/suicide-in-the-us-statistics-and-prevention.shtml.

Patterson, W.M., Dohn, H.H., Bird, J., et al. (1983). Evaluation of suicidal patients: The SAD PERSONS scale. *Psychosomatics, 24,* 343-349.

Qin, P. (2003). The relationship of suicide risk to family history of suicide and psychiatric disorders. *Psychiatric Times, 20*(13).

Roy, A., Segal, N.L., Centerwall, B.S., & Robinette, C.D. (1991). Suicide in twins. *Arch Gen Psychiatry 48*(1): 29-32.

Ryan, S. (2006). Cutting and other self-injurious behaviors. *Program and abstracts of the Pediatric Societies' 2006 Annual Meeting,* April 2006, San Francisco, CA.

Sadock, B.J., & Sadock, V.A. (2007). *Kaplan & Sadock's synopsis of psychiatry,* 10th ed, Philadelphia: Wolters Kluwer/Lippincott Williams & Wilkins.

Silverman, M.M. (2005). *Suicide assessment, intervention and prevention.* Retrieved March 19, 2007, from www.thedoctorwillseeyounow.com/articles/behavior/suicide_13.

Thompson, R. (1996). *Post-traumatic loss debriefing: Providing immediate support for survivors of suicide and sudden loss.* Ann Arbor, MI: Erie Clearinghouse on Counseling and Personal Services.

CHAPTER 21

Anger and Aggression

Elizabeth M. Varcarolis and Carrol Alverez

Key Terms and Concepts

aggression, p. 425
anger, p. 425
catastrophic reaction, p. 437
critical incident debriefing, p. 435

de-escalation techniques, p. 429
restraint, p. 434
seclusion, p. 434
violence, p. 425

Objectives

1. Discuss the interplay of genetic, biological, and sociological influences on the propensity toward violence for an individual.
2. Summarize the physical indicators for a patient who is escalating out of control.
3. Compare and contrast interventions for a patient who is angry and loud in the pre-escalation phase and one who is escalating to the aggressive phase.
4. Explain the principles of de-escalation.
5. Identify criteria for the use of seclusion or restraint.
6. Discuss the purpose and content of critical incident debriefing.
7. List the areas for which the nurse must provide written information when violence was averted or actually occurred.

For additional resources related to the content of this chapter, visit the Evolve website at http://evolve.elsevier.com/Varcarolis/essentials.

- Chapter Outline
- Chapter Review Answers

- Nurse, Patient, and Family Resources
- Concept Map Creator

Edited by Verna Benner Carson in the fifth edition of
Foundations of Psychiatric Mental Health Nursing

Anger is a primal—and not always logical—human emotion. It varies in intensity from mild irritation to intense fury and rage (APA, 2007). **Aggression** is harsh physical or verbal action that reflects rage, hostility, and potential for physical or verbal destructiveness and can be directed at others or oneself.

Anger may arise as a response to feelings of vulnerability and uneasiness because of a frustration of desire, a threat to one's needs (emotional or physical), or a challenge. Anger is an unplanned reaction to a stressor. When managed in a constructive manner (e.g., assertive communication), anger can help keep people safe and meet needs. When managed in a destructive manner (e.g., aggression), anger may meet needs but at the expense of causing emotional or physical harm to ourselves or others.

Aggression is a hostile reaction that occurs when control over anger is lost. It is used in an attempt to regain control over the stressor or flee the situation. **Violence** is a term that is uniquely associated with human beings and refers specifically to physical aggression. Anger and aggression can lead to a physical loss of control resulting in violence and harm. Control of violence in the health care setting becomes a top priority to maintain the milieu, and safety on the psychiatric unit is the number one concern. Fortunately, patients usually communicate increasing anxiety before it escalates to anger, aggression, or violence. Nurses can recognize the early escalation of anger and intervene appropriately.

PREVALENCE AND COMORBIDITY

Anger and violence are common aspects of social interaction and occur in all environments. Of the 1.6 million violent deaths in the United States in 2000, half were suicides, almost one third were homicides, and approximately one fifth were casualties of war. See Chapters 18 and 19 for information on the prevalence of child abuse, elder abuse, intimate partner violence (IPV), and sexual assault.

Workplace violence in the health care system is notably higher than for private sector industries and is not confined to the United States. Workplace-related violence against nurses is a major international occupational health problem (Alexy & Hutchins, 2006). Violence can occur anywhere in the hospital, but is most frequent in psychiatric units, emergency departments (EDs), waiting rooms, and geriatric units.

Although anger is a universal emotion, not everyone responds to anger with aggression and violence. Although most people who have **psychiatric disorders** are not violent, those who have a psychiatric disorder are five times more violent than those who do not. For example, there is evidence that anger coexists with attention deficit hyperactivity disorder, oppositional defiant disorder, and impulsivity in children, especially male children. Anger is a common response in people with dementia as they mourn the loss of independence and reject the help of others. In addition, anger frequently co-occurs with depression, attempted suicide, posttraumatic stress disorder, mania, psychotic disorders with paranoid delusions, conduct disorders, and personality disorders (Sadock & Sadock, 2004).

Numerous **medical and neurological** causes of organic brain syndrome can result in agitated, aggressive, or violent behavior. For example, certain brain tumors, Alzheimer's disease, temporal lobe epilepsy, and traumatic injury to certain parts of the brain result in changes to personality that includes increased violence. Other medical conditions that may affect an individual's control of violence are infections, subdural hemotomas, Tourette's disease, degenerative disorders, endocrine-metabolic imbalances, and intoxication.

THEORY

Anger biologically stimulates the hypothalamus, causing the body to react to the anticipation of harm. There is some indication that heredity may be involved in individual reactions to this biological process. Males with an XYY chromosome are more likely to have problems with aggression. Socially, angry reactions are learned and reinforced through the family and societal norms.

Selye's general adaptation syndrome describes the process as the fight-or-flight syndrome. *Freud's ego defense mechanisms* suggest that the mind can channel anger into more socially acceptable ways. Freud also stated that anger cannot be suppressed and will eventually express itself in some form (somatoform illnesses, defense mechanisms, maladaptive behaviors, etc.).

Clearly, some individuals are biologically more predisposed than others to respond to life events with irritability, easy frustration, and anger. This predisposition may be a function of genetics or of neurological development that occurs in infancy and childhood. Lewis (2005) states that perhaps the most important contributor to the genesis of violent behaviors is early and ongoing physical, sexual, or emotional abuse.

Neurobiological Factors
Brain Structure
One site known to be associated with aggression is the limbic system, which mediates primitive emotion and behaviors that are necessary for survival. The limbic system

EXAMINING THE EVIDENCE   Managing the Variables of Violence

I will be doing my psychiatric rotation in a state hospital that has a forensic population of about 25%. Although other students in my class seem to be a little nervous about working with "criminals," I am actually looking forward to the challenge and am even considering forensics as a career. At the same time, I want to be safe. Can you give me any advice?

You're among a growing number of nurses who are interested in forensic nursing, a subspecialty in graduate nursing in which the focus is, in part, perpetrators of criminal activity and violence. This increased popularity may be a result of the influence of such shows as *Crime Scene Investigation* portraying elite professionals carrying out exciting and often dangerous investigations. The reality of forensic nursing is likely less glamorous, but certainly challenging!

To answer your question, a multitude of factors pertaining to inpatient violence are studied by researchers. Patient, unit, and staff factors are all variables influencing the possibility for acting-out (Johnson, 2004). Patient variables are probably the most studied, and we know that particular characteristics raise red flags for aggression. According to Daffern and colleagues (2005), patients are more likely to act out if they have been violent before, recently used substances, been antisocial, or are experiencing psychosis (disturbed thought and auditory hallucinations).

Environmental circumstances may also predispose individuals toward violence. Crowding is one problem. Imagine how you feel when you're stuck in a crowded auditorium or go shopping the day after Thanksgiving. Now imagine what it would be like to be in too close quarters when you're already severely depressed or have disturbed thinking. Indeed, several studies found crowding on psychiatric units to be related to increased aggression, especially verbal aggression, but caution that it's not just the high number; it's a high number of *acutely* ill patients (Chou et al., 2002; Ng et al., 2001).

Staffing variables are complex, but researchers often examine such things as gender, experience, and staff satisfaction (Johnson, 2004). Regarding gender, there are two schools of thought. One is that females are less likely to bring about aggression because they are not considered as threatening. Another is that males provide an air of authority that reduces acting-out. Studies support both conclusions.

Regarding staff experience, intuitively experience would seem to be a plus, and it is. Research supports experience along with training as contributory to decreased patient aggression (Owen et al., 1998). Staff job satisfaction has been found to be correlated with aggression, suggesting that the more satisfied the staff were, the less likely the patients were to be aggressive (Morrison, 1998). It makes one wonder, however, if cause and effect are reversed, that is, less aggressive units create more satisfied staff.

A final staff variable relates to interaction style. As a new staff nurse working 3 to 11 PM, I noticed that every time I followed Cherie, the day shift nurse, I began my shift hearing about the terrible behavior of the patients, occasionally learning she'd been assaulted, and frequently reassessing the patients she'd put in seclusion and usually taking them out. Cherie was controlling, demanding, and confrontational. Not surprisingly, studies indicate that this coercive style of interaction is associated with more frequent aggressive behavior (Duxbury, 2002; Morrison, 1998).

Finally, research aside, my advice to you is to get to know your patient and the unit as much as possible before beginning your assignment. Ask if there is anything important for you to know about your patient and the unit. Be sure to review the process of handling disruptive behavior. In the end, trust your instincts. If you feel uncomfortable or uncertain, remove yourself from the situation and seek the advice of your instructor or staff. Your innate skills combined with these strategies should virtually ensure a worthwhile learning experience.

Chou, K.R., Lu, R.B, & Mao, W.C. (2002). Factors relevant to patient assaultive behavior and assault in acute inpatient psychiatric units in Taiwan. *Archives of Psychiatric Nursing, 16*(4), 187-195.

Daffern, M., Howells, K., Ogloff, J., & Lee, J. (2005). Individual characteristics predisposing patients to aggression in a forensic psychiatric hospital. *Journal of Forensic Psychiatry and Psychology, 16*(4), 729-746.

Duxbury, J. (2002). An evaluation of staff and patient views of and strategies employed to manage inpatient aggression and violence on one mental health unit: A pluralistic design. *Journal of Psychiatric and Mental Health Nursing, 9*, 325-337.

Johnson, M.E. (2004). Violence on inpatient psychiatric units: State of the science. *Journal of the American Psychiatric Nurses Association, 10*(3), 113-121.

Morrison, E. (1998). The culture of caregiving and aggression in psychiatric settings. *Archives of Psychiatric Nursing, 12*, 21-31.

Owen, C., Tarantello, C., Jones, M., & Tennant, C. (1998). Violence and aggression in psychiatric units. *Psychiatric Services, 49*, 1452-1457.

Ng, B., Kumar, S., Ranclaud, M., et al. (2001). Ward crowding and incidents of violence on an acute psychiatric inpatient unit. *Psychiatric Services, 52*, 521-525.

contains several structures that appear to have a role in the production of aggression. The area of the brain called the *amygdala* mediates anger experiences, judging events as either aversive or rewarding. For example, in animal studies stimulation of the amygdala produces rage responses, whereas lesions in the same structure produces docility.

The temporal lobe of the brain shares some structures with the limbic system. In the temporal lobe, memory is thought to be integrated; memory of previous insult is important in the cognitive appraisal of threat in the face of new stimuli. This lobe is also the source of complex partial seizures, which may give rise to aggressive behavior. Interestingly, high violence scores correlate with computed tomography (CT) scans and electroencephalography (ECC) abnormalities in the temporal lobes of patients in maximum security (Kavoussi et al., 1997).

Neurotransmitters

It is thought that cholinergic and catecholaminergic mechanics are involved with stimulating and maintaining predatory aggression. The serotonergic system and γ-aminobutyric acid (GABA), on the other hand, see to modulate effective aggression. Also, dopamine appears to facilitate aggression; but on the other hand, norepinephrine and serotonin are thought to inhibit aggression (Sadock & Sadock, 2007).

Studies have shown a relationship among impulsive aggression, history of suicide, and low levels of cerebrospinal fluid (CSF) 5-HIAA (the neurotransmitter serotonin) (Kavoussi et al., 1997). It is unclear, however, if the low CSF 5-HIAA is a marker for impulsivity or a certain kind of aggression. To date, no single neurotransmitter or lack thereof has been identified as a contributing factor for violence.

Genetic Factors

Twin studies have indicated that there is a genetic component in the etiology of violence. Research findings indicate that violence is a function of both genetics and childhood environment. Although there seems to be genetic contributions to aggression, most scientists agree that genetic characteristics alone do not account for the complexities of human behavior (Lewis, 2005). For example, researchers have noted that family dynamics affect the dispositions of infant members; disorganized, unpredictable families, or those high in conflict, tend to have more irritable infants than families that are stable (Brackbill et al., 1990; Eisenberg et al., 1997). Similarly, anger in toddlers has been seen to be related to childrearing variables in their mothers; nonconflictual parent-child relationships are most highly correlated with low toddler anger (Brook, Whiteman, &

Brook, 1999). Of course, family dynamics may themselves reflect genetic variables.

Filley and colleagues (2001) conclude that a study of the neurobehavioral aspect of violence, particularly frontal lobe dysfunction, altered serotonin metabolism, and the influence of heredity will lead to a deeper understanding of factors in the genesis of violence. They emphasize that social and evolutionary factors also play a role.

CULTURAL CONSIDERATIONS

Violence is a complex issue. Socioeconomic issues as well as medical and psychiatric issues are all contributing factors. The differing rates of violent crime among societies and within subcultures plays up the importance of social factors in the genesis of violence. For example, the rates of violent death in poorer and lower middle-income communities are twice as high as those in wealthier communities (Lewis, 2005). Substantial correlations have been found between environmental factors and aggression (e.g., poverty, disruption of marriages, unemployment, poor family cohesiveness, and difficulty maintaining social control).

Males in general are far more violent than females. Individuals with the highest prevalence of violence appear to be lower-class men with substance abuse disorders or major mental disorders. A subculture that supports the use of intimidation and aggression as an acceptable way of problem solving and achieving social status can reinforce the use of violence as acceptable behavior. This is particularly true in an environment where healthy, appropriate, and effective ways of dealing with frustration, anger, and aggression are not modeled.

Application of the Nursing Process

ASSESSMENT

Accurate and early assessment can usually identify patient anxiety before it escalates to anger and aggression. Always try to identify the problem causing the patient's increase in anxiety. Such assessment also leads directly to appropriate nursing diagnosis and intervention.

Patient expressions of anxiety and of anger generally look similar. Both may involve increased demands, irritability, frowning, redness of the face, pacing, twisting of the hands, or clenching and unclenching of the fists. Changes in mood and behavior from quiet to talkative and loud, from talkative to silent and withdrawn, from calm to angry, from depressed to elated also may occur. Box 21-1 identifies signs and symptoms that indicate the risk of escalating anger, which may in turn lead to aggressive behavior. Simple observation of these signs, however, does not provide

BOX 21-1

Some Predictive Factors of Violent Outcomes*

1. Signs and symptoms that usually (but not always) precede violence:†
   a. Angry, irritable affect
   b. Hyperactivity: most important predictor of imminent violence (e.g., pacing, restlessness, slamming doors)
   c. Increasing anxiety and tension: clenched jaw or fist, rigid posture, fixed or tense facial expression, mumbling to self (patient may have shortness of breath, sweating, and rapid pulse)
   d. Verbal abuse: profanity, argumentativeness
   e. Loud voice, change of pitch, or very soft voice forcing others to strain to hear
   f. Intense eye contact or avoidance of eye contact
2. Recent acts of violence, including property violence
3. Stone silence
4. Suspiciousness or paranoid thinking
5. Alcohol or drug intoxication
6. Possession of a weapon or object that may be used as a weapon (e.g., fork, knife, rock)
7. Milieu characteristics conducive to violence:
   a. Loud
   b. Overcrowding
   c. Staff inexperience
   d. Provocative or controlling staff
   e. Poor limit setting
   f. Staff inconsistency (e.g., arbitrary revocation of privileges)

*Violent outcomes include screaming, cursing, yelling, spitting, biting, throwing objects, hitting, and punching at self or others.
†Sometimes violence may be perceived to come from "out of the blue."

the information necessary to drive the appropriate intervention. Taking an accurate history of the patient's background and usual coping skills, as well as determining the patient's perception of the issue (if possible), are required.

On admission, take a comprehensive history of the patient gathered from a variety of sources (e.g., patient when calm, previous staff notes, family and friends). Patient history is a good predictor of risk for violence. The importance of gathering complete history in predicting violence was highlighted in a violence reporting program established at the Veterans Administration Medical Center in Portland, Oregon. Patients with a history of violence were identified in a computerized database. This program helped reduce the number of violent attacks by 91.6% by alerting staff to take additional safety measures when serving these patients (CDC, 2002).

VIGNETTE

A male abuser has been admitted to the unit for spousal and child abuse. He is considered a high risk for violent acting-out behaviors. Violence can be anticipated to be toward female authority figures and female staff members.

An intoxicated, homophobic male is admitted to the unit for detoxification. Violence can be anticipated if an all-male team is brought together to escort the patient to a quiet room.

Assessment Guidelines

Anger and Aggression

1. A history of violence is the single best predictor of future violence.
2. Patients who are hyperactive, impulsive, or predisposed to irritability are at higher risk for violence.
3. Assess patient risk for violence:
   • Does the patient have a wish or intent to harm?
   • Does the patient have a plan?
   • Does the patient have means available to carry out the plan?
   • Does the patient have demographic risk factors, including male gender, ages 14 to 24 years, low socio-economic status, and low support system?
4. Aggression occurs most often in the context of limit-setting by the nurse.
5. Patients with a history of limited coping skills, including lack of assertiveness or use of intimidation, are at higher risk of using violence.
6. Assess self for personal triggers and responses likely to escalate patient violence, including patient characteristics or situations that trigger impatience, irritation, or defensiveness.
7. Assess personal sense of competence when in any situation of potential conflict; consider asking for the assistance of another staff member.

DIAGNOSIS

The safety of patients and others is always the first priority. When anxiety levels escalate to levels at which there is a threat of harm to self or others, *Risk for self-directed violence* and *Risk for other-directed violence* are primary. If a patient is escalating and not amenable to early nursing interventions, and if de-escalating techniques are not effective, psychopharmacological means or restraints may be necessary to ensure the safety of patients and staff.

Initially, when anxiety begins to escalate and there is a potential for aggression, *Ineffective coping* (overwhelmed or maladaptive) is a likely nursing diagnosis. Patients may have coping skills that are adequate for day-to-day events in their lives but are overwhelmed by the stresses of illness or hospitalization. Other patients may have a pattern of maladaptive coping that is marginally effective and consists of a set of coping strategies that have been developed to meet unusual or extraordinary situations (e.g., abusive families). Ideally, intervention occurs at the point of *Ineffective coping.*

Nurses can teach patients ways of coping that will decrease anxiety and distress. However, patient behavior may escalate quickly, or the patient may mask early signs of distress. Nurses may be distracted and may miss those early signs, even when they are visible. Other nursing diagnoses may include *Confusion, Disturbed thought processes, Disturbed sensory perception,* and others.

OUTCOMES IDENTIFICATION

Short-term or intermediate outcomes goals may include, Patient will:

- Display nonviolent behaviors toward self and others (by *date*)
- Recognize when anger and aggressive tendencies begin to escalate and employ at least one new tension-reducing behaviors at that time (time outs, deep breathing, talking to a previously designated person, employing an exercise such as jogging) (by *date*)
- Make plans to continue with long-term therapy (individual, family, group) to work on violence-prevention strategies and increase coping skills (by *date*)

Long-term outcomes goals may include:

- Patient and others will remain free from injury.
- Hostile and abusive behavior toward others, property, animals, etc. will cease.
- Use of assertive and healthy behaviors to get needs met is in constant evidence.
- A variety of healthy anxiety reduction techniques to keep anger in check will be used.
- Impulses will be controlled.

PLANNING

Planning interventions necessitates having a sound assessment, including history (previous acts of violence, comorbid disorders), present coping skills, and willingness and capacity of the patient to learn alternative and nonviolent ways of handling angry feelings. However, among the most important aspect of planning is consistency of approach among staff. A clear management approach to dealing with violent situations and individuals includes staff well-versed in unit protocols and well-trained in **de-escalation techniques**. The following questions help determine appropriate planning.

Does the patient have:

- Good coping skills but is presently overwhelmed?

- Marginal coping skills?
- Use anger or violence as a way to cover other feelings and gain a sense of mastery or control?
- A neuropsychotic or chronic psychotic disorder?
- A tendency toward violence?
- Cognitive deficits (in the form of misinterpretation of environmental stimuli) that predispose to anger?

Does the situation call for:

- Psychotherapeutic approaches to teach the patient new skills for handling anger?
- Immediate intervention to prevent overt violence (de-escalation techniques, restraints or seclusion, or medications)?

Does the environment provide:

- A safe, therapeutic milieu?
- Privacy for the patient?
- Enough space for patients, or is there overcrowding?
- A healthy balance between structured time and quiet time?

Do the skills of the staff call for:

- Additional education in verbal de-escalation techniques?
- Counseling interventions because of punitive and arbitrary approaches to patients?
- Additional training in restraint techniques?

Planning also involves attention to the numbers of personnel who are available to respond to a potentially violent situation.

IMPLEMENTATION
Ensuring Safety

Safety is always a first consideration. **Ensure your safety first.** You must feel safe to be able to communicate in a calm manner. Staff and other personel should be alerted in case reinforcement is needed. The goals are that no one will become hurt, and the patient will experience the least restrictive interventions. The following is a list of specific interventions for working with a potentially angry, aggressive, or violent patient:

1. All patients should be searched for contraband and dangous objects when admitted to the unit and after visits.
2. In some cases supervised visits are advised.
3. Give the patient space. Always minimize personal risks. Stay at least one arm's length away from patient. Give more if patient is anxious or if you want more space. *Always trust your instincts.*
4. Give adequate space for the patient and staff to ensure easy withdrawal from an escalating situation.
5. Know where panic buttons or alarms are located. Sometimes it is necessary to wear a body alarm to ensure safety.

BOX 21-2

Setting Limits

1. Set limits in only those areas in which a clear need to protect the patient or others exists.
2. Establish realistic and enforceable consequences of exceeding limits.
3. Make patient aware of limits and the consequences of not adhering to the limits before incidents occur. The patient should be told in a clear, polite, and firm manner what the limits and consequences are, and should be given the opportunity to discuss any feelings or reactions to them.
4. All limits should be supported by the entire staff, written in the care plan, and communicated verbally to all involved.
5. When a decision to discontinue the limits is made by the entire staff, the decision is based on consistent desired behavior, not promises or sporadic efforts.
6. The staff should formulate their own plan to address their own difficult in maintaining consistent limits.

Adapted from Chitty K.K., & Maynard, C.K. (1986). Managing manipulation. *Journal of Psychosocial Nursing and Mental Health Services, 24*(6).

6. Exit strategies apply to both the nurse and the patient. The nurse should be positioned between the patient and the door, but not directly in front of the patient or in front of the doorway. Not only can this position be interpreted as confrontational, but it can also make the patient feel trapped. It is better to stand off to the side and encourage the patient to have a seat.
7. Set limits at the outset (Box 21-2).
   • Direct approach: "Violence is unacceptable." Describe the consequences (restraints, selcusion). Best for confused or psychotic patients.
   • Use indirect approach if patient is not confused or psychotic. Give patient a choice. "You have a choice. You can take this medication and go into the interview room (or hallway, etc.) and talk, or you can sit in the seclusion room until you feel less anxious."
8. When interviewing a patient whose behavior begins to escalate:
   • Provide feedback about what you observe: "You seem to be very upset." Such an observation allows exploration of the patient's feelings and may lead to de-escalation of the situation.
   • If the patient's behavior continues to escalate, end the interview and assure the patient that the staff will provide for the patient's, as well as everyone else's safety, and leave.

9. Having enough staff is essential for a show of strength and is often enough to head off confrontation. Only one person should talk to the patient, but staff need to maintain an unobtrusive presence in case the situation escalates.
10. Give the patient the opportunity to voluntarily walk to the quiet room without assistence when team interventions seem appropriate.
11. Do not touch the patient unless the team is with you and you are ready for a possible restraint situation.
12. In the event of a restraint or seclusion situation, the team functions as a single unit, with each member assigned a limb or a function as previously practiced according to unit protocols and policy.
13. Avoid wearing dangling earrings, necklaces, or ponytails. The patient may become focused on these and grab at them, causing serious injury. This is a serious danger.

Stages of the Violence Cycle

When interventions to prevent or deal with patient violence are considered, it is important to take into account the stages of the violence. These stages include the preassaultive stage, the assaultive stage, and the postassaultive stage when the patient returns to baseline. See Chapter 8 for nursing interventions for moderate levels of anxiety that escalates to severe and panic levels.

Preassaultive Stage: De-escalation Approaches

During the preassaultive stage, the patient becomes increasingly agitated. Staff requires training in both verbal techniques of de-escalation and physical techniques to restrain without harm. The better trained the staff, the less chance that either staff or patient will be injured. Frequently verbal interventions are sufficient during this stage. Interventions at this stage are listed in Table 21-1.

Throughout these procedures, maintain the patient's self-esteem and dignity. Linehan (1993) states that respect can be maintained if the nurse operates from the following assumptions:
   • Patients are doing the best they can
   • Patients want to improve
   • Patient's behaviors make sense within their worldview

The use of empathic statements such as, "It sounds like you are in pain and confused," "You're here to get help, and we're going to try to figure out what's going on," and "Let us help you, don't be afraid" can aid in reducing anxiety and anger. These statements reinforce the feeling that the person is in a safe environment and that everyone is there to help in his or her treatment (Petit, 2005).

TABLE 21-1   Interventions for the Preassaultive Stage

Intervention	Rationale
1. Pay attention to angry and aggressive behavior. Respond as early as possible (e.g., Box 21-1).	1. Minimization of angry behaviors and ineffective limit setting are the most frequent factors contributing to the escalation of violence.
2. Assess for and provide for personal safety.	2. Pay attention to the environment. • Leave door open or use hallway. Choose a quiet place, but one that is visible to staff. • Have a quick exit available. • If you are uncomfortable, have other staff nearby. • The more anrgy the patient, the more space needed to feel comfortable. • Never turn your back on an angry patient • If *on home visit,* go with a colleague. • Leave immediately if there are signs that behavior is escalating out of control.
3. Appear calm and in control.	3. The perception that someone is in control can be comforting and calming to an individual who is beginning to lose control.
4. Speak softly in a nonprovocative, nonjudgmental manner	4. When tone of voice is low and calm and the words are spoken slowly, anxiety levels in others may decrease.
5. Demonstrate genuineness and concern.	5. Even the most psychotic schizophrenic individual may respond to nonprovocative interpersonal contact and expressions of concern and caring.
6. Set clear, consistent, and enforceable limits on behavior (Box 21-2) (e.g., "It's okay to be angry with Tom, but it is not okay to threaten him. If you are having trouble controlling your anger we will help you").	6. Gives patient understanding of expectations and consequences of not adhering to those behaviors.
7. If patient is willing, both nurse and patient should sit at a 45-degree angle. Do not tower over or stare at the patient.	7. Sitting at a 45-degree angle puts you both on the same level but allows for frequent breaks in eye contact. Towering over or staring can be interpreted as threatening or controlling by paranoid individuals.
8. When patient begins to talk, listen. Use clarification.	8. Allows patient to feel heard and understood, help builds rapport, and energy can be channeled productively.
9. Acknowledge the patient's needs regardless of whether the expressed needs are rational or irrational, possible or impossible to meet.	9. Contributes to patient's perception that the nurse is trying to understand, and allows for problem solving how some of the patient's needs can be met in appropriate ways.

VIGNETTE

A 21-year-old male who was in an automobile accident is bedridden with a pelvic fracture. During his first day of admission, he yells at each nurse who walks by his room, using expletives in his demands that the nurse enter the room.

Intervention

The nurse who is assigned to the patient for the evening stops in his doorway after he yells at her. She asks in a calm, nonsarcastic manner showing mild disbelief, "Is this working for you? Do nurses really come in here when you yell at them that way?" The patient responds sullenly, justifying his behavior by complaining about his care. The nurse responds by saying, "It seems to me that you need to feel you can get care when you need it." The patient responds in a loud voice that he has been waiting 20 minutes for a bedpan and how would she like it? The nurse gets him his bedpan, and he has calmed down somewhat. The nurse's challenge has caught his attention. The nurse then goes on to suggest (i.e., teach) alternative strategies for contacting her and other nurses. The strategies are immediately put into use by the patient.

When health care personnel can teach patients alternate strategies and healthier ways to get their needs met, the patients have more choices and thus more control over their situation.

APPLYING THE ART   A Person with Anger and Aggression

SCENARIO: I'd just attended group on the forensic unit where the group leader had to set limits with 23-year-old Hector. During our initial one-to-one, Hector had been almost overly polite in contrast with his abrasiveness with some of the other patients in group. I followed Hector out of the group room.

THERAPEUTIC GOAL: By the end of this interaction, Hector will identify at least one incident where a person can demonstrate an action of kindness or caring towards another and still see self as manly.

Student-Patient Interaction	Thoughts, Communication Techniques, and Mental Health Nursing Concepts
Hector: *In harsh loud voice.* "Bunch of losers." **Student's feelings:** *I was taken aback and intimated by how lightening-fast Hector's anger arose when some other guys took the seats that Hector had chosen for us during group.*	He went from being friendly with me this morning to this abrupt outburst of anger.
Student: "You're talking about what just happened in group." *I walked towards the seating area closest to the nursing station.* **Student's feelings:** *After Hector's bullying episode in group, I feel safer in plain view.*	I *validate* to make sure I understand his reference. I'm beginning to realize that Hector's earlier politeness and charm might have to do with his *personality disorder.*
Hector: *In a loud and angry voice.* "Just because I made those guys get out of those seats. What did you think? You think that's such a big deal?"	
Student: "But why did you have to yell and scream at them? I remember some yelling and swearing." **Student's feelings:** *I didn't think this through with all his anger coming out. I am reacting defensively, and I'm feeling like I am in way over my head. I feel like I need a break.*	Asking a why question is nontherapeutic for sure. He will take it as criticism. I hope he doesn't get any angrier.
Student: "What were you feeling when you saw they were in the seats you wanted?" **Student's feelings:** *I hope he focuses on his feelings rather than my accusatory "why" question.*	I attempt to *translate* into feelings. When in doubt, always go for feelings.
Hector: "Look, I always get a raw deal. The leader likes those guys better than me."	After all this I don't think I will be going with him to *occupational therapy.* That way, I'll get to consult my instructor to check if I'm on the right track.
Student: "But when this happened, you were feeling. . . . what?" **Student's feelings:** *It really is okay to take care of myself. Knowing I can access my teacher soon lets me refocus and attend to Hector's needs.*	I again ask him to *focus* on his feelings.
Hector: "Nothing. Never mind."	I wonder what makes Hector unable to look at his feelings at all. He refers to the leader like he's competing for attention. Almost like *sibling rivalry.* Perhaps all that macho talk hides *low self-esteem.*

APPLYING THE ART   A Person with Anger and Aggression—cont'd

Student-Patient Interaction	Thoughts, Communication Techniques, and Mental Health Nursing Concepts
Student: "I think I'd feel frustrated when directed to give the other patients their original chairs back. Maybe even a little embarrassed."	I *give information* about self but really the intent serves to *reflect* Hector's possible feelings.
Hector: *Avoids eye contact.* "My dad would've pounded the ____ out of me for letting those guys win."	
Student: "You are able to say how your dad taught lessons with his fists. I'm guessing any little boy would feel enormous pressure when interacting with others means either you win or you get pounded." ***Student's feelings:*** *I'm beginning to see how powerless Hector must feel somewhere inside all that bravado. I am beginning to feel some compassion for him.*	I give *support* by using the words "you are able to" in order to encourage Hector to recognize a link between his current responses and past abusive experiences.
Hector: "He was just teaching me how to be a man."	He justifies his father pounding on him. A *history of violence* is the best *predictor of violence*. Hector defines how to be a man the same way his father did. Does he know other ways exist?
Student: "I wonder if a person can be a man in other ways besides winning or losing. This morning I saw you help when someone bumped the patient carrying breakfasts back for those who eat on the unit." ***Student's feelings:*** *My belief in my nursing self fluctuates. But I do feel some rapport exists between us.*	I use an *indirect question* and make an *observation* of his recent behavior. I know that when a person feels comfortable with you, even if one uses "nontherapeutic techniques" a person will often understand the intent behind the words.
Hector: "What a mess."	
Student: "And you helped anyway. Then when the patient apologized so much, you told him, 'It's okay. Accidents happen.' "	I *make observations* describing Hector's healthier behaviors, like spontaneously helping another.
Hector: "Others helped too."	Hector excels at generating *negative attention*. He does not know what to do with *positive feedback*.
Student: "You also spoke kindly to him."	Again I *make an observation* and give my attention to *positively reinforcing* his kind act.
Hector shrugs.	
Student: "Sometimes it seems manliness and kindness might coexist in one person."	I deliberately link Hector's kind words with his earlier idea of manhood.
Hector: *Nods slightly.* "I need a drink of water." *Goes to water fountain.* ***Student's feelings:*** *I feel glad that he nods even slightly. I find it difficult to make even small changes, like regularly flossing my teeth. What must Hector's world be like? I have people who care about me. Who does he have for support . . . especially since he's an expert at pushing others away?*	His *intermittent explosive disorder* is most likely connected to his repeated abusive "lessons" equating any vulnerability or even a kindness as weakness. Hector nods showing *partial understanding* that showing kindness is okay for a man, although it appears to make him anxious as he uses physical withdrawal (getting a drink) to protect himself (fight-or-flight).

Assaultive Stage: Medication, Seclusion, Restraint

If the patient progresses to the assaultive stage, the staff must respond quickly. Generally, a team approach with at least five staff members is advisable to restrain a resistant patient, but the team may be larger if the patient requires it. One leader speaks to the patient and instructs members of the team. Only the leader will communicate with the patient. The interventions include the use of medications and seclusion or physical restraints.

Seclusion refers to "the involuntary confinement of a patient alone in a room, which the patient is prevented from leaving" (HCFA, 1999). The goal of seclusion should never be punitive. Rather, the goal is safety of the patient and others. **Restraint** refers to "any manual method, or mechanical device, material or equipment attached or adjacent to the patient's body that he or she cannot easily remove that restricts freedom of movement or normal access to one's body" (HCFA, 1999). When applying the rule of thumb, the least restrictive means of restraint for the shortest duration, seclusion, or physical restraint is used only after alternative interventions have been attempted (e.g., medications, verbal interventions, decrease in sensory stimulation, removal of a particular problematic stimulus, presence of a significant other, frequent observation, and use of a sitter who provides 24-hour one-to-one observation of the patient).

Seclusion or restraint is used in the following circumstances (APNA, 2000):

- The patient presents a clear and present danger to self.
- The patient presents a clear and present danger to others.
- The patient has been legally detained for involuntary treatment and is thought to pose an escape risk.
- The patient requests to be secluded or restrained.

Prior to the development of psychotropic medications, seclusion and restraint were extremely common methods of managing aggressive behavior. In the past half century their use has decreased dramatically as a result of effective medications, as well as concern that such restriction was overused, abusive, and dangerous. All facilities that use seclusion and restraint have strict regulatory policies, and students should be familiar with their institutions' policies.

A patient may not be held in seclusion or restraint without a physician's order, although that order may be received *after* employing one of these methods. Once in restraint, a patient must be protected from all sources of harm. Each team member is trained in the correct use of physical restraining maneuvers as well as the use of physical restraints. The team is organized before approaching the patient so that each team member knows his or her individual responsibility regarding limb securing. Before approaching the patient, the team is prepared with the correct number and size of restraints and with medication, if ordered. The team leader explains to the patient in a matter-of-fact manner exactly what the team is about to do and why. If restraints are to be used, the patient is informed at this point of the team's intent and the reason for the team's actions. Sometimes, the patient is ready to cooperate and moves to the seclusion room, where either four-point or two-point restraints may be used.

Once the patient is restrained, the nurse might administer an intramuscular injection of an antipsychotic or an antihistamine, depending on the physician's order. The nurse's role is to provide an explanation to the patient for the medication and to make sure that the patient is properly restrained so that the medication can be safely administered. Throughout this time, the team leader continues to relate to the patient in a calm, steady voice, communicating decisiveness, consistency, and control.

While the patient is restrained and in seclusion, staff closely monitor the patient to determine the patient's ability to reintegrate into the unit activities. Reintegration is gradual and is geared to the patient's ability to handle increasing amounts of stimulation. If the reintegration proves to be too much for the patient and results in increased agitation, the patient is returned to the room or another quiet area.

Generally a structured reintegration is the best approach. For instance, reintegration can begin by reducing four-point restraints to two-point restraints. Once the patient no longer requires the locked seclusion room, the patient may be given specified time-out periods to leave the room and move slowly into the milieu of the unit. The time-out periods are gradually lengthened until the patient is able to maintain control within the unit.

VIGNETTE

A 19-year-old male has a 2-year history of quadriplegia. This patient also has a history of drug abuse that began in grade school, an inability to set or work toward long-term goals, and a primary coping style of anger and intimidation. The patient is admitted to an inpatient psychiatric unit because of increasing suicidal ideation. He clearly communicates to staff that his preferred means of coping with anger is to "cuss people out" and run into them with his wheelchair. However, in the hospital, the consequence of wheelchair assaults is that the patient is secluded in his room, which he finds intolerable. The patient asks the staff to help him manage his anger.

Intervention

The nurse assigned to this young man sets aside time to interview him regarding the triggers for his anger. He identifies

continued

several issues that "make him angry." These typically relate to feeling unheard and controlled by the staff. Together the nurse and patient examine alternative ways for him to deal with these situations, such as telling the staff that he does not feel that they are listening to him and letting them know that he needs to be involved in the planning of his care to increase his sense of control. The patient and nurse role-play a situation in which the patient is told by a staff member that he must attend a group session. Such a situation would usually result in the patient's becoming angry and aggressive, but in the role-play he is willing to "try out" alternative communication techniques to communicate his feelings to the staff member and thus to handle his anger. In addition, the patient is willing to enter into a behavioral contract with the nurse who states that he will not curse at staff or assault anyone with his wheelchair. Instead, he will let the staff know when he is feeling angry and what the triggering issue is so that a nonaggressive resolution can be found.

Response

Because this patient is motivated to gain increased personal control, he responds positively to these suggestions. In addition, once it becomes clear that issues of feeling unheard and out of control underlies most episodes of anger, the patient is able to target these issues for problem solving. He rapidly develops effective and appropriate ways to make himself heard and understood. He also becomes adept at communicating when he feels out of control and at finding ingenious ways of negotiating control on issues that are particularly important to him. The patient's suicidal impulses, which occur when he is frustrated, also diminish.

Postassaultive Stage

Once the patient no longer requires seclusion or restraints, the staff should review the incident with the patient as well as among themselves. Discussion with the patient is an important part of the therapeutic process. Going over what has occurred allows the patient to learn from the situation, identify the stressors that precipitated the out-of-control behavior, and plan alternative ways of responding to these stressors in the future.

Critical Incident Debriefing

Staff analysis of an episode of violence, referred to as **critical incident debriefing**, is crucial for a number of reasons. *First,* a review is necessary to ensure that quality care was provided to the patient. Staff members need to critically examine their response to the patient. Questions to be answered include the following:

- Could we have done anything that would have prevented the violence?
- If yes, then what could have been done, and why wasn't it done in this situation?

- Did the team respond as a team? Were team members acting according to the policies and procedures of the unit? If not, why not?
- Is there a need for additional staff education regarding how to respond to violent patients?
- How do staff members feel about this patient? About this situation? Feelings of fear and anger must be discussed and handled. Otherwise, the patient may be dealt with in a punitive and nontherapeutic manner.

Second, the profound effects of workplace violence do not, unfortunately, disappear after the incident is over, and the harm is not only to the individual assaulted. Clements and colleagues (2005) state that some nurses will internalize (depression, avoidance, withdrawal) and others will externalize (anger, outbursts, fluctuating mood) emotional and behavioral responses. These are normal response to an abnormal event. However, agencies need to provide support and debriefing to prevent long-term psychological sequelae for all types of workplace violence (Alexy & Hutchins, 2006). Employee morale, productivity, use of sick leave, transfer requests, and absenteeism are affected by patient violence, especially if a staff member has been injured. Staff members must feel supported by their peers as well as by the organizational policies and procedures established to maintain a safe environment.

Documentation of a Violent Episode

Most facilities provide standardized seclusion and restraint records. There are a number of areas in which the nurse *must* provide documentation in situations in which violence was either averted or actually occurred:

- Assessment of behaviors that occurred during the preassaultive stage *(time)*
- Nursing interventions and the patient's responses *(time)*
- Evaluation of the interventions used
- Detailed description of the patient's behaviors during the assaultive stage
- All nursing interventions used to defuse the crisis
- Patient's response to those interventions
- Who was called to assess the patient and order and any medications, seclusion, and or restraints *(time)*
- Time patient put in restraints or seclusion
- Observations of and interventions performed while the patient was in restraints or seclusion *(food, toileting, vital signs, verbatim statements, and general behaviors) (15 to 30 minutes depending on state law)*
- Any injuries to staff or patient
- The way in which the patient was reintegrated into the unit milieu *(time and behavior)*

See Chapter 26 for more definitive legal and procedural guidelines.

Anticipating Increased Anxiety and Anger in Hospital Settings

Hospitals can be lonely, scary places for many people. Patients often feel that they are not being heard, and they may feel vulnerable, discounted, frightened, out of control of their situation, and tired. Some patients may have specific vulnerabilities for responding to their increasing anxiety and loss of autonomy through the use of violence. Therefore some patients with poor coping skills or mental or neurological problems may resort to anger, intimidation, or violence to obtain their short-term goals of feelings of control or mastery. For others, the anger occurs when limited or primitive attempts at coping are unsuccessful and alternatives are unknown. For these patients, anger and violence are particular risks in inpatient settings.

This is especially true for hospitalized patients with chemical or alcohol dependency that may be anxious about being cut off from their substance of choice; they may have well-founded concerns that any physical pain will be inadequately addressed. Many patients with marginal coping also have personality styles that externalize blame. That is, they see the source of their discomfort and anxiety as being outside themselves; relief must therefore also come from an outside source (e.g., the nurse, medication).

Interventions begin with attempts to understand and meet the patient's needs. For instance, baseline anxiety can be moderated by the provision of comfort items before they are requested (e.g., decaffeinated coffee, deck of cards); this can build rapport and acts symbolically to reassure. Anxiety also can be minimized by reducing ambiguity. This strategy includes clear and concrete communication. An interaction providing clarity about what the nurse can and cannot do is most usefully ended by offering something within the nurse's power to provide (i.e., leaving the patient with a "yes").

Interventions for anxiety might also include the use of distractions, such as magazines, action comics, and video games. Generally, distractions that are colorful and do not require sustained attention work best, although this varies according to the patient's interests and abilities. Finally, patients with a high level of baseline anxiety and limited coping skills are helped when their interactions with the treatment team are predictable; this might include speaking with the physician at a specific time each day or having the patient see a single spokesperson from the treatment team each day.

Because some patients have limited coping skills, once anxiety is moderated, nursing interventions include teaching alternative behaviors and strategies. With increased tools to deal with anxiety and frustration, patients have the opportunity have choices and increase a sense of control over their behaviors.

Often, anger may be communicated via verbal abuse directed at the nurse. If attempts to teach alternatives have not been successful, three interventions can be used:

1. The first is to leave the room as soon as the abuse begins; the patient can be informed that the nurse will return in a specific amount of time (e.g., 20 minutes) when the situation is calmer. This is said in a matter-of-fact manner. If the nurse is in the middle of a procedure and cannot leave immediately, the nurse can break off conversation and eye contact, completing the procedure quickly and efficiently before leaving the room. Note that the nurse avoids chastising, threatening, or responding punitively to the patient.

2. Withdrawal of attention to the abuse is successful only if a second intervention is also used. This step requires attending positively to, and thus reinforcing, nonabusive communication by the patient. Interventions can include discussing non–illness-related topics, responding to requests, and providing emotional support.

3. Patients who are regularly verbally abusive may respond best to the predictability of routine, such as scheduled contacts with the nurse (e.g., every 30 minutes or every 60 minutes) as long as the patient's behavior is not abusive. Such a contract works only to the extent that the nurse maintains the scheduled contacts as agreed on and other staff members must be informed of the care plan and remain consistent so that they do not inadvertently sabotage it by responding to incidental requests by the patient. If the patient's illness or injury requires nursing care outside the scheduled contact times, these visits can be carried out in a calm, brief manner. This contract is negotiated with the patient and addresses the patient's anxiety about getting needs met and being heard.

Implementing appropriate interventions can be difficult when the nurse is feeling threatened. Remaining matter-of-fact with patients who habitually use anger and intimidation can be difficult because these people are often skillful at making personal and pointed statements. It is important for the nurse to remember that patients do not know their nurses personally and thus, have no basis on which they can make accurate judgments. Nurses can also vent their own responses elsewhere, with other staff or family members, or via critical incident debriefing.

Anxiety Reduction Techniques

There are a number of strategies that nurses can teach and individuals can learn to help control anxiety and minimize anxiety escalation, including relaxation training, deep breathing exercises, journaling, meditation, learning more effective problem-solving techniques, learning to listen rather than jump impulsively, taking time out, and physical exercise. Sometimes people need more in-depth teaching, in which case a trained anger management therapist is indicated.

Interventions for Patients with Cognitive Deficits

Patients with cognitive deficits are particularly at risk for acting aggressively. Such deficits may result from delirium, dementia (e.g., Alzheimer's disease, multi-infarct dementia), or brain injury. Traditional approaches to disorientation and to the agitation that it can cause have relied heavily on reality orientation and medication. Reality orientation consists of providing the correct information to the patient about place, date, and current life circumstances. For some patients, orientation does not work. Because of their cognitive disorder, they can no longer "enter into our reality," and they become frightened and agitated and may become aggressive.

Sedating medication may calm agitation, but in some cases the risks may outweigh the benefits. Sedation only further clouds a patient's sensorium, which makes disorientation worse and increases the risks of falls and injuries. It is better to examine alternative interventions.

Sometimes the patient with a cognitive disorder experiences such severe agitation and aggression that it is referred to as a **catastrophic reaction.** The patient may scream, strike out, or cry because of overwhelming fear. Adopting a calm and unhurried manner is the best response. The steps for making contact with a patient experiencing a catastrophic reaction are listed in Box 21-3.

To respond effectively to episodes of agitation, it is crucial to identify the antecedents, or what preceded the episode, and the consequences of such episodes. Once antecedents are understood, interventions are often obvious. Consequences of agitation also may be a factor if they serve to reinforce the behaviors. For example, an older man who loves ice cream and becomes calm when it is given to him becomes agitated more often when ice cream is routinely used to stop his angry behaviors.

Finally, patients who misperceive their setting or life situation may be calmed by validation therapy (Feil, 1992). Some disoriented patients believe that they are young and feel the need to return to important tasks that were a

---

BOX 21-3

Cognitive Deficits and the Catastrophic Reaction: Making Contact

Cognitive deficits result in:
- A decreased ability to interpret sensory stimuli.
- A decreased ability to tolerate sensory stimuli.

Striking out represents fear or the feeling that the environment is out of control.

Presence of a second agitated person (e.g., staff member) leads to increased agitation; therefore:

1. Face the patient from within 2 feet, remaining as calm and unhurried as possible.
2. Say the patient's name.
3. Gain eye contact.
4. Smile.
5. Repeat (2) through (4) several times if necessary, to gain and maintain contact.
6. Use gentle touch and keep voice soft (the person often matches this tone and lowers his or her voice also).
7. Ask the patient if there's a need to use the bathroom.
8. Help the patient regain a sense of control—ask what is needed.
9. Validate the patient's feelings: "You look upset. This can be a confusing place."
10. Use short, simple sentences. Complex explanations just represent more noise.
11. Decrease sensory stimulation.
12. Get the patient to use rhythmic sources of self-stimulation (e.g., humming, a rocking chair).

Adapted from Rader, J., Doan, J., & Schwab, M. (1985). How to decrease wandering, a form of agenda behavior. *Geriatric Nursing, 6*(4), 196-199.

---

significant part of their earlier years. For example, an older woman may insist that she must go home to take care of her babies. Telling the patient that her babies have grown up and there is no home to return to is not only cruel but nontherapeutic and will result in increased agitation. It is often more helpful to reflect back to the patient the feelings behind her demand and to show understanding and concern for her worry.

Rather than attempting to reorient the patient, the nurse asks him or her to further describe the setting or situation that the patient has reported to be a problem (e.g., the need to return home). During the conversation, the nurse can comment on what appears to be underlying the patient's distress, thus validating it. For example, the woman who believes that she needs to return home to care for her children is asked to tell the nurse more about her children. The nurse may note that the patient misses her children and may be lonely: "Mrs. Green, you miss your children, and the hospital can be a lonely place."

As the nurse shows interest in aspects of the patient's life, the nurse establishes himself or herself as a safe, understanding person who can be trusted. In turn, the patient often becomes calmer and more open to redirection. As patients reminisce in this fashion, they often bring themselves into the present: "Of course, they're all grown and doing well on their own now." See Chapter 15 for more on interventions for people with cognitive impairments.

VIGNETTE

An 81-year-old female with Alzheimer's disease always becomes agitated during her morning care; this comes to be a time dreaded by her caregivers. Careful observation of the antecedents to episodes of agitation reveals a natural course to the morning problems. The patient is initially calm when care begins. However, one staff person gives morning care to the patient and her roommate at the same time, moving between the two. Observation of the process reveals that the patient becomes distracted by cues being given to her roommate and often startles when the caregiver returns to her. As this process continues over several minutes, the patient becomes increasingly distressed and then agitated. When a change is made so that the patient's care is provided by one person who remains with her throughout the process, the patient's morning agitation ends.

Psychotherapy

Management of chronic aggression requires comprehensive neuropsychological testing and cognitive-behavioral assessment to establish the appropriate treatment approach for each individual. Besides psychopharmacological treatment, individual therapies may include behavioral management, cognitive-behavioral techniques, family interventions, and psychosocial supports (Sanders, 2004).

The cognitive-behavioral assessment includes determining the psychotherapeutic approach most appropriate for a chronically aggressive patient. Data are obtained as to the type of aggressive behavior, psychiatric diagnosis, and patient's intellectual ability. For example, individuals with schizophrenia and those with organic brain disease (mental retardation, dementias, autism, brain injury) who experience a marginal response to medications, might do well with behavioral techniques. People with personality disorders whose aggression is secondary to difficulties in

regulating emotional states, are often more effectively treated with cognitive-behavioral techniques (Alpert & Spillmann, 1997). It should be noted that anger treatment is *not* indicated for those who cannot control their violent behavior or whose violent behavior fits their own personal goals and is experienced in a positive or satisfactory manner by the violent individual (Quanbeck, 2006).

Behavioral interventions are based on social learning theory. This theory supports the belief that social behaviors are learned and acquired over time through two mechanisms: (1) experiencing success or failure as a result of one's own actions, and (2) observing the positive and negative consequences of others' behaviors (Quanbeck, 2006). The goal of behavioral intervention is to restructure the consequences of a person's actions so that the link between aggressive behavior and its reinforcers are weakened, while the link between alternative, more socially acceptable behaviors is reinforced.

One such behavioral strategy is the **token economy.** In this behavioral approach, a person earns a "token" when socially acceptable behaviors are demonstrated. This token can be accumulated and traded in for privileges (games, TV time, or snacks) (Quanbeck, 2006). Often social skills training is used in conjunction with behavioral programs, teaching the individual alternative and effective behaviors for getting needs met. Patients often learn assertive and self-control skills in an individual or a group setting.

Cognitive-behavioral approaches are based on anger management techniques. Novaco's (1997) cognitive-behavioral model of anger asserts that anger and aggression are mediated by a person's perception of threat from others and an ability to formulate strategies for managing conflict in a nonaggressive manner. Anger management skills training programs teach participants the following key components:

- Stress inoculation (imagining angry scenarios and using relaxation techniques to decrease arousal)
- Identifying and challenging cognitive distortions (misattributing the intentions of others as hostile)
- Identifying their own unique early signs of anger so they are more aware when they need to use anger management skills
- Early recognition of potentially provocative situations and implementation of nonaggressive responses (problem solving)
- Providing a person with behavioral skills for managing conflict, such as walking away

Dialectical behavioral therapy (DBT) (Linehan) is effective in people with borderline personality disorders and has also been found useful to treat violence and anger in male forensic patients (Evershead et al., 2003).

Pharmacological, Biological, and Integrative Therapies

Medications for Acute Aggression

Medications that are most frequently used in emergency violent situations are **atypical antipsychotics** (e.g., intramuscular [IM] risperidone, olanzapine, ziprasidone) or high-potency **typical neuroleptics** (e.g., IM haloperidol). They are both first-line treatments for acute aggression and psychosis-induced violence. **Benzodiazepines** (e.g., lorazepam) are often the first choice for acute aggressive episodes, especially in episodic dyscontrol and incipient rage episodes (Maxmen & Ward, 2002).

Atypical antipsychotics have fewer side effects, although most do not have short-acting IM injectable if the patient refuses to take oral medication. Olanzapine short-acting IM has many caveats for use and should be used only if a person has had previous dystonic or severe extapyramidal symptoms from IM haloperidol, or needs an antipsychotic but has preexisting stable cardiac disease, or there has been no response an hour after giving IM lorazepam (Gaskell, 2006).

Among the typical antipsychotics, haloperidol is usually the first choice. It is sedating, can be given in higher doses, and is less likely to cause orthostatic hypotension. However, there are risks for hypotension in large doses, oversedation, and acute dystonic reactions.

Lorazepam is often a first choice of among the benzodiazepines. Violence, aggression, and suicidality associated with panic or anger attacks are responsive to benzodiazepines.

Medications for Chronic Aggression

Chronic aggression is a common problem in psychiatry, and aggression can be diminished only after a therapeutic dose of the appropriate medication is used for 4 to 8 weeks. Carbamazepine is useful for intermittent explosive disorder, borderline personality disorder, posttraumatic stress disorder, and schizophrenia. Beta blockers (e.g., propranolol, nadolol, pindolol) and buspirone (BuSpar) are helpful in organically based violence (e.g., dementias, head injuries, stroke). Beta blockers are useful in decreasing aggressive behavior in schizophrenia. Lithium is effective in a wide range of Axis I and II disorders (e.g., bipolar disorder, borderline personality disorder, conduct disorder, and episodic dyscontrol). Anticonvulsants (e.g., phenytoin, carbamazepine) have been shown to reduce impulsive rage reactions in individuals with antisocial and borderline personality disorders, substance use disorder, attention deficit disorder, and intermittent explosive disorder.

EVALUATION

Evaluation of the care plan is essential for patients who are angry and aggressive. A well-considered plan has specific outcome criteria. Evaluation provides information about the extent to which the interventions have achieved the outcomes. If the outcomes have not been achieved, the plan must be revised. Revision focuses on all aspects of the nursing process:

- Was the assessment accurate and thorough?
- Were the nursing diagnoses applicable to the assessment data?
- Did the nursing diagnoses accurately drive nursing interventions?
- Was the plan comprehensive and individualized?
- Were interventions appropriate?
- Were interventions carried out properly?

For instance, the initial plan may have included assessment of the environmental stimuli that precede a patient's agitation. Once these are identified the plan provides interventions that are specific to those stimuli. However, the plan can work only if staff members evaluate the effectiveness of the approach by noting the extent to which agitation is decreased. Evaluation may reveal that the patient's agitation has decreased except in specific situations. The plan is then revised to include these situations.

KEY POINTS TO REMEMBER

- Angry emotions and aggressive actions are difficult targets for nursing intervention.
- Nurses benefit from an understanding of how the angry and aggressive patient should be approached.
- Understanding patient cues to escalating aggression, appropriate goals for intervention for individuals in a variety of situations, and helpful nursing interventions is important for nurses in any setting.
- The roles of sociocultural influences and neurobiological vulnerabilities are intertwined in a person's propensity for violence.
- Cues to assess when anger is escalating (verbal and nonverbal, including facial expression, breathing, body language, and posture) are provided.
- Assess patient's history. A patient's past aggressive behavior is the most important indicator of future aggressive episodes.
- Many approaches are effective in helping patients de-escalate and maintain control.
- The general hierarchy of interventions for coping with aggression is verbal intervention, psychopharmacology, seclusion, and then restraint.

KEY POINTS TO REMEMBER—cont'd

- Different interventions are used depending on the patient's level of anger.
- Guidelines for de-escalation of patient behavior are given.
- Specific medications such as antipsychotics, lithium, and antianxiety medications may be useful.
- Seclusion or restraints may be needed to ensure the safety of the patient as well as the safety of other patients and the staff.

- Each unit has a clear protocol for the safe use of restraints and for the humane management of care during the time the patient is restrained, as well as clear guidelines for understanding and protecting the patient's legal rights.
- Careful documentation throughout any incidence of escalating violence, especially leading to seclusion or restraints according to the laws of your state.

CRITICAL THINKING

1. Mr. Arnold, a 24-year-old with mania, is admitted to an inpatient unit. Staff note that the patient is agitated and irritable and has a history of assault. He shouts at the nurse in a loud piercing voice that she is a "slut, a mut, tut-tut." He is pacing back and forth pointing his finger at the staff.
   A. What are the appropriate nursing diagnoses for him at this time?
   B. What interventions would most likely be effective at this time?
   C. Role-play verbal techniques you could use during any other interventions being initiated at this time.

2. In the morning 2 days later, Mr. Arnold comes to the nurses' desk and asks for a pass. When told that it was up to the physician to write an order, who wouldn't be in until the afternoon, Mr. Arnold becomes verbally loud, demanding that the nurse phone the physician "right this minute to get that pass."
   A. What interventions do you think most appropriate to start at this time?
   B. Role-play your verbal techniques.
3. Write a summary of the protocol for intervening with irate patients as found in the hospital procedure manual.

CHAPTER REVIEW

Choose the most appropriate answer.
1. Which is a clinical example of "predictability of routine" that can be used with an angry, verbally abusive patient who has underlying anxiety about getting needs heard and met?
   1. The nurse refocuses conversation to minimize patient tangentiality.
   2. The nurse empathizes with the patient's underlying fear and anxiety.
   3. The nurse agrees to meet with the patient for 10 minutes every 2 hours.
   4. The nurse teaches the patient techniques to manage auditory hallucinations.
2. In planning intervention for an angry patient, the nurse must understand that withdrawal of attention to verbally abusive behaviors works only if the strategy is accompanied by:
   1. attending positively to nonabusive communication.
   2. requiring the patient to wait before granting requests.
   3. giving large doses of antipsychotic medication.
   4. using empathic communication.

3. To help prevent displays of anger and aggression, the nurse must understand that anger and aggression are preceded by feelings of:
   1. vulnerability.
   2. depression.
   3. elation.
   4. isolation.
4. Which of the following is most useful to the nurse planning intervention for an angry patient?
   1. Creative, individualized approaches to the patient's behavior by staff members
   2. The availability of group therapy sessions focused on cathartic expression of emotion
   3. An understanding of the patient's medical diagnosis
   4. Consistency of approach to the patient by staff members
5. The nurse should understand that encouraging a patient to vent anger:
   1. is a strategic nursing intervention.
   2. should always be taught as a beneficial anger management technique.
   3. is not always useful.
   4. is useful only in a well-controlled inpatient setting.

REFERENCES

Alexy, E.M., & Hutchins, J.A. (2006). Workplace violence: A primer for critical care nurses. In H.J. Thompson & E.M. Alexy (Eds.), *Violence, injury and trauma*. Philadelphia: Saunders.

Alpert, J.E., & Spillmann, M.K. (1997). Psychotherapeutic approaches to aggressive and violent patients. *Psychiatric Clinics of North America, 20*(2), 453-472.

American Psychiatric Nurses Association. (2001). *Position statement on the use of seclusion and restraint. Journal of the American Psychiatric Nurses Association, 7*, 130-133.

American Psychological Association. (2007). Controlling anger—before it controls you. Retrieved March 15, 2007, from http://apa.org/topics/controlanger.html.

Brackbill, Y., White, M., Wilson, M., et al. (1990). Family dynamics as predictors of infant disposition. *Infant Mental Health Journal, 11*(2), 113-126.

Brook, J., Whiteman, M., & Brook, D. (1999). Transmission of risk factors across three generations. *Psychological Reports, 85*(1), 227-241.

Centers for Disease Control and Prevention, National Institute for Occupational Safety and Health. (2002). *Violence: Occupational hazards in hospitals* (DHHS [NIOSH] Publication 2002-101). Retrieved March 7, 2005, from www.cdc.gov/niosh/2002-101.html.

Clements, P.T., DeRanieri, J.T., Clark, K., et al. (2005). Workplace violence and corporate policy for health care settings. *Nursing Economics, 23*(3), 119-124.

Eisenberg, N., Fabes, R.A., Shepard, S.A., et al. (1997). Contemporaneous and longitudinal prediction of children's social functioning from regulation and emotionality. *Child Development, 68*(4), 642-664.

Evershed, S., Tennant, A., Boomer, D., et al. (2003). Practice-based outcomes of dialectical behavior therapy (DBT) targeting anger and violence, with male forensic patients: A pragmatic and non-contemporaneous comparison. *Criminal Behavior and Mental Health, 13*(3), 198-213.

Feil, N., & de Klerk-Rubin, V. (1992). *V/F validation: The Feil method*. Cleveland, OH: Edward Feil Productions.

Filley, C.M., Price, B.H., Neil, V.D., et al. (2001). Toward an understanding of violence: neurobehavioral aspects of unwarranted physical aggression: Aspen neurobehavioral conference consensus statement. *Cognitive and Behavioral Neurology, 14*(1), 1-14.

Gaskell, C. (2006). Guidelines for the management of acute behavioural disturbance in adult and older peoples inpatient wards. Cambridge and Peterborough Mental Health Partnership NHS Trust: A Cambridge University Teaching Trust. Retrieved July 11, 2007, from www.cambsmh.nhs.uk/documents/Clinical/Rapid_Tranquillisation_Guidelines14122005.pdf.

Health Care Financing Administration, Centers for Medicare & Medicaid Programs (HCFA). (1999). *Hospital conditions of patient's rights: Interim final rule*. Washington, DC: Author.

Kavoussi, R., Armstead, P., & Coccaro, E. (1997). The neurobiology of impulsive aggression. *Psychiatric Clinics of North America, 20*(2), 395-403.

Lewis, D.O. (2005). Adult antisocial behavior, criminality, and violence. In B.J. Sadock & V.A. Sadock (Eds.), *Kaplan & Sadock's comprehensive textbook of psychiatry* (8th ed.). Philadelphia: Lippincott Williams & Wilkins.

Linehan, M. (1993). *Cognitive-behavioral treatment of borderline personality disorder*. New York: Guilford Press.

Maxmen, J.S., Ward, N.G., Dubovsky, S.L., et al. (2002). *Psychotropic drugs: fast facts* (3rd ed.). New York: Norton.

Novaco, R.W. (1997). Remediating anger and aggression with violent offenders. *Legal and Criminological Psychology, 2*, 77-88.

Petit, J.R. (2005). Management of the acutely violent patient. *Psychiatric Clinics of North America, 28*(3), 701-711.

Quanbeck, C. (2006). Forensic psychiatric aspects of inpatient violence. *Psychiatric Clinics of North America, 29*(3), 743-760.

Sadock, B.J., & Sadock, V.A. (2004). *Kaplan & Sadock's concise textbook of clinical psychiatry* (2nd ed.). Philadelphia: Lippincott Williams & Wilkins.

Sadock, B.J., & Sadock, V.A. (2007). *Kaplan & Sadock's synopsis of psychiatry* (10th ed.). Philadelphia: Lippincott Williams & Wilkins.

Sanders, K.M. (2004). The violent patient. In T.A. Stern, J.B. Herman, & P.L. Slavin (Eds.), *Massachusetts General Hospital guide to primary care psychiatry* (2nd ed). New York: McGraw-Hill.

CHAPTER 22

Grief and Loss

Elizabeth M. Varcarolis

Key Terms and Concepts

Objectives

1. Differentiate between the terms *bereavement* and *mourning*.
2. Compare the characteristics of normal bereavement with those of complicated grieving.
3. Summarize the similarities among the frameworks (models) of understanding loss through stages (Kübler-Ross, Parkes, Engel, Lindemann, Bowlby, etc.).
4. Discuss the behavioral outcomes that indicate a successful bereavement.
5. Describe situations and circumstances that could affect a person's coming to terms with loss.

For additional resources related to the content of this chapter, visit the Evolve website at http://evolve.elsevier.com/Varcarolis/essentials.

- Chapter Outline
- Chapter Review Answers

- Nurse, Patient, and Family Resources
- Concept Map Creator

Loss is part of the human experience, and grief and bereavement are the normal responses to loss. We grieve on a recurring basis as we face the commonplace losses in our lives, be they loss of a relationship (divorce, separation, death, abortion), health (a body function or part, mental or physical capacity), friendship, status, prestige, or security (occupational, financial, social, cultural). Some losses may be even more intangible such as the loss of a projected future or dreams. Normal losses include changes in circumstances, such as retirement, promotion, marriage, and aging.

The course of our lives depends on how we adapt to losses and how we use change as a vehicle for growth. Changes that we do not adapt to—or fully mourn—may negatively affect our lives by sapping energy and impairing ability to connect (Volkan & Zintl, 1993).

Loss through death is a major life crisis. People grieve because they have become attached and deeply committed to the dying person. To sever that bond is to do without shared joy, security, satisfaction, growth, and comfort (Tschudin, 1997). On the whole, this is a physically painful process. Simone Weil (1998) described grief as an "almost biological disorder caused by the brutal unloosing of an energy hitherto absorbed by an attachment and now left undirected." Losses of this kind can hurt and diminish the part of life that is shared with and related to others, but it can also hurt and diminish one's inner life, which is not so readily shared (Tschudin, 1997).

It is well known and documented that the sequelae of grief for some may result in morbidity and mortality. Williams's (2002) extensive review of the literature substantiated that grieving spouses are far more likely to experience cardiovascular death and depression than are their peers not experiencing grief. The *Diagnostic and Statistical Manual of Mental Disorders* (*DSM-IV-TR*) places bereavement in "Additional Conditions That May Be a Focus of Clinical Attention."

Grief is the reaction to loss. Normal grief reactions include depressed mood, insomnia, anxiety, poor appetite, loss of interest, guilt, dreams about the deceased, and poor concentration. Psychological states include shock, denial, anger, and yearning and searching for the deceased. Anger is related to feelings of being abandoned and left alone without the love and support of the loved one. As common as it is in the normal process of mourning, some individuals react uncomfortably when these intense feelings emerge. The acute grief reaction typically lasts from 4 to 8 weeks, the active symptoms of grief usually last from 3 to 6 months, and the work of mourning may take from 1 to 2 years or more to complete.

Bereavement is the social experience of dealing with the death of a loved one. It refers to the event of losing an important person to death and is derived from the Old English word *berafian,* meaning "to rob." People react within their own cultural patterns and their own value and personality structure as within their own social environment. Most of us are programmed in our responses to death. **Mourning** refers to culturally patterned expressions of bereavement and grief. Sensitivity to the ethnic, cultural, spiritual, and religious beliefs of a diverse cultural population can help nurses more effectively identify a person's needs (Bateman, 1999).

Denial and fear of death are strong in the American culture, which affects the ways in which the bereaved, family, and those who support the family experience and express grief. Advances in medicine have fed the cultural expectation that only the old will die, and little attention is paid to coping with grief throughout the life span. Geographic mobility has eroded communities that used to provide a context for grief support. Mourning and bereavement have been deritualized in economically developed countries, which further reduces cultural comfort with mourning (Cable, 1998).

Nurses are affected by cultural myths and conditions in the same way the rest of society is; when they are faced with a person who is dying, nurses may feel uncomfortable and unequipped to face the loss. They may remember their own losses that have not been fully grieved. Difficult memories and unresolved feelings are often awakened. When staff members have not been able to resolve their own conflicts with loss, their ability to help others is minimized. Psychological support and education should be available to help staff better understand the grieving process. When nurses examine their own feelings and their personal experiences of loss, verbal and nonverbal clues to the needs of grieving family members of a dying patient become more apparent (Marks, 1976).

Sometimes nurses grieve with family members at the death of a person they have cared for and become fond of. Sometimes, an entire staff may mourn the death of a patient. After patients die, nurses may be faced with managing their own tasks of mourning, such as making sense of the death, dealing with mild to intense emotions, and realigning relationships. Albert (2001) states that "in the face of overwhelming, unending death, health care workers may come to question their deepest values, the meaning of their existence, and the value of the work they do." Losses such as these are often complicated and may come under the heading of disenfranchised grief. Disenfranchised grief and grief engendered by public tragedy are two specific types of grief worth examining here.

DISENFRANCHISED GRIEF

There are circumstances under which an individual experiences an intense loss that is not congruent with a socially recognized and sanctioned role; for example, the role of lover, neighbor, foster parent, in-law, caregiver, roommate, co-worker, counselor, or health care worker (Albert, 2001). Often these mourners do not have the opportunity to publicly grieve the loss. Doka (1989) refers to these experiences as **disenfranchised grief**—"the grief a person experiences when they [sic] incur a loss that is not and cannot be openly acknowledged, publicly mourned, or socially supported." Thus health care workers may experience real grief over the loss of a patient, a grief that may not be recognized or acknowledged by others. This grief may be solitary and uncomforted (Albert, 2001) and may be difficult to resolve.

GRIEF ENGENDERED BY PUBLIC TRAGEDY

Another kind of loss can be caused by public tragedies. **Public tragedies** involve a loss whose effect is felt broadly across a community or the general public. Because of the scale of the loss, many are affected, and the events often involve strong elements of surprise and shock (Corr, 2003). The media bring pictures and coverage of devastating events right into our home, and often the coverage is repeated over and over, allowing us to witness these tragedies secondhand and, in so doing, making the devastation more immediately real to us. Common public tragedies include, among others:

- Terrorist assaults (e.g., the terrorist attacks on September 11, 2001)
- Assassinations
- Tornados, earthquakes, flooding, or hurricanes (e.g., Katrina)
- Large-scale wildfires
- Well-publicized kidnappings of children who are later found to have been assaulted or killed
- School shootings (e.g., Columbine, Virginia Tech, Northern Illinois University)

Responses to a public tragedy encompass two ongoing processes (Corr & Doka, 2001):

1. Coping with loss, grief, and trauma
2. Finding ways to adapt to a changing world

After a public tragedy, life has forever changed for many of those involved. As an example, since the September 11, 2001, terrorist attacks, life will never be the same for most of us in the United States, certainly for those who lost loved ones, for the first responders, and for all those living in New York City at that time.

THEORY

Grieving is a psychological process that involves disengaging strong emotional ties from a significant relationship and reinvesting the energy once given to the deceased into a new and productive direction over a period of time. This reinvestment of emotional energy into new relationships or creative activities is necessary for a person's mental health and ability to function in society. It does not necessarily mean that a relationship with the deceased has ended, when ties were strong the experience of the relationship remains after the physical presence of the person has long since departed.

Studies of grief and loss by Parkes (1970, 1975), Caplan (1974), Engel (1964), Kübler-Ross (1969), and others postulated various phases of bereavement that proceed in orderly sequences within certain time frames. In reality, these phases overlap, and regression to previous phases is common and usually marked by erratic peaks and valleys. The distinct phases of human response to death and dying identified by Kübler-Ross (denial, anger, bargaining, depression, and acceptance) do not occur in a specific order; instead, an individual might go through all phases in the space of a few minutes, in varying order (Tschudin, 1997).

The various frameworks for grieving and phases of grief are useful models for helping people to normalize the deeply felt and disturbing phenomena they experience when they confront profound loss. Denial and shock, anger and guilt, emotional turmoil, disorganization, panic, depression, loneliness, and, eventually, acceptance of the loss are common during bereavement. Models and frameworks help organize the experience of loss, but models do not provide the focus of care when facilitating the process of mourning.

Some of the most widely known grief theorists are George Engel, Colin Parkes, Erich Lindemann, John Bowlby, and Edgar Jackson. Although each theorist uses different terminology, the process all of them outline is fundamentally the same. Each describes commonly experienced psychological and behavioral phenomena. However, we now know that these phenomena do not always follow a pattern of response. The following are common phenomena a person may experience at some point in the grief process:

1. Shock and disbelief
2. Denial
3. Sensation of somatic distress

EXAMINING THE EVIDENCE   Grieving: The Case Against Closure

My 80-year-old patient just lost his wife of 45 years to a devastating throat cancer 2 months ago. The tumor was so far advanced when they found it that they had to remove her vocal cords, and the experience was horrifying for him. He thinks about her all the time and feels guilty that she died and he lived when she was such a beautiful person. He stares at the floor, is barely eating, and doesn't want to attend activities. I don't know what to say to help bring him closure.

Few people get through life without experiencing significant loss. In a perfect world we'd view grief as a positive outcome of having caring and being cared for. However, grief can be devastating and become a permanent and lasting part of the life of a person. It can also lead to suicide, substance abuse, anxiety, and depression. You are right to be concerned about your patient's mood and health. According to research, older adults are at a much higher risk of death in the 6 months following the loss of a spouse, particularly men. This is especially true for men who watch their wives suffer before they die (Richardson & Balaswamy, 2001).

Research indicates that people believe that there is a "formula" for grieving that ultimately results in goodbye, resolution, and moving on (Moules et al., 2004). This belief in formula undoubtedly came out of the work of Elisabeth Kübler-Ross (1969), who provided clinicians and the masses with orderly steps for grieving, steps that ultimately result in the aesthetically pleasing concept of acceptance, also known as closure.

We as caregivers, understandably, want to prevent the pain of complicated grieving. We may also have difficulty in witnessing the process—so much so that we push for closure, a word that Sheehy (2003) refers to as "the dirtiest word in the lexicon of trauma victims" because it seems to dictate that the missing and longing end at some given point. Moules and colleagues (2004) emphasize that it is crucial to understand that grief is not saying goodbye but maintaining a relationship with the deceased partner. This is especially true among older adults. According to Costello and Kendrick (2000) in the first year following the death of a spouse, it is normal for older adults to focus on and also modify the emotional relationship they had with their deceased partner.

Right now your patient's history, sense of self, and meaning are inextricably bound to his wife who is gone. He may never experience acceptance and closure in the way that we wish he would. In the meantime, research by Kaunonen and colleagues (1999) supports letting him "disorganize safely" by providing a safe environment and support, thereby increasing his chances of healing and finding new meaning for his life. Your role can be to assist your patient's journey through grief, one that "is a graceful, periodic, deliberate walk backwards while keeping a sure foot in living forward" (Moules et al., 2004, p. 99).

Kaunonen, M., Tarkka, M.T., Paunonen, M., et al. (1999). Grief and social support after the death of a spouse. *Journal of Advanced Nursing, 30,* 1304-1311.

Costello, J., & Kendrick, K. (2000). Grief and older people: The making or breaking of emotional bonds following partner loss in later life. *Journal of Advanced Nursing, 32,* 1374-1832.

Moules, N.J., Simonson, K., Prins, M. et al. (2004). Making room for grief: Walking backwards and living forward. *Nursing Inquiry, 11,* 99-107.

Richardson, V.E., & Balaswamy, S. (2001). Coping with bereavement among elderly widowers. *Omega, 43,* 129-144.

Sheehy, G. (2003). *Middletown, America: One town's passage from trauma to hope.* New York: Random House.

4. Preoccupation with the image of the deceased
5. Guilt
6. Anger
7. Change in behavior (e.g., depression, disorganization, or restlessness)
8. Reorganization of behavior directed toward a new object or activity

Shock and Disbelief

The bereaved person's first response is that of **denial.** The person is emotionally unable to accept his or her painful loss. Denial functions as a buffer against intolerable pain and allows the person slowly to acknowledge the reality of death. The mourner may appear to be functioning like a robot. Often, the bereaved person feels numb. A death may be accepted intellectually during this stage—"It's just as well, she was suffering"—although the emotional responses are still repressed. Denial is a needed defense that lasts for a few hours or a few days. Denial that persists longer than a few days may become complicated, making it difficult to move through the process of mourning.

Development of Awareness

As denial fades, painful feelings begin to surface. The finality of the loved one's death becomes more of a reality. Waves of anguish and pain are experienced and may be localized in the chest or the epigastric area. **Anger** often surfaces at this time. Doctors and nurses are often the objects of blame. Awareness by staff that anger is often displaced onto people in the hospital environment may decrease defensive staff behaviors. **Guilt** is often experienced, and the bereaved blames him- or herself for taking or for failing to take specific actions. Impulsive and self-destructive acts by the mourner may occur, such as smashing a hand through a window or beating the head against a wall.

Crying is a common phenomenon during this stage. "It is during this time that the greatest degree of anguish or despair, within the limits imposed by cultural patterns, is experienced or expressed" (Engel, 1964). Crying can afford a welcome release from pent-up anguish and tension. Assessment of cultural patterns is important in making clinical judgments about the appropriateness of the bereaved's behavior. Failing to cry can be the result of cultural influences or environmental restraints. The person may cry in private. Inability to cry, however, may be the result of a high degree of ambivalence toward the deceased. A person who is unable to cry may have difficulty in successfully completing the work of mourning.

Restitution

Restitution is the formal, ritualistic phase of mourning during the acute stage. It is the institutionalization of mourning: it brings friends and family together in the rites of the funeral service and serves to emphasize the finality of death. The viewing of the body, the lowering of the casket or scattering of ashes, and the various religious and cultural rituals all help the bereaved shed any residual denial in an atmosphere of support. Every human society has its own moral and cultural standards according to which the rituals of mourning take place. The gathering in ritualistic farewell to the deceased provides support and sustenance for the family.

After the acute stage has been completed, the main work of mourning goes on intrapsychically during the long-term stage, which lasts for 1 to 2 years or longer. Various phenomena experienced during bereavement are described in Table 22-1.

In truth, we know that these phases are not all encompassing. Some people experience all the phenomena mentioned in the preceding text, and some do not, and few will reach acceptance. In a study of the grief responses of older adult widows, Hegge and Fischer (2000) found that the grief work followed an erratic cycle, with peaks and valleys, spurts and relapses, through the various phases of loss and bereavement mentioned in the literature.

Zisook and Zisook (2005) state that people may use other coping methods such as terror, humor, or compassion to offset each stage. Because the roles of religion, spiritual beliefs, and culture play a profound role in the process of death and dying and how we grieve, there are other models of grief and mourning that recognize individual differences in ways people and groups may experience grief. For example, Worden (2002) and Doka (2006) propose more current models of grief and mourning that tend to see the process of grief as a series of processes or tasks. These tasks include:

1. Acknowledging the reality of the loss
2. Expressing manifest and latent emotions associated with the loss
3. Adjusting to a life without the deceased
4. Rebuilding faith or philosophical systems challenged by the loss

Strobe and Schut (1999) describe grief as "dual processes." That is, a bereaved individual oscillates between a **loss-oriented** and **restoration-oriented** process. The loss-oriented processes are those that deal with recognizing the loss, whereas the restoration-oriented processes aim at re-creating a new life (Doka, 2006). In this way, the successful griever is able to use distraction to focus on more positive emotions, and essentially control the amount of grief he or she is able to bear.

Application of the Nursing Process

ASSESSMENT

Most bereaved people come to terms with their losses with support from family and friends. However, more than 30% may require professional support (Lloyd-Williams, 1995). As mentioned, unresolved grief reactions over a lifetime have been called the hidden disease and may account for many of the physical symptoms seen in doctors' offices and hospital units. Suicide is higher among people who have had a significant loss, especially if losses are multiple and grieving mechanisms are limited.

In some cases, bereaved persons become disorganized, neglect themselves, do not eat, use alcohol or drugs, and are susceptible to physical disease. Several studies have shown that the health of widows and close relatives of the deceased declines within 1 year of bereavement, and medical and psychiatric problems increase (Bowlby & Parkes, 1970; Carr, 1985). Health care workers are not immune to grief reactions. A study by Feldstein and Gemma (1995) found that oncology nurses scored higher than other nurses in despair, social isolation, and somatization.

Often a history of an individual can alert health care personnel to signs or symptoms of potential difficulty a person may encounter during a time of mourning. The following questions identify risk factors that may complicate the successful completion of mourning:

1. Do any of the following factors relate to the bereaved?
   - Was the bereaved heavily dependent on the deceased?
   - Were there persistent, unresolved conflicts with the deceased?
   - Was the deceased a child? (Perhaps the most profound loss of all)

TABLE 22-1 Phenomena Experienced During Bereavement

Symptoms	Examples
Sensations of Somatic Distress The bereaved may experience tightness in the throat, shortness of breath, sighing, mental pain, or exhaustion; food tastes like sand; things feel unreal. Pain or discomfort may be identical to the symptoms experienced by the dead person. Normally, symptoms are brief.	A woman whose husband died of a stroke complains of weakness and numbness on her left side.
Preoccupation with the Image of the Deceased The bereaved brings up, thinks, talks about numerous memories of the deceased. The memories are positive. This process goes on with great sadness. The idealization of the deceased lets the bereaved relive the gratifications associated with the deceased and helps resolve any guilt the bereaved feels concerning the deceased. The bereaved may also take on many of the mannerisms of the deceased through identification. Identification serves the purpose of holding on to the deceased. Preoccupation with the dead person can continue for many months before it lessens.	A man whose wife has very recently died states, "I just can't stop thinking about my wife. Everything I see reminds me of her. We picked up this seashell on our honeymoon. I remember every wonderful moment we had together. The pain is so great, but the memories just keep coming." His friends notice that when he talks, his hand gestures and expressions are very like those of his recently deceased wife.
Guilt The bereaved reproaches himself or herself for real or fancied acts of negligence or omissions in the relationship with the deceased.	"I should have made him go to the doctor sooner." "I should have paid more attention to her, been more thoughtful."
Anger The anger the bereaved experiences may not be toward the object that gives rise to it. Often the anger is displaced onto the medical or nursing staff. Often it is directed toward the deceased. The anger is at its height during the first month but is often intermittent throughout the first year. The overflow of hostility disturbs the bereaved, resulting in the feeling that he or she is "going insane."	"The doctor didn't operate in time. If he had, Mary would be alive today." "How could he leave me like this . . . how could he?"
Change in Behavior: Depression, Disorganization, Restlessness A person may exhibit marked restlessness and an inability to organize his or her behavior. A depressive mood during routine activities is common, decreasing as the year passes and the intensity of the grief declines. Absence of depression is more abnormal than its presence. Loneliness and aimlessness are most pronounced 6 to 9 months after the death. Reorganization of behavior directed toward a new object or activity gradually occurs. The person renews his or her interest in people and activities. The grieving thus releases the bereaved from one interpersonal relationship, and new ones are free to take its place.	Six months after her husband died, Mrs. Faye states, "I just can't seem to function. I have a hard time doing the simplest tasks. I can't be bothered with socializing. I feel so down . . . so, so empty." Twenty months after her husband's death, Mrs. Faye tells a friend, "I'll be away this weekend. I am going fishing with my brother and his friend. This is the first time I've felt like doing anything since Harry died."

- Does the bereaved have a meaningful relationship or support system?
- Has the bereaved experienced a number of previous losses?
- Does the bereaved have sound coping skills?

2. Was the deceased's death associated with a cultural stigma (e.g., acquired immunodeficiency syndrome [AIDS], suicide, homicide)?
3. Has the bereaved had difficulty resolving past significant losses?
4. Does the bereaved have a history of depression, drug or alcohol abuse, or other psychiatric illness?
5. If the bereaved is young, are there indications for special interventions?
6. Was the deceased a veteran or victim of war?

Acute grief can bring on an exacerbation of any preexisting medical or psychiatric problems. And, of course, a history of depression, substance abuse, or posttraumatic stress disorder can complicate grief. Complicated grieving essentially means that the grief work is unresolved. Prolonged depression is the most common response to unresolved grief. Disturbances in mood are associated with biological changes in the body during stress-related depressive illness. Some examples include electrolyte disturbance, nervous system alterations, and faulty regulation of the autonomic nervous system. Always assess the potential for suicide. Someone who is having difficulty negotiating the work of mourning and is suffering can benefit from counseling, as mentioned earlier.

Assessment Guidelines

Grieving and Complicated Grieving

1. Identify whether the individual is at risk for complicated grieving (see assessment history).
2. Identify the bereaved person's cultural beliefs, length of typical grieving, and mourning rituals.
3. Evaluate for psychotic symptoms, agitation, increased activity, alcohol or drug abuse, and extreme vegetative symptoms (anorexia, weight loss, not sleeping).
4. Do not overlook people who do not express significant grief in the context of major loss. These individuals might have an increased risk of subsequent complicated or unresolved grief reactions.
5. Complicated grief reactions require significant interventions. Suicidal or severely depressed people might require hospitalization. Always assess for **suicide** with signs of depression or other dysfunctional signs.
6. Assess support systems. If support systems are limited, find bereavement groups in the community.
7. When grieving is stalled or complicated, a person is at high risk for major depression or other mental illnesses.

There are a variety of therapeutic approaches that have proved beneficial. Make referrals.
8. Grieving can bring with it severe spiritual anguish. Assess whether spiritual counseling or a specific counselor would be useful for the bereaved.

Table 22-2 presents a comparison between the symptoms of a "normal" mourning process and those of a complicated grief reaction.

DIAGNOSIS

Three nursing diagnoses that apply to grief are *Grieving, Complicated grieving,* and *Risk for complicated grieving.* During the time of grief, especially if the grieving process is prolonged or symptomatic (e.g., profound depression or disorganization), other nursing diagnoses may come into play. *Ineffective coping, Compromised family coping, Disturbed sleep pattern, Risk for spiritual distress, Disturbed thought processes, Chronic sorrow,* and *Social isolation* are examples.

Grieving

Grieving is a normal process in which people come to terms with losses that are actual, perceived, or anticipated. These responses affect the whole person and are experienced emotionally, physically, spiritually, socially, and intellectually. Grief is felt emotionally through anger, blame, despair, relief, pain, distress, and suffering. Physically, loss can result in altered immune and neuroendocrine function, and bring about sleep disturbances. Significant loss commonly results in spiritual uncertainty as questions such as, "How could God let that happen?" arise. Socially, people often become temporarily isolative and detached as they integrate the meaning of the loss. Loss can also have positive outcomes as the grieving process results in personal growth.

When a loved one is ill over a long period of time, many people will experience what is known as *anticipatory grieving* toward the end of life. It was previously believed that anticipatory grief could help minimize the ensuing grief reaction, but research has found that the intensity of the grief reaction is not altered or influenced by whether the loss is anticipated or not (Doka, 2006). However, the same research studies did find that unanticipated death often overwhelms defenses and challenges the capacity of an individual(s) to adapt to the loss.

Complicated Grieving or Risk for Complicated Grieving

Complicated grieving occurs when individuals have difficulty coming to terms with their loss and experience

TABLE 22-2	Common Responses and Pathological Intensification During Grief
Typical Response	**Pathological Intensification**
Dying	
Emotional expression and immediate coping with the dying process	Avoidance; feeling of being overwhelmed, dazed, confused; self-punitive feelings; inappropriately hostile feelings
Death and Outcry	
Outcry of emotions with news of the death and turning for help to others or isolating self with self-soothing	Panic; dissociative reactions, reactive psychoses, suicidal ideation
Warding Off (Denial)	
Avoidance of reminders and social withdrawal, focusing elsewhere, emotional numbing, not thinking of implications to self or of certain themes	Maladaptive avoidance of confronting the implications of death through drug or alcohol abuse, promiscuity, fugue states, phobic avoidance, feeling of being dead or unreal
Reexperience (Intrusion)	
Intrusive experiences, including recollections of negative experiences during relationship with the deceased, bad dreams, reduced concentration, compulsive reenactments	Flooding with negative images and emotions; uncontrolled ideation, self-impairing compulsive reenactments, night terrors, recurrent nightmares, distraught feelings resulting from the intrusion of anger, anxiety, despair, shame, or guilt; physiological exhaustion resulting from hyperarousal
Working Through	
Recollection of the deceased and a contemplation of self with reduced intrusiveness of memories and fantasies and with increased rational acceptance, reduced numbness and avoidance, more "dosing" of recollections, and a sense of working it through	Feeling of inability to integrate the death with a sense of self and continued life; persistent warding-off themes that may manifest as anxious, depressed, enraged, shame-filled, or guilty moods, self-injurious behaviors and psychophysiological syndromes
Resolution	
Reduction in emotional swings and a sense of self-coherence and readiness for new relationships; ability to experience positive states of mind	Failure to negotiate the process of mourning, which may be associated with inability to work or create, or to feel emotion or positive states of mind

From Horowitz, M.J. (1990). A model of mourning: Change in schemas of self and other. *Journal of the American Psychoanalytic Association, 38*(2), 297-324.

phenomena outside the normal grief reaction, which impairs their ability to function. The *DSM-IV-TR* identifies a number of symptoms that are not characteristic with normal mourning, which include:

1. Guilt about things other than actions taken or not taken by the survivor at the time of death
2. Thoughts of death other than the survivor feeling that he or she would be better off dead or should have died with the deceased person
3. Morbid preoccupation with worthlessness
4. Marked psychomotor retardation
5. Prolonged and marked functional impairment
6. Hallucinatory experiences other than thinking that he or she hears the voice of, or transiently sees the image of, the deceased person

OUTCOMES IDENTIFICATION

Ideally, successful outcomes would include the following. An individual:

- Can tolerate intense emotions
- Reports decreased preoccupation with the deceased (loss)
- Demonstrates increased periods of stability
- Tends to previous responsibilities
- Takes on new roles and responsibilities
- Has energy to invest in new endeavors
- Expresses positive expectations about the future
- Remembers positive as well as negative aspects of the deceased loved one

PLANNING

Nurses constantly encounter people who are faced with loss, although that loss might not be the reason they come into the medical or psychiatric health care system. In hospital settings, grief is expressed when there is a loss besides death; for example, loss of a limb from amputation or a breast after surgery for breast cancer. Sometimes simple active listening can go a long way in offering comfort and respite from loneliness, or perhaps a referral to a grieving support group is indicated. Still at other times, the nurse may realize that even though individuals present with a medical or emotional problem, they are also undergoing a profound loss; therefore the nurse might suggest the need for a referral for grief counseling, re-grief work, or psychotherapy. As mentioned, physical or emotional symptoms may be related to a complicated grief reaction.

IMPLEMENTATION

The nurse's focus when facilitating bereavement is on helping the bereaved deal with the most important issues emerging at a particular time. Often the nurse or other caregiver can best serve the grieving person simply by being present, listening with interest, and encouraging talking and the recounting of meaningful stories. Table 22-3 provides guidelines for helping people grieve.

Communication Guidelines

Because we know that prolonged and serious alterations in social adjustment, as well as medical diseases, may develop if the phases of mourning are interrupted or if needed support is not available, listening may be the most important support for acute grief. The helping person should keep his or her own talking to a minimum. Telling the story

---

TABLE 22-3   Interventions for Helping People in Acute Grief

Intervention	Rationale
1. Use methods that can facilitate the grieving process (Robinson, 1997).	
a. Give your full presence: use appropriate eye contact, attentive listening, and appropriate touch.	a. Talking is one of the most important ways of dealing with acute grief. Listening patiently helps the bereaved express all feelings, even ones he or she feels are "negative." Appropriate eye contact helps to convey the awareness that you are there and are sharing the person's sadness. Suitable human touch can express warmth and nurture healing. Inappropriate touch can leave a person confused and uncomfortable.
b. Be patient with the bereaved in times of silence. Do not fill silence with empty chatter.	b. Sharing painful feelings during periods of silence is healing and conveys your concern.
2. Know about and share with the bereaved information about the phenomena that occur during the normal mourning process, because they may concern some people (intense anger at the deceased, guilt, symptoms the deceased had before death, unbidden floods of memories). Give the bereaved support during the occurrence of these phenomena and a written handout to refer to.	2. Although the knowledge won't eliminate the emotions, it can greatly relieve a person who is thinking there is something wrong with having these feelings.
3. Encourage the support of family and friends. If no supports are available, refer the patient to a community bereavement group. (Bereavement groups are helpful even when a person has many friends or much family support.)	3. Friends can help with routine matters. For example: • Getting food into the house • Making phone calls • Driving to the mortuary • Taking care of the kids or other family members
4. Offer spiritual support and referrals when needed.	4. Dealing with an illness or catastrophic loss can cause the most profound spiritual anguish.
5. When intense emotions are in evidence, show understanding and support (see Table 22-4).	5. Empathic words that reflect acceptance of a bereaved individual's feelings are healing (Robinson, 1997).

over and over is therapeutic for the bereaved but needs to alternate with periods activities that offer distraction from the loss.

Listening actively, not just listening to the words but to the whole person, can assist in healing. Tschudin (1997) states that "listening and not talking, not interrupting, being comfortable with silence when indicated, and using prompts like 'go on,' etc., to encourage the person to continue talking" are the most helpful behaviors. When appropriate, validating the individual's feelings is also helpful.

Talking can release negative emotions. When a person is faced with loss, strong feelings of anger, guilt, and hate are normal reactions that must be expressed to facilitate the process of mourning. It is important that someone listen and encourage the expression of feelings surrounding the person's loss or anticipated loss.

Banal advice and philosophical statements are useless. Unhelpful responses by others, such as "He's no longer suffering" or "You can always have another child" or "It's better this way" can lead the bereaved to believe that others do not understand the acute pain being suffered and that the personal impact of the loss is being minimized. Such statements can compound feelings of isolation. Such statements can emphasize feelings of isolation and reinforce misunderstanding promoting isolation.

More helpful responses include "His death will be a terrible loss" or "No one can replace her" or "He will be missed for a long time." Statements such as these validate the bereaved person's experience of loss and communicate the message that the bereaved is understood and supported. Table 22-4 offers communication guidelines for what to say to a person suffering a profound loss.

Psychotherapy

Grief is a process that most of us negotiate with the help of family, friends, and staying connected in the community activities. Some people find comfort and support in grief counseling or support groups. Six to 10 sessions of psychotherapy have been found to be helpful during the crisis period. At a later stage, the use of 15 sessions or more has a good outcome.

For people at risk for complicated grief reactions (history of mental illness, loss by suicide or homicide, facing multiple simultaneous losses, loss of a child), brief and time-limited psychotherapy may be indicated. According to Zisook and Zisook (2005), effective short-term therapies include:

1. **An educational component:** Helping people to know what to expect and to normalize their confusing feelings and behaviors
2. **Encouragement of full expression of emotions and affect:** May include writing letters to deceased, role-playing, looking at pictures
3. **An attempt to help bereaved come to peace with a new relationship to the deceased:** This involves the process integrating the loss of the deceased into current reality.

More complicated or pathological patterns of grief may require special techniques, such as re-grief work. When a major depression or other mental health illness is involved, psychotherapeutic techniques geared to grief work as well as addressing the individual's mental health issues, can help greatly in improving the person's quality of life. At times psychobiological interventions may be needed (e.g., antidepressants). Box 22-1 offers guidelines that can help people and their families cope with catastrophic loss.

EVALUATION

Worden (2002) developed a model that describes the tasks involved in the process of mourning:

Text continued on p. 455

TABLE 22-4   Guidelines for Communicating with a Bereaved Person

Situation	Sample Response
When you sense an overwhelming *sorrow*	"This must hurt terribly."
When you hear *anger* in the bereaved person's voice	"I hear anger in your voice. Most people go through periods of anger when their loved one dies. Are you feeling angry now?"
If you discern *guilt*	"Are you feeling guilty? This is a common reaction many people have. What are some of your thoughts about this?"
If you sense a *fear* of the future	"It must be scary to go through this."
When the bereaved seems *confused*	"This can be a confusing time."
In almost any *painful situation*	"This must be very difficult for you."

Adapted from Robinson, D. (1997). *Good intentions: The nine unconscious mistakes of nice people* (p. 249). New York: Warner Books.

BOX 22-1

Guidelines for Dealing with Catastrophic Loss

Take the time you need to grieve. The hard work of grief uses psychological energy. Resolution of the numb state that occurs after loss requires a few weeks at least. A minimum of 1 year, to cover all the birthdays, anniversaries, and other important dates without your loved one, is required before you can learn to live with your loss.

Express your feelings. Remember that anger, anxiety, loneliness, and even guilt are normal reactions and that everyone needs a safe place to express them. Tell your personal story of loss as many times as you need to—this repetition is a helpful and necessary part of the grieving process.

Establish a structure for each day and stick to it. Although it is hard to do, keeping to some semblance of structure makes the first few weeks after a loss easier. Getting through each day helps restore the confidence you need to accept the reality of loss.

Don't feel that you have to answer all the questions asked you. Although most people try to be kind, they may be unaware of their insensitivity. Down the road you may want to read books about how others have dealt with similar circumstances. They often have helpful suggestions for a person in your situation.

As hard as it is, try to take good care of yourself. Eat well, talk with friends, get plenty of rest. Be sure to let your primary care clinician know if you are having trouble eating or sleeping. Make use of exercise. It can help you let out pent-up frustrations. If you are losing weight, sleeping excessively or intermittently, or still experiencing deep depression after 3 months, be sure to seek professional assistance.

Expect the unexpected. You may begin to feel a bit better, only to have a brief emotional collapse. These are expectable reactions. Moreover, you may find that you dream about, visualize, think about, or search for your loved one. This, too, is a part of the grieving process.

Give yourself time. Don't feel that you have to resume all of life's duties right away.

Make use of rituals. Those who take the time to say goodbye at a funeral or a viewing tend to find that it helps the bereavement process.

If you do not begin to feel better within a few weeks, at least for a few hours every day, be sure to tell your doctor or primary care practitioner. If you have had an emotional problem in the past (e.g., depression, substance abuse), be sure to get the additional support you need. Losing a loved one puts you at higher risk for a relapse of these disorders.

From Zerbe, K.J. (1999). *Women's mental health in primary care* (pp. 207-208). Philadelphia: Saunders.

APPLYING THE ART   A Person Experiencing Grief

SCENARIO: I met 19-year-old Monica during her brief hospitalization to stabilize her insulin-resistant (type 1) diabetes. Under her veneer of sarcasm, I sensed depression as she talked about her pledging a sorority, too much partying, failing grades, and her diabetes raging out of control.

THERAPEUTIC GOAL: By the conclusion of this interaction, Monica will make at least one decision to break out of her self-destructive cycle and deal with the issue(s) and feelings she is pushing down.

Student-Patient Interaction	Thoughts, Communication Techniques, and Mental Health Nursing Concepts
Monica: "You're back again. Couldn't find anything better to do?" ***Student's feelings:*** *Monica's sarcasm tends to disconcert me until I remind myself that fear and loss fuel her anger.*	
Student: "Hi, Monica. I will be working with you again today. How are you?"	I ignored her comment, which *non-reinforces* the sarcasm. I'm willing myself to not take it personally.

APPLYING THE ART   A Person Experiencing Grief—cont'd

Student-Patient Interaction	Thoughts, Communication Techniques, and Mental Health Nursing Concepts
Monica: "Fine. The doctor just yelled because my right heel has a sore on it that I've ignored. If I fail one more class, I go on academic probation and finals start next week. Yeah, I'm doing just great."	I forgot that using a social greeting like, "How are you?" typically elicits an automatic "fine." Using a *broad opening* like "What's been happening with you since we talked yesterday?" would better let Monica know that I really want her to share.
Student: *Leaning in.* "Somehow your 'just great' doesn't sound so great." **Student's feelings:** *I feel overwhelmed listening to her. Because I carry a heavy academic load, I identify with her struggles. Yet I feel some frustration that Monica does not seem to take charge of her life.*	I make an observation then use attending body language to show empathy. Is that countertransference? Isn't that my own fear that I will lose control of all the pieces I juggle?
Monica: "No use worrying." *Leaning in and speaking quietly.*	
Student: "And yet somehow the worry creeps back in. Sometimes the worry looks like sadness or even anger. Sometimes it shows up as a blood sugar that refuses to stabilize." **Student's feelings:** *I hope I'm not pushing her too much. We have some rapport and she lets herself vent with me.*	I refer to "the worry" and "a blood sugar" to depersonalize the reference, yet still allow Monica to choose insight, if possible.
Monica: *Nods.*	
Student: "You feel overwhelmed."	
Monica: "The doctor yelling about my foot! Wish I could hide in some hole where no one could ever find me or tell what I should be doing."	In *crisis terms* the doctor "yelling" likely acted as the *precipitating event.*
Student: "I wonder what pressures you the most."	I ask Monica an indirect question to help her identify stress. Should I have instead attempted to translate into feelings? For example, "You're discouraged and having a hard time believing in yourself."
Monica: "The feeling that no matter what I do it isn't enough. It isn't good enough. I'm not good enough."	
Student: "You say you aren't good enough—for who?"	I am assessing a *balancing* factor in *crisis* when I help Monica talk about her *perception of the event* and most significantly, her perception of self.
Monica: "Since I was diagnosed when I was 6, my mother insisted I was the same as everybody else; 'The diabetes doesn't change anything, Monica. You can do anything!' So I pledge a sorority, go with the flow, ignoring what I should or shouldn't eat or drink. Then I stay out late and screw up my sleep and my blood sugar goes haywire. I feel bad, so I don't study."	Monica *projects* the blame for her trouble onto her Mother. *What must it be like for a person to deal with diabetes since 6 years old?*

Continued

APPLYING THE ART   A Person Experiencing Grief—cont'd

Student-Patient Interaction	Thoughts, Communication Techniques, and Mental Health Nursing Concepts
Student: "So in trying to prove the diabetes does not matter, it ends up influencing major areas of your life. What does your mother say now?"	I *clarify* to try to understand Monica's meaning. I also *gather information.*
Monica: "Nothing. She doesn't know I'm in here."	Monica independently brought up the subject of her mother, so I will listen to see if her mother is a *situational support,* a *second balancing factor* in crisis.
Student: "She doesn't know?"	I *restate* to say, "Go on."
Monica: "I thought I could put it off until after finals, but my life is falling apart."	
Student: "Put what off, Monica?" *Student's feelings: Did I do this the right way? I probably should have helped her talk about her life falling apart but I am also curious about what she has put off.*	I still do not understand about "put off" so, I ask an *indirect question.*
Monica: *Sobbing.* "She's dying. My mother is dying. She's survived the cancer so long that I never thought she'd actually die. She has maybe 2 months."	She's been grieving losing her mother.
Student: "Oh! I'm so sorry. You've been holding this pain inside, trying to put off . . . ?" *Student's feelings: My feelings of sorrow came out without my thinking first.*	
Monica: "No one knows. My friends don't even know." *Student's feelings: I feel compassion for her. She must feel so alone.*	
Student: "I wonder what telling others would mean to you."	
Monica: "That I can't make it by myself. That it's real. She's going to die. I can't do my life without her." *Crying.* *Student's feelings: I am picking up some of her feelings of aloneness and powerlessness with the impending death of her mom. I have to watch that I don't get sucked into these feelings but rather focus on Monica's feelings and thoughts.*	I wonder if *unconsciously* Monica's noncompliance with her diabetes and even doing poorly at school has to do with *acting out* her belief that "I can't do my life without her." I know how devastated I would be to lose my mother.
Student: "Monica, what are you saying, that you don't want to live?"	Is she saying she cannot live without her mother? Is this a covert message about suicide?
Monica: "I wouldn't do anything to hurt myself, but I already feel so lonely, like she's gone already." *Student's feelings: I feel relieved that she chooses to not hurt herself, though her lifestyle choices aren't healthy.*	She describes *anticipatory grief.* However, Edwin Shneidman might refer to her behavior as subintentional suicide.

APPLYING THE ART   A Person Experiencing Grief—cont'd

Student-Patient Interaction	Thoughts, Communication Techniques, and Mental Health Nursing Concepts
Student: "You feel lonely. You miss her already. In what ways have you been able to let your mother know what she means to you?" ***Student's feelings:*** *Helping Monica look at saying goodbye makes me think about telling the people I love how much they mean to me.*	I validate to be sure I understand. Again, I need to assess for countertransference and keep the pace at Monica's comfort level, not my own.
Monica: "I haven't gone home all semester. I barely talk when she calls. I guess if I go home I can't pretend that it's not happening anymore."	Monica uses the word *pretend*. The *denial* stage of grief plays a part, too.
Student: "It's natural to feel afraid. It's scary to let yourself experience this pain of saying goodbye." *She nods.* "I wonder what you think might happen." ***Student's feelings:*** *I feel good that Monica is working with me to think through how she will handle talking to her mother.*	I give *support* and ask an *indirect question*.
Monica: "Maybe I won't be strong. I'll break down."	
Student: "And then?"	I help Monica *problem-solve* by anticipating what will likely happen with each step, in order to decrease her *anxiety*. Being able to predict meets *safety needs*.
Monica: "My mom will cry, too."	
Student: "You will cry together." *Monica nods.*	
Monica: "I need to talk to her. Will you stay with me while I call?"	
Student: "Yes." ***Student's feelings:*** *I feel honored that Monica is reaching out to me and has at least made a decision to be with her mom and share their losses together.*	Our talking together highlighted the third crisis *balancing factor*, namely *situational support*. Before we terminate today, I want to help Monica think about who can lend support as she juggles school, her diabetes, and the *grief* of losing her mother. Monica's decision to call her mother means she is *working through the denial stage* of the grief process and she is ready to go through the painful process of saying goodbye.

1. Accept the reality of the loss.
2. Work through the pain of grief. (Sharing with others can facilitate this task.)
3. Adjust to an environment in which the deceased is missing.
4. Restructure the family's relationship with the deceased and reinvest in other relationships and life pursuits.

Evaluation should address whether these tasks have been accomplished. The work of mourning is over when the bereaved can remember realistically the pleasures and the disappointments of the relationship with the lost loved one. Brief periods of intense emotions may still occur at significant times, such as holidays and anniversaries, but the person or family members have energy to reinvest in new relationships that bring shared joys, security, satisfaction, and comfort. If, after a normal period (12 to 24 months), a person has not been able to find pleasure, satisfaction, and comfort in their life, then reassessment and reevaluation are indicated.

KEY POINTS TO REMEMBER

- Bereavement is a series of psychological processes and the normal reaction to a loss, real or perceived, including the loss of a person, security, self-confidence, or a dream. Essentially, a loss results in a change in self-concept.
- Acute grief may last from 4 to 8 weeks; the complete process of mourning may take a year or two or longer.
- Common phenomena are evident during the experience of grief, and people usually show similar patterns of grief and mourning within their cultural norms. Culture greatly affects the patterns of response to death and dying in patients as well as nurses.
- Grief, when experienced by health care workers, can reactivate distressing feelings related to previous losses. If nurses have unresolved issues of grief and depression, their ability to help others is greatly minimized, so it is important to recognize that staff members need psychological support when they work with people who are grieving.
- Many people are experts on loss but not on coping with loss. Health care workers can use a number of coping skills to help comfort the bereaved and facilitate mourning. Actively listening to a grieving person's story without offering banal or philosophical responses can assist in healing. Short-term grief counseling and groups are often helpful.
- Indicators of the potential for complicated or unresolved grief include social isolation, extensive dependency on the deceased person, unresolved interpersonal conflicts, loss of a child, violent and senseless death, or a catastrophic loss. A history will often reveal potential risks for complicated grieving.
- Grief work is successful when the relationship to the deceased person has been restructured and energy is available for new relationships and life pursuits. The work of mourning is complete when the bereaved person or persons can remember realistically both the pleasures and the disappointments of the lost relationship. Outcomes for successful grief work have been identified.

CRITICAL THINKING

1. What are some concrete ways in which you can help another to cope with a loss? Identify specific components in the following areas:
   A. How can you let the person tell his or her story?
   B. What is the potential therapeutic value of doing so?
   C. Avoiding banal advice, what are some things you might say that could offer comfort? Use the guidelines in Table 22-3 and Table 22-4 to describe how you would help a person who is suffering a profound loss.

CHAPTER REVIEW

Choose the most appropriate answer(s):

1. Grief is best described as:
   1. a normal response to a significant loss.
   2. a mild to moderately severe mood disorder.
   3. the display of feelings associated with death.
   4. denial of the reality of the loss of a significant person, object, or state of being.

2. Which statement indicates that a patient has successfully mourned a loss in his or her life?
   1. "She was so strong after her husband died. She never cried the whole time. She kept a stiff upper lip."
   2. "She was a wreck when her sister died. She cried and cried. It took her about a year before she resumed her usual activities with any zest."
   3. "You know, he still talks about his mother as if she were alive today, and she's been dead for 4 years."
   4. "He never talked about his wife after she died. He just picked up and went on life's way."

3. K., 34 years of age, is single and has very few close friends and relatives. He was very dependent on his mother before her death, although he often complained about their arguing over her intrusiveness. What statement best describes his risk for problems in resolving his grief?
   1. He is at no particular risk because the death of parents is an expected event in one's life.
   2. He is at low risk because the task of young adulthood is to develop independence from the family of origin.
   3. He is at moderate risk.
   4. He is at high risk because he was dependent on his mother, demonstrated unresolved conflicts with her, and has a limited support system.

4. Which statement represents a loss that involves "disenfranchised grief"?
   1. Dorothy has lost her husband of 15 years in an auto accident.
   2. Robert is grieving the loss of his business as a result of a fire.
   3. Allison is grieving the loss of her therapist after 2 years of psychotherapy work ended.
   4. Richard is grieving the loss of his mother, who was 90 and lived 600 miles from him.

CHAPTER REVIEW—cont'd

5. Which responses of a child to a father's untimely death represent an early stage of normal grieving? Select all that apply.
   1. The child lies in bed, banging his head against the mattress, shouting, "No, no, no!"
   2. The child refuses to go to school 2 weeks after his father's funeral, claiming "aches and pains all over my body."

3. The child begins to obsessively attend to his game card collection and spends hours sorting and ordering cards for the first month after his father's death.
4. The child repeatedly comes home from school and reports "seeing Dad" around a corner, but then "he just disappears."

REFERENCES

Albert, P.L. (2001). Grief and loss in the workplace. *Progress in Transplantation, 11*(3), 169-173.

Bateman, A.L. (1999). Understanding the process of grieving and loss: A critical social thinking perspective. *Journal of the American Psychiatric Nurses Association, 5*(5), 139-147.

Bowlby, J., & Parkes, C.M. (1970). Separation and loss within the family. In E.J. Anthony & C. Koupernik (Eds.), *The child in his family.* New York: Wiley.

Cable, D. (1998). *Grief in the American culture.* In K.J. Doka & J.D. Davidson (Eds.), *Living with grief: Who we are, how we grieve.* Philadelphia: Brunner/Mazel.

Caplan, G. (1974). *Support systems and community mental health. Lectures on concept development.* New York: Behavioral Publications.

Carr, A.C. (1985). Grief, mourning, and bereavement. In H.I. Kaplan & B.J. Sadock (Eds.), *Comprehensive textbook of psychiatry* (4th ed.). Baltimore: Williams & Wilkins.

Corr, C.A. (2003). Loss, grief and trauma in public tragedy. In M. Lattanzi-Light & K. J. Doka (Eds.), *Living with grief: Coping with public tragedy.* Washington, DC: Hospice Foundation of America.

Corr, C.A., & Doka, K.J. (2001). Master concepts in the field of death, dying, and bereavement: Coping versus adaptive strategies. *Omega, 43,* 183-199.

Doka, K. (1989). *Disenfranchised grief: Recognizing hidden sorrow.* New York: Lexington Books.

Doka, K.J. (2006). Grief: The constant companion of illness. In J.R. Gavin (Guest Ed). Anesthesiology Clinics, 2006, *24*(1), 205-212. Philadelphia: Saunders.

Engel, G.L. (1964). Grief and grieving. *American Journal of Nursing, 64*(9), 93-98.

Feldstein, M.A., & Gemma, P.B. (1995). Oncology nurses and chronic compounded grief. *Cancer Nursing, 18*(3), 228-236.

Hegge, M., & Fischer, C. (2000). Grief responses of senior and elderly widows: Practice implications. *Journal of Gerontological Nursing, 26*(2), 35-43.

Kübler-Ross, E. (1969). *On death and dying.* New York: Macmillan.

Lloyd-Williams, M. (1995). Bereavement referrals to a psychiatric service: An audit. *European Journal of Cancer Care, 4*(1), 17-19.

Marks, M.J.B. (1976). The grieving patient and family. *American Journal of Nursing, 76,* 1488-1491.

Parkes, C.M. (1970). The first year of bereavement: A longitudinal study of the reaction of London widows to the death of their husbands. *Psychiatry, 33*(4), 444-467.

Parkes, C.M. (1975). *Bereavement: Studies of grief in adult life.* Harmondsworth, England: Penguin.

Robinson, D. (1997). *Good intentions: The nine unconscious mistakes of nice people.* New York: Warner Books.

Stroebe, M., & Schut, H. (1999). The dual process model of coping with bereavement: Rationale and description. *Death Studies, 23,* 197-224.

Tschudin, V. (1997). *Counselling for loss and bereavement.* London: Baillière Tindall.

Volkan, V.D., & Zintl, E. (1993). *Life after loss: The lessons of grief.* New York: Simon and Schuster.

Weil, S. (1998). *Simone Weil: Writings selected with an introduction by Eric Springsted.* New York: Orbis Books.

Williams, J.R. (2002). Effects of grief on survivor's health. In K. Doka (Ed.), *Living with grief: Loss in later life.* Washington, DC: The Hospice Foundation of America.

Worden, W. (2002). *Grief counseling and grief therapy: A handbook for the mental health practitioner* (3rd ed.). New York: Springer.

Zisook, S., & Zisook, S.A. (2005). Death, dying and bereavement. In B.J. Sadock & V.A. Sadock (Eds.), *Kaplan & Sadock's comprehensive textbook of psychiatry* (8th ed, vol 11, pp. 2367-2392). Philadelphia: Lippincott, Williams & Wilkins.

Communicating with and Planning Care for Patients with Discrete Needs

CHAPTER 23

Children and Adolescents

Cherrill W. Colson

Key Terms and Concepts

Asperger's syndrome, p. 464
attention deficit hyperactivity disorder (ADHD),
   p. 467
autistic disorder, p. 464
bibliotherapy, p. 471
conduct disorder, p. 468
dramatic play therapy, p. 472
mental retardation, p. 463
mental status assessment, p. 462
mood disorders, p. 467
movement and dance therapy, p. 472
music therapy, p. 472
oppositional defiant disorder, p. 468

pervasive developmental disorder (PDD), p. 463
play therapy, p. 471
posttraumatic stress disorder (PTSD), p. 465
recreational therapy, p. 472
resilient child, p. 461
separation anxiety disorder, p. 465
social phobia, p. 465
temperament, p. 461
therapeutic drawing, p. 471
therapeutic games, p. 471
therapeutic holding, p. 471
time-out, p. 471
Tourette's disorder, p. 470

Objectives

1. Discuss the various factors and influences involved with the development of child and adolescent disorders.
2. Describe the components of a holistic assessment to determine the characteristics of mental health or mental illness in children and adolescents.
3. Identify the clinical features and behaviors of child and adolescent psychiatric disorders and the appropriate nursing assessment guidelines.

4. Analyze medical and nursing diagnoses and the overall nursing interventions for the various disorders.
5. Compare and contrast treatment modalities for children and adolescents, being mindful of developmental stages.

evolve

For additional resources related to the content of this chapter, visit the Evolve website at
http://evolve.elsevier.com/Varcarolis/essentials.

- Chapter Outline
- Chapter Review Answers

- Nurse, Patient, and Family Resources
- Concept Map Creator

PREVALENCE AND COMORBIDITY

About one half of all Americans will meet the criteria for a DSM-IV disorder at sometime during their life. The first onset will most likely occur in early childhood or early adolescence (Kessler et al., 2005).

One in five children and adolescents in the United States suffers from a major psychiatric disorder that causes significant impairments at home, school, and with peers. An estimated two thirds of all young people with mental health problems are not getting the help they need. Mental illness can continue into adulthood, as evidenced by the fact that 74% of 21-year-olds with mental disorders have had previous problems. Approximately 60% of all children in out-of-home care have moderate to severe mental health problems. Suicide is now the third leading cause of death among youth ages 15 to 24 years and the sixth leading cause of death for 5- to 14-year-olds (Mental Health America, 2006). Although the general suicide rate has decreased over the last 25 years, the rate has tripled for those between 15 and 24 years of age (FAS, 2007).

The federal government's recognition of these mental health problems and efforts toward effective treatments were identified in *Mental Health: A Report of the Surgeon General* (USDHHS, 1999). Identified barriers to assessment and treatment remain: (1) lack of clarity about why, when, and how children should be screened; (2) lack of coordination of multiple systems with different funding streams and eligibility requirements; (3) lack of resources; (4) lack of mental health providers; and (5) inadequate reimbursement (Children's Defense Fund, 2004).

Children with mental illness often meet the criteria for more than one diagnostic category. For example, attention deficit hyperactivity disorder (ADHD) occurs in 60% to 90% of individuals with juvenile-onset bipolar disorder. Conduct disorders are associated with later substance use disorder, elevated rates of mood disorders, oppositional defiant disorder, and ADHD (Sadock & Sadock, 2007). Children with depression have a significant incidence of conduct or oppositional disorders, anxiety disorders, and symptoms of ADHD (Inder, 2000).

THEORY

A child's vulnerability to psychopathology is the result of complex interactions between biological, psychological, genetic, and environmental variables (Popper et al., 2002). Younger children are harder to diagnose than older children, as the boundaries between normal and abnormal behaviors are less distinct. Intervention may be delayed until the child reaches school age to see whether a symptom is the result of a developmental lag or something more serious.

Genetic Factors

Genetic factors have been implicated in a number of mental disorders, including autism, bipolar disorders, schizophrenia, ADHD, and mental retardation (Sadock & Sadock, 2004). According to the *Diagnostic and Statistical Manual of Mental Disorders (DSM-IV-TR),* some disorders have a direct genetic link, such as the mental retardation in Tay-Sachs disease, phenylketonuria, and fragile X syndrome.

Temperament, the style of behavior habitually used to cope with demands of the environment, is a constitutional factor thought to be genetically determined. It may be modified by the parent-infant relationship. In the case of the difficult-child temperament, if the caregiver is unable to respond positively to the child, there is an increased risk of insecure attachment, developmental problems, and mental disorders.

Biochemical Factors

Biochemical factors in childhood psychopathology include alterations in neurotransmitters with decreases in norepinephrine and serotonin levels related to depression and suicide. In ADHD, a misfiring in the brain's executive function is thought to result in the behavior problems in this disorder (Bush et al., 2005).

Environmental Factors

Environmental factors put stress on children and adolescents and shape their development. Any type of abuse (physical, emotional, sexual) and neglect increases a child's risk for developing psychopathology. Familial characteristics that correlate with child psychiatric disorders are (1) severe marital discord, (2) low socioeconomic status, (3) large families and overcrowding, (4) parental criminality, (5) maternal psychiatric disorders, and (6) foster care placement. Stressful life events are known to relate to anxiety, posttraumatic stress disorder, conduct disorders, delinquency, impaired social and cognitive function, depression, and suicidal behaviors.

RESILIENCY

Not all vulnerable children develop mental disorders. It is assumed that constitutional resilience and a supportive environment play roles in keeping disorders from developing. Studies have shown that a **resilient child** has the following characteristics: (1) a temperament that can adapt to changes in the environment, (2) the ability to form nurturing relationships with other adults when a parent is not available, (3) the ability to distance himself or herself from the emotional chaos of the parent or family, (4) social intelligence, and (5) the ability to use problem-solving skills.

MENTAL HEALTH ASSESSMENT

The type of data collected to assess mental health depends on the setting, the severity of the presenting problem, and the availability of resources. The nurse is often the first health care professional to have contact with the child and completes a holistic assessment including the presenting problem, medical and developmental issues, family history, and a mental status assessment. In all cases, a physical examination is part of a complete workup.

A **mental status assessment** in children and adolescents provides information about problems with thinking, feeling, and behaving (Box 23-1). This assessment is similar to that in adults except that the developmental level is considered. A **developmental assessment** provides information about

---

BOX 23-1

Child/Adolescent Mental Status Assessment

General Appearance
Size: height and weight
General health and nutrition
Dress and grooming
Distinguishing characteristics
Gestures and mannerisms
Looks or acts younger or older than chronological age

Activity Level
Hyper- or hypoactivity
Tics, other body movements
Autoerotic and self-comforting movements (thumb sucking, ear or hair pulling, masturbation)

Speech
Rate, rhythm, intonation
Pitch and modulation
Vocabulary and grammar appropriate to age
Mute, hesitant, talkative
Articulation problems
Other expressive problems
Unusual characteristics (pronoun reversal, echolalia, gender confusion, neologisms)

Coordination or Motor Function
Posture
Gait
Balance
Gross motor movement
Fine motor movement
Writing and drawing skills
Unusual characteristics (bizarre postures, banging, and hand biting)
Tiptoe walking, hand flapping, head

Affect
Predominant emotion
Kinds of feelings expressed
Feelings appropriate to the situation
Range and stability of feelings

Intensity of feelings
Unusual characteristics (apathy, sulking, oppositional behavior)

Manner of Relating
Eye contact
Ability to separate from caregiver, be independent
Attitude toward interviewer
Behavior during interview (tolerance, impulsive, aggressive, ability to have fun or play, low frustration)

Intellectual Functions
Fund of general information
Ability to communicate (follow directions, answer questions)
Memory
Creativity
Sense of humor
Social awareness
Learning and problem solving
Conscience (sense of right and wrong, accepts guilt and limits)

Thought Processes and Content
Orientation
Attention span
Self-concept and body image
Fantasies and dreams
Ego-defense mechanisms
Perceptual distortions (hallucinations, illusions)
Preoccupations, concerns, unusual ideas
Sex role, gender identity

Characteristics of Child's Play
Age-appropriate use of toys
Themes of play
Imagination and pretend play
Role and gender play
Age-appropriate play with peers
Relationships with peers (empathy, sharing, waiting for turns, best friends)

the child's current maturational level that, when compared with the child's chronological age, identifies developmental lags and deficits. One popular assessment tool that provides this comparison is the Denver II Developmental Screening Test for infants and children up to 6 years of age.

Methods of collecting data include interviewing, screening, testing (neurological, psychological, intelligence), observing, and interacting with the child or adolescent. Histories are taken from parents, caregivers, the child (when appropriate) or adolescent, and other family members. Structured questionnaires and behavior checklists can be completed by parents and teachers.

The observation or interaction part of a mental health assessment begins with a semistructured interview in which the child or adolescent is asked about life at home with parents and siblings and life at school with teachers and peers. Because the interview is not structured, children are free to describe their current problems, even giving information about their own developmental history. Activities such as games, drawings, puppets, and free play are used for younger children who cannot respond to a direct approach. An important part of the first interview is observing the interactions between the child or adolescent, the caregiver, and siblings (if available).

MENTAL RETARDATION

Mental retardation is the most common developmental disorder (CDC, 2005). Mental retardation affects approximately 1% of the population, and in 30% to 40% of the cases the etiology is unknown (APA, 2000). A lack of intellectual development impairs adaptive function, learning, communication, interpersonal skills, and social adjustment. The degree of impairment is determined by assessing the intelligence quotient (IQ) with standardized tests such as the Wechsler Intelligence Scales for Children.

Causes may be a result of heredity (Tay-Sachs, fragile X syndrome), alterations in early embryonic development (Down syndrome, fetal alcohol syndrome), pregnancy and perinatal problems (fetal malnutrition, prematurity, hypoxia, infections), and other factors such as trauma and poisoning.

Mild retardation constitutes 85% of the individuals with mental retardation. Their IQ level is 50 to 70. These children develop communication and social skills during childhood with minimal sensorimotor impairment and can be indistinguishable from children with normal IQs. They may be able to acquire up to sixth-grade academic skills and vocational skills as late teenagers. They may be capable of independent living or do better in a group home.

Moderate retardation constitutes 10% of the individuals with mental retardation. Their IQ level is 35 to 49. These children develop communication and social skills during childhood but may only be able to acquire second-grade academic skills. They benefit from vocational training and can perform semi-skilled work with supervision. As teenagers they have difficulty following social conventions, and this interferes with peer relationships. They do well in the community while living at home or in a supervised setting.

Severe retardation constitutes 3% to 4% of the individuals with mental retardation. Their IQ level is 20 to 34. They acquire little or no speech during early childhood but may learn to talk and carry out basic self-care skills at a later age. They can be taught to carry out simple tasks with close supervision. They can be managed living at home or in a supervised setting.

Profound retardation constitutes 1% to 2% of the individuals with mental retardation. Their IQ level is less than 20. These individuals usually have an identified neurological disorder causing the retardation. They have considerable sensorimotor impairments and may only develop minimal communication and self-care skills with constant supervision in a highly structured setting.

DIAGNOSIS

The child with mental retardation may have impairments in communication skills, social interactions, self-care abilities, and disruptive behaviors depending on the severity of the retardation and other neurological conditions. There is no list of specific behaviors to assess as there are for other mental disorders. A psychiatric diagnosis of mental retardation is made on the basis of IQ testing and assessment of developmental milestones. The nursing diagnoses will relate to the problems identified in a child/adolescent mental status assessment guide. Appropriate nursing diagnoses and guidelines for nursing interventions are spelled out in the later sections Pervasive Developmental Disorders, Attention Deficit Hyperactivity Disorder, and Disruptive Behavior Disorders.

PERVASIVE DEVELOPMENTAL DISORDERS

A **pervasive developmental disorder (PDD)** is characterized by severe and pervasive impairment in reciprocal social interaction and communication skills, usually accompanied by stereotyped behavior, interests, and activities (APA, 2000). Mental retardation is often evident in these disorders. The latest diagnostic refinement in the *DSM-IV-TR* identifies two of the most common subtypes as autistic disorder and Asperger's syndrome.

AUTISTIC DISORDER

Autistic disorder is a behavioral syndrome resulting from abnormal brain function of unknown etiology. Problems with language, logic and reasoning, impaired arousal with oversensitivity or indifference to stimuli are evident, whereas music and visuospatial activities may be enhanced as in savant syndrome (Popper et al., 2002).

Autistic disorder is usually observed before 3 years of age when the child fails to interact with others or be socially responsive through eye contact, facial expressions, and language. The prognosis for this disorder is related to the child's overall intellectual level, the development of social and language skills, as well as early intervention (APA, 2000). Few autistic individuals are able to live and work independently, and only about one-third can achieve partial independence.

ASPERGER'S SYNDROME

Asperger's syndrome differs from autistic disorder in that it appears to have a later onset, and it does not cause a delay in cognitive and language development (APA, 2000). As with autism, the etiology is unknown and there appears to be a familial pattern. Also like autism, restricted and repetitive behaviors and idiosyncratic interests may develop. Problems with empathizing and modulating social relationships become more noticeable when the child enters school and may continue in adulthood. In the movie *Rain Man*, Dustin Hoffman portrayed a man with Asperger's syndrome who was mathematically gifted.

ASSESSMENT

In assessing for autism, **three presenting characteristics** are examined (APA, 2000). The first is impairment in communication and imaginative activity. Autism may result in delay or total absence of language, immature grammatical structure, pronoun reversal, inability to name objects, and stereotypical or repetitive use of language. While most children like to pretend to be things they are not, such as pretending to be a dog and barking, autistic children have a lack of spontaneous make-believe play or imaginative play and a failure to imitate.

A second characteristic of autism is impairment in social interactions. This impairment manifests itself in lack of responsiveness to and interest in others, lack of eye-to-eye contact and facial responses, indifference or aversion to affection and physical contact, failure to cuddle or be comforted, and lack of friendships.

A final characteristic of autism is markedly restricted and stereotyped behaviors, interests, and activities. People with autism seem to need rigid adherence to routines and rituals, and respond catastrophically to minor changes. Stereotypical and repetitive motor mannerisms, such as rocking, are common. Autistic individuals are often preoccupied with specific objects (buttons, parts of the body, wheels on toys) and repetitive activities.

Assessment Guidelines

Pervasive Developmental Disorders

1. Assess for developmental spurts or lags, uneven development, or loss of previously acquired abilities.
2. Assess the quality of the relationship between the child and parent or caregiver for evidence of bonding, anxiety, tension, and difficulty-of-fit between the parent and child's temperament.
3. Be aware that children with behavioral and developmental problems are at risk for abuse.

DIAGNOSIS

There are several nursing diagnoses appropriate for children and adolescents with pervasive developmental disorders, including *Defensive coping*, *Ineffective coping*, *Delayed growth and development*, *Personal identity disturbed*, *Impaired verbal communication*, *Risk for impaired parent/child attachment*, *Fear*, *Risk for injury*, *Risk for self-mutilation*, *Risk for self-directed violence*, *Risk for other-directed violence*, *Impaired social interaction*, and *Self-care deficit*.

IMPLEMENTATION

Children with PDD are treated in therapeutic nursery schools, day treatment programs, and special education classes in public schools, as their education or treatment is mandated under the Children with Disabilities Act. Treatment plans include working with parents, who are taught how to modify the child's behavior and to foster the development of skills when the child is home. Pharmacological agents such as antipsychotics, selective serotonin reuptake inhibitors (SSRIs), and propranolol have been used with some success.

The ultimate *long-term outcome* is to help children with PDD reach their full potential by fostering developmental competencies and coping skills. The following guidelines for nursing interventions are useful with all children in all settings:

1. Increase the child's interest in reciprocal interactions.
2. Foster the development of social skills.
3. Facilitate the expression of appropriate emotional responses, including the development of trust, empathy, shame, remorse, anger, pride, independence, joy, and enthusiasm.
4. Foster the development of reciprocal communication, especially language skills.
5. Provide for the development of psychomotor skills in play and activities of daily living (ADL).
6. Facilitate the development of cognitive skills (attention, memory, cause and effect, reality testing, decision making, and problem solving).
7. Foster the development of self-concepts (identity, self-awareness, body image, and self-esteem).
8. Foster the development of self-control, including impulse control, tolerance of frustration and delay gratification.

ANXIETY DISORDERS

Anxiety becomes a problem when the child or adolescent fails to move beyond the fears associated with certain developmental stages or when anxiety interferes with normal functioning.

Anxiety disorders are the most common mental disorders of childhood and adolescence, affecting 13% of youth between the ages of 9 and 17 (USDHHS, 1999). There may be a genetic vulnerability to anxiety disorders, which seem to run in families. Anxiety disorders can develop in response to physical or psychosocial stressors and trauma. Cognitive theorists propose that anxiety is the result of dysfunctional efforts to make sense of life's events.

The characteristics of anxiety in children or adolescents are basically the same as those in adults. The one anxiety disorder specific to a child or adolescent is separation anxiety. Those that can be applied to both preadults and adults are identified as agoraphobia, generalized anxiety disorder, panic disorder, specific phobia and **social phobia**, obsessive-compulsive disorder, and posttraumatic stress disorder (PTSD). Separation anxiety and PTSD are discussed here as they relate to children and adolescents.

SEPARATION ANXIETY DISORDER

Children and adolescents with **separation anxiety disorder** become excessively anxious when separated from or antici-

pating a separation from their home or parental figures (APA, 2000). This disorder may develop after a significant stressful event. The prevalence of the disorder in children is estimated to be 4%, with a higher incidence in females and first-degree biological relatives. Although the remission rates are high, the disorder can persist and lead to **panic disorder with agoraphobia.** A **depressed mood** often accompanies the anxiety.

The *DSM-IV-TR* characteristics of separation anxiety disorder are:

- Excessive distress when separated from or anticipating separation from home or parental figures
- Excessive worries about being lost or kidnapped or that parental figures will be harmed
- Fear of being home alone or in situations without other significant adults
- Refusal to sleep unless near a parental figure and refusal to sleep away from home
- Refusal to attend school or other activities without a parental figure
- Physical symptoms such as a response to anxiety

POSTTRAUMATIC STRESS DISORDER

Posttraumatic stress disorder (PTSD) can occur at any age and has now been recognized in children. Rather than reliving the traumatic event as an adult might, younger children with PTSD tend to react with behaviors indicative of internalized anxiety. In older children and adolescents the anxiety is more often externalized.

Preschool children generally internalize PTSD behaviors and exhibit the following responses:

- Agitated and disorganized behavior
- Separation anxiety
- Sleep difficulties (including falling or staying asleep, sleeping alone)
- Nightmares or night terrors with unknown content, or changing to dreams of monsters
- Reliving the trauma in repetitive play of the event
- Increase in specific fears, especially those related to the trauma stimuli (storms, noise, a specific place)
- Irritability, whining, angry outbursts, temper tantrums
- Regression or loss of previously learned skills
- Somatic complaints
- Withdrawal from activities

School-age children generally externalize PTSD behaviors and exhibit the following responses:

- Sleep difficulties, especially nightmares of monsters, rescuing others, or being threatened

- Irritability and increased fighting with friends and siblings
- Difficulty concentrating, with impaired academic performance
- Repetitive playing out of the traumatic event
- Feeling jumpy and hypervigilant and having an increased startle response
- Belief that their lives will be short
- Belief that they can foresee untoward events in the future ("omen formation")
- Somatic complaints

ASSESSMENT

Assessment Guidelines

Anxiety Disorders

1. Assess the quality of the child-parent-caregiver relationship for evidence of anxiety, conflicts, or difficulty-of-fit between child and parent temperaments.
2. Assess for recent stressors and their severity, duration, and proximity to the child.
3. Assess the parent's or caregiver's understanding of developmental norms, parenting skills, and handling of problematic behaviors (lack of knowledge contributes to increased anxiety).
4. Assess the developmental level and whether regression has occurred.
5. Assess for physical, behavioral, and cognitive symptoms of anxiety.

Separation Anxiety Disorder

1. Assess the child's previous and current ability to separate from parent or caregiver. (The separation or individuation process may not be completed or the child may have regressed.)
2. Assess for presence of anxiety problems in the parent or caregiver. (In addition to genetic issues, anxiety and depression can be "contagious.")
3. Assess parental response to the child's anxiety. (Increased attention reinforces behavior.)

Posttraumatic Stress Disorder

1. Assess for personal exposure to an extreme traumatic stressor or event.
2. Assess for evidence of internalized or externalized anxiety symptoms.

DIAGNOSIS

There are several nursing diagnoses appropriate for children and adolescents with anxiety disorders, including *Anxiety*,

Fear, *Delayed growth and development*, *Impaired parenting*, *Ineffective coping*, and *Post-trauma syndrome*.

IMPLEMENTATION

Children and adolescents with anxiety disorders are most often treated on an outpatient basis with cognitive behavioral therapies in individual, group, or family modalities. Medications such as antihistamines, antianxiolytics, and antidepressants are also used; selective SSRIs have proven most effective. Cognitive therapy focuses on the underlying fears and concerns, and behavior modification is used to reinforce self-control behaviors. Children who refuse to start primary school are introduced gradually into the school environment with a parent or caregiver present for support for part of the day. When adolescents develop school phobia, the goal is to return them to the classroom at the earliest possible date and to give parents support in setting limits on truancy.

The following are guidelines for nursing interventions for children with anxiety disorders:

1. Help the child or adolescent reach full potential by fostering developmental competencies and coping skills.
2. Protect from panic levels of anxiety by acting as a parental surrogate and providing for biological and psychosocial needs.
3. Accept regression, but give emotional support to help the child progress again.
4. Increase self-esteem and feelings of competence in the ability to perform, achieve, or influence the future.
5. Help the child or adolescent accept and work through traumatic events or losses.

MOOD DISORDERS

It was once believed that children did not suffer from the same type of depression that adults did, and that a child's sadness in reaction to an event or situation would be short-lived. However, symptoms of depression in children and adolescents may be similar to adult symptoms, with feelings of sadness, pessimism, hopelessness, anhedonia, social withdrawal, and thoughts of suicide.

Children are more apt to have somatic complaints, be critical of themselves and others, and feel unloved. Adolescents are more apt to have psychomotor retardation and hypersomnia (APA, 2000). Depressive symptoms tend to be expressed as irritability and can lead to aggressiveness. They are less likely than adults to have psychotic symptoms, and auditory hallucinations are more common than delusions. The acting-out behaviors of children and adolescents, once considered symptoms of masked depression, can clearly be related to the presence of **mood disorders.** These signs of depression may involve risk taking, drug or alcohol use, running away or truancy, misuse of sex, and interest in morbid music and literature.

Factors associated with child and adolescent depression are physical and sexual abuse, neglect, homelessness, marital discord between parents, death, divorce, separation of parents, separation from parents, learning disabilities, chronic illness, conflicts with family or peers, and rejection by family or peers. The complications of depression are school failure and dropping out, drug and alcohol abuse, sexual promiscuity, pregnancy, running away, illegal and antisocial behavior, and suicide.

Rates of suicide in childhood are increasing, and suicide is the third leading cause of death in adolescence (Sadock & Sadock, 2007), second only to accidental death and homicide. There has been a decrease of adolescent suicide in the past 15 years, both completed suicide and suicidal ideation. The decrease coincides with the increase of SSRIs prescribed to adolescents with mood and behavioral symptoms (Sadock & Sadock, 2007). Currently, depression is being treated with psychotherapy and medication rather than letting it run its course. The most frequently diagnosed mood disorders are major depressive disorder, dysthymic disorder, and bipolar disorder.

ASSESSMENT

Assessment Guidelines

Mood Disorders

1. Assess for changes in mood or affect, cognition, social behavior, and physical status.
2. Assess for major life-changing events, stressors or losses.
3. Assess the child's or adolescent's maturational level including lags or regressions
4. Assess the quality of the relationship with the parent or caregiver and current conflict issues.
5. Assess the parent's or caregiver's understanding of growth and development, parenting skills, and handling of problematic behaviors.
6. Assess for family history of mood disorders and suicide.

DIAGNOSIS

There are several nursing diagnoses appropriate for children and adolescents with mood disorders, including *Grieving,*

Hopelessness, Ineffective coping, Risk for injury, Risk for violence, Self-esteem disturbance, and *Social isolation.*

IMPLEMENTATION

Suicidal children and adolescents are hospitalized for evaluation and treatment with psychotherapy and antidepressants or mood stabilizers. Individual, group, and family therapies are used to relieve the distress; correct self-appraisals and improve self-esteem; and promote problem-solving and adaptive coping skills. Tricyclic antidepressants (TCAs) are still used but only with careful monitoring for cardiac effects. The atypical antidepressants in the form of SSRIs have proven very effective for many children and adolescents with mood disorders, despite the controversy.

The overall *long-term outcome* is to help the child or adolescent with a mood disorder reach his or her full potential by fostering the development of competencies and coping skills. The following are guidelines for nursing interventions for children with mood disorders:

1. Provide for biological and psychosocial needs by acting as a parental surrogate.
2. Protect the child from aggressive and self-destructive impulses.
3. Help the child to explore and reality test thoughts, feelings, and life events.
4. Help the child develop and use cognitive skills.
5. Increase the child's self-esteem, and social skills through activities and a caring relationship.
6. Help the child accept and work through losses and limitations.

ATTENTION DEFICIT HYPERACTIVITY DISORDER AND DISRUPTIVE BEHAVIOR DISORDERS

ATTENTION DEFICIT HYPERACTIVITY DISORDER

Children with **attention deficit hyperactivity disorder (ADHD)** show an inappropriate degree of inattention, impulsiveness, and hyperactivity. ADHD is difficult to diagnose before 4 years of age. ADHD often manifests as excessive gross motor activity that becomes less pronounced as the child matures. The disorder is most often identified when the child has difficulty adjusting to elementary school. The attention problems and hyperactivity contribute to low tolerance for frustration, temper outbursts, labile moods, poor academic performance, rejection by peers, and low self-esteem (Sadock & Sadock, 2007). An increased incidence of nocturnal or daytime enuresis, disruptive behavior disorders, and Tourette's disorder has been associated with ADHD (Popper et al., 2002).

Symptoms of ADHD include the following:

Inattention
- Has difficulty paying attention in tasks or play
- Does not seem to listen, follow through, or finish tasks
- Does not pay attention to details and makes careless mistakes
- Is easily distracted, loses things, and is forgetful in daily activities

Hyperactivity
- Fidgets, is unable to sit still or stay seated in school
- Runs and climbs excessively in inappropriate situations
- Acts as if "driven by a motor" constantly "on the go"
- Talks excessively

Impulsivity
- Blurts out answer before question is completed
- Has difficulty waiting his or her turn
- Interrupts, intrudes in others' conversations and games

DISRUPTIVE BEHAVIOR DISORDERS

Oppositional Defiant Disorder

Oppositional defiant disorder is a recurrent pattern of negativistic, disobedient, hostile, and defiant behavior toward authority figures without seriously violating the basic rights of others (APA, 2000). Such children exhibit persistent stubbornness, argumentativeness, testing of limits, unwillingness to give in or negotiate, and refusal to accept blame for misdeeds. This behavior is evident at home but may not be present elsewhere. These children and adolescents do not see themselves as defiant; instead, they feel they are responding to unreasonable demands or situations. This disorder is usually evident before 8 years of age and is more common in males until puberty when the incidence is equal.

Conduct Disorder

Conduct disorder is characterized by a persistent pattern of behavior in which the rights of others and age-appropriate societal norms or rules are violated. The *DSM-IV-TR* identifies four types of behaviors: (1) aggression toward people and animals, (2) destruction of property, (3) deceit-

fulness or theft, and (4) serious violations of rules. If the conduct disorder persists into adulthood, it may result in the diagnosis of antisocial personality disorder.

Predisposing factors are ADHD, oppositional child behaviors, parental rejection, inconsistent parenting with harsh discipline, out-of home placements, frequent shifting of parental figures, large family size, absence of father or alcoholic father, antisocial and drug-dependent family members, and association with a delinquent group.

Childhood onset conduct disorder occurs mainly in males before age 10 years. These children are physically aggressive, have poor peer relationships with little concern for others, and lack feelings of guilt or remorse. To make matters worse, they misperceive the intentions of others as being hostile and believe their aggressive responses are justified. Although they try to project a tough image, they have low self-esteem, have low tolerance for frustration, show irritability, and have temper outbursts.

Adolescent-onset conduct disorder results in less aggressive behaviors and more normal peer relationships. These preadults tend to act out their misconduct with their peer group (e.g., truancy, early-onset sexual behaviors, drinking, substance abuse, and risk-taking behaviors). Males are more apt to fight, steal, vandalize, and have school discipline problems, whereas girls lie, run away, and engage in prostitution. Conduct disorders lead to academic failure and school dropouts, juvenile delinquency, and the need for the juvenile court system to assume responsibility for youths who cannot be managed by their parents. Other psychiatric disorders frequently coexist with conduct disorders such as anxiety, mood disorders, learning disorders, and ADHD.

ASSESSMENT

Assessment Guidelines

Attention Deficit Hyperactivity Disorder and Disruptive Behavior Disorders

1. Assess the quality of child-parent-caregiver relationship for evidence of bonding, anxiety, tension, and difficulty-of-fit between parent's and child's temperament, which can contribute to the development of disruptive behaviors.
2. Asses the parent's or caregiver's understanding of growth and development, parenting skills, and handling of problematic behaviors; lack of knowledge contributes to the development of these problems.
3. Assess cognitive, psychosocial, and moral development for lags or deficits; immaturity in developmental competencies results in disruptive behaviors.

Attention Deficit Hyperactivity Disorder

1. Observe the level of physical activity, attention span, talkativeness, and ability to follow directions and control impulses. Medication is often needed to ameliorate problems in these areas.
2. Assess difficulty in making friends and performing in school. Academic failure and poor peer relationships lead to low self-esteem, depression, and further acting-out.
3. Assess for problems with enuresis and encopresis.

Oppositional Defiant Disorder

1. Identify issues that result in power struggles, when they begin, and how they are handled.
2. Assess the severity of the defiant behavior and its effect on life at home, at school, and with peers.

Conduct Disorder

1. Assess the seriousness of the disruptive behavior, when it started, and what has been done to manage it. Hospitalization or residential placement may be necessary in addition to medication.
2. Assess the levels of anxiety, aggression, anger, and hostility toward others and ability to control impulses.
3. Assess moral development for the ability to understand the effect of hurtful behavior on others, to empathize with others, and to feel remorse or guilt.

DIAGNOSIS

There are several nursing diagnoses appropriate for children and adolescents with attention deficit hyperactivity disorder and disruptive behavior disorders, including *Risk for other-directed violence, Risk for caregiver role strain, Defensive coping, Risk for injury, Impaired social interaction, Ineffective coping, Chronic low self-esteem,* and *Disturbed thought processes.*

IMPLEMENTATION

Nursing interventions are directed at changing or modifying the specific behaviors that cause the problems with families, peers, and authorities and impede the normal development of the child or adolescent. The *long-term outcome* for all these disorders is to help the child or adolescent reach full potential by fostering developmental competencies and coping skills.

The following are guidelines for nursing interventions for children and adolescents with ADHD and disruptive behavior disorders:

1. Protect the child or adolescent from harm and provide for biological and psychosocial needs while acting as a parental surrogate and role model.
2. Increase the child's or adolescent's ability to trust and use interpersonal skills to maintain satisfying relationships with adults and peers.
3. Increase the child's or adolescent's ability to control impulses, tolerate frustration, and modulate the expression of affect.
4. Foster the child's or adolescent's identification with positive role models so that positive attitudes and moral values can develop that enable the youth to experience feelings of empathy, remorse, shame, and pride.
5. Foster the development of a realistic self-identity and self-esteem based on achievements and the formation of realistic goals.
6. Provide support, education, and guidance for parents or caregivers.

The **interventions for ADHD** are behavior modification and pharmacological agents for the inattention and the hyperactive or impulsive behaviors, special education programs for the academic difficulties, and psychotherapy and play therapy for the emotional problems that develop as a result of the disorder. Psychostimulants are used to treat ADHD as a sluggish frontal lobe is thought to be causative of the disorder. Methylphenidate (Ritalin) is the most widely used stimulant because of its safety and simplicity of use. It is available orally and as a transdermal patch (Daytrana). Concerta is an extended-release Ritalin that allows once-daily dosing. Adderall is a newer psychostimulant that contains dextroamphetamine and amphetamine. Research on alternative drugs is ongoing because 30% of children with ADHD do not respond to stimulants or cannot tolerate the side effects (Harvard Mental Health Letter, 2006).

Interventions for oppositional defiant and conduct disorder focus on correcting the child's or adolescent's faulty personality (ego and superego) development, which involves developing more mature and adaptive coping mechanisms. This is a gradual process not amenable to brief treatment. Conduct disorders may require inpatient hospitalization for crisis intervention, evaluation, and treatment planning, as well as transfer to therapeutic foster care or long-term residential treatment. Youths with oppositional defiant disorder are generally treated as outpatients, with much of the focus on parenting issues. Multisystemic therapy is an evidence-based model that emphasizes the home environment and empowering families through several hours of treatment each week.

To control **aggressive behaviors**, a wide variety of pharmacological agents have been tried, including antipsychotics, lithium carbonate, anticonvulsants, antidepressants, and β-adrenergic blockers. Cognitive-behavioral therapy is used to change the pattern of misconduct by fostering the development of internal controls, both cognitive and emotional. Problem solving, conflict resolution, empathy, and social interaction skills are important components of the treatment program.

Families are involved in therapy and are given support in parenting skills designed to help them provide nurturance and set consistent limits. They are the key players in carrying out the treatment plan, using behavior modification techniques at home, monitoring the medication's effect, collaborating with the teacher to foster academic success, and setting up a home environment that promotes the achievement of normal developmental tasks. When families are abusive, drug dependent, or highly disorganized, the child may benefit from out-of-home placement.

The following are nursing interventions for working with parents or caregivers of children and adolescents with ADHD and disruptive behavior disorders:

1. Assess parent's or caregiver's knowledge of the disorder and the related behaviors and provide needed information.
2. Explore the effect of the behaviors on family life.
3. Assess the family's or caregiver's support system.
4. Discuss realistic behavioral goals and how to set them.
5. Give parents or caregivers support as they learn to apply techniques.
6. Provide educational information about medications.
7. Refer parent or caregiver to an appropriate support group.

TOURETTE'S DISORDER

Tourette's disorder involves motor and verbal tics that cause marked distress and significant impairment in social and occupational function (APA, 2000). Tics may appear as early as 2 years of age, but the average age of onset is 7 years. The duration of the disorder is usually lifelong, but there can be periods of remission, and the symptoms often diminish during adolescence or sometimes disappear by early adulthood. Motor tics usually involve the head but can also involve the torso or limbs, and they change in location, frequency, and severity over time. In half of the cases, the first symptom is a single tic, most often eye blinking. Other motor tics are tongue protrusion, touching, squatting, hopping, and retracing steps. Vocal tics include words and sounds (barks, grunts, yelps, clicks, snorts, sniffs, coughs). Coprolalia (uttering obscenities), although a color-

ful subject of films (such as *What About Bob*) and mainstream culture, is present in less than 10% of cases.

Tourette's disorder affects 4 or 5 individuals per 10,000 and is more common in males. There is a familial pattern in about 90% of cases. Vulnerability is transmitted in an autosomal dominant pattern, with 70% of females and 99% of males who have inherited the gene developing the disorder. "Nongenetic" Tourette's disorder often coexists with PDD or a seizure disorder.

ASSESSMENT

Symptoms associated with Tourette's disorder are obsessions, compulsions, hyperactivity, distractibility, and impulsivity. In addition, the child or adolescent with tics has low self-esteem from feeling ashamed, self-conscious, and rejected by peers. The fear of having tic behavior in public situations causes the individual to limit activities severely. Central nervous system (CNS) stimulants increase the severity of the tics, and therefore children with coexisting ADHD must have their medication carefully monitored.

DIAGNOSIS

There are several nursing diagnoses appropriate for children and adolescents with Tourette's disorder, including *Anxiety*, *Impaired social interaction*, *Chronic low self-esteem*, and *Social isolation*.

IMPLEMENTATION

The focus of treatment is on helping the child, family, and school understand and cope with the tic behaviors. This disorder is treated on an outpatient basis unless there are severe tics or obsessive-compulsive behaviors that severely impair the child's function at home and in school. Sometimes inpatient or day hospitalization is needed for a complete evaluation and pharmacological intervention. The tricyclic antidepressant clomipramine (Anafranil) is currently the drug of choice for this disorder.

THERAPEUTIC MODALITIES FOR CHILD AND ADOLESCENT DISORDERS

Parental involvement is recognized as important in the supportive and educative system for the child or adolescent. In addition to therapy with a single family, multiple-family therapy can be used to engage families as co-therapists to help them learn to (1) like and respect others, (2) capitalize on strengths and accept shortcomings, (3) develop insight and improve judgment, (4) use new information, and (5) develop lasting and satisfying relationships.

Group therapy for younger children takes the form of play. For grade school children, it combines playing and talking about the activity. For adolescents, it involves more talking, and focuses largely on peer relationships as well as specific problems. A challenge of using groups when working with children and adolescents lies in the contagious effect of disruptive behavior.

Groups have been used effectively to deal with specific issues in the life of a youth (e.g., bereavement, physical and sexual abuse, substance abuse, sexuality and dating, teenage pregnancy, chronic illnesses, depression, suicidal ideation).

Milieu therapy is a philosophical basis for structuring inpatient, residential, and day treatment programs. The nurse collaborates with other health care providers in structuring and maintaining a therapeutic environment which facilitates the individual's growth and positive behavioral change. The physical milieu is designed to provide a safe, comfortable place to live, play, and learn, with areas for group activity as well as private time. There may be a gym, outdoor playground, swimming pool, garden, cooking or other recreational facilities, and even pets. The daily schedule structures the activities (e.g., school, therapy sessions, group activities and outings, family visits).

Behavior modification is based on the principle that rewarded behavior is more likely to be repeated. Developmentally appropriate behaviors are normally rewarded with validation by a significant adult in the child's life, so modifying behavior in this manner is a standard parenting technique. To extinguish undesirable behavior, either the behavior is ignored or, if it is too disruptive or dangerous, limits that have specified consequences are set. A proactive approach to dealing with disruptive behavior includes increasing the structure of a group activity, increasing staff presence, and anticipating the contagious effects by means of "antiseptic bouncing" of a disruptive child from the activity.

One common method is the point and level system, in which points are awarded for desired behaviors, and increasing levels of privileges can be earned. Points are given for behaviors such as dressing, attending school and activities on time and without being disruptive, and demonstrating social skills. Each level has increasing privileges such as going off the unit with a staff member, or later bedtime on weekends. At the highest level, the privilege might be to leave the unit unescorted. Earned points and level status are recorded daily. Points are collected and used to obtain specific rewards.

Removal and restraint are controversial treatment modalities for children. Seclusion may bring about superficial compliance, but has little to do with real behavioral change. The child or adolescent will usually perceive seclusion as punishment, and the experience of being overpowered by adults is terrifying, especially for one who has been abused.

Instead of seclusion, a unit may have an unlocked **quiet room** for a youth who needs to be removed from the situation for either self-control or control by the staff. Other approaches include the feelings room or the freedom room with objects that can be punched, kicked, and thrown. The youth is encouraged to express and work through feelings in private or with staff support.

Time-out is a common method for intervening in disruptive or inappropriate behaviors. Time-out procedures are designed so that staff can be consistent in their interventions. The child's individual behavioral goals are considered in setting limits on behavior and using time-out periods. If they are overused or used as an automatic response to a behavioral infraction, time-outs lose their effectiveness.

A youth's behavior can sometimes be so destructive that physical restraint is needed. Although a mechanical restraint such as a helmet for head banging may be used, **therapeutic holding** is a long-established practice for the control of destructive behaviors. This intervention requires prompt, firm, nonretaliatory protective restraint that is gently applied and leads to a reduction in the youth's distress, greater relaxation, a return of self-control, and trust in the staff.

Cognitive-behavioral therapy helps to change both cognitive processes and behaviors, thereby reducing the frequency of maladaptive responses and replacing them with new competencies. This therapy is carried out in individual or group sessions that teach youth how to cope with problems and stressors through a series of cognitive-behavioral activities (e.g., cognitive rehearsal, positive affirmations, role-playing social skills and assertiveness, and relaxation techniques).

Play therapy is based on the notion that play is the work of childhood and the way a child learns to master impulses and adapt to the environment. Play is also the language of childhood and the communication medium for assessing developmental and emotional status, determining diagnosis, and instituting therapeutic interventions. There are many forms of play therapy that can be used individually or in groups. Playrooms are equipped with art supplies and a variety of toys including hand puppets, dolls, and action figures. These toys provide the child with opportunities to act out conflicts and stressful situations, to work through feelings, and with the help of the therapist to develop more adaptive ways of coping.

Dramatic play therapy is a treatment modality that uses dramatic techniques to act out emotional problems, examine subjective experience, develop new perspectives, and try out new behaviors. This modality may be used with groups of verbal children and adolescents. If they are psychotic, reality-based role plays are substituted for fantasies. Dramatic play is a form of psychodrama. Hand puppets and puppet shows are a favorite way to act out problems and solutions. Uninhibited children and adolescents enjoy acting roles in dramas that they have created spontaneously or scripted. The dramas can be videotaped for reviewing the experience and facilitating new learning.

Therapeutic games are an ideal treatment modality for children who may have difficulty talking about their feelings and problems while developing rapport with health care workers. The game might be as simple as checkers, but therapeutic games are more effective in eliciting children's fears and fantasies. A well-known game by Gardner is the *Talking, Feeling, and Doing Game* (1986), a board game appropriate for latent and preadolescent children. The player draws a talking, feeling, or doing card, which gives instructions or asks a question, "All the girls in the class were invited to a birthday party except one. How did she feel?" If this game is played with a group, additional responses can be elicited.

Bibliotherapy involves using children's literature to help the child express feelings in a supportive environment, gain insight into feelings and behavior, and learn new ways to cope with difficult situations. Children unconsciously identify with the characters in the story, so the books selected should reflect the situation or feeling that is problematic for the child. It is important to assess the child's readiness for the particular topic and the child's level of understanding.

Therapeutic drawing allows children to spontaneously express themselves in artwork capturing thoughts, feelings, and tensions they may be unable to express verbally. When drawing any human figure, children leave an imprint of the inner self, revealing personality traits, strengths, weaknesses, behaviors, and interpersonal relationships including attitudes and values of the family and cultural group. Drawings are most reliable after children are able to create objective representations of what is seen (usually between 5 and 7 years of age). Often children draw human figures,

and the following characteristics are general indicators of children's emotions and are not necessarily indicative of psychopathology.

- Size of figures: very large (aggression, poor impulse control); very small (shyness, insecurity)
- Emphasis on and exaggeration of body parts: large heads (desire to be smarter), large mouths (speech problems), large arms (desire for strength and power)
- Omissions of body parts: hands (trauma, insecurity), arms (inadequacy), legs (lack of support), feet (insecure, helpless), mouth (difficulty expressing self or relating to others)
- Facial expressions: personal mood and affect
- Integration of body parts: scattered or disorganized parts indicate cognitive or psychological problems or both

Music therapy brings about changes in both the physiology of the body systems and social interactions. Music therapy may incorporate recorded music, songs, song writing, or use of a musical instrument. Children love to use simple noisemakers for the expression of feelings, for the development of coordination and rhythm, and as an opportunity for social interactions. Music on inpatient units is often used to create a relaxing mood for rest periods and bedtime.

Movement and dance therapy is a direct expression of the self that helps the youth get in touch with feelings and thoughts, work off tensions, develop greater body awareness, improve or correct a distorted body image, improve coordination, and increase social interactions. The type of movement used with children can be as simple as a game of "Follow the Leader" or it can be creative, free-form movements to the mood of the music. For older children and adolescents, more formal classes in exercise, karate, or the latest dance craze may be of interest.

Recreational therapy generally takes place off the unit and is often conducted by a recreational therapist with assistance from the nursing staff. Activities can be organized around a game that teaches psychomotor and social skills, or they can be individual activities (e.g., riding a bike, learning to swim). Special field trips and "outings" give children the opportunity to do what other children are doing and to act appropriately in public situations. The communicated expectation is that the children's behavior will be within normal limits, and this becomes a self-fulfilling prophecy leading to increased self-control and self-esteem.

KEY POINTS TO REMEMBER

- Between 12% and 22% of children and adolescents are estimated to have emotional problems, and only a small percentage of these youths actually receive treatment.
- Risk factors known to contribute to the development of mental and emotional problems in children and adolescents include genetic, biochemical (pre- and postnatal), temperament-based, psychosocial developmental, social or environmental, and cultural factors.
- Resiliency in a preadult includes an adaptable temperament, the ability to form nurturing relationships with surrogate parental figures, the ability to distance the self from emotional chaos in parents and family, and good social intelligence and problem-solving skills.
- The most commonly diagnosed child psychiatric disorders are mood disorders, anxiety disorders, ADHD, adjustment reactions, and conduct and oppositional disorders. The PDDs are rarer.

- Treatment of childhood and adolescent disorders requires a multimodal approach. Close work with schools, the availability of remediation services, and the incorporation of behavior modification techniques should be part of the intervention.
- Cognitive-behavioral therapies, social skills groups, family therapy, parent training in behavioral techniques, and individual therapy have been found useful. Skills training may focus on a variety of areas, depending on the child's or adolescent's presenting symptoms.
- Child and adolescent psychiatric nurses are increasingly becoming aware of the need to educate the family and involve the members in the treatment process. The family remains an integral part of the supportive and educative system for the child and adolescent.

CRITICAL THINKING

1. T.S., a 4-year-old boy, has been diagnosed with a PDD—autism.
   A. Describe the specific behavioral data you would find on assessment in terms of (1) communication, (2) social interactions, and (3) behaviors and activities.
   B. Name at least six realistic outcomes for a child with PPD.
   C. Which interventions do you think are the most important for a child with PDD? Identify at least six.
   D. What kinds of support should the family receive?
2. N.T. is a 7-year-old girl who has been diagnosed with ADHD.
   A. This child is in second grade. What clinical behaviors might she be exhibiting at home and in the classroom?

   Give behavioral examples for her (1) inattention, (2) hyperactivity, and (3) impulsivity.
   B. Identify at least six intervention strategies one might use for her. What medications might help her?
   C. Describe the concept of time-out.
3. J.F. is an 8-year-old boy who has been diagnosed with conduct disorder.
   A. Explain to one of J.F.'s classmates his probable behaviors in terms of (1) aggression toward others, (2) destruction of property, (3) deceitfulness, and (4) violation of rules.
   B. What are the outcomes for this child? What is the overall prognosis for children with this disorder?
   C. What are at least seven ways you could support J.F.'s parents? Where could you refer this family within your own community?

CHAPTER REVIEW

Choose the most appropriate answer(s).
1. Which of the following should not be identified by the nurse as a risk factor associated with child psychiatric disorders?
   1. Separation from extended family through relocation across the county
   2. Severe marital discord
   3. Low socioeconomic status
   4. Maternal psychiatric disorder
2. The nurse working in the emergency department usually assesses adult patients, but tonight she is responsible for

assessing the suicide potential of a 13-year-old child. Which topic must be explored in this assessment of a child that is different from such an assessment in an adult?
   1. The presence of distorted perceptions about suicide and death.
   2. The presence of ideas about hurting self seriously or causing death.
   3. Circumstances at the time suicidal thoughts are experienced.
   4. Identification of feelings such as depression, anger, guilt, and rejection.

CHAPTER REVIEW—cont'd

3. G.L., age 5 years, has been diagnosed by a psychiatrist as having a PDD. Which of the following disorders could also be correct medical diagnoses for the child? Select all that apply.
    1. Asperger's syndrome
    2. Autistic disorder
    3. Attention deficit hyperactivity disorder
    4. Posttraumatic stress disorder

4. Which topic would be least relevant as a focus during the assessment of a 12-year-old with suspected ADHD?
    1. Effect of impulsive behavior on the child's life at home and school

2. The child's level of physical activity and attention span
3. The child's ability to pay attention and perform in school
4. The child's progress with toilet training and self-care habits

5. A method of modifying the disruptive behavior of a child that will be perceived by the child as punishment is:
    1. therapeutic holding.
    2. planned ignoring.
    3. restructuring.
    4. seclusion.

REFERENCES

American Psychiatric Association. (2000). *Diagnostic and statistical manual of mental disorders (DSM-IV-TR)* (text rev, 4th ed.). Washington, DC: Author.

Bush, G., Valera, E., & Seidman, L. (2005). Functional neuroimaging of attention-deficit/hyperactivity disorder: A review and suggested future directions. *Biological Psychiatry, 57,*1273-1284.

Centers for Disease Control and Prevention (CDC). (2005). *Developmental disabilities: Retardation.* Retrieved January 10, 2007 from www.cdc.gov/ncbddd/dd/mr3.htm.

Children's Defense Fund. (2004). Newsletter from Marian Wright Edelman. Washington, DC.

FOCUS Adolescent Services (FAS). (2007). Retrieved February 17, 2008 from http://focusas.com/Suicide.html.

Gardner, R.A. (1986). The talking, feeling and doing game. In C.E. Schaefer & S.E. Reid (Eds.), *Game play: Therapeutic use of childhood games* (pp. 41-72). New York: John Wiley.

Harvard Mental Health Letter (2006). ADHD update: New data on the risks of medication (attention deficit hyperactivity disorder). October, 2006.

Kessler, R.C., Berglund, P., Demler, O., et al: (2005). Lifetime prevalence and age-of-onset distributions of *DSM-IV* disorders in the National Comorbidity Survey Replication. *Arch Gen Psychiatry, 62*(6), 593-602.

Inder, T. (2000). *Advances and application of psychopharmacology in pediatrics.* Paper presented at Advancing Children's Health 2000: Pediatric Academic Societies, Boston, MA., May 12-14, 2002, and (PAS) and the American Academy of Pediatrics (AAP) yearly joint meeting.

Popper, C.W., Gammon, G.D., West, S.A., & Bailey, C.F. (2002). Disorders usually first diagnosed in infancy, childhood, or adolescents. In R.F. Hales & S.C. Yudofsky (Eds.), *The American Psychiatric Publishing Textbook of clinical psychiatry* (4th ed.). Washington, DC: American Psychiatric.

Sadock, B.J., & Sadock, V.A. (2004). *Kaplan and Sadock: Comprehensive textbook of psychiatry* (8th ed.). Philadelphia: Lippincott, Williams & Wilkins.

Sadock, B.J., & Sadock, V.A. (2007). *Kaplan & Sadock's synopsis of psychiatry* (10th ed.). Philadelphia: Lippincott, Williams & Wilkins.

U.S. Department of Health and Human Services (USDHHS). (1999). *Mental health: A report of the surgeon general—Executive summary.* Rockville, MD: Author.

Adults

Edward A. Herzog

Key Terms and Concepts

Objectives

1. Discuss ways in which severe mental illness affects society.
2. Understand issues or problems commonly experienced by those living with severe and persistent mental illness.
3. Describe evidence-based treatments for severe and persistent mental illness.
4. Describe impulse control disorders and their implications for society.
5. Understand nursing interventions appropriate for people with impulse control disorders.
6. Describe sexual disorders and their implications for society.
7. Discuss the forms of treatment for sexual disorders.
8. Understand the indicators or symptoms suggestive of adult attention deficit hyperactivity disorder.

evolve

For additional resources related to the content of this chapter, visit the Evolve website at http://evolve.elsevier.com/Varcarolis/essentials.

- Chapter Outline
- Chapter Review Answers
- Case Study
- Nurse, Patient, and Family Resources
- Concept Map Creator

This chapter focuses on mental health issues and needs affecting primarily the adult population. We will look at what it is like to have a **severe and persistent mental illness (SPMI)**, the issues and challenges faced by those diagnosed with these illnesses, and resources and treatment programs available for illness management. Other adult mental issues examined in this chapter include disorders involving impulse control, sexual functioning, and maintaining appropriate attention and activity levels.

SEVERE AND PERSISTENT MENTAL ILLNESS

You are a 19-year-old nursing student working as a nursing assistant. One night you're sitting alone in your dorm studying when you hear someone call your name. No one is there, and you attribute it to lack of sleep. However, over the coming weeks this happens repeatedly, and the voices begin to comment on what you are doing, criticize you, and tell you what to do. You have trouble concentrating. Your schoolwork suffers and your grades begin to drop. You feel that people know what is happening inside your head. You become uncomfortable being around others, begin to skip classes, avoid friends, and quit work.

Distracted by the now ever-present voices, you step into the street and are knocked off your feet by a car. A policeman comes to your aid, but you believe he wants to kill you and you try to run, only to be caught and restrained. The next few days are a confusing, frightening blur of doctors, nurses, injections, and restraints. You are on a psychiatric unit and told that you have something called a schizophreniform disorder.

Medications push the voices into the background, but you feel disconnected, like you are wrapped in layers of cotton. Just as you begin to attend groups and trust some of the staff, you are discharged with an appointment to see a new doctor in a mental health center far from your neighborhood. At the mental health center people look and act very strangely; some are mumbling to themselves, some get too close to you, and some pull away when you walk by. You think, "This can't be happening to me," and wonder what your future will be like.

UNDERSTANDING SEVERE AND PERSISTENT MENTAL ILLNESS

Categorizing mental illness according to levels of severity has tremendous implications for setting mental health policy, establishing insurance reimbursement standards, and facilitating access to appropriate care (Peck & Scheffler, 2002). In the United States each state determines how to classify mental illness for the purpose of insurance coverage. The definitions used by the states generally fall into one of three categories. "Broad-based mental illness" refers to any diagnosis found within the *Diagnostic and Statistical Manual of Mental Disorders (DSM-IV-TR)*, whereas "serious mental illness" and "biologically based mental illness" refer to a limited number of *DSM* diagnoses.

The federal government's classifications of "serious mental illness" (SMI) and "severe and persistent mental illness" (SPMI) refer to those most deeply affected by psychiatric disorders. SMI includes 5.4% of all adults and refers to disorders that somehow interfere with social functioning. In this chapter, the focus is on SPMI, which affects about half of the people in the SMI group, or 2.6% of all adults. SPMI refers to significant impairment of global functioning that may be continuous or episodic and results in disability in 30% to 50% of cases. Disorders that fall into this category include severe forms of depression, panic disorder, obsessive-compulsive disorder, schizophrenia, and bipolar disorder.

Individuals with SPMI usually have difficulties in multiple areas, including activities of daily living (cooking, hygiene), relationships, social interaction, task completion, communication, leisure activities, safe movement about the community, finances and budgeting, health maintenance, vocational and academic activities, and coping with stressors. Associated issues for those with SPMI include poverty, stigma, unemployment, and inadequate housing.

Extent of the Problem

Effect on the Individual

Individuals with SPMI often fall significantly short of their potential, experiencing significantly less academic, vocational, relational, and other forms of success than they likely would have achieved had they not been affected by severe mental illness. People with SPMI often experience stigmatization and discrimination. They are more likely to be victims of crime, be medically ill, have undertreated or untreated physical illnesses, die prematurely, be homeless, be incarcerated, be unemployed or underemployed, engage in binge substance abuse, be living in poverty, and report lower quality of life than those without such illnesses (Aquila & Emanuel, 2003; Glied, 2007).

Effect on Families, Caregivers, and Significant Others

The role of caregivers varies considerably, from substantial (providing housing, clothing, food, social support, transportation, health care access, housekeeping, and financial support) to simply providing periodic contact and interpersonal support. The burden on caregivers is also affected by their own coping abilities, support systems, and financial and other resources. Caregivers may not have an adequate understanding of the mental illness, how to cope with it, or how to help, and they may not be in communication with the health care providers, leaving them feeling frustrated and powerless. Caregiving demands that are chronic and exceed their coping abilities can result in burnout and withdrawal from the patient, or even rejection or abuse (Cuijpers & Stam, 2000; Harrison et al., 1998). Caregivers may be stigmatized by association as if they were somehow tainted by the relationship with the SPMI person (Mehta & Farina, 1988). Fear of this response often results in keeping the problem a secret, thus increasing isolation.

Effect on Society

Most mental health treatment (57%) is paid for with public dollars rather than private insurance as compared with 46% for overall health care expenditures (President's New Freedom Commission on Mental Health, 2003). It has been estimated that untreated and inadequately treated mental illness leads to decreased productivity and other losses that cost our society more than $113 billion per year (National Mental Health Association, 2001). Thirty-five percent of Supplemental Security Income (SSI) and 28% of Social Security Disability Income (SSDI) (both providing income to disabled individuals) go to assist people with SMIs (NAMI, 2004).

Issues Facing Those with Severe and Persistent Mental Illness

Even with successful treatment, people with SPMI often have **residual symptoms,** which are milder, leftover symptoms of the disorder. These remaining symptoms can lead to frustration and hopelessness that they will not get better and that the medications and treatments are not working. In turn, the patient may decide to discontinue treatment, ironically worsening the course of the illness.

Medication side effects, particularly for the typical antipsychotic medications, can produce a wide range of distressing symptoms, including sedation, visual blurring, involuntary movements, weight gain, sexual dysfunction, and increased risk of medical disorders such as diabetes. It is important to educate patients about these side effects because some are amenable to treatment, such as extrapyramidal side effects being managed with anticholinergics. Others are not treatable, although in many cases they diminish over time or can be compensated for by changes in lifestyle or behavior (e.g., learning to change position slowly to prevent dizziness from orthostatic hypotension, or calorie reduction to reduce weight gain and metabolic syndrome). Side effects are an essential issue to address in treatment because, if not managed, they may impair one's quality of life or cause (or provide a justification for)

discontinuing treatment. See Chapter 14 for a more extensive discussion of medications used to treat psychotic disorders.

Relapse, chronicity, and loss may occur despite adherence to medications and therapy (Doering et al., 1998). Disorders such as schizophrenia are for the most part chronic illnesses, and as with other chronic illnesses, living with them requires more effort and psychic energy than required of people without these illnesses.

Depression and suicide may be the result of a profound sense of loss of pre-illness life and potential. If at one point you are a successful premed student, and 3 years later you are unemployed and living in a group home, there is a significant disconnect between your original life trajectory and where you are now. This loss, along with the chronicity of the illness and its demands and effect on daily life, can contribute to despair, depression, and risk of suicide (about 5% to 10% of those with SPMI commit suicide) (Pompili et al., 2007).

Co-occurring medical illnesses occur more frequently with SPMI, particularly hypertension (22%), obesity (24%), cardiovascular disease (21%), diabetes (12%), chronic obstructive pulmonary disease (COPD) (10%), and trauma (6%) (Miller et al., 2007). Risk of premature death (about 28 years) from these disorders is 1.6 to 2.8 times greater than in the general population. People with SPMI may not provide for their own health needs and may not receive adequate care due to costs, difficulty accessing health care, or stigma or stereotyping (e.g., emergency department [ED] personnel assuming that because a person is psychotic that person's chest pain is not real). In some cases psychiatric presentation might influence the quality of health care provided to a person whose presenting complaint is expressed in a bizarre manner.

Unemployment and poverty contribute to poor self-esteem and lack of identity. Eighty-five percent of people with SMIs are unemployed, and disability entitlements received by 50% of those with SMIs do not provide much income: On average, a person with SPMI who is disabled will receive perhaps $700 per month from SSDI or $400 from SSI (NAMI, 2000). However, it can be difficult to find an employer open to hiring a person with a mental illness, and laws to prevent discrimination do not guarantee a job. Even if patients find a job, the income could cause them to become ineligible for health care coverage, forcing them to pay for medications out-of-pocket, in turn likely reducing adherence to medications (and contributing to the problem of decreased access to health care in general) (Rosenheck et al., 2006).

Housing instability can contribute to stress for individuals with SPMIs. If patients cannot afford a car, they need to live near public transportation. To get a cheap apartment they may have to live where gunshots are heard most nights—not a good situation for anyone, let alone a person overwhelmed by mental illness. An ill-timed episode of inappropriate behavior could also lead to eviction, and once known in the circle of local landlords, could mean closed doors in the neighborhood and no references to help the patient move somewhere else.

Stigma for mental illness is a significant problem in our society. It causes others to assume that people with mental illness are less than human, dangerous, and even somehow responsible for their condition. It can leave the affected person feeling ashamed or angry, pushing him or her further away from others and reducing access to potential support systems. Stigma is perpetuated by stereotypical images or language in the media, thoughtless comments by everyday people or celebrities, and a thousand other sources. NAMI and other advocacy groups, mental health consumers and professionals, and many others are working to reduce stigma in the same way that was once necessary for developmentally disabled people. At present, many people have not yet come to see the problem in calling mentally ill people crazy, which is the equivalent of calling someone with mental retardation a "retard."

Anosognosia is the inability of a person to recognize deficits *from* the illness due *to* the illness. With mental illness it's the brain that is sick, the same organ needed for insight and decision making. It is an extremely frustrating Catch-22, and one that is at the heart of treatment nonadherence and all its attendant problems (Amador, 2007). Would you take medicine for an illness you do not believe you have?

Social isolation and loneliness are significant issues for many people with chronic illnesses, not just those with SPMIs. Stigma and social stratification contribute to reduced social contact with "out" groups, such as severely mentally ill individuals. Factors, such as poor self image, poverty (which interferes with access to and participation in social or recreational social activities), passivity, impaired hygiene, and anxiety also reduce interaction and interfere with relationships. As a result many people with SPMIs are socially isolated and experience significant amounts of loneliness.

Medication may reduce the libido or the ability to function sexually and interfere with intimate physical relationships. Negative self image and delusional thinking may place additional barriers to close interpersonal connections. People with SPMIs may be taken advantage of sexually or make ill-advised choices regarding sexual partners or practices, which can increase the risk of STDs and unplanned pregnancies (Torkelson & Dobal, 1999).

NAMI estimates that up to half of all people with mental illnesses are receiving **inadequate treatment** that does not match treatment guidelines, is not supported by research, or is outmoded (NAMI, 2000). Some of the most recent medications or other treatments that are most supported by research are excluded from formularies or unapproved by third-party payers. Treatment innovations and changing standards of practice can be slow to be incorporated into practice (President's New Freedom Commission on Mental Health, 2003).

Atypical antipsychotic medications can be **extremely expensive**. McCombs and colleagues (2000) documented an average cost of more than $25,000 per year. Even with Medicaid one might have a copay or a spend-down (a need to exhaust one's own funds each month in order to reestablish Medicaid eligibility) in order to obtain medications. People with insurance may find their share of costs to be prohibitively high, or that their insurance company has restrictions that end their care before they are clinically ready—or do not cover it at all.

Some estimate that co-occurring **substance abuse** can be found in 50% of those with a SPMI (NAMI, 2007). One theory is that it is a form of self-medication, a way of countering the dysphoria or other symptoms caused by one's illness, or the sedation caused by one's medications. Nicotine use has always been higher in the SPMI population and is not declining as it has been in the general population. Substance abuse contributes to co-occurring physical health problems, reduced quality of life, risk of incarceration, risk of relapse, and reduced effectiveness of psychotropic treatments (McCloughen, 2003).

Victimization is more common among mentally ill people by a factor of two and one-half times (Hiday et al., 1999). Sexual victimization, such as assault or coerced sexual activity, also occurs in this vulnerable population (e.g., a patient whose boyfriend "loaned" her sexually to peers in return for drugs, compelling her to cooperate in return for housing). Factors such as impaired judgment, impaired interpersonal skills (e.g., unknowingly acting in ways that might provoke others, such as standing too close or not leaving when told to), passivity, poor self-esteem, dependency, living in urban or high-crime neighborhoods, and seeming more vulnerable to criminals may contribute to this significant problem. Drug abuse and transient living conditions have been shown to be strong predictors of victimization in the population (Hiday et al., 1999).

Issues Affecting Society and the Individual

Involuntary treatment involves treatment mandated by a court order and delivered without the patient's consent. **Outpatient commitment** was designed to provide mandatory treatment in a less restrictive setting, typically after the patient leaves the hospital or prison. Some consider it a form of assisted treatment in that it helps people who do not realize they are mentally ill to maintain the best mental health status possible (Torrey & Zdanowicz, 2001).

Criminal offenses and incarceration may be the result of desperation, impaired judgment, or impulsivity. Most often they are nonviolent crimes such as trespassing or petty theft. Patients with SPMIs may also become public nuisances, cannot be persuaded to accept treatment, and do not meet criteria for involuntary treatment because they are not an imminent danger to self or others. An example might be a man with SPMI and impaired judgment who does not dress adequately for cold weather and hangs out in laundromats and libraries for warmth. When expelled, the man is at risk of hypothermia, and in such cases loved ones or police may seek the person's arrest simply to get him or her off the streets. Efforts to improve responses to SPMI include **educating police** to identify mental illness and distinguish it from criminal intent, and providing people with help instead of jailing them. **Mental health courts** are designed to assist people whose crimes are secondary to mental illness, and divert people with SPMIs to treatment instead of imprisonment.

Transinstitutionalization is the shifting of a person or population from one form of institution to another, such as from state hospitals to jails, prisons, nursing homes, or the street. Although **deinstitutionalization** has given the appearance of providing care in less restrictive settings and provided for financial savings, in a large number of cases the new setting is in fact more restrictive, and the costs have simply been transferred to another provider (Torrey, 1997).

Application of the Nursing Process
ASSESSMENT

Assessment involves observation for signs of risk to self or others, including suicidality or homicidality; depression or hopelessness; signs of relapse, especially increased impulsivity or paranoia, diminished reality testing, increased delusional thinking, or command hallucinations; and inadequate attention to one's needs for proper nutrition, clothing, or medical care. Impaired judgment and psychosis increase the risk of intentionally and unintentionally dangerous behaviors. Such patients may start fires by leaving pots on the stove and becoming distracted or falling asleep. They may begin to respond to command hallucinations or paranoid ideation, which indicates that another person is a threat to them.

It is essential to observe for signs of treatment nonadherence and impending relapse. Correcting non-

adherence helps reduce relapse, and early detection of relapse reduces its intensity and duration. Assess for physical health problems such as tumors or metabolic disorders, which cause psychiatric symptoms and may be mistaken for mental illness or relapse (White, 2003). Monitor comorbid illnesses to ensure that the patient provides adequate self-care and receives adequate health care for such disorders.

DIAGNOSIS

Nursing diagnoses for SPMI include *Impaired adjustment; Compromised family coping; Ineffective coping; Ineffective health maintenance; Risk for loneliness; Noncompliance; Bathing/hygiene and Dressing/grooming Self-care deficit; Chronic low self-esteem; Chronic sorrow;* and *Disturbed thought processes.* See Table 24-1 for interventions to be used with patients who have an SPMI.

OUTCOMES IDENTIFICATION

The following are examples of potential outcome measures:
- Patient identifies "voices" as hallucinations.
- Patient demonstrates three adaptive responses when faced with hallucinations.
- Patient remains free from police involvement.
- Patient maintains stable housing.
- Patient remains free from harm.
- Patient demonstrates consistent treatment adherence.

IMPLEMENTATION

The following are interventions to be used to improve adherence with treatment:
1. Monitor side effects to avert or minimize patient distress, which encourages nonadherence.
2. Simplify treatment regimens to make them more acceptable to the patient (e.g., once-per-day dosing instead of twice daily).
3. Tie treatment adherence to achieving the patient's goals (not the doctor's or society's) to increase patient motivation. Point out and reinforce improvements, connecting them to the patient's treatment adherence.
4. Facilitate referrals for assistance with treatment costs and access to improving treatment adherence.
5. Provide psychoeducation regarding SPMI and the role of treatment in recovery to improve insight and motivation.

TABLE 24-1   Interventions for Severe and Persistent Mental Illness

Intervention	Rationale
1. Mutually develop incremental, patient-centered goals and interventions that will help a patient achieve the desired quality of life, rather than on symptom reduction.	1. Patient involvement in goal-setting and treatment selection builds the therapeutic alliance and increases the likelihood of treatment adherence and success.
2. Enhance and promote **reality testing** (e.g., teaching a patient, when he or she hears voices, to scan the immediate environment to see if anyone else seems to be hearing the voices; if not, encourage the patient to label it as a hallucination and to distract self from it or disregard it).	2. Impaired reality testing is the hallmark of SPMI, and impairments in this ability contribute to hallucinations and delusional thinking. Training and encouraging the patient to verify whether experiences are real can help the patient manage symptoms of the illness.
3. Provide psychoeducation, guidance, support, and reinforcement for actions that help patients manage their symptoms of SPMI (see Box 14-3 on page 293). Include the family in psychoeducational activities as tolerated and possible.	3. Whistling or other simple auditory distractions can reduce auditory hallucinations; gaining mastery over symptoms improves function, reduces disruption, and provides one with a sense of control and confidence.
4. Reduce loneliness and isolation by interacting frequently with the patient, supporting opportunities for interaction (e.g., day programs, social, and recreational events), helping the patient to manage social anxiety, helping the patient who does not want to socialize to identify and use alternative resources (e.g., pets, stuffed animals), and involving the patient in social skills training.	4. SPMIs decrease sociability and predispose individuals to isolation as a result of stigma, loss of social skills, and social discomfort. Activities that increase skill and comfort with interaction, especially with supportive people and positive role models, such as other patients who are farther along in recovery, contribute to improved functioning and a higher quality of life.
5. Encourage involvement of patients and their loved ones in NAMI and similar support meetings.	5. NAMI members "have been there" and can provide support, socialization, and practical suggestions for issues and problems facing patients and significant others; involvement in such groups is also empowering for the patient.
6. Provide education and support regarding making sound decisions regarding interpersonal relations, STD prevention, and family planning.	6. People with SPMI may have impaired judgment, feel isolated, and have other vulnerabilities that increase their risk for victimization, STDs, and undesired pregnancies; patients seeking to have families may benefit from genetic counseling regarding their disorders.
7. Connect the patient with case managers and other personnel who are likely to be able to work with him or her for extended periods and who are skilled at developing and maintaining therapeutic relationships.	7. Trusting and therapeutic relationships are key resources for achieving treatment adherence, and SPMI patients often require extended periods of working together with staff to form these connections.
8. Actively promote treatment adherence.	8. Treatment adherence reduces relapse and improves the long-term prognosis and quality of life.
9. Provide supportive psychosocial interventions.	9. This aids in maintaining therapeutic rapport and helps the patient to maintain a positive self-esteem, and to cope effectively rather than maladaptively.
10. Provide for regular and frequent contact with the patient, but not so much that it overstimulates the patient or contributes to paranoid ideation.	10. Ongoing contact promotes therapeutic alliances and allows for monitoring so relapse or nonadherence can quickly be intercepted.
11. Educate, guide, support, and reinforce behaviors that prevent or control actual or potential medical comorbidities; act as an advocate as needed to ensure adequate health care for SPMI patients.	11. SPMI patients have higher burdens of physical illness, poorer hygiene and health practices, less access to effective medical treatment, and more premature mortality than the general population.
12. Involve persons with co-occurring substance abuse or addiction to Alcoholics Anonymous or Narcotics Anonymous (AA or NA) and dual diagnosis (substance abuse/mental illness [SAMI]) services.	12. Substance abuse rates are high in SPMI populations, increase relapse, and interfere with recovery; achieving sobriety is most associated with AA and integrated treatment programs.

NAMI, National Alliance on Mental Illness; *STDs*, sexually transmitted diseases; *SPMI*, severe and persistent mental illness.

6. Assign consistent, committed caregivers who have (or are skilled at building) positive therapeutic bonds with the patient.

7. Involve the patient in support groups that have members who have greater insight and a first-hand experience with illness and treatment that the patient may be more likely to accept.

8. Provide culturally sensitive care. Cultural beliefs and practices of a patient (such as suspicious attitudes toward health care and authority figures, or valuing of self-sufficiency or privacy above health care) may be crucial in treatment adherence.

9. Consider judicious use of medication decreases or discontinuation to control side effects or improve the therapeutic alliance (Weiden, 2007).

10. As indicated, and when other interventions have not been successful, use medication monitoring and long-acting forms of medication (depot injections or sustained-release formats), to maximize the benefits of medication.

11. Never reject, blame, or shame the patient when nonadherence occurs; instead, label it as simply an issue for continuing focus, often requiring numerous tries.

Pharmacological, Biological, and Integrative Therapies

State hospitals and psychiatric units in general hospitals provide inpatient care. Outpatient care for SPMI are the **community mental health centers (CMHCs)**, private providers (primarily psychiatrists, psychologists, therapists, social workers, and advanced-practice nurses), and private and governmental agencies. Community-based services vary with local needs and resources. It may also be difficult to "work the maze" of multiple agencies and services. See Chapter 27 for a full discussion of mental health treatment settings.

Rehabilitation Versus Recovery

Until recently the **rehabilitation model** has been the dominant paradigm in mental health care. It focuses on deficits, symptoms, and stability rather than on quality of life and cure. It has been criticized for emphasizing dependence on health care providers, with staff essentially functioning as parents and the patient as the dependent child. A new model of care developed out of the consumer movement—a movement that emphasizes choices and empowerment—is called the **recovery model**. It is promoted by the **National Alliance on Mental Illness (NAMI)**, a leading advocacy organization. The recovery model involves a partnership between care providers and the patient, with patients having an active role in choosing and directing their treatment (Frese et al., 2001). It is a positive, hopeful, empowering strength-focused model wherein staff are in an assistive role and the consumer uses his or her strengths to achieve the highest quality of life possible (Mulligan, 2005).

Evidence-Based Treatment Approaches and Services

The following evidence-based treatment approaches are recommended for use for SPMI and available in a variety of settings in many communities.

Programs of assertive community treatment (PACT) have been shown to improve symptoms of SMI and to decrease inpatient admissions, incarceration, and homelessness among people with mental illness (Coldwell & Bender, 2007). Rather than going to multiple departments or agencies, a consumer works with a set team of professionals who provide a comprehensive array of services.

Cognitive-behavioral therapy (CBT) has been effective in helping individuals with SMIs reduce and cope with symptoms such as auditory hallucinations (Sensky et al., 2000). The cognitive component of CBT helps patients perceive circumstances more accurately and in a more positive light by guiding them to reconsider their perceptions and restructure their thinking to be more in line with reality. The behavioral component uses natural consequences and positive reinforcers (rewards) to shape the person's behavior in a more positive or adaptive manner.

Promotion of family support and partnerships is based on the premise that that having sound support systems is one of the strongest predictors of recovery, and that treatment is enhanced when treatment providers work as empathic partners with patients and significant others (Farhall et al., 1998; NAMI, 2007). An example of this partnership is NAMI's Family-to-Family program, a psychoeducational program focusing on the skills families need to cope with their loved one's illness and to promote recovery (NAMI, 2007).

Social skills training focuses on teaching persons with SPMI a wide variety of social skills. Social deficits cause both direct and indirect functional impairment; people unable to respond assertively, for example, may instead respond aggressively or fail to get their needs met. Complex interpersonal skills (such as negotiating or resolving a conflict) are broken down into subcomponents that are then taught in a stepwise fashion.

Supportive psychotherapy focuses on supporting the individual here and now, rather than on a more complex insight-oriented therapy in which change and growth are the goals. It stresses empathic understanding, improved coping, and anxiety reduction; is informal in style; can be used by any member of the treatment team and in combination with other modalities; and has been shown to enhance the therapeutic alliance and improve long-term recovery prospects in patients with SMIs (Hellerstein et al., 1998).

Vocational rehabilitation and supported employment enhances self-esteem, improves organizational abilities, and increases socialization and income. Vocational rehabilitation has been used for many years and stresses prevocational training, employment in a sheltered setting (e.g., a consumer-run business), and competitive employment in the general business world. **Supported employment** focuses on rapid employment and on-the-job training, thereby providing competitive employment from the onset, and ongoing supports (Cook et al., 2005).

Other Potentially Beneficial Approaches or Services

Although not yet evidence based to the extent of the preceding approaches, research supports potential benefits from use of the following.

Advance directives are legal documents provided for by law in certain states that—when the patient's illness is under control and informed decisions are possible—give the patient the opportunity to direct how future relapses and treatment needs should be managed. For example, a patient can give consent to hospitalization or forced antipsychotic medications and specify when these responses may be used, minimizing the patient's loss of control over his or her treatment and avoiding the need for involuntary admission and related court involvement.

Peer support and consumer-run programming range from informal "clubhouses" that offer socialization, recreation, and sometimes other services to competitive businesses, such as snack bars or janitorial services that provide needed services and consumer employment while encouraging independence and building vocational skills.

Technology holds the potential to reduce treatment costs, improve treatment access, and improve outcomes. Electronic records available in multiple locations via wireless technologies can assist in assessments or service delivery anywhere in the community. Service providers in remote locations are using "teletherapy," speaking with patients by phone or closed-circuit television when patients cannot otherwise find transportation to distant services; this can also save transit time for providers (Dunn et al., 2007).

IMPULSE CONTROL DISORDERS

Sarah, 76, is shopping in a pharmacy when she notices the lipstick display. She rarely wears lipstick, but for some reason she is drawn to the display and feels the urge to take one. She sup-

presses the urge, but it grows stronger and harder to resist. She ultimately snatches the lipstick and puts it in her purse. She feels a sense of relief, and an odd sort of pleasure. Over time she finds that this urge to steal things is repeatedly happening. Most of the time she cannot resist, and she sometimes takes ridiculous chances by taking things. However, later she feels ashamed and consumed with remorse and even returns the items or throws them away. Despite being caught once and threatened with jail, she continues to steal.

The problem in **impulse control disorders** involves a decreased ability to resist an impulse (or a drive) to perform certain acts that are potentially harmful to self or others. In most cases the pattern is one of increasing tension that builds until a particular action is taken. The actions may be impulsive (e.g., stealing) or involve considerable planning (e.g., fire setting). The tension reduction reinforces the action and makes future resistance more difficult. Except for pathological gambling, these disorders are considered to be relatively rare.

THEORY
Biological Factors

The causes underlying impulse control disorders are not clearly established. Certain disorders or abnormalities of the brain seem to reduce one's ability to resist impulses. Violent people often show electroencephalographic variations and may have higher cerebrospinal fluid (CSF) serotonin metabolite levels (Moeller et al., 2001). Frontotemporal dementia or tumors (especially those most prominently affecting the right hemisphere), Parkinson's disease, and even multiple sclerosis have been documented as contributing to impulsivity in general, as have traumatic brain injury and substance abuse, but there is not a clear link between such pathology and these disorders.

Genetic Factors

A gene associated with impulsive violence is suspected of weakening the brain's impulse control circuitry (NIMH, 2005). Although the incidence of some impulse disorders is greater within families (e.g., trichotillomania), neither this gene nor others have been linked causally to these disorders.

Psychological Factors

Theories regarding psychological causes of these disorders include an impaired ability to manage anxiety, wherein the person might be defending against (coping with) anxiety by subconsciously choosing an action that gives a sense of control over the anxiety. This theory is supported by a pattern of increased incidence of acts during periods of high stress. Some of these disorders may be a variant, or an expression, of anxiety disorders such as obsessive-compulsive disorder (OCD) or posttraumatic stress disorder (PTSD). There is also a parallel to addictive behaviors in that the patient may experience craving for the act and relief upon achieving it, supporting an addictions-based etiology (Chamberlain et al., 2007).

CLINICAL PICTURE

The *DSM-IV-TR* (APA, 2000) identifies six impulse control disorders. In all cases, the diagnosis of these disorders requires elimination of all other medical and psychiatric causes—such as antisocial personality disorder or substance abuse—of the behavior in question, as well as ruling other causations outside the arena of psychological functioning, such as seeking profit or attaining revenge. Judgment is intact and psychotic elements are absent in all the following disorders.

Intermittent explosive disorder involves a recurrent failure to resist aggressive impulses, resulting in serious assaults or property destruction. The aggressive act is greatly out of proportion to any precipitating factors or provocations, and people with this disorder may experience the acts as "spells" that begin with a buildup of tension and followed by a sense of release or relief. They may feel angry or enraged preceding the event (or chronically), and depressed or remorseful afterward. They may face recrimination, arrest, civil actions, and loss of relationships and employment as a result of their actions. It is considered a rare disorder, and is more common in men. The onset, course, and prognosis are highly variable.

Kleptomania is a disorder wherein individuals repeatedly steal items that they do not need and that are not of value to them, accompanied by rising tension before the act and tension release afterward. The disorder may begin at any age, and two thirds of the people with this disorder are women. The behavior may occur at widely scattered intervals or be more regular and protracted. The acts are perceived as illogical and wrong.

Pyromania involves repeated, purposeful fire-setting that is preceded by arousal or tension and results in relief or psychological gratification. The act does not have a criminal motive. The disorder is often accompanied by a fascination with fire and fire-related phenomena, such as firefighting apparatus or organizations. People with this disorder may also cause false alarms or even become firefighters for psychological gratification. It is a rare disorder usually found in men and usually begins in adulthood. It follows a variable course and may result in criminal prosecution.

Pathological gambling is characterized by recurrent gambling behavior that is progressive and maladaptive, ultimately causing significant personal disruption of one's family, finances, work, and other aspects of one's life. People with this disorder are preoccupied with gambling, feel aroused and positive when engaging in the behavior, and feel they cannot relieve tension without it. The behavior continues despite social consequences and the person's own efforts to curtail it. Pathological gamblers may lie, rationalize, manipulate others, and conceal their behavior in order to maintain it. In severe cases, work and social function may be disrupted and compromised. Most people with this disorder are men, and the incidence of this disorder is about 1% (Grant et al., 2005) but may be higher in settings where gambling opportunities are more varied and easily accessed and within families in which other members also have the disorder.

Trichotillomania is a disorder involving pulling out one's hair in order to relieve tension. The person may pull out his or her hair episodically for brief periods, or may engage in protracted periods of the behavior, lasting hours or longer in some cases. It tends to worsen under stress but also occurs when the person is calm, sometimes in an almost absent-minded fashion. In some cases, the hair is ingested and can produce "hairballs" similar to those seen in animals. Hair loss can significantly affect one's appearance, causing distress and social discomfort. The incidence is much higher in adult women than adult men, but about equal among boys and girls. It may be self-limited or continue for decades.

Impulse control disorders not otherwise specified (NOS) includes other disorders of impulse control that do not meet the criteria of any of those previously mentioned. It includes skin picking, compulsive Internet use, hoarding, and compulsive shopping.

Effect on Individuals, Families, and Society

People with these disorders are often confused and troubled by them, feeling embarrassment, shame, or guilt. Usually they realize that the acts are illogical or wrong, but despite their best efforts, the urge to act overwhelms them. Shame and distress accumulating from the unacceptable behaviors increase the risk of developing depression and of committing suicide (Petry & Armentano, 1999). They may find themselves socially isolated or stigmatized.

Kleptomania is estimated to account for between 4% and 10% of all shoplifting losses (Koran et al., 2007). Gambling can cause tremendous financial losses, disrupt families, reduce job productivity, and cause loss of status, housing, cars, jobs, and marriages. Intermittent explosive disorder and pyromania can cause injury or even death to others, and can put the patient at risk of being sued for damages or injured by the victim's defensive response. When criminal offenses are involved, society can bear the costs of prosecution, incarceration, and forensic treatment, and the individual may lose civil rights (e.g., the right to vote) or private or governmental entitlements (e.g., eligibility for federal housing assistance, ability to hold a professional license or work in a particular field).

Application of the Nursing Process

ASSESSMENT

Information suggesting the presence of an impulse control disorder is often minimized, withheld, or concealed by the patient or overlooked by staff; therefore, careful assessment is important, and self-assessment is essential. The nurse's beliefs and attitudes about the behavior in question may compromise his or her ability to perceive the disorder or remain objective about it. For example, if the nurse believes that setting fires is simply criminal behavior and does not believe that there could be a mental disorder that causes this behavior, the nurse is not likely to see opportunities for helping the patient or intervene to help the patient control these impulses.

Because the actions associated with impulse control disorders may be embarrassing or even criminal in nature, building trust and conveying empathy and acceptance are key to helping the patient disclose these problems. Significant others who may be less reluctant to share information can also help identify concealed concerns. Nurses should look for patterns of recurrent loss of control in the patient's oral responses and history and should observe for signs suggesting these disorders (e.g., fascination with fire, unusual familiarity with gambling terminology, patches where hair is thin, pulling at or chewing on hair, etc.).

It is helpful to ask about circumstances that increase the patient's tension, as well as ways the patient reduces this tension. Empathic prompting can be helpful here, such as, "Sometimes people find themselves feeling tense and having urges to do different things to release the tension. Can you tell me about times when this may have happened to you?" Frank, direct questioning may set a tone for openness and prompt greater frankness in the patient's responses, for example, "Tell me about times when you've hit someone or come close to losing control."

A patient's legal history may also be suggestive of these disorders. Recurrent assaults or any episodes of fire setting should merit further psychiatric assessment. In some cases, the patient may be dealing with concurrent depression or be sufficiently distressed to be considering self-harm. Assess-

ment for these risks is essential. Finally, it is always important to assess how the disorder has impacted the patient and significant others, as well as the patient's knowledge of the disorder and ways of reducing or coping with it.

DIAGNOSIS

A variety of diagnoses may apply to people with impulse control disorders, including *Impaired adjustment*, *Anxiety*, *Compromised family coping*, *Ineffective coping*, *Risk for injury*, *Low self-esteem*, and *Social isolation* (NANDA-I, 2007). Nursing interventions for these disorders vary with the particular disorder being addressed, but some general interventions likely to fit most related circumstances are listed in Table 24-2.

OUTCOMES IDENTIFICATION

Expected outcomes vary with the disorder but typically focus on reducing the problematic acts and substituting more adaptive means to reduce tension. Examples of desired outcomes include "Patient does not set fires," "Hair loss is reduced by 20%," "Patient substitutes corrective self-talk when experiencing impulses to act inappropriately," "Patient demonstrates use of three or more tension reduction strategies," and "Patient rates anxiety as 5 or less on a 1 to 10 scale."

IMPLEMENTATION
Pharmacological, Biological, and Integrative Therapies

Treatment strategies for impulse control disorders in most cases focus on a combination of psychotherapy and medication. Because people with these disorders usually do not manifest an imminent risk to themselves or others, or present with emergent needs, treatment is usually provided on an outpatient basis.

Psychopharmacology

Psychopharmacological interventions presently dominate in the treatment of some impulse control disorders. Selective serotonin reuptake inhibitors (SSRIs), the antidepressant bupropion (Dannon et al., 2005), and opioid antagonists (e.g., naltrexone) (Grant & Kim, 2002) are used in the treatment of kleptomania, trichotillomania, and pathological gambling. Lithium and the antipsychotic risperidone have shown to have efficacy in conduct disorder, a child-adolescent disorder with certain similarities to intermittent explosive disorder (Ipser & Stein, 2007), and adult studies of lithium and SSRIs suggest efficacy for reducing violence (Moeller et al., 2001).

TABLE 24-2   Interventions for Impulse Control Disorders

Intervention	Rationale
1. Guide the patient to understand and practice tension reduction and stress control strategies such as stress avoidance, correction of negative self-talk, and breathing control exercises.	1. Tension usually precedes and contributes to impulsive actions; tension reduction and adaptive tension management can reduce the incidence of impulsive behavior.
2. Suggest and facilitate the progressive substitution of alternate, less-maladaptive responses to tension, such as applying pressure to one's scalp with a thumb rather than pulling out one's hair.	2. Impulse control disorders involve maladaptive behaviors, some of which are criminal offenses; substitution of more adaptive responses can prevent negative consequences.
3. Assist the patient to explore feelings preceding or associated with the impulses, such as shame, fear, or guilt, and to manage these feelings adaptively.	3. Negative emotions contribute to stress and tension, features associated with maladaptive impulsive behaviors.
4. Promote effective communication by guiding the patient to master and demonstrate assertive communication skills.	4. Assertive communication can improve the patient's ability to meet his or her needs effectively, prevent misunderstandings, and reduce conflict and tension.
5. Assist the patient to identify the consequences of his or her actions, e.g., ask: "How do other people respond when you _____?"; "Tell me what things are like the day after you've set a fire"; or "Imagine you set the fire: what do you think will happen in the days and weeks that follow?" (anticipatory fantasy).	5. Identifying consequences can help the patient become more empathic to his or her effect on others, and increase motivation to refrain from problematic behaviors. Anticipatory fantasy guides the patient to imagine the consequences of his or her behavior, serving to dampen urges to act on impulses.
6. Educate the patient that drugs and alcohol may increase impulsive behavior through disinhibition or impairment of judgment; educate the patient regarding the effect of "triggers," i.e., circumstances hat evoke tension or impulses (e.g., going to bars).	6. Disinhibiting drugs and exposure to triggers that evoke impulsive behavior increase the frequency of impulsive actions; reducing disinhibition and exposure to such triggers can reduce the frequency and intensity of the impulsive actions.
7. Pathological gamblers may respond well to group therapy; organizations such as Gamblers Anonymous (www.gamblersanonymous.org) provide significant assistance through support, education, and practical tips on managing gambling impulses and other concerns.	7. 12-step programs have been shown to be of significant help in reducing activities that have a compulsive or addictive component; peer support groups are effective for confronting defenses and rationalization that the patient uses to support the gambling.
8. Trichotillomania patients can benefit from special hair styling, hair weaves, or other cosmetology assistance; they may require considerable support in order to access such resources, however, because of embarrassment.	8. Hair loss can create a significant cosmetic defect, resulting in impaired self-esteem and further dysfunctional coping; compensating cosmetically for such defects can enhance the person's self-image and self-esteem.

Antidepressants and mood stabilizers have been used for this class of disorders with varying results. Opioid antagonists such as nalmefene may be of particular benefit in pathological gambling (Grant et al., 2006). Anticonvulsants, along with propranolol and similar β-adrenergic antagonists, may be useful for reducing aggression, particularly in individuals whose impulse control problems seem to stem from organic disorders such as dementia (Moeller et al., 2001).

Nonpharmacological Treatments

Nonpharmacological treatments include a variety of approaches. Hypnotherapy may be of benefit in some cases, and cognitive-behavioral approaches such as habit reversal have found success in disorders such as trichotillomania (Bruce et al., 2005). Using cognitive techniques is an evidence-based practice. By modifying thinking patterns and reducing thinking distortion, patients can also change their actions. Behavioral conditioning through the use of positive rewards and negative consequences is research-supported for reducing problematic habitual behaviors (Moeller et al., 2001). Group psychotherapy provides for therapeutic confrontation from peers and tends to be particularly helpful for people who have poor insight or difficulty accepting responsibility for their behavior.

SEXUAL DISORDERS

Sexual disorders are disorders involving sexual function and identity. **Gender identity disorder**, formerly known as transsexualism, is a rare disorder involving a persistent, strong cross-gender identification wherein a person feels he or she should actually be a member of the opposite gender. It often first becomes apparent in childhood or adolescence, and people with this disorder may alter their dress, use hormonal medications, and even pursue surgery in order to make their appearance as congruent as possible with their desired gender (Wylie, 2004). Other sexual disorders not discussed in this chapter are the various sexual dysfunctions (e.g., alterations in one's sexual desire and sexual response cycle, including difficulties achieving the sexual act or deriving the expected level of pleasure from it).

Paraphilias are psychological disorders in which the patient has a preoccupation with sexual fantasies and related sexual urges that focus on nontraditional and socially unacceptable sexual "targets" such as children, animals, or objects. People with a paraphilia may or may not act on their urges.

As a result of divergent religious and cultural expectations, there is a degree of conflict within our society about how to define appropriate sexual behavior. For example, opinions can vary widely in terms of what is an appropriate age for the onset of sexual relations, whom one should be able to choose as a sexual partner (based on gender, age, or race, for example), and whether such relations should occur before or outside of marriage. It is difficult to measure the incidence of paraphilias because of reluctance of those affected to disclose this information as a result of stigma, the potential for prosecution, and other concerns.

THEORY
Biological Factors

The cause of gender identity disorder is unknown, but theories include abnormalities in sexual hormone and related neurodevelopment in utero or development aberrations in early life (Wylie, 2004). The causes underlying paraphilias have not yet been determined. As with impulse disorders, certain disorders or abnormalities of the brain seem to increase impulsiveness or reduce one's ability to resist impulses, and frontotemporal dementia, tumors, and Parkinson's disease have been documented as contributing to paraphilias such as pedophilia (Mendez et al., 2000). Increased sympathetic activity and reduced serotonergic activity have been implicated in pedophilia (Fagan et al., 2002). Traumatic brain injuries are also associated with sexual offenses, although not necessarily sexual disorders; for example, Langevin (2006) surveyed sexual offenders (not pedophiles per se) and found that 49% had received head trauma sufficient to cause loss of consciousness.

Psychological Factors

Theories regarding **psychological causes** of these disorders include failure to develop appropriate attachments in early childhood, resulting in inadequate or inappropriate attachments at later developmental stages (Sawle & Kear-Colwell, 2001). Another theory is that the disorders are learned responses to inappropriate sexual role models, causing the children to later develop an inappropriate "love map" (Fagan et al., 2002). Research also suggests that the paraphilias may be caused by one's own sexual victimization, a notion supported by the fact that 30% to 60% of pedophiles were themselves sexually abused as children. A confounding factor limiting our understanding of these disorders is that funding agencies and research institutions, perhaps because of the sometimes controversial aspects of these disorders, are sometimes reluctant to fund or support research related to the causes and treatment of such disorders (Arehart-Treichel, 2006).

For the most part we do not have any pathophysiological correlates for these disorders and there is no laboratory test, scan, or other widely accepted objective means of detecting them. Instead they are diagnosed based the characteristic patterns of behavior that are the symptoms of these disorders.

CLINICAL PICTURE

The *DSM-IV-TR* (APA, 2000) criteria for gender identity disorder include persistent discomfort with one's present gender assignment and related roles and a strong and persistent desire to assume the characteristics (e.g., dress and mannerisms) and roles of the opposite or desired gender. These features are sufficient to cause significant distress and role impairment (e.g., social, vocational).

The *DSM-IV-TR* distinguishes the following types of paraphilias. In all cases, the diagnosis of these disorders first requires eliminating all other medical and psychiatric causes of the behavior in question (e.g., criminal intent, manic episodes, dementia, substance abuse, schizophrenia, or any disorder that causes disinhibition or impairs judgment or impulse control). Psychotic elements are absent in all the following described forms, and most have their onset during adolescence. Most people with paraphilias are male. Finally, to be diagnosed with a paraphilia, the features must have been present for at least 6 months (i.e., occasional experiences of gratification through paraphilic-like experiences would not meet the criteria to be diagnosed with that paraphilia).

Exhibitionism is a disorder wherein a person derives sexual pleasure and gratification by exposing his or her genitalia to others. The person has strong, recurrent fantasies or acts involving exposing genitalia and must also have either experienced significant distress related to the fantasies or enacted these fantasies by exposing himself or herself. Exhibitionism seems to begin in adolescence but can begin at any age, and the incidence seems to taper by age 40.

Fetishism involves experiencing recurrent, intensely arousing fantasies, sexual urges, or behaviors involving the use of nonliving objects for sexual gratification. These fantasies or behaviors must cause significant distress or significantly impair role functioning (e.g., as a spouse or employee), and the objects are not those typically used to cause or enhance sexual arousal. Examples of objects that are commonly the focus of fetishes include women's undergarments, rubber items, and shoes.

Frotteurism is touching or rubbing against a nonconsenting person in order to achieve sexual gratification. To receive this diagnosis, one has to either act on the impulses or experience marked distress or interpersonal difficulties as a result of the impulses or behavior.

Pedophilia involves fantasized or actual sexual activity with a prepubescent child (usually defined as younger than 14 years) as the object of sexual gratification. A pedophile must either have acted on the fantasies or experienced significant distress or interpersonal difficulties as a result of the fantasies. The person must also be at least 16 years of age and at least 5 or more years older than the object of fantasy. Individuals with pedophilia may focus on children of the same, opposite, or both genders, although most are heterosexually focused. They may be focused on children exclusively or may have a sexual interest in adults as well. Some people with pedophilia focus their activities on relatives (incestual form), others on non-family members, and some on both.

Sexual masochism and **sexual sadism** involve deriving sexual gratification from the suffering caused by receiving, or the pleasure caused by creating, psychological and physical abuse, respectively. Masochism can include bondage, verbal abuse, electrical shocks, whipping, being urinated on, and being forced to humiliate oneself. Sadism includes inflicting such acts on a (usually masochistic) partner, and often involves the theme of having complete psychological and physical control over one's partner. In some cases, the partner may be nonconsenting to the sadistic acts.

Transvestic fetishism involves deriving sexual gratification by dressing as a person of the opposite gender, specifically a male dressing as a female. The diagnosis is not applicable if the crossdressing occurs as part of a gender identify disorder or in the course of transsexualism.

Voyeurism involves deriving sexual gratification from fantasies or actions that focus on observing unsuspecting persons in sexually arousing situations (e.g., undressing or engaging in sexual activity).

Paraphilias not otherwise specified (NOS) include other unusual sexual preoccupations not addressed in the preceding text. Examples include foot fetishes, necrophilia (sexual behavior involving corpses), being aroused by enemas, and deriving sexual pleasure from exposure to excrement or urine.

Although not paraphilias, sexual addiction and other forms of distress or dysfunction related to sexuality can be diagnosed as sexual disorder NOS. Other disorders related to sexuality, although not covered in this chapter or classified as sexual disorders, include those relating to chromosomal abnormalities (e.g., Klinefelter's syndrome), head trauma or other organic disorder, and those arising from SPMIs that affect impulse control and social and sexual interaction (e.g., schizophrenia).

Effect on Individuals, Families, and Society

Gender identity disorder can be accompanied by significant embarrassment, shame, discrimination, and social isolation because many people in our society do not understand the disorder and react with repugnance. The effect of paraphilias may be relatively minor and limited to the individual with the diagnosis (e.g., a person with transvestic fetishism). When people with paraphilias engage sexually with unwilling partners (e.g., frotteurism or voyeurism), victims may feel violated and experience significant and protracted psychological distress.

Pedophilic offenders may injure or kill their victims, and even when the child victim survives or is physically uninjured, there is virtually always significant, protracted, and sometimes disabling psychological damage. Victims are at increased risk of disorders such as PTSD, depression, anxiety, and substance abuse disorders (Fagan et al., 2002). Families, loved ones, and the general community are often traumatized and left unable to feel fully secure in the future.

Patients with these disorders may be distressed by them, overwhelmed with shame or guilt. Others are indifferent or blasé about their paraphilia, or may attempt to justify their actions through rationalization or other means. Some even lobby to decriminalize acts such as sexual relations with children. Even those who never enact their fantasies may find themselves socially isolated or stigmatized as a result of these irresistible yet unacceptable preoccupations. Disorders such as sexual addiction (which affects more than 20 million Americans) can contribute to guilt, marital discord, low self-esteem, and sexually transmitted diseases (Coleman-Kennedy & Pendley, 2002).

Sexual abuse is a significant problem in our society. For example, 12% of men and 17% of women report being sexually touched as children (Fagan et al., 2002). However, only a portion of this abuse involves persons with pedophilia. Furthermore, parents and caregivers commit more than 90% of the sexual abuse of children in the United States (strangers account for less than 5% of child sexual offenses) (Fagan et al., 2002). The **recidivism** (repeating of a previous offense) rates for untreated child sexual offenders (both pedophilic and non-pedophilic combined) are relatively high. Up to 80% of 18- to 24-year-old offenders and up 50% for those 25 to 60 re-offend within 5 years of their release from prison or hospitals, although the rate drops to almost zero for those older than 60 years (Thornton, 2006).

Application of the Nursing Process
ASSESSMENT

Self-assessment is essential because the nurse's beliefs and attitudes about these unusual (from the nurse's perspective) or sometimes abhorrent behaviors may compromise objectivity. In cases in which the nurse has been a victim of sexual abuse, treating perpetrators can be difficult and even traumatic, requiring additional support (e.g., clinical supervision to help the nurse recognize and deal with responses to the patient; counseling to help cope with reawakened memories of earlier abuse). As with impulse control disorders, actions associated with paraphilias may be embarrassing or even criminal in nature, making building trust and conveying empathy and acceptance essential. Patients often conceal or deny paraphilic thoughts and behavior, making careful assessment and validation of the patient's reports important.

Written assessment questionnaires can elicit possibly embarrassing information without the tension of a face-to-face interview, and can form the basis of a more focused interview thereafter. Significant others who may be less reluctant to share information can also help identify concealed issues. For example, it is not unusual for children of individuals with pedophilia to report inappropriate sexual contact during their childhood. In some cases, the patient may be dealing with concurrent depression or be sufficiently distressed as to be considering self-harm, making assessment for this risk essential. This is especially true for those who recently have been accused of (or publicly exposed in reference to) sexual offenses involving children, and who face considerable shame and even hostilities within their families and communities as a result. Finally, it is always important to assess how the disorder has affected the patient and significant others, as well as the patient's knowledge of the disorder and ways of reducing or coping with it.

DIAGNOSIS

A variety of diagnoses may apply to individuals with gender identity disorder and paraphilias, including *Impaired adjust-*

ment, Anxiety, Compromised family coping, Ineffective coping, Risk for injury, Low self-esteem, Sexual dysfunction, Ineffective sexuality pattern, Risk for other-directed violence, and Social isolation (NANDA-I, 2007). Nursing interventions for these disorders vary with the disorder and its expression in a particular patient, and are affected by any comorbid mental health disorders. Some general interventions likely to fit most related circumstances are listed in Table 24-3.

OUTCOMES IDENTIFICATION

Expected outcomes vary with the disorder but typically focus on reducing the problematic acts and substituting more adaptive means to meet sexual needs. Examples of desired outcomes include "Patient reports ability to fantasize about adults as well as children," "Patient does not go to locations where children are likely to be found," "Patient does not touch any child for 6 months," and "Patient rates urge to have contact with children a 5 or less on a 1 to 10 scale."

IMPLEMENTATION
Pharmacological, Biological, and Integrative Therapies

People with sexual disorders may seek treatment when sufficiently distressed by their disorder, or when compelled to do so in order to address the concerns of spouses, significant others, or officers of the court. Individuals with gender identity disorder may choose sexual reassignment, which involves a period of counseling to assist the person in fully considering and preparing for this somewhat drastic intervention. This is followed by living for 1 to 2 years as a member of the opposite or desired gender (to help ensure readiness), hormonal therapy to suppress undesired physical characteristics and elicit desired sexual characteristics (e.g., to diminish facial hair and cause breast enlargement), and, finally, surgical intervention to alter their genitalia to match that of the desired gender.

People with paraphilias who commit criminal offenses may be court-ordered to submit to treatment. Except for criminal offenders with comorbid SPMIs, treatment is almost always on an outpatient basis. In some states, sexual offenders may be held in inpatient psychiatric treatment settings (usually state forensic hospitals) for extended periods, where they receive ongoing treatment, sometimes even if clinicians do not believe their behavior is a result of a paraphilia. This "preventive psychiatric incarceration" is controversial within the mental health field, and some feel it is an abuse of psychiatry to hold a person who does not require that level of clinical care (an inpatient setting), or to hold people in psychiatric settings when there may be

TABLE 24-3   Interventions for Sexual Disorders

Intervention	Rationale
1. Use inclusive language, set and convey a tone of acceptance, normalize disclosure pertaining to sexuality, and provide active support.	1. These actions promote free and open disclosure and discussion of patient behavior and needs (Huygen, 2006).
2. Assist individuals with gender identity disorders to connect with peers and professionals who are supportive and receptive to their needs, and to access resources such as www.wpath.org and www.transgenderlaw.org, which can be good starting points for people dealing with these disorders.	2. Stigma and discrimination can result in isolation and hopelessness; connecting with others and pursuing educational resources for the patient and significant others can enhance understanding and acceptance.
3. Maintain and reinforce appropriate interpersonal boundaries with people with sexual disorders.	3. Role modeling of appropriate boundaries allows the patient to identify and adopt more effective ways of relating to others, and maintains an effective nurse-patient relationship.
4. Mutually set, track, revise, and reinforce incremental goals, along with related actions that will meet those goals.	4. Mutual goal-setting increases patient "buy-in"; incremental goals are easier to attain, reducing discouragement from unmet goals and providing a series of successes that reinforce patient efforts.
5. Guide the patient to understand and practice tension reduction and stress control strategies such as stress avoidance, correction of negative self-talk, and breathing control exercises.	5. High levels of stress and tension, especially when coupled with a limited or ineffective repertoire of coping strategies, increase the chance of maladaptive stress reduction behaviors.
6. Educate the patient (and, as applicable, involved support people and personnel from the criminal justice system) regarding his or her disorder: its causes, treatments, and especially, ways to cope with and control symptoms and maladaptive behaviors.	6. Understanding the psychological and psychiatric aspects of one's disorder, as well as available ways to cope with or reduce symptoms, can decrease guilt and powerlessness, instilling hope and improving the patient's sense of control over his or her situation.
7. Assist the patient to identify and explore feelings preceding or associated with the target behavior, such as excitement, shame, or guilt.	7. Covert sensitization—guiding the patient to connect an undesired behavior with negative consequences—diminishes unacceptable behaviors; unresolved feelings can cause desperation and lead to acting-out or loss of control.
8. Assist the patient to identify the consequences of his or her actions, e.g., ask: "How do other people seem to feel about your behavior?" or "What tends to happen when you go where children play?"	8. Insight that develops from within tends to be more accepted than feedback provided externally.
9. Address comorbid disorders and mental health needs such as substance abuse or a history of sexual victimization during the patient's youth.	9. Depression and other mental disorders further impair problem-solving and coping abilities, and drain the patient's energy for addressing the target problems.
10. If available, involve the patient in group therapy with others with paraphilias; a mixture of new and recovered members is desirable.	10. Group psychotherapy allows for frank feedback and therapeutic confrontation by those who've "been there" and are thus difficult to manipulate; a mix of new and recovered members provides positive role models for the new members.

no known (or further) psychiatric treatment available for their particular situation.

Treatment of pedophilia usually involves medications and psychotherapy. The medications typically interfere with the production or action of male sexual hormones and in effect produce varying degrees of **chemical castration** (e.g., depot-leuprolide, medroxyprogesterone acetate [MPA, an analog of progesterone], cyproterone acetate [CPA, Depo-Provera], or analogs of gonadotropin-releasing hormone).

Other potentially helpful drugs include those that reduce compulsive or impulsive behavior (e.g., naltrexone, carbamazepine, clonazepam, and SSRIs). These drugs are also used to treat other paraphilias and sexually inappropriate behavior in other medical or psychiatric conditions, such as dementia (Light & Holroyd, 2005). They can have multiple and significant side effects, including feminization, weight gain, clotting disorders, thromboembolism, decreased fertility and sexual dysfunction, depression, and hypertension (Almeida et al., 2003; Kafka, 1996). Side effects frequently discourage use of the antiandronergic drugs in particular, and often these are used under court order and in depot (long-acting injectable) forms to ensure adherence. In rare cases, surgical castration may be pursued by the patient in lieu of drugs.

Psychotherapeutic treatments include group and one-to-one psychotherapy and psychoeducational interventions. Cognitive-behavioral therapies in particular are believed to be helpful. For people with gender identity disorder, counseling can help patients compare and choose various paths they might take, including sexual reassignment, and cope with their feelings and society's responses to this disorder.

Behavioral approaches for paraphilias can include desensitization techniques to reduce sexual responsiveness to undesired stimuli. In some cases, patients are guided to fulfill their gratification needs in non-socially offensive ways, such as via masturbatory reconditioning and "fantasy sex." Twelve-step programs also have been effective, and treatment of comorbid disorders, particularly those that impair impulse control (e.g., substance abuse), can reduce the risk of recidivism or conversion to criminal behavior (Marshall, 2006).

ADULT ATTENTION DEFICIT HYPERACTIVITY DISORDER

Andrea, a 32-year-old graduate student in psychology, presents at the student health center concerned that she might have attention deficit hyperactivity disorder (ADHD) after reading a magazine article about it. She reports that throughout her life teachers and others told her she was extremely bright, but that somehow this was not reflected in her grades, which were Bs and Cs. She notes that she has difficulty maintaining concentration, often "tuning out" during lectures and having to regularly reread parts of her assignments, and that it is difficult for her to effectively organize her work and studies.

Andrea has difficulty sitting still, frequently changing position and sometimes walking about the room. She interrupts other speakers regularly and then apologizes but has difficulty regaining her train of thought. Distraction, worry, and irritability are frequent. She often loses track of belongings, spends much time looking for misplaced items, forgets appointments, and frequently overlooks tasks she had intended to do.

Other psychiatric and physical problems are ruled out. After treatment with methylphenidate and counseling, Andrea reports that she was able to finish a major written assignment in about one third the time, and with much less stress than usual. She is happy with the improvement and hopeful regarding further improvement. She says that friends have commented on the improvement, saying she seems more at ease and less scattered. She agrees to join an ADHD support group on campus and go to a 6-week follow-up appointment.

PREVALENCE AND COMORBIDITY

ADHD involves a persistent pattern of inattention, impaired ability to focus and concentrate, or hyperactivity and impulsivity that are more noticeable and more severe than would otherwise be seen at a given developmental level. It has its onset in childhood, usually peaking between the ages of 5 and 10 years. It is typically considered a disorder primarily of children and adolescents. However, there is a concern that the apparent decrease in ADHD by adulthood is really a result of using inadequate criteria for adult diagnosis and the enhanced ability of adults to compensate for or conceal their symptoms. ADHD clearly exists in, or persists into, adulthood, albeit in many cases with a somewhat different feel or appearance compared with its expression in children (Spencer et al., 2007).

Estimates for the incidence in children range from 3% to 10% (some research suggests up to 19%), and it is more common in males (2 : 1 to 9 : 1 males to females, depending on the study). The incidence in adults has not been well established, but is likely in nearly the same range as for children; however, as hyperactivity decreases over time, fewer males remain diagnosed with ADHD in adulthood, and the adult ADHD incidence is more evenly split between males and females (Greydanus et al., 2007).

ADHD contributes to a wide variety of interpersonal, social, academic, and vocational problems, and can significantly limit or disrupt a person's ability to function and negatively affect health habits and educational or socioeconomic achievement well into adulthood. It is also a controversial diagnosis in the eyes of some laypeople and health professionals, who feel the disorder, especially in children, is too readily and too subjectively diagnosed, and too quickly addressed through medications rather than non-pharmacological treatments. Some even feel it is not a true disorder, but simply a more severe presentation of inattentiveness and hyperactivity that to some extent exists in most children (*Lancet*, 2003).

Psychiatric comorbidity is common in ADHD, with upward of 80% of child ADHD patients having at least one other diagnosis, and 67% having two other diagnoses. Conduct and oppositional defiant disorders, anxiety disorders, and learning disorders are common co-occurring disorders in children, and depression and antisocial personality disorder are relatively common co-occurring disorders in adults with ADHD (with antisocial elements tending to be more common in those with the combined type of ADHD) (Spencer et al., 2007). **Co-occurring physical health disorders** include Tourette's disorder and other tics, substance abuse, sexually transmitted diseases, traumatic brain injuries, and general trauma (Greydanus et al., 2007).

THEORY
Genetic Factors

Multiple causes and contributing factors seem to play a part in ADHD. There appears to be a strong genetic and familial component; for example, if one identical twin has the disorder, depending on the subtype involved, there is an 80% to 98% chance that its sibling will as well, and parents of ADHD children themselves often have features of ADHD.

Biological Factors

Alterations in the neurotransmitters norepinephrine and dopamine also have been implicated. Research suggests that the key brain areas involved in ADHD are the frontal lobe, the basal ganglia, and their connections to the cerebellum; imaging studies show diminished activity (Brassett-Harknett & Butler, 2007) and relatively smaller areas of brain matter in these areas in people with ADHD. "Biological adversity" (biological challenges) is another possible factor: fetal distress, low birth weight, prematurity, maternal bleeding, and maternal smoking and drug abuse are implicated as contributing to ADHD, as is exposure to toxins such as lead (Spencer et al., 2007).

Psychological Factors

Theories regarding **psychological causes** suggest that intra-familial conflict and distress are causative for, and a creation of, ADHD. The disorder appears to be at least aggravated by familial, social, and environmental factors. Some research suggests that the strong familial nature (increased likelihood of occurrence within a family) argues for family dysfunction being a significant contributing factor (Biederman, 2004).

CLINICAL PICTURE

ADHD tends to be underappreciated and underdiagnosed in adults. The diagnosis of ADHD is complicated by the complexity and varied presentation of the disorder. Because of the high percentage of patients with co-occurring mental disorders and the complexity of ADHD, a complete mental health assessment, and in complicated cases, an ADHD specialist, is highly recommended. There is no laboratory test, scan, or other objective means for detecting it. Instead, ADHD is diagnosed based the characteristic patterns of behavior and organizational and attentional dysfunction, which are the symptoms of these disorders.

The *DSM-IV-TR* (APA, 2000) requires that six or more symptoms of inattention and six or more symptoms of hyperactivity-impulsivity be present in order to diagnose ADHD in children (see Chapter 23). To be diagnosed under current criteria, the symptoms must have been present before the age of 7 years, must be present in at least two different settings (i.e., not just in school alone), must be sufficient to significantly impair functioning (academic, social, occupational), and cannot be a consequence of other disorders.

The *DSM* does not have separate diagnostic criteria for the disorder in adults, although some experts believe separate diagnostic criteria and tools should exist. People who have some of the diagnostic elements of ADHD but who do not meet the full criteria may be diagnosed with ADHD in partial remission (if originally diagnosed as a child), or as having ADHD not otherwise specified (e.g., if the disorder was not present before the age of 7, or if the person meets other criteria but has hypoactivity instead of hyperactivity). Some experts believe that childhood ADHD does not go away as once thought, and that if properly assessed, many adults who had ADHD as children would at least merit one of these lesser ADHD diagnoses. Research suggests that persistence of significant ADHD symptomatology and related impairment into adulthood may range up to 80% (Faraone et al., 2000).

Effect on Individuals, Families, and Society

The effect of ADHD on individuals is significant, not only while it is active (e.g., during childhood) but also even when it has diminished or resolved by adulthood. Adults diagnosed with ADHD as children tend to achieve lower socio-economic status, complete fewer years of school, are more likely to smoke and to abuse alcohol and drugs, are more likely to have traffic incidents (e.g., road rage, accidents, speeding offenses), have more contact with police, are at greater risk of sexually transmitted diseases, change jobs more frequently, report more interpersonal and relational difficulties, and have higher rates of depression than people without ADHD (Brassett-Harknett & Butler, 2007;

Spencer et al., 2007). ADHD is also significantly more prevalent in incarcerated populations, suggesting a contributing role to criminal activity.

The effect on society is less well established. ADHD inhibits academic achievement at all ages, and it is theorized that the disorder reduces work productivity and increases costs significantly in the criminal justice system, but hard data do not yet exist.

Application of the Nursing Process

ASSESSMENT

Assessment is based on patient reports, nursing observation, and when available, reports of employers, family members, and other third parties. It should focus on behaviors supportive of the diagnosis as well as on indicators of the patient's present knowledge of and ability to cope with the disorder. Support systems play a major role in the patient's achieving successful outcomes and are another key element for assessment.

If the patient is experiencing significant distractibility or has difficulty processing complex statements, keep comments and questioning concise and clear and choose interview spaces that are relatively quiet and devoid of distractions. If needed, prompts can help the patient organize responses and stay on track. Observe for indications of disorganization, distractibility, irritability, impulsive comments or behavior, difficulty processing information or following instructions, difficulty achieving at the expected level in social and vocational settings, and hyperactivity (excess or nonpurposeful motor activity). Substance abuse, particularly of methamphetamine and other stimulants, can mimic ADHD and should be ruled out.

DIAGNOSIS

Nursing diagnoses for ADHD include *Impaired social interaction*, *Defensive coping*, *Compromised family coping*, *Impaired adjustment*, *Sleep pattern disturbance*, *Anxiety*, and *Personal identity disturbance* (NANDA-I, 2007). Nursing interventions focus on symptom management and coping with chronic illness (Table 24-4). As a general rule, the interventions for adults are different from those for children.

OUTCOMES IDENTIFICATION

Examples of potential outcome measures include "Patient demonstrates ability to stay on task by completing one task before starting another;" "Patient discusses three techniques to reduce environmental distractions," and "Patient rates concentration as a 5 or greater on a 1 to 10 scale."

IMPLEMENTATION
Pharmacological, Biological, and Integrative Therapies

Medications are a well established and researched treatment modality for ADHD. The same drugs used to treat children are also used, in most cases, to treat adults. Stimulants are the most widely used medication for ADHD, and they show a high degree of efficacy, with 75% to 95% reporting improvement from methylphenidate (e.g., Ritalin, which comes in many different forms and formulations) and amphetamine variants (e.g., Adderall). Stimulant medications are thought to augment dopamine and/or norepinephrine neurotransmission that serves to regulate prefrontal cortex activities critical for modulation of behavior, attention, and cognition. It might seem counterintuitive for stimulants to help hyperactivity, but they all in some way promote enhanced dopamine and norepinephrine functioning.

Stimulants are available in short-, intermediate-, and long-acting forms, some with sustained-release technology. Longer-acting and timed-release forms allow patients to take the medicines once or twice per day before and after (rather than during) school or work, and are popular for this convenience. This feature probably improves compliance because inattentiveness and other features of ADHD tend to interfere with adherence to drug therapy. Clonidine and a variety of antidepressants also have shown efficacy for ADHD (Greydanus et al., 2007). Atomoxetine, a nonstimulant drug (a selective norepinephrine reuptake inhibitor with antidepressant activity), enhances norepinephrine function and allows for a once-daily regimen (Scahill, 2004).

Psychotherapy

Psychotherapeutic treatments are of equal importance in managing ADHD. Cognitive therapy is helpful for correcting distortions in self-image and improving focus and concentration, and counseling can be important in addressing co-occurring issues such as marital discord and coping with chronic illness. Psychoeducation about the disorder, its treatment, and techniques for managing and coping with symptoms, are essential and may be done individually or in a group setting. Support groups can be helpful for addressing self esteem and anxiety issues, can be excellent sources of helpful hints for day-to-day management of the disorder, and can be helpful in aiding the patient who is adjusting to life with ADHD.

TABLE 24-4   Interventions for Adult Attention Deficit Hyperactivity Disorder

Intervention	Rationale
1. Educate the patient and significant other(s) regarding attention deficit hyperactivity disorder (ADHD): its causes, treatments, and especially, ways to cope with and control its symptoms.	1. Understanding the psychological and psychiatric aspects of one's disorder, as well as available ways to cope with or reduce symptoms, can decrease powerlessness, instill hope, and improve patient's sense of control.
2. Guide the patient to understand and practice stimulation reduction strategies such as environmental structuring (reducing auditory and visual distraction in the environment).	2. Distractions in the environment make concentration, already impaired in ADHD, more difficult.
3. Mutually set, track, revise, and reinforce incremental goals, along with related actions that will meet those goals.	3. Mutual goal-setting increases patient "buy-in"; incremental goals are easier to attain, reducing discouragement from unmet goals and providing successes that reinforce patient efforts.
4. Guide the patient to identify and use enhanced organizational skills; many techniques exist to increase organization and efficiency in completing tasks, from simple techniques such as reminder lists to the use of PDAs to track appointments.	4. Enhancements in organization can improve functioning and promote a positive self-image as the patient experiences increased task success; Internet resources and a large variety of published materials can be readily accessed for this purpose.
5. Guide the patient to identify and use enhanced time management skills (e.g., structured priority setting wherein the patient asks self "What will happen if I do not do this task next?" then uses those responses to determine which task to tackle next).	5. Better time management can improve functioning and reduce stress; Internet resources and a large variety of published materials on this topic can be readily accessed.
6. Assist the patient to identify and explore feelings pertaining to ADHD and its effect on his or her life, and to correct any distorted self-talk pertaining to self-image.	6. ADHD may contribute to feelings of frustration or impair one's self-esteem because of day-to-day challenges and, in the longer term, one's unmet potential; people with ADHD may be critical of themselves and use negative "self-talk" (e.g., "I am so stupid; why can't I do this? What is wrong with me!").
7. Encourage participation in ADHD support groups when accessible, and of vetted online support resources such as ADHD blogs.	7. Support groups and online resources can provide pragmatic "helpful hints" from peers and support from an "I've been there" perspective.
8. Address comorbid disorders and mental health needs such as substance abuse.	8. Depression and other disorders further impair problem-solving and coping abilities; substance abuse can significantly worsen impulsivity and concentration.

KEY POINTS TO REMEMBER

• Severe and persistent mental illnesses are persistent or recurrent and likely to be highly disruptive or disabling.
• Stigma and chronicity present many challenges to coping and contribute to a variety of other social, physical health, and mental health problems such as increases in a variety of other areas (substance abuse, poverty and unemployment, comorbid physical illnesses and premature mortality, arrest, depression, and suicide risk).
• Impulse control disorders involve impulsive behaviors that are disruptive and serve to relieve psychological tension. These disorders include impulsive thefts, setting fires, sudden assaults or property destruction, hair pulling, and pathological gambling.
• Impulse control disorders are treated primarily through psychotherapy and sometimes with antidepressant or anticompulsive medications.
• Sexual disorders include gender identity disorder and the paraphilias. A person with gender identity disorder believes his or her biological gender is incorrect, and that he or she should be the opposite gender.
• People with gender identity disorder may be subject to ridicule and harassment and may experience significant distress

KEY POINTS TO REMEMBER—cont'd

related to their gender dissatisfaction. One intervention is gender reassignment, which involves counseling, practice living as the opposite gender, use of hormones, and surgical reassignment.

• Paraphilias are disorders in which sexual gratification is obtained in atypical and often socially unacceptable ways.

• Pedophilia includes having sexual fantasies or contact with young children. This disorder stirs strong feelings in staff and society.

• The causes of paraphilias are not clearly established, but neurological dysfunction may be a contributing factor.

• Medications that improve neurological dysfunction or reduce sexual drive may improve paraphilias.

• Psychotherapy and medication to reduce sexual drive and function can reduce offensive sexual behavior in pedophiles.

• ADHD is associated with childhood but may continue into or first be diagnosed in adulthood. In adults it is characterized by difficulty maintaining focus and organization, and can be disruptive to task completion, employment, relationships, and other key areas of functioning.

• ADHD often goes undiagnosed in adults, who may try to compensate for its symptoms. It is treated with a combination of counseling and stimulants (or sometimes other drugs).

CRITICAL THINKING

1. You are working with a patient who has recently been diagnosed with adult ADHD. He is very impulsive and frequently makes comments to you and others that are inappropriate and rude. You find yourself avoiding him and feeling angry toward him. Describe the approaches you could use to intervene in a therapeutic manner with this patient.

2. Are you comfortable with your own sexuality? With that of others? Are you judgmental? Could you be helpful to someone who has a sexual disorder? What factors have influenced your beliefs and values regarding sexuality? What do you think is the effect of sexually explicit television, music videos, and movies on your sexual attitudes, values, and beliefs?

CHAPTER REVIEW

Choose the most appropriate answer(s).

1. Federal and state categorization of mental illnesses according to levels of severity has tremendous implications for which of the following? Select all that apply.
    1. Providing a standard, nationally based medical classification to facilitate diagnosis
    2. Setting mental health policy
    3. Facilitating access to appropriate care
    4. Providing employers with the basis to understand work capacities for mentally ill employees

2. NAMI has been developed to:
    1. regulate neurotransmission along critical pathways involved in schizophrenia.
    2. provide social and employment opportunities for patients with mental health disorders through partial hospitalization programs.
    3. provide a structured, phased approach for improved management of ADHD symptoms.
    4. offer support and education for patients and families of patients with mental health disorders.

3. Which of the following are accurate statements about impulse control disorders? Select all that apply.
    1. Causes of impulse control disorders are not clearly understood.

2. Genetic factors are not considered to contribute to impulse control disorders.
    3. Anxiety may play an important role in impulse control disorders.
    4. Impulse control disorders are frequently associated with depression.

4. Which sexual disorder is illegal?
    1. Fetishism
    2. Transvestism
    3. Pedophilia
    4. Gender dysphoria

5. Which of the following nursing interventions would not be considered essential when working with an adult with ADHD?
    1. Establishing a regular exercise regimen to provide physical release and daily structure
    2. Guiding the patient to identify and use enhanced organizational skills
    3. Educating the patient's significant others about causes, treatments, and ways to cope with its symptoms
    4. Guiding the patient in understanding and practicing stimulation reduction strategies

REFERENCES

Almeida, O.P., Waterreus, A., Spry, N., et al. (2003). One year follow-up study of the association between chemical castration, sex hormones, beta-amyloid, memory and depression in men. *Psychoneuroendocrinology, 29*, 1071-1081.

Amador, X. (2007). *I am not sick, I don't need help!* (2nd ed.) Peconic, NY: Vida Press.

American Psychiatric Association (APA). (2000). *Diagnostic and statistical manual of mental disorders (DSM-IV-TR)* (4th ed., text rev.) Washington, DC: Author.

Aquila, R., & Emanuel, M. (2003). *Managing the long-term outlook of schizophrenia.* Retrieved July 1, 2007, from www.medscape.com/viewprogram/2680_index.

Arehart-Treichel, J. (2006). Pedophilia often in headlines, but not in research labs. *Psychiatric News, 41*(10), 37-39.

Brassett-Harknett, A., & Butler, N. (2007). Attention-deficit/hyperactivity disorder: An overview of the etiology and a review of the literature relating to the correlates and lifecourse outcomes for men and women. *Clinical Psychology Review, 27*, 188-210.

Bruce, T.O., Barwick, L.W., & Wright, H.H. (2005). Diagnosis and management of trichotillomania in children and adolescents. *Pediatric Drugs, 7*(6), 365-376.

Chamberlain, S.R., Menzies, L., Sahakian, B.J., et al. (2007). Lifting the veil on trichotillomania. *American Journal of Psychiatry, 164*(4), 568-574.

Coldwell, C.M., & Bender, W.S. (2007). The effectiveness of assertive community treatment for homeless populations with severe mental illness: A meta-analysis. *American Journal of Psychiatry, 164*(3), 393-399.

Coleman-Kennedy, C., & Pendley, A. (2002). Assessment and diagnosis of sexual addiction. *Journal of the American Psychiatric Nurses Association, 8*(5), 143-151.

Cook, J.A., Leff, H.S., Blyler, C.R., et al. (2005). Results of a multisite randomized trial of supported employment interventions for individuals with severe mental illness. *Archives of General Psychiatry, 62*, 505-512.

Cuijpers, P., & Stam, H. (2000). Burnout among relatives of psychiatric patients attending psychoeducational support groups. *Psychiatric Services, 51*(3), 375-379.

Dannon, P.N., Lowengrub, K., Musin, E., et al. (2005). Sustained-release bupropion versus naltrexone in the treatment of pathological gambling: A preliminary blind-rater study. *Journal of Clinical Psychopharmacology, 25*(6), 593-596.

Doering, S., Müller, E., Köpcke, W., et al. (1998). Predictors of relapse and rehospitalization in schizophrenia and schizoaffective disorder. *Schizophrenia Bulletin, 24*(1), 87-98.

Dunn, J.A., Arakawa, R., Greist, J.H., et al. (2007). Assessing the onset of antidepressant-induced sexual dysfunction using interactive voice response technology. *Journal of Clinical Psychiatry, 68*(4), 525-532.

Fagan, P.J., Wise, T.N., Schmidt, C.W., et al. (2002). Pedophilia. *Journal of the American Medical Association, 288*, 2458-2465.

Faraone, S.V., Biederman, J., Spencer, T., et al. (2000). Attention-deficit/hyperactivity disorder in adults: An overview. *Biological Psychiatry, 48*, 9-20.

Farhall, J., Webster, B., Hocking, B., et al. (1998). Training to enhance partnerships between mental health professionals and family caregivers: A comparative study. *Psychiatric Services, 49*(11), 1488-1490.

Frese, F.J., Stanley, J., Kress, K., et al. (2001). Integrating evidence-based practices and the recovery model. *Psychiatric Services, 52*, 1462-1468.

Glied, S. (2007). *Better but not well: Mental health policy in the United States since 1950.* Presented at the Eighth Annual All Ohio Institute on Community Psychiatry. Beachwood, OH, 16 March 2007.

Grant, J.E., Potenza, M.N., Hollander, E., et al. (2006). Multicenter investigation of the opioid antagonist nalmefene in the treatment of pathological gambling. *American Journal of Psychiatry, 163*, 303-312.

Grant, J.E., Levine, L., Kim, D., et al. (2005). Impulse control disorders in adult psychiatric inpatients. *American Journal of Psychiatry, 162*, 2184-2188.

Grant, J.E., & Kim, S.W. (2002). Effectiveness of pharmacotherapy for pathological gambling: A chart review. *Annals of Clinical Psychiatry, 14*(3), 155-161.

Greydanus, D.E., Pratt, H.D., & Patel, D.R. (2007). Attention deficit hyperactivity disorder across the lifespan: The child, adolescent and adult. *Disease-a-Month, 53*(2), 70-131.

Harrison, C.A., Dadds, M.R., & Smith, G. (1998). Family caregivers' criticism of patients with schizophrenia. *Psychiatric Services, 49*, 918-924.

Hellerstein, D.J., Rosenthal, R.N., Pinsker, H., et al. (1998). A randomized prospective study comparing supportive and dynamic therapies: Outcome and alliance. *Journal of Psychotherapy Practice and Research, 7*, 261-271.

Hiday, V.A., Swartz, M.S., Swanson, J.W., et al. (1999). Criminal victimization of persons with severe mental illness. *Psychiatric Services, 50*, 62-68.

Huygen, C. (2006). Understanding the needs of lesbian, gay, bisexual, and transgender people living with mental illness. *Medscape General Medicine, 8*(2), 29-31.

Kafka, M.P. (1996). Therapy for sexual impulsivity: The paraphilias and paraphilia-related disorders. *Psychiatric Times, 13*(6).

Koran, L.M., Aboujaoude, E.N., & Gamel, N.N. (2007). Escitalopram treatment of kleptomania: An open-label trial followed by double-blind discontinuation. *Journal of Clinical Psychiatry, 68*(3), 422-427.

Lancet. (2003). Promoting optimum management for ADHD (editorial). *Lancet, 369*(9565), 880.

Langevin, R. (2006). Sexual offenses and traumatic brain injury. *Brain &Cognition, 60*(2), 206-207.

Light, S.A., & Holroyd, S. (2005). The use of medroxyprogesterone acetate for the treatment of sexually inappropriate behaviour in patients with dementia. *Journal of Psychiatry Neuroscience, 31*(2), 132-134.

Marshall, W.L. (2007). Diagnostic issues, multiple paraphilias, and comorbid disorders in sexual offenders: Their incidence and treatment. *Aggression and Violent Behavior, 12*(1), 16-35.

McCloughen, A. (2003). The association between schizophrenia and cigarette smoking: A review of the literature and implications for mental health nursing practice. *International Journal of Mental Health Nursing, 12*, 119-129.

McCombs, J.S., Nichol, M.B., Johnstone, B.M., et al. (2000). Antipsychotic drug use patterns and the cost of treating schizophrenia. *Psychiatric Services, 51*, 525-527.

Mehta, S., & Farina, A. (1988). Associative stigma: Perceptions of the difficulties of college-aged children of stigmatized fathers. *Journal of Social and Clinical Psychology, 7*, 192-202.

Mendez, M.F., Chow, T., Ringman, J., et al. (2000). Pedophilia and temporal lobe disturbances. *Journal of Neuropsychiatry and Clinical Neuroscience, 12*, 71-76.

Miller, B.J., Paschall, C.B., & Svendsen, D.P. (2007). *Mortality and medical comorbidity among patients with serious mental illness.* Poster presented at the Eighth Annual All Ohio Institute on Community Psychiatry, Beachwood, OH. 16 March 2007.

Moeller, F.G., Barratt, E.S., Dougherty, D.M., et al. (2001). Psychiatric aspects of impulsivity. *American Journal of Psychiatry, 158,* 1783-1793.

Mulligan, K. (2005). Recovery model seeks more than symptom relief. *Psychiatric News, 40*(18), 6.

NANDA International (NANDA-I). (2007). *NANDA nursing diagnoses: Definitions and classification 2007-2008.* Philadelphia: Author.

National Alliance on Mental Illness (NAMI). (2004). *Statement of Margaret Stout on behalf of NAMI before the U.S. House of Representatives, Committee on Appropriations, Subcommittee on Labor-HHS-Education and Related Agencies.* Retrieved July 2, 2007, from www.nami.org/Content/ContentGroups/Policy/Issues_Spotlights/NAMI_Presses_Congress_for_FY_2005_Funds_for_Mental_Illness_Research_and_Services.htm.

National Mental Health Association. (2001). *Labor Day 2001 report: Untreated and mistreated mental illness and substance abuse costs U.S. $113 billion a year: The 'dollars and sense' case for increased investments in mental health and substance abuse.* Alexandria, VA: Author.

Peck, M.C., & Scheffler, R.M. (2002). An analysis of the definitions of mental illness used in state parity laws. *Psychiatric Services, 53,* 1089-1095.

Pompili, M., Amador, X.F., Girari, P., et al. (2007). Suicide risk in schizophrenia: Learning from the past to change the future. *Annals of General Psychiatry, 6,* 10. Retrieved July 2, 2007, from www.annals-general-psychiatry.com/content/6/1/10.

President's New Freedom Commission on Mental Health. *Report of the President's New Freedom Commission on Mental Health: Achieving the promise: transforming mental health in America: Executive summary.* (2003). Retrieved June 28, 2007, from www.mentalhealthcommission.gov/reports/FinalReport/FullReport.htm.

Rosenheck, R., Leslie, D., Keefe, R., et al. (2006). Barriers to employment for people with schizophrenia. *American Journal of Psychiatry, 163,* 411-417.

Sawle, G.A., & Kear-Colwell, J. (2001). Adult attachment style and pedophilia: A developmental perspective. *International Journal of Offender Therapy and Comparative Criminology, 45*(1), 32-50.

Scahill, L., Carroll, D., & Burke, K. (2004). *Methylphenidate: Mechanism of action and clinical update.* Retrieved June 29, 2007, from http://findarticles.com/p/articles/mi_qa3892/is_200404/ai_n9356900.

Sensky, T., Turkington, D., Kingdon, D., et al. (2000). A randomized controlled trial of cognitive-behavioral therapy for persistent symptoms in schizophrenia resistant to medication. *Archives of General Psychiatry, 57,* 165-172.

Spencer, T.J., Biederman, J., & Mick, E. (2007). Attention-deficit/hyperactivity disorder: Diagnosis, lifespan, comorbidities, and neurobiology. *Journal of Pediatric Psychology, 32*(6), 631-642.

Thornton, D. (2006). Age and sexual recidivism: A variable connection. *Sexual Abuse: Journal of Research and Treatment, 18*(2), 123-135.

Torkelson, D.J., & Dobal, M.T. (1999). Sexual rights of people with serious and persistent mental illness: Gathering evidence for decision making. *Journal of the American Psychiatric Nurses Association, 5*(5), 150-161.

Torrey, E.F. (1997). *A well-intentioned disaster: The fallout from releasing the mentally ill from institutions.* Retrieved July 2, 2007, from http://chronicle.com/che-data/articles.dir/art-43.dir/issue-40.dir/40b00401.htm.

Torrey, E.F., & Zdanowicz, M. (2001). Outpatient commitment: What, why and for whom. *Psychiatric Services, 52,* 337-341.

White, S. (2003). Personal accounts: Mistaken identity. *Psychiatric Services, 54,* 479-481.

Weiden, P.J. (2007). Discontinuing and switching antipsychotic medications: Understanding the CATIE schizophrenia trial. *Journal of Clinical Psychiatry, 68*(Suppl 1), 12-19.

Wylie, K. (2004). Gender related disorders. *BMJ, 329,* 615-617.

CHAPTER 25

Older Adults

Elizabeth M. Varcarolis and Sally K. Holzapfel

Key Terms and Concepts

advance directives, p. 511
ageism, p. 498
chemical restraints, p. 510
directive to physician, p. 511
durable power of attorney for health care, p. 511

elderspeak, p. 501
living will, p. 511
Omnibus Budget Reconciliation Act (OBRA), p. 510
Patient Self-Determination Act (PSDA), p. 511
physical restraints, p. 510

Objectives

1. Summarize the facts and myths about aging.
2. Describe the effect of ageism in providing care to older adults.
3. Analyze how ageism affects attitudes and willingness to care for older adults.
4. Compare the different group interventions commonly used with older adults.
5. Defend the importance of a comprehensive geriatric assessment including assessment guidelines for an older adult.
6. Compare and contrast depression and suicide in the older adult population and with that of the younger adult population.

7. Identify the risk factors for elder suicide and the nurse's role in prevention of suicide.
8. Compare the physiological effects of alcohol use on an older individual to that of a younger adult.
9. Delineate the requirements for the use of physical and chemical restraints.
10. Discuss institutional requirements related to the Patient Self-Determination Act (1990).
11. Compare living wills, directives to physicians, and durable power of attorney for health care.

evolve

For additional resources related to the content of this chapter, visit the Evolve website at http://evolve.elsevier.com/Varcarolis/essentials.

- Chapter Outline
- Chapter Review Questions

- Concept Map Creator

Edited by Evelyn Yap in the fifth edition of
Foundations of Psychiatric Mental Health Nursing.

The increasing proportion of older adults within the population has altered the socioeconomic condition in America and at the same time is transforming the practice of health care. By the year 2030, 23% of the U.S. population will consist of individuals older than 65 years of age. Among older adults, the fastest-growing subgroups are minorities, the poor, and those aged 85 years and older. By 2050, the population of seniors 65 years of age and older will double, and the number of those 85 years and older will quadruple (Henderson, 2003).

As people live longer they are more likely to experience chronic illness, disability, and mental health issues (Miller, 2004). On average, an older adult has three or four chronic illnesses and a nearly 20% annual risk of hospitalization (Narang & Sikka, 2006). After age 85, there is a one-in-three chance of developing dementia, immobility, incontinence, or another age-related disability.

Women generally outlive men. Because husbands more often predecease (die before) their spouses, they benefit from the support of their wives to help with health-related issues. On the other hand, many older women lack this type of support. Women's greater longevity has significant ramifications for society at large and for the health care system in particular.

Chronological age is considered an arbitrary indicator of function because there are significant variables that contribute to the capabilities of older adults. Surveys focusing on how they see themselves reveal that nearly half of people 65 years and older consider themselves to be middle-aged or young. Only 15% of people 75 years and older consider themselves "very old" (Ebersole et al., 2004). However, current standards (Hogstel & Weeks, 2000) classify people into the following age categories:

- **Young old**: 65 to 74 years of age
- **Middle old**: 75 to 84 years of age
- **Old old**: 85 to 94 years of age
- **Elite old**: 95 years or older

There are noticeable differences between individuals in their 60s and people in their 80s. Whereas those in the younger group are relatively healthy, those in the older group are much more vulnerable, frail, and at risk for visual problems, cognitive impairment, and falls. They also have more limited economic resources and community supports, and are more affected by the chronic diseases and disorders of aging (Ebersole et al., 2004).

AGEISM

Ageism has been defined as a bias against older people because of their age; it is a system of destructive, erroneous beliefs. In essence, ageism represents a dislike by the young of the old, reflecting the disparaging effects of society's attitudes toward older adults. This age prejudice is based on the notion that aging makes people increasingly unattractive, unintelligent, asexual, unemployable, and senile.

Ageism is not limited to the way the young may look at the old. It is also seen in the views of older people, who tend to be critical about themselves and their peers. Indeed, the attitudes of older adults toward their peers, particularly those with mental disabilities, are often more negative than the views held by the young (although this is not always the case). The threat of social contagion by association with the frail and infirm may simply be too strong to bear. Age proximity raises feelings of vulnerability. This may explain why older adults often do not like to be referred to as "old." By seeing themselves as "young" rather than "old," they adjust better to their advancing years.

Ageism differs from other forms of discrimination in that it cuts across gender, race, religion, and national origin. In our culture, old age does not award a desirable status or membership in a sought-after club; rather, it is a social category with negative connotations. Today a new form of ageism puts the older adult in a no-win situation: those who are well-to-do are envied for their economic progress, those who are middle-class are blamed for making Social Security too costly, and those who are poor are resented for being tax burdens.

The results of ageism can be observed throughout every level of society. Even health care providers are not immune to its effects. Negative values can surface in myriad ways in the health care system. Financial and political support for programs for older adults is difficult to obtain; their needs are addressed only after those of younger, albeit smaller, population groups. The Gray Panthers and the American Association of Retired Persons (AARP), however, are powerful lobbying groups that are fighting to change this trend.

Ageism Among Health Care Workers

Health care personnel do not always share medical information, recommendations, and opportunities with the older adult. Studies show that older adults receive less information and sometimes less care than those who are younger. Ageism is also reflected in public policy, which leads to discrimination against older adults (Hooyman, 2003; Nelson, 2002).

Health care workers who deal on a daily basis with the confused, ill, and frail older adult may tend to develop a somewhat negative and biased view of them. The negative attitudes of most health care workers are often a reflection of the views of society, which again are most often characterized by negativism and stereotyping. The rendering of medical care to older adults has been burdened with pessimism, defeatism, and professional aversion. Unfortunately, such thinking can be found among professionals as well as among ancillary personnel working in nursing homes and other institutional settings.

Negative views of the older adult are frequently held by nurses. Studies have found that recruits to nursing hold ageist views, which has significant implications for practice, education, and research (Lueckenotte, 2000). Positive attitudes toward older adults and their care need to be instilled during basic nursing education. If the goal of nursing programs is to prepare students to practice in the future, then preparing students to care for older adults in a wide variety of settings is mandatory, because that *is* the future (Lueckenotte, 2000). Educational programs must include the following:

- Information about the aging process
- Discussion of attitudes relating to the care of the older adult
- Sensitization of participants to their patients' needs
- Exploration of the dynamics of nurse-patient and staff-patient interactions

Box 25-1 lists some facts and myths about aging.

ASSESSMENT AND COMMUNICATION STRATEGIES

Nurses who work with the older adult benefit from specific knowledge about normal aging, drug interactions, and chronic disease. **Geropsychiatric nurses** are those who work with older adult patients who have mental health problems. Geropsychiatric nurses have special skills in interviewing and assessing, specific knowledge of effective treatment modalities, the normal aging process, and sociocultural influences on older adults and their families.

The National Institutes of Health recommend a comprehensive geriatric assessment to evaluate and manage the care and progress of all older adult patients. A comprehensive geriatric assessment includes a mental status exam, a focus on physical health; functional, economic, and social status; and environmental factors that might impinge on the older adult patient's well-being (Dharmarajan & Norman, 2003). Figure 25-1 provides an example of a comprehensive geriatric assessment. (Refer to the inside back cover for an example of a mental status exam.)

An examination and interview of an older adult conducted in unfamiliar surroundings will most likely produce anxiety. Unlike younger patients, who may be comfortable discussing personal issues such as family conflicts, feelings of sadness, sexual practices, finances, and bodily functions, older adults are part of a generation that viewed these topics

---

BOX 25-1

Facts and Myths About Aging

Facts

- The senses of vision, hearing, touch, taste, and smell decline with age.
- Muscular strength decreases with age. Muscle fibers atrophy and decrease in number.
- Regular sexual expressions are important to maintain sexual capacity and effective sexual performance.
- At least 50% of restorative sleep is lost as a result of the aging process.
- Older adults are major consumers of prescription drugs because of the high incidence of chronic diseases in this population.
- Older adults have a high incidence of depression.
- Many individuals experience difficulty when they retire.
- Older adults are prone to become victims of crime.
- Older widows appear to adjust better than younger ones.

Myths

- Most adults past the age of 65 years are demented.
- Sexual interest declines with age.
- Older adults are not able to learn new tasks.
- As individuals age, they become more rigid in their thinking and set in their ways.
- Older adults are well off and no longer impoverished.
- Most older adults are infirm and require help with daily activities.
- Most older adults are socially isolated and lonely.
- All older adults are significantly hard of hearing and should be spoken to in a loud voice.

---

as private, and as a result, they may be uncomfortable discussing these personal matters. Although the more recent baby boom generation of older adults may come from a more open and so called "sophisticated" age, it is important to respect these feelings in everyone while reviewing essential history. Older adults will guide you as to their level of comfort with personal information. The following are basic rules of thumb:

- Conduct the interview in a private area.
- Introduce yourself and ask the patient what he or she would like to be called.
- Establish rapport and put the patient at ease by sitting or standing at the same level.
- Ensure that lighting is adequate and noise level is low in recognition of the fact that hearing and vision may be impaired in the older adult patient.
- Use touch to convey warmth while at the same time respecting the older adult's comfort level with personal touch.

COMPREHENSIVE GERIATRIC ASSESSMENT				
Name:		**Date of birth:**		**Gender:**
Physical Health				
Chronic disorder				
Vision	Adequate Inadequate	Eyeglasses: Y N		Needs evaluation
Hearing	Adequate Inadequate	Hearing aids: Y N		
Mobility	Ambulatory: Y N	Assistive device:		
	Falls: Y N			Needs evaluation
Nutrition	Albumin:	TLC:	HCT:	
	Weight:	Weight loss or gain: Y N		Needs evaluation
Incontinence	Y N	Treatment: Y N		Needs evaluation
Medications	Total number:	Reviewed & revised: Y N		
	Adverse effects/allergy:			
Screening	Cholesterol:	TSH:	B12:	Folate:
	Colonoscopy: Date:		N/A	
	Mammogram: Date:		N/A	
	Osteoporosis: Date:		N/A	
	Pap smear: Date:		N/A	
	PSA: Date:		N/A	
Immunization	Influenza: Date:			
	Pneumonia: Date:			
	Tetanus: Date:		Booster:	
Counseling	Diet	Exercise	Calcium	Vitamin D
	Smoking	Alcohol	Driving	Injury prevention
Mental Health				
Dementia	Y N MMSE score:	Date:	Cause (if known):	
Depression	Y N GDS score:	Date:	Treatment: Y N	
Functional Status				
ADL	Bathing: I D	Dressing: I D	Toileting: I D	
	Transferring: I D	Feeding: I D	Continence: Y N	

Figure 25-1 ▪ Comprehensive geriatric assessment. *ADL,* Activities of daily living; B_{12}, vitamin B_{12}; *D,* dependent; *GDS,* Geriatric Depression Scale; *HCT,* hematocrit; *I,* independent; *MMSE,* Mini-Mental State Examination; *N,* no; *PSA,* prostate-specific antigen; *TLC,* total lymphocyte count; *TSH,* thyroid-stimulating hormone; *Y,* yes.

TABLE 25-1	Comparison of Delirium, Dementia, and Depression		
	Delirium	**Dementia**	**Depression**
Onset	Sudden, over hours to days	Slowly, over months	May have been gradual with exacerbation during crisis or stress
Cause or contributing factors	Hypoglycemia, fever, dehydration, hypotension; infection, other conditions that disrupt body's homeostasis; adverse drug reaction; head injury; change in environment (e.g., hospitalization); pain; emotional stress	Alzheimer's disease, vascular disease, human immunodeficiency virus infection, neurological disease, chronic alcoholism, head trauma	Lifelong history, losses, loneliness, crises, declining health, medical conditions
Cognition	Impaired memory, judgment, calculations, attention span; can fluctuate throughout the day	Impaired memory, judgment, calculations, attention span, abstract thinking; agnosia	Difficulty concentrating, forgetfulness, inattention
Level of consciousness	Altered	Not altered	Not altered
Activity level	Can be increased or reduced; restlessness, behaviors may worsen in evening (sundowning); sleep-wake cycle may be reversed	Not altered; behaviors may worsen in evening (sundowning)	Usually decreased; lethargy, fatigue, lack of motivation; may sleep poorly and awaken in early morning
Emotional state	Rapid swings; can be fearful, anxious, suspicious, aggressive, have hallucinations and delusions	Flat; delusions	Extreme sadness, apathy, irritability, anxiety, paranoid ideation

- Summarize the interaction and invite feedback from the patient.
- Assess the cognitive, behavioral, and emotional status of the older adult—this is very important in managing the nursing care of the patient and is particularly vital for detecting delirium, dementia, and depression (Table 25-1) because their prevalence increases with age (Dharmarajan & Norman, 2003). In addition to depression, suicide and alcohol/substance abuse are major health problems among older adults.
- Evaluate any indications of abuse (physical, sexual, neglect, financial) in a discreet manner (see Chapter 18).

People talk to older adults differently. Anyone who has visited a nursing home, hospital unit with older adult patients, or even a grocery store can attest to a pernicious and condescending method of communicating with the older adult. **Elderspeak** is manifested by health care workers talking to patients as if they were small children. They use terms of endearment (e.g., honey, sweetie), overly simple sentences, an increased volume and pitch, and collective pronouns (do "we" want a bath?) (Williams et al., 2003). Generally, this style of speech is meant to convey caring and nurturance (and it may do just that with family members and same-age acquaintances); however, it implies that the older adult person is incompetent and inferior.

Another related communication problem is when health care workers dismiss the presence of older adults in the room and speak about them rather than to them. Nursing students should consciously avoid using elderspeak. Address the older adult when asking a question, and when necessary, ask the family member or other health care worker(s) if they have anything to add. Box 25-2 provides helpful communication and interview techniques.

PSYCHIATRIC DISORDERS IN OLDER ADULTS

Not only are older adults with mental disorders less likely to be accurately diagnosed, they are more likely to receive inappropriate or inadequate treatment compared with younger adults (Bartels & Drake, 2005). This is especially true for individuals with depression and anxiety. In this age of emerging evidence-based practice (EBP), there is a huge lack of evidence-based literature and studies dealing with geriatric anxiety disorder, bipolar disorders, geriatric

---

BOX 25-2

Communication Guidelines for Interviewing the Older Adult

1. Gather preliminary data before the session and keep questionnaires relatively short.
2. Ask about often-overlooked problems, such as difficulty sleeping, incontinence, falling, depression, dizziness, or loss of energy.
3. Pace the interview to allow the patient to formulate answers; resist the tendency to interrupt prematurely.
4. Use yes-or-no or simple choice questions if the older patient has trouble coping with open-ended questions.
5. Begin with general questions such as, "How can I help you most at this visit?" or "What's been happening?"
6. Be alert for information on the patient's relationships with others, thoughts about families or co-workers, typical responses to stress, and attitudes toward aging, illness, occupation, and death.
7. Assess mental status for deficits in recent or remote memory, and determine if confusion exists.
8. Be aware of all medications the patient is taking and assess for side effects, efficacy, and possible drug interactions.
9. Determine how fast the condition of the patient has been changing to assess the extent of the patient's concerns.
10. Include the family or significant other in the interview process for added input, clarification, support, and reinforcement.

From National Institute on Aging. *Working with your older patient: A clinician's handbook.* Bethesda, MD: Author.

---

schizophrenia, or geriatric alcohol use disorders (Bartels & Drake, 2005). Primary mental health issues affecting the older adult are depression, suicide, and alcohol and drug use. Elder abuse is also a great national concern. Elder abuse and *Caregiver role strain* are covered in more detail in Chapter 18.

DEPRESSION

Depression is the most common psychiatric disorder in the older adult. The prevalence of major depressive disorder is up to 5% of elders living in the community, with an 8% to 27% prevalence for minor depression. Major depression was found to be up to 27% of older adults in a screening of emergency department (ED) participants. Unfortunately, only about half of all older adults who suffer from depressive symptoms are identified as depressed (Piechniczek-Buczek, 2006).

Depression in the older adult community is a serious public health problem. Health care providers frequently misinterpret clinical depression in older adults as a normal part of aging (Henderson, 2003). Even when those are detected and treated, the effectiveness of the available interventions is modest. And if acute phase treatment is effective, the chances or relapse or recurrence is high. Therefore prevention of depression is a priority (Cole, 2005).

Depression is often confused with dementia, and a careful, systematic assessment is necessary to properly distinguish between the two. Unlike dementia, depression is treatable with medication and other interventions. In the older adult, symptoms of memory loss and other intellectual impairments or asocial or agitated behavior are generally associated with dementia but may actually be caused by depression. At times, dementia may be masked by the more frank symptoms of delirium. A careful assessment is needed to distinguish among delirium, dementia, and depression because presenting symptoms can be similar, or two or more may coincide. (See Table 25-1 for a comparison of dementia and depression.) Chapter 15 gives thorough assessment guides and interventions for a patient experiencing delirium or dementia.

In making an assessment, the nurse needs to be familiar with the symptoms of later-life depression (NIMH, 2004), which include one or more of the following:

- Changes in sleep patterns (insomnia)
- Changes in eating patterns (loss of appetite)
- Loss of interest or pleasure in usual activities (anhedonia)
- Excessive fatigue (anergia)
- Increased concern with bodily functions
- Feelings of depression
- Apprehension and anxiety without any cause
- Low self-esteem (feelings of insignificance or pessimism)

A careful evaluation of the cause of the depression is necessary. A variety of biological and psychosocial risk factors have been identified (e.g., medical illness, functional disability, social isolation, accumulation of life stressors, losses, and genetic vulnerabilities) (Charney et al., 2003). Depression can be caused by drugs (e.g., reserpine and other *Rauwolfia* derivatives, steroids, phenothiazines), by metabolic and endocrine disorders (e.g., hepatitis and adrenal and thyroid insufficiency), and by acute medical events such as cerebrovascular accident or myocardial infarction. Depression also can augment suicide potential. Thorough assessment for any medical or drug-induced side effects should be performed, as well as psychosocial and medical assessment. (See Figure 25-2 for the Geriatric Depression Scale.)

Depressed older adults are at high risk for physical decline. Prevention and treatment of depression are practical interventions to reduce physical decline in later years.

Geriatric Depression Scale (Short Form)

	Yes	No
1. Are you basically satisfied with your life?	○	○
2. Have you dropped many of your activities and interests?	○	○
3. Do you feel that your life is empty?	○	○
4. Do you often get bored?	○	○
5. Are you in good spirits most of the time?	○	○
6. Are you afraid that something bad is going to happen to you?	○	○
7. Do you feel happy most of the time?	○	○
8. Do you often feel helpless?	○	○
9. Do you prefer to stay at home, rather than going out and doing new things?	○	○
10. Do you feel you have more problems with memory than most?	○	○
11. Do you think it is wonderful to be alive now?	○	○
12. Do you feel pretty worthless the way you are now?	○	○
13. Do you feel full of energy?	○	○
14. Do you feel that your situation is hopeless?	○	○
15. Do you think that most people are better off than you are?	○	○

Figure 25-2 ■ Geriatric Depression Scale (Short Form). (From Sheikh, J.I., & Yesavage, J.A. (1986). Geriatric Depression Scale (GDS): Recent evidence and development of a shorter version. In T.L. Brink (Ed.), *Clinical gerontology: A guide to assessment and intervention* (pp. 165-173). New York: Haworth Press.)

Patient and family education is an important component of successful management.

Antidepressant Therapy

In choosing a drug to treat depression in the older adult, primary emphasis is placed on avoidance of possible side effects rather than on efficacy. When antidepressant therapy is initiated, low dosages (usually half the routine recommended dosage) are suggested, and the dosage is then slowly and gradually increased if needed (Doddi, 2003). If the individual is at risk for suicide, then caregivers must be aware that as the depression begins to lift, there is a greater chance that the individual will complete the suicide.

Selective serotonin reuptake inhibitors (SSRIs) are the first-line antidepressants for older adults because of their more benign side effects and their lack of toxicity when taken in overdose (Ebersole et al., 2004; NIMH, 2004). The SSRIs are also helpful for those older adults with conduction

defects, ischemic heart disease, glaucoma, and prostate disease (Rueben et al., 2003). However, SSRIs may also cause some problems, especially for older adults who are more sensitive to medications and are therefore at greater risk for drug interactions (Schatzberg & Nemeroff, 2004). Caution must be taken with older adults using SSRIs because it appears that SRRIs may double the risk of bone fractures (Richards et al., 2007). The risk is two-fold, as clinical fractures can occur from falls as well as stress put on the bones by even minor activity (e.g., walking or standing).

Fluvoxamine (Luvox) and paroxetine (Paxil) can cause symptoms of central nervous system stimulation, including increased awakenings, reduced time in rapid eye movement sleep, and insomnia. Age does not appear to affect the pharmacokinetics of sertraline. However, the metabolism of fluoxetine and paroxetine is impaired in the older adult, which results in higher plasma levels. This makes sertraline (Zoloft) a good choice among the SSRIs for antidepressant therapy. Among the tricyclic antidepressants, which are less expensive and are the TCAs recommended by the American Academy of Family Physicians, are desipramine (Norpramin), and nortriptyline (Pamelor). These appear to be the best tolerated by older adults although TCAs are often avoided because of their anticholinergic side effects.

Psychotherapy

Nurse clinicians may provide individual or group psychotherapy to the depressed patient. Groups can diminish social isolation and loneliness and help the members understand that they are not alone in their situation. Group members can learn creative ways to raise their mood and increase quality of life. A number of different kinds of groups are useful for older adults (Table 25-2).

Evidence-based studies suggest that cognitive therapy, behavioral therapy, and brief dynamic therapy are effective treatments of elder depression (Mackin & Arean, 2005). It is believed that best outcomes often result from combining some kind of therapy with medication. Preliminary studies support this, but more studies are needed.

SUICIDE

Although suicide is often associated with the young, the suicide rates among older adults in the United States are the highest of any age-group—it is now one of the top 10 causes of death. Although older adults account for only 13% of the population, they are disproportionately affected by suicide: 20% of all suicides are committed by individuals 65 years of age or older (Luggen, 2004; McAndrews, 2001). Nationally, the highest rates of suicide are found in individuals older than age 65 (Ingram, 2001).

In older adults, suicide is most closely associated with untreated depression (National Center for Injury Prevention and Control, 2003). As the most frequent functional psychiatric disorder of later life, depression accounts for up to 70% of late-life suicides. Research has shown that most

TABLE 25-2	**Useful Group Therapy Modalities for Older Adult Patients**	
Remotivation Therapy	**Reminiscence Therapy (Life Review)**	**Psychotherapy**
Purpose of Group		
Resocialize regressed and apathetic patients	Share memories of the past	Alleviate psychiatric symptoms
Reawaken interest in the environment	Increase self-esteem	Increase ability to interact with others in a group
	Increase socialization	Increase self-esteem
	Increase awareness of the uniqueness of each participant	Increase ability to make decisions and function more independently
Format		
Groups are made up of 10 to 15 people.	Groups are made up of 6 to 8 people.	Group size is 6 to 12 members.
Meetings are held once or twice a week.	Meetings are held once or twice weekly for 1 hour.	Group members should share similar:
Meetings are highly structured in a classroom-like setting.	Topics include holidays, major life events, birthdays, travel, and food.	• Problems
Group uses props.		• Mental status
Each session discusses a particular topic.		• Needs
		• Sexual integration
		Group meets at regularly scheduled times (certain number of times a week, specific duration of session) and place.
Desired Outcomes		
Increase participants' sense of reality	Alleviate depression in institutionalized older adult	Decrease sense of isolation
Offer practice of health roles	Through the process of reorganization and reintegration, provide avenue by members	Facilitate development of new roles and reestablish former roles
Realize more objective self-image than older adult can	Achieve a new sense of identity.	Provide information for other group
	Achieve a positive self-concept.	Provide group support for effecting changes and increasing self-esteem

From Matteson, M.A., & McConnell, E.S. (Eds.). (1988). *Gerontologic nursing: Concepts and practice* (p. 80). Philadelphia: Saunders.

older adults who commit suicide suffer from the most treatable kind of depression and yet do not receive needed mental health services (NIMH, 2004). Early identification of and treatment for depression, therefore, are key measures for suicide prevention. Piechniczek-Buczek (2006) states that efforts need to be made, especially in the emergency department (ED) and primary care setting to identify risk factors, clues, and signs of imminent threats of late life suicide. This is doable since perhaps as many as 70% of elder individuals who committed suicide visited their physicians within a week to a month of their deaths (Andersen et al., 2000; Piechniczek-Buczek, 2006).

Even though the suicide rate among older adults is high, suicides in this group are probably underreported. Suicide is often not listed on the death certificate, even if it is suspected. The numbers also do not reflect those who passively or indirectly commit suicide by abusing alcohol, starving themselves, overdosing or mixing medications, stopping life-sustaining drugs, or simply losing the will to live.

The highest prevalence of suicide occurs in older white males accounting for 81% of completed suicide in late life (Szanto et al., 2001). One explanation for the high rate may lie in changes of occupational status and measures of success in men at the time of retirement and thereafter (Ebersole et al., 2004). With retirement, a man may lose status, influence, and contact with fellow workers in the community. On the other hand, the older woman retains many of her earlier activities and roles. It remains to be seen whether women and other groups who have become more active in the workforce will experience the same effects as men on retirement. The Protestant white male older than 85 years of age living alone in his home is at highest risk. Although such a person appears neat and calm, he is often taking either antianxiety or antipsychotic medication (Hogstel & Weeks, 2000).

Other factors that can lead to suicide are feelings of hopelessness, uselessness, and despair. For older adults, suicide may be seen as a final gesture of control at a stage when independence is at risk or activities are limited. Severe medical illness, functional disability, alcohol abuse, history of suicide attempts, comorbid anxiety, and psychotic depression are added risk factors for suicide (Dharmarajan & Norman, 2003). For this reason, the suicide attempts of the older adult are more likely to succeed. Unlike younger people, whose suicidal gestures may be intended to draw attention to their problems, those of older adults do not signify a call for help but rather a desire to die.

Financial need is another risk factor contributing to the high suicide rate. Federal reductions in programs such as Medicare, Medicaid, and food stamps, along with state-ordered cuts in medical care, cause many older Americans to worry about their future. An inverse relationship between economic conditions and suicide rate has been identified.

Assessment of Suicide Risk

The assessment of older patients must include attention to the high-risk factors that potentially contribute to suicide, such as widowhood, acute illnesses and intractable pain, status change, chronic illness, family history of suicide, chronic sleep problems, alcoholism, depression, and losses (Hogstel & Weeks, 2000). Losses may be personal (death of a family member or close friend), economic (loss of earnings or job), or social (loss of prestige or position). Multiple losses accompany the aging process, increasing stress at a time when the older adult may be the most vulnerable and least able to cope with stress, thus precipitating a depressive state. Nevertheless, many older adults are able to function despite their losses. Those who give in may do so because of hopelessness.

The nurse must remain vigilant for possible suicidal tendencies in patients later in life. In assessing suicide risk, the health care provider must examine previous suicidal behavior, seriousness of the intent, presence of active plans, availability of the means to commit the act, lethality of the method chosen, and the specific details of the plan. Compared to those in younger age-groups, older adults are less likely to communicate their suicidal thoughts and plans (Hogstel & Weeks, 2000). Nurses play a vital role in the prevention of older adult suicide because of their presence in every care setting. Attention must be focused on building awareness and use of community resources in the high-risk population. Screening for depression and suicidal thinking in the older adult should be standard and can save lives.

The nurse is professionally obligated to respond and intervene with the older adult patient in crisis, especially when the patient believes that the willful destruction of life is the only option available. It is therefore very important to maintain a sensitive, compassionate, and therapeutic approach with the patient. Communication with the older adult patient must be skillful, clear, direct, and respectful of the individual's rights. For some people, these interventions may restore a sense of self and purpose so that life may be preserved (Ebersole et al., 2004). Questions such as the following may be asked in suicide assessment:

- What kinds of thoughts do you have about a person's right to take his or her own life?
- What advantage does ending one's life offer?
- What is the most important thing you have to live for?
- Have you thought of taking your life?

Refer to Chapter 20 for the SAD PERSONS scale, which is an appropriate suicide assessment tool for older as well as younger adults.

Right to Die

One concern of nursing is the question of whether older adults have the right to end their life by way of physician-assisted suicide (PAS) or taking their own life. Suicide in any manner always raises spiritual and moral issues. However, there are some in society who believe that older adults with terminal illnesses or who suffer intractable pain, should be able to control their own deaths. If an alert older adult patient is confronted with an intractable, lingering, and painful illness, with no hope of relief except through death, either by PAS or suicide, is such an intervention justifiable?

The American Nurses Association (ANA) advises nurses not to participate in assisted suicide. It is a violation of the ANA *Code of Ethics for Nurses* to participate in assisted suicide; however, this does not mean that patients who want their life terminated should be abandoned. The ANA (1992) takes the position that nurses ethically support the provision of compassionate and dignified end-of-life care no matter what decision is made, including the withholding of withdrawing life-sustaining treatment (Provision 1.3). This emotionally debated issue raises religious, cultural, and "right to self-determination" issue that will most likely continue as our population ages and more members of society will face painful terminal illnesses. Refer to Chapter 20 for a brief discussion of PAS and right-to-die issues.

Although suicide is discussed in Chapter 20, specific factors that concern older adults are noted here, such as retirement-related difficulties, physical illness, economic problems, loneliness, social isolation, multiple losses, and ageism. Innovative methods to deal with these factors need to be developed for the older adult. Education of the public in general—and health care providers, in particular—is necessary to raise the level of awareness of this geriatric problem.

ALCOHOLISM AND SUBSTANCE ABUSE

The American Medical Association has termed alcohol and substance abuse among older adults a hidden epidemic. Substance abuse and dependence in the geriatric population have been identified as the fastest growing health problem in the country (Piechniczek-Buczek, 2006). This is predominately a result of the greater life-time rates of drug use of the baby-boom generation, which suggests that the large size of the generation now entering their sixties will further increase the number of people using drugs in the next two decades (Colliver et al., 2006). Identifying alcohol and substance abuse is often difficult because personality and behavioral changes frequently go unrecognized and health care providers seldom assess the older adult for these problems (Riger, 2000). Let us first examine alcoholism.

Alcoholism

Epidemiological studies suggest that alcohol dependence is present in up to 4% of community-dwelling older adults. This prevalence is on the rise, and has been recognized as a major public health problem (Oslin, 2005). Unfortunately, most (85%) receive no treatment. There are two major types of abusers: (1) the early-onset alcoholic or aging alcoholic, and (2) the late-onset alcoholic or geriatric problem drinker. The aging alcoholic has generally had alcohol problems intermittently throughout life, with a regular pattern of alcohol abuse starting to evolve in late middle age or later. The geriatric problem drinker, on the other hand, has no history of alcohol-related problems but develops an alcohol abuse pattern in response to the stresses of aging (Wagenaar et al., 2001).

The stressful or reactive factors that precipitate late-onset alcohol abuse are often related to environmental conditions and may include retirement, widowhood, and loneliness. These stressors in the older adult, who may have retired, may not drive, and may be isolated from family and friends, are often greater than the problems faced by the middle-aged adult, who has to manage a job or career and care for a family and household. Work and family responsibilities may help keep a potential alcoholic from drinking too much. Once these demands are gone and the structure of daily life is disrupted, there is little impetus to remain sober.

Alcohol and Aging

Excessive consumption of alcohol can create particular problems for older adults. They have an increased biological sensitivity to (a decreased tolerance for) the effects of alcohol. The decreased tolerance is related to the stomach, and an increased sensitivity to alcohol in the brain. As people age there is also a decline in lean tissue and an increase in fatty tissue that can contribute to increased blood alcohol levels (BAL) (Offsay, 2007). This diminished resistance, combined with age-related changes such as weakened manual dexterity, balance, and postural flexibility, can increase the likelihood of falls, burns, or other accidents (Wagenaar et al., 2001).

Some drinkers, as they get older, note changes in their response to alcohol, such as the occurrence of headaches, reduction in mental abilities with memory losses or lapses, and feelings of malaise rather than well-being. These problems start to occur at lower levels of consumption than was the case in earlier years. Older adults are likely to drink more frequently but in lesser quantities than younger individuals, who tend to drink larger amounts less often. Thus the possibility of alcohol abuse in cases of only moderate ingestion by older adults often is not recognized by the alcoholic's friends or family.

With aging, the body becomes less resilient; healing from injury or infection is slower, and stress is more likely to cause a loss of physiological equilibrium. As the proportion of fatty tissues to lean body mass increases with age, the individual's metabolic rate usually slows down, which increases the amount of time it takes the body to eliminate drugs (Wagenaar et al., 2001).

Alcohol and Medication

The interaction of drugs and alcohol in the older adult can have serious consequences. There is a decreased functioning of the liver enzymes that break down the alcohol, which on a short-term basis has the effect of prolonging the action of many medications, potentiating their effect. On the other hand, chronic ingestion of alcohol speeds up the metabolism of many drugs (Wagenaar et al., 2001).

Older individuals can expect to reach higher blood alcohol levels than younger people with an equivalent intake of alcohol. The effects of alcohol on the brain may be one reason that alcohol abuse sometimes mimics or exacerbates normal changes of aging, because even a moderate intake of alcohol can impair the cognition and coordination skills that are already decreased with age.

Extreme care is required when treating the older alcoholic with medication. Central nervous system toxicity from psychoactive drugs increases with aging. Ingestion of antidepressants or tranquilizers can be particularly harmful because their effect is further potentiated by alcohol. The toxicity of other drugs (e.g., acetaminophen) is enhanced by alcohol-associated malnutrition and reduced stores of detoxifying substances such as glutathione.

Alcohol consumption produces a change in sleep patterns, particularly in older adults. Unlike younger individuals, older adults take longer to fall asleep and do not sleep as restfully. Although alcohol may decrease the time it takes to fall asleep, this benefit is offset by frequent awakenings during the night caused by alcohol (Luggen, 2004).

Symptoms of Elder Dependence

Health practitioners need to be concerned with, and sensitive to, possible alcohol abuse among their older patients. Signs of alcohol abuse in younger individuals (e.g., alcohol-induced pancreatitis or liver disease, blackouts, major

trauma) occur infrequently in older adults. Instead, the older alcoholic displays vague geriatric syndromes of contusions, malnutrition, self-neglect, impaired cognition, sleep disturbances, depression, and falls (Offsay, 2007). Also present may be symptoms of diarrhea, urinary incontinence, a decrease in functional status, failure to thrive, and apparent dementia. Symptoms of poor coordination or visual changes may also mimic the normal aging process but actually be a result of excessive drinking. Although confusion and disorientation in an older patient are often associated with dementia or Alzheimer's disease, they could be caused by other factors, including alcohol abuse. Assessment of these conditions is necessary to differentiate the normal physiological changes of aging from those due to excessive drinking.

Whenever there is a suspicion or indication that an older adult is abusing alcohol, the health care provider should conduct a screening test. The CAGE-AID screening tool (see Box 16-5) or the MAST-G (Figure 25-3) is commonly used to assess alcohol problems (Menninger, 2004).

Treatment of the Older Adult Alcoholic

Because many older adults do not live in big families or have work-related contacts, they are less likely to be referred for treatment than are younger drinkers. Too often, by the time the older adult alcoholic comes to the notice of any treatment agencies, the patient's support systems and resources are severely decreased or depleted. Declining social, physical, and psychological performance is frequently found, which exacerbates the difficulties of loneliness, depression, monotony, accidents, social conflict, loss, and the physiological changes of aging (Wagenaar et al., 2001).

Ageism has deterred the development of treatment programs designed specially for the older adult. Beliefs that they are too isolated, too embedded in denial of their illness, and too old to function have been detrimental to encouraging health professionals to work with chemically dependent seniors. Another factor that may play a role is that older adults often try to hide alcohol dependence because they consider such abuse sinful or feel they can handle any problems themselves (Ebersole et al., 2004).

Treatment plans for the older problem drinker should emphasize social therapies. Older adult alcoholics tend to be more passive than younger alcoholics and may benefit from interpersonal involvement with professional health care personnel—many respond to emotional and social support. Family therapy should be encouraged. Group therapy with other middle-aged and older alcoholics as well as self-help groups like Alcoholics Anonymous can be effective.

Michigan Alcoholism Screening Testing—Geriatric Version (MAST-G)

Please answer yes or no to each question by marking the line next to the question. When you finish answering the questions, please add up how many "yes" responses you checked and put that number in the space provided at the end.

	Yes	No
1. After drinking have you ever noticed an increase in your heart rate or beating in your chest?	○	○
2. When talking to others, do you ever underestimate how much you actually drank?	○	○
3. Does alcohol make you sleepy so that you often fall asleep in your chair?	○	○
4. After a few drinks, have you sometimes not eaten or been able to skip a meal because you didn't feel hungry?	○	○
5. Does having a few drinks help you decrease your shakiness or tremors?	○	○
6. Does alcohol sometimes make it hard for you to remember parts of the day or night?	○	○
7. Do you have rules for yourself that you won't drink before a certain time of the day?	○	○
8. Have you lost interest in hobbies or activities you used to enjoy?	○	○
9. When you wake up in the morning, do you ever have trouble remembering part of the night before?	○	○
10. Does having a drink help you sleep?	○	○
11. Do you hide your alcohol bottles from family members?	○	○
12. After a social gathering, have you ever felt embarrassed because you drank too much?	○	○
13. Have you ever been concerned that drinking might be harmful to your health?	○	○
14. Do you like to end an evening with a nightcap?	○	○
15. Did you find your drinking increased after someone close to you died?	○	○
16. In general, would you prefer to have a few drinks at home rather than go out to social events?	○	○
17. Are you drinking more now than in the past?	○	○
18. Do you usually take a drink to relax or calm your nerves?	○	○
19. Do you drink to take your mind off your problems?	○	○
20. Have you ever increased your drinking after experiencing a loss in your life?	○	○
21. Do you sometimes drive when you have had too much to drink?	○	○
22. Has a doctor or nurse ever said they were worried or concerned about your drinking?	○	○
23. Have you ever made rules to manage your drinking?	○	○
24. When you feel lonely, does having a drink help?	○	○
TOTAL	_____	

Scoring: A score of 3 points or less is considered to indicate no alcoholism; a score of 4 points is suggestive of alcoholism; a score of 5 points or more indicates an alcohol problem.

Figure 25-3 ■ Michigan Alcoholism Screening Testing—Geriatric Version (MAST-G). (© The Regents of the University of Michigan, 1991.)

The prognosis for the geriatric problem drinker—a person who had lived to this point without recourse to alcohol and whose drinking is caused by losses and stress—is excellent. This individual often responds very positively to brief alcohol counseling or an alcoholic recovery program, especially if it is accompanied by environmental interventions. It is important that health care providers recognize this recovery potential. Proper education and awareness of a positive outcome for the geriatric problem drinker can increase the availability of resources; if the prognosis is good, providers and agencies should be more willing to spend resources on treatment.

For those elderly with long histories of alcohol use and who meet the criteria for alcohol abuse or dependence, a more rigorous treatment plan is required. This regimen needs to include detoxification, often in a 5-7 day inpatient unit (Offsay, 2007). Medications may also play a part in longer term treatment. Naltrexone has evidence-based efficacy and at 50 mg/day is thought to be safe for the elderly when used along with ongoing blood work for hepatic enzymes (Offsay, 2007).

Considering the magnitude of the problems and the likelihood that the number of older abusers will continue to increase, efforts need to be intensified to identify the causes of alcohol dependence and to develop appropriate interventions for treating it. If not, such dependence can overwhelm those charged with meeting the health and social service needs.

Substance Abuse

Illegal Drug Use

Currently the prevalence of illicit drug use among those 65 or older is low, about 1% (SAMHSA, 2006). However, there is real concern that this will change dramatically as baby boomers move into old age. Among older adults 50 to 59, the rate has increased from 2.7% to 4.4% between 2002 and 2005 (SAMHSA, 2006). It is estimated that the number of older adults (aged 50 or older) in need of substance abuse support will increase from 1.7 million in 2000 and 2001 to about 4.4 million in 2020 (Gfroerer et al., 2003). Treatment need is defined as *DSM-IV-TR* alcohol or illicit drug use in the past year. The sheer numbers of aging baby boomers threaten to overwhelm treatment resources. Today most substance abuse treatment is geared to the young abuser; major changes will need to occur to manage a large number of older adult abusers.

Prescription and Over-the-Counter Drug Use and Abuse

Because older adult patients use both prescription and over-the-counter drugs at a higher rate than the general population, it is difficult to accurately estimate the extent to which these drugs are abused or misused. The high exposure to medications coupled with age-related physiological changes, including decreased metabolism, increased accumulation, and, in the case of long-acting benzodiazepines and anticholinergics, increased sensitivity, raises the likelihood of medication-related adverse events such as increased sedation, delirium, confusion, and falls, resulting in hip fractures (Patterson et al., 1999). To compound the problem, often the older adult will abuse two or more drugs (polypharmacy, polydrug use), increasing the likelihood of medical or physical complications.

ACQUIRED IMMUNODEFICIENCY SYNDROME AND AIDS-RELATED DEMENTIA

Dementia is often a sequela in people with human immunodeficiency virus (HIV) infection, and AIDS is rising faster among the older population than among those 24 years old and younger (Goodroad, 2003). AIDS-related dementia often has a rapid onset and is often mistaken for symptoms of depression.

Butler and Lewis (2002) indicate that 10% of people older than age 50 have active AIDS; one fourth of those are older than 60 years and 4% are older than 70 years. Blood transfusions are no longer the main cause for the spread of AIDS in the older adult. Research shows that elders are sexually active and thus at risk for HIV and AIDS because of failure to practice safe sex; those who received blood transfusions before 1985 are also at risk. In addition, diagnosis and treatment of HIV and AIDS in the older adult are delayed because health care providers believe that this population is not sexually active. In general, lack of adequate knowledge about HIV and AIDS among older adults, coupled with denial that this illness occurs in their generation, increases their risk for HIV infection and AIDS.

Older women who are sexually active are at higher risk for HIV and AIDS from an infected partner than are older men. Changes in vaginal tissue caused by the aging process can lead to tears in the vaginal mucosa during intercourse that allows HIV to penetrate. In addition because pregnancy is no longer a threat, use of condoms in this age-group is uncommon. This puts the older woman at greater risk of exposure (Hess, 2004).

Dementia caused by AIDS and that caused by Alzheimer's disease can be easily confused. Therefore a careful assessment and workup are required. Health care providers must be aware that AIDS can occur in the older adult. Because AIDS-related dementia has such a rapid onset and may mimic symptoms of Alzheimer's disease (confusion, forgetfulness, leg tremors, progressive weakness, apathy, fatigue, weight loss, and neurological abnormalities), a thorough workup should be conducted (Hess, 2004). See Chapter 15 for a comprehensive discussion of Alzheimer's disease.

Generally, health care providers have directed their educational efforts in HIV prevention toward the younger age-group. The potential for exposure to HIV exists among sexually active older adults; therefore educational programs need to address prevention strategies for both the older adult and health care providers.

LEGAL AND ETHICAL ISSUES THAT AFFECT THE MENTAL HEALTH OF OLDER ADULTS

Many subjects might be included here. Among the most important for practicing nurses in any setting to be familiar with are the following:

1. Use of restraints
2. Decision making about health care

Elder abuse, another serious problem for the older adult, is addressed in Chapter 18.

USE OF RESTRAINTS

The use of restraints is an ethical, legal, and safety concern. Restraints can be both physical and chemical. **Physical restraints** are any manual methods or mechanical devices, materials, or equipment that inhibit free movement. Examples include tightening a bedsheet to limit movement; side rails; Posey belt; leg, arm, and mitt restraints; or wheelchairs positioned against the wall restricting movement. Wrist bands or devices on clothing that trigger an alarm to notify staff that an older adult is leaving a room or an area should **not** be considered restraints. **Chemical restraints** are drugs given for the very specific purpose of inhibiting a certain behavior or movement.

Physical Restraints

Whether health care providers have the right to restrain another individual physically has always been a question. Being physically restrained can be a humiliating and demoralizing experience. Older adults have responded to such action with anger, fear, anxiety, depression, and stress-related syndromes (Meiner & Miceli, 2000). Surveys undertaken by the state and federal authorities in the United States between the 1970s and 1980s revealed levels of physical restraint use as high as 75% in some facilities and levels

of psychotropic drug use as high as 90% (Marchello, 2003). Physical restraints have traditionally been used with hospitalized confused patients primarily to prevent disruption of medical therapies and to prevent falls. Paradoxically, they are perceived as a form of physical and psychological abuse by the patient and often the family.

In addition to the risk of falls, physical restraints pose a risk of death through strangulation or asphyxiation (Dharmarajan & Norman, 2003). Side effects directly related to the use of restraints include incontinence, increased agitation, weak muscles, pressure sores, loss of mobility, and increased illness to name a few (CANHR, 2004). The current standard of care is to maintain a restraint-fee policy (Park et al., 2005).

More and more facilities are using electronic sensing systems to alert staff if a resident is about to stand up or try to get out of a bed or wheelchair. Restraints should never be used as a means of controlling behavior or as a punishment. Physical restraints should be used for emergency purposes only when there is a threat to the safety of the resident or others. Physical restraints are used as a last resort and other methods used to calm the resident and prevent harm have been used and documented.

Residents in restraint-free facilities have experienced fewer injuries from falls than those in facilities using restraints. A study by Neufield and colleagues (1999) found that serious injuries declined significantly when restraint orders were discontinued. The researchers concluded that restraint-free care is safe when a comprehensive assessment is performed and alternatives to restraints are used.

The **Omnibus Budget Reconciliation Act (OBRA)** of 1990 declares that each nursing home resident has the right to be free from unnecessary drugs and physical restraints. In addition, each resident must be provided with treatment to reduce dependency on chemical and physical intervention (Hogstel & Weeks, 2000). The Nursing Home Reform Amendment in OBRA details the regulatory framework governing the use of restraints in all states (Marchello, 2003).

The Joint Commission (TJC) developed recommendations on the use of physical restraints (JCAHO, 1999). Derived from OBRA regulations, TJC guidelines for physical restraints include the following:

1. A physician's order must be obtained.
2. Restraint application must be time limited.
3. Attempts at alternative approaches must be documented.
4. Ongoing observation and assessment of the patient must be documented.
5. Care interventions (e.g., provision of food and fluids, toileting, help with activities of daily living, and response to attempted release) must be documented.

Nurses can avoid liability by knowing the law, knowing the laws of their state, adhering to the policies and procedures of the institution at which they work, and using good nursing judgment. All nursing homes and hospitals should have written restraint procedures and policies available to all health care providers. If restraints are used, the nurse is responsible for the patient's safety. The patient should be restrained only for a minimal time and for a valid purpose. Use of restraints does not enhance patient care. Creative nursing skills and interventions are frequently more beneficial.

Chemical Restraints

Drugs considered to be chemical restraints include antipsychotics, antianxiety drugs, minor tranquilizers, sedatives, hypnotics, and antidepressants (Ebersole et al., 2004). The National Citizens' Coalition for Nursing Home Reform (1991) wrote guidelines for the use of antipsychotic drugs in certain circumstances. For example, when a person with a cognitive disorder or dementia (with associated psychotic or agitated features) presents a danger to self or to others, and when psychotic symptoms cause the nursing home resident "frightful distress," the use of these drugs is considered medically appropriate and necessary. It is important for nurses to be aware that using chemical restraints increases the risk of falls.

CONTROL OF THE DECISION-MAKING PROCESS
Patient Self-Determination Act

Since the 1960s, the public's desire to participate in decision making about health care has increased. This interest in patient advocacy was recognized when Congress passed the **Patient Self-Determination Act (PSDA)** in 1990, requiring that health care facilities provide clear written information for every patient regarding his or her legal rights to make health care decisions, including the right to accept or refuse treatment. It also establishes the right of a person to provide directions for clinicians to follow in the event of a serious illness. Increasing numbers of older adults are creating written directives.

An **advance directive** is a term used to describe living wills, durable powers of attorney for health care, and health care surrogate appointments (Ebersole et al., 2004). Health care institutions that receive federal funds are required to provide to each patient at the time of admission written information regarding his or her right to execute advance directives and are required to inquire if such directives have been made by the patient. The patient's admission records should state whether such directives exist. The ANA (1992) recommends that specific questions be part of every nurse's admission assessment. Box 25-3 reproduces these questions and describes the responsibilities of health care workers under the PSDA.

Such a directive indicates preferences for the types of medical care or amount of treatment desired. The directive comes into effect should physical or mental incapacitation prevent the patient from making health care decisions. These wishes can be communicated through one or more of the following: (1) a living will, (2) a directive to physician, and (3) a durable power of attorney for health care. These documents must be in writing and the patient's signature must be witnessed; depending on state and institutional provisions, notarization may be required.

Living Will
A **living will** is a personal statement of how and where one wishes to die (Ebersole et al., 2004). It is activated only when the person is terminally ill and incapacitated. A competent patient may alter a living will at any time. The question of whether an incompetent person can change a living will is addressed on a state-by-state basis. Executing a living will does not always guarantee its application.

Directive to Physician
In a **directive to physician**, a physician is appointed by the individual to serve as proxy. Many of the features of a directive to physician parallel those of a living will, such as activation only when a terminal illness is present, need for verification of the terminal illness by the physician, and requirement for patient competency at the time of signing. The directive to physician designating the physician as surrogate can be particularly useful in cases of terminal illness when an individual has no family. The physician must agree in writing to be the patient's agent and must be one of the two physicians who made the original determination that the patient is terminally ill. Unlike the living will, the directive to physician can be revoked orally at any time without regard to patient competency.

Durable Power of Attorney for Health Care
The **durable power of attorney for health care** differs from living wills and directives to physicians in that a person other than a physician is appointed to act as the patient's agent. The patient must be competent and of age when making the appointment and must be competent in order to revoke the power. Individuals do not have to be terminally ill or incompetent to allow the empowered individual to act on their behalf. No physician's certification is required.

BOX 25-3

Nurses' Responsibilities and the Patient Self-Determination Act (1990)

Part of Nursing Admission Assessment

- Nurses should know the laws of the state in which [they] practice and should be familiar with the strengths and limitations of the various forms of advance directive.
- The ANA recommends that the following questions be part of the nursing admission assessment:
  1. Do you have basic information about advance directives, including living wills and durable power of attorney?
  2. Do you wish to initiate an advance directive?
  3. If you have already prepared an advance directive, can you provide it now?
  4. Have you discussed your end-of-life choices with your family or designated surrogate and health care workers?

Responsibilities of Health Care Workers Under the Patient Self-Determination Act of 1990

- Hospitals, skilled nursing facilities, home health agencies, hospice organizations, and health maintenance

organizations serving Medicare and Medicaid patients must:

1. Maintain written policies and procedures for providing information to their patients for whom they provide care.
2. Give written material to patients concerning their rights under state law to make decisions about medical care, including the right to accept or refuse surgical or medical care and to formulate advance directives and provide written policies and procedures for the realization of these rights.
3. Document in patients' records whether they have advance directives.
4. Not discriminate in care or in other ways against patients who have or have not prepared advance directives.
5. Make sure that policies are in place to ensure compliance with state laws governing advance directives.

Data from Schlossberg, C., & Hart, M.A. (1992). Legal perspectives. In M.M. Burke & M.B. Walsh (Eds.), *Gerontologic nursing: Care of the frail elderly* (p. 469). St. Louis: Mosby; and American Nurses Association. (1992). *Position statement: Nursing and the patient self-determination act.* Washington, DC: Author.

Nursing Role in the Decision-Making Process

The nurse explains the ethics and legal policies of the institution to both the patient and family and helps them understand the concepts behind advance directives. The nurse explains that the family need not feel morally obligated to provide for all possible medical care when such care will only extend the suffering of a loved one. This is especially true when such extraordinary measures do not represent the person's values and beliefs. The nurse serves as an advocate and a knowledgeable resource person for the older adult patient and family. The patient is encouraged to verbalize his or her feelings and thoughts during this sensitive time of decision making. In addition, nurses are responsible for being knowledgeable about the state regulations on advance directives as well as the potential obstacles in completing the directives for the state in which they practice. Maintaining an open and continuing dialogue among patient, family, nurse, and physician is of principal importance. The nurse supports any surrogates appointed to act on the patient's behalf and seeks consultation for ethical issues the nurse feels unprepared to handle.

Every health care facility receiving federal funds is required to have written policies, procedures, and protocols in compliance with the PSDA. Nurses must prepare themselves to deal with the legal, ethical, and moral issues involved when counseling about advance directives. The law does not specify who should talk with patients about treatment decisions, but in many facilities nurses are being asked to discuss this issue with the patient. If the advance directive of a patient is not being followed, the nurse intervenes on the patient's behalf. If the problem cannot be resolved with the physician, the facility's protocol providing for notification of the appropriate supervisor is followed.

Although nurses, especially in nursing homes, may discuss options with their patients, they may not assist patients in writing advance directives because this is considered a conflict of interest. The existence of an advance directive serves as a guide to health care providers in advocating for the older adult patient's rightful wishes in this process.

KEY POINTS TO REMEMBER

- The older adult population continues to increase exponentially.
- The increase in the number of older adults poses a challenge not only to nurses but also the entire health care system to be prepared to respond to the special needs of this population.
- Attitudes toward the older adult are often negative, reflecting ageism Posey belt a bias based solely on age.
- Ageism is found at all levels of society and even among health care providers, which affects the way we render care to our older adult patients.
- Nurses who care for older adults in various settings may function at different levels. All should be knowledgeable about the process of aging and be cognizant of the differences between normal and abnormal aging changes.

- Older adults face increasing problems of alcoholism, abuse and misuse of prescription and over-the-counter drugs, and suicide.
- OBRA established guidelines and a philosophy of care that call for patients to be free from unnecessary use of drugs and physical restraints.
- Nurses working with the mentally ill patient must know psychotherapeutic approaches relevant for older adults, such as remotivation and reminiscence therapy. Nurse clinicians may offer psychotherapy groups geared toward the special needs of this population.
- When it comes to dying and death, older adults' wishes and those of their families are frequently ignored. The implementation of the PSDA, passed in 1990, can afford some patients autonomy and dignity in death.

CRITICAL THINKING

1. Mr. Lopez is 70 years old and has been admitted to the intensive care unit with a diagnosis of alcohol withdrawal delirium. He is confused and combative, and threatens to strike the nurse who is trying to render care to him unless he is allowed to leave. The nurse applies wrist restraints to keep Mr. Lopez from striking her and leaving the room. What are the mandates of OBRA (1990) regarding the use of restraints?

2. Mr. Lopez has received treatment for alcohol withdrawal. He appears very quiet, refuses to eat, does not sleep at night,

admits to thoughts of desperation, and wishes he could die. He also confides that he attempted suicide when his wife died 5 years earlier and at that time he started drinking heavily. Which is the appropriate depression assessment tool to use in assessing the severity of Mr. Lopez's condition? Explain your answer.

   A. Michigan Alcoholism Screening Test
   B. Geriatric Depression Scale
   C. Mini-Mental State Examination
   D. Patient Self-Determination Act

CHAPTER REVIEW

Choose the most appropriate answer.

1. For conducting a comprehensive nursing assessment of an older adult patient, which of the following would provide the broadest perspective from which to understand his needs? The nurse's knowledge of:
   1. the normal aging process.
   2. drug interactions.
   3. chronic diseases that affect older adults.
   4. community supports specific to the patient.
2. Which of the following psychiatric disorders is found most frequently among older adults?
   1. Depression
   2. Dementia
   3. Anxiety
   4. Social phobia
3. Which statement regarding the use of restraints is true?
   1. Restraint-free care appreciably diminishes the overall safety of any older adult patient compared with the use of physical or chemical restraints.
   2. The nurse is responsible for patient safety during the time the patient is restrained.
   3. Chemical restraint presents less potential for patient harm than physical restraint.

   4. Restraint may be used to prevent extubation if a nursing protocol exists.
4. Which of the following health problems of older adults is increasing faster than any other?
   1. Suicide
   2. Cancer
   3. Alzheimer's disease
   4. Substance abuse and dependence
5. In carrying out patients' wishes and directives as a nurse, which of the following is an unethical action for the nurse?
   1. Ignoring a "Do not resuscitate" order for an older adult patient in the intensive care unit
   2. Implementing a physician's order to withhold artificial hydration from an older adult patient in irreversible coma
   3. Adhering to the choices made for an older adult patient by the individual with durable power of attorney for health care
   4. Advocating for an older adult patient in the terminal stage of cancer who wishes to discontinue chemotherapy

REFERENCES

American Nurses Association (ANA). (1992). Position statement on nursing and the patient self-determination act. Washington, DC: Author.

Andersen, U.A., Andersen, M., Rosholm, J.U., et al. (2000). Contacts to the health care system prior to suicide: A comprehensive analysis using registers for general and psychiatric hospital admissions, contacts to general practitioners and practising specialists, and drug prescriptions. *Acta Psychiatrica Scandinavia, 102*(2), 126-134.

Bartels, S.J., & Drake, R.E. (2005). Evidence-based geriatric psychiatry: An overview. *Psychiatric Clinics of North America, 28*(4), 763-784.

Butler, R., & Lewis, M. (2002). *The new love and sex after 60.* New York: Ballantine.

California Advocates for Nursing Home Reform (CANHR) (2004). Restraint-free care. Retrieved February 19, 2008, at www.canhr.org/factsheets/fs_RestraintFreeCare.htm.

Charney, D.S., Reynolds, C.F., Lewis, L., et al. (2003).Depression and bipolar support alliance consensus statement on the unmet needs in diagnosis and treatment of mood disorders in late life. *Archives of General Psychiatry, 60*(7), 664-672.

Cole, M.G. (2005). Evidence-based review of risk factors for geriatric depression and brief preventive interventions. *Psychiatric Clinics of North America, 28*(4), 785-803.

Colliver, J.D., Compton, W.M., Gfroerer, J.C., et al (2006). Projecting drug use among aging baby boomers in 2020. *Annals of Epidemiology, 16*(4), 257-265.

Dharmarajan, T.S., & Norman, R.A. (Eds.). (2003). *Clinical geriatrics.* New York: Parthenon.

Doddi, S.R. (2003). Depression in older adults. In T.S. Dharmarajan & R.A. Norman (Eds.), *Clinical geriatrics.* New York: Parthenon.

Ebersole, P., Hess, P., & Luggen A. (2004). *Toward healthy aging: Human needs and nursing response* (6th ed.). St. Louis: Mosby.

Gfroerer, J., Penne, M., Pemberton, M., & Folsom, R. (2003). Substance abuse treatment need among older adults in 2020: The impact of the aging baby-boom cohort. *Drug and Alcohol Dependence, 69*, 127-135.

Goodroad, B.K. (2003). HIV and AIDS in people older than 50: A continuing concern. *Journal of Gerontological Nursing, 29*(4), 18-24.

Gurvich, T., & Cunningham, J.A. (2000). Appropriate use of psychotropic drugs in nursing homes. *American Family Physician, 61*, 1437-1446.

Henderson, J.N. (2003). Aging and public health. In T.S. Dharmarajan & R.A. Norman (Eds.), *Clinical geriatrics.* New York: Parthenon.

Hess, P. (2004). Intimacy, sexuality, and aging. In P. Ebersole, P. Hess, & A.S. Luggen (Eds.), *Toward healthy aging: Human needs and nursing response.* St. Louis: Mosby.

Hogstel, M.O., & Weeks, S.M. (2000). Mental health. In A.G. Lueckenotte (Ed.), *Gerontologic nursing* (2nd ed.). St. Louis: Mosby.

Hooyman, N. (2003). Todd Nelson: Ageism: Stereotyping and prejudice against older persons.—ed—book review [Review of the book *Ageism: Stereotyping and Prejudice Against Older Persons*]. *Journal of Sociology and Social Welfare, 30*(2), 18.

Ingram, T.N. (2001). Risk for violence: Self-directed or directed at others. In M. Maas, K.C. Buckwalter, and M. Hardy, et al. (Eds.), *Nursing care of older adults: Diagnoses, outcomes, and interventions.* St. Louis: Mosby.

Joint Commission on Accreditation of Healthcare Organizations (JCAHO). (1999). *Standards for behavioral health care.* Oakbrook, IL: Author.

Lueckenotte, A.G. (2000). Gerontologic assessment. In A.G. Lueckenotte (Ed.), *Gerontologic nursing* (2nd ed.). St. Louis: Mosby.

Luggen, A.S. (2004). Mental wellness and disturbances. In P. Ebersole, P. Hess, & A.S. Luggen (Eds.), *Toward healthy aging: Human needs and nursing response.* St. Louis: Mosby.

Mackin, R.S., & Areán, P.A. (2005). Evidence-based psychotherapeutic interventions for geriatric depression. *Psychiatric Clinics of North America, 28*(4), 805-820.

Marchello, V. (2003). Long-term care. In T.S. Dharmarajan & R.A. Norman (Eds.), *Clinical geriatrics.* New York: Parthenon.

McAndrews, M.M. (2001). Lighting the darkness. *Advance for Long-Term Care Management, 4*(5), 40.

Meiner, S.E., & Gray-Miceli, D. (2000). Safety. In A.G. Lueckenotte (Ed.), *Gerontologic nursing* (2nd ed.). St. Louis: Mosby.

Menninger, J.A. (2002). Assessment and treatment of alcoholism and substance-related disorders in the elderly. *Bulletin of the Menninger Clinic, 66*(2), 166-183.

Miller, C. (2004). *Nursing for wellness in older adults: Theory and practice* (4th ed.). Philadelphia: Lippincott Williams & Wilkins.

Moscicki, E.K., & Caine, E.D. (2004). Opportunities of life: Preventing suicide in elderly patients. *Archives of Internal Medicine, 164*, 1171-1172.

Narang, A.T., & Sikka, R. (2006). Resuscitation of the elderly. *Emergency Medicine Clinics of North America, 24*(2), 261-272.

National Center for Injury Prevention and Control. (2003). *Suicide: Fact sheet.* Retrieved April 6, 2005, from www.cdc.gov/ncipc/factsheets/suifacts.htm.

National Citizens' Coalition for Nursing Home Reform. (1991). *Nursing home reform law: The basics.* Washington, DC: Author.

National Institute of Mental Health (NIMH). (2004). *Older adults: Depression and suicide facts.* Washington, DC: Author. Retrieved March 21, 2005, from www.nimh.nih.gov/publicat/elderlydepsuicide.cfm.

Nelson, T.D. (2002). *Ageism: Stereotyping and prejudice against older persons.* Cambridge, MA: MIT Press.

Neufeld, R.R., Libow, L.S., Foley, W.J., et al. (1999). Restraint reduction reduces serious injuries among nursing home residents. *Journal of the American Geriatrics Society, 47*, 1202-1207.

Offsay, J. (2007). Treatment of alcohol-related problems in the elderly. *Annals of Long-Term Care, 15*(7), 39-44.

Oslin, D.W. (2005). Evidence-based treatment of geriatric substance abuse. *Psychiatric Clinics of North America, 28*(4), 897-911.

Park, M., Hsiao-Chen Tang, J., & Ledford, L. (2005). *Changing the practice of physical restraint use in acute care.* Iowa City, IA: University of Iowa Gerontological Nursing Interventions Research Center, Research Translation and Dissemination Core.

Patterson, T.L., Lacro, J.P., & Jeste, D.V. (1999). Abuse and misuse of medications in the elderly. *Psychiatric Times, 16*(4), 54-57.

Piechniczek-Buczek, J. (2006). Psychiatric emergencies in the elderly population. *Emergency Medicine Clinics of North America, 24*(2), 467-490.

Reuben, D.B., Roth, C., Kamberg, C., et al. (2003). Restructuring primary care practices to manage geriatric syndromes: The ACOVE-2 intervention. *Journal of the American Geriatrics Society, 51*(12), 1787-1793.

Richards, J.B., Papaioannou, A., Adachi, J.D., et al. (2007). Effect of selective serotonin reuptake inhibitors on the risk of fracture. *Archives of Internal Medicine, 167*(2), 188-194.

Rigler, S.K. (2000). Alcoholism in the elderly. *American Family Physician, 61,* 1710-1716.

Salisbury, S. (1999). Alcoholism. In J. Stone , J. Wyman, S. Salisbury, *Clinical gerontological nursing.* Philadelphia: Saunders.

Schatzberg, A.F., & Nemeroff, C.B. (2004). *Textbook of psychopharmacology* (3rd ed.). Washington, DC: American Psychiatric Publishing.

Sheikh, J.I, & Yesavage, J.A. (1986). Geriatric Depression Scale (GDS): Recent evidence and development of a shorter version. In T.L. Brink (Ed.), *Clinical gerontology: A guide to assessment and intervention.* New York: Haworth Press.

Substance Abuse and Mental Health Service Administration (SAMHSA). (2006). Results from the 2005 National Survey on Drug Use and Health: National findings (Office of Applied Studies, NSDUH Services ^-30, D1-1 1-15 publication No SMAAA 06-4194). Rockville, Md.

Szanto, K., Prigerson, H.G., & Reynolds, C.F. (2001). Suicide in the elderly. *Clinical Neuroscience Research, 1*(5), 366-376.

Wagenaar, D.B., Mickus, M.A., & Wilson, J. (2001). Alcoholism in late life: Challenges and complexities. *Psychiatric Annals, 31*(11), 665-672.

Williams, K., Kemper, S., & Hummert, M.L. (2003). Improving nursing home communication: An intervention to reduce elderspeak. *The Gerontologist, 43,* 242-247.

Caring for Patients Within the Context of the Mental Health Care System

CHAPTER 26

Legal and Ethical Basis
for Practice

Penny Simpson Brooke

Key Terms and Concepts

Objectives

1. Compare and contrast the different admissions procedures including admission criteria.
2. Summarize patients' rights as they pertain to the patient's (a) right to treatment, (b) right to refuse treatment, and (c) right to informed consent.
3. Delineate the steps nurses are advised to take if they suspect negligence or illegal activity on the part of a professional colleague or peer.
4. Discuss the legal considerations of patient privilege (a) after a patient has died, (b) if the patient tests positive for human immunodeficiency virus, or (c) if the patient's employer states a "need to know."
5. Summarize situations in which health care professionals have a duty to break patient confidentiality.
6. Discuss a patient's civil rights and how they pertain to restraint and seclusion.
7. Discuss in detail the balance between the patient's rights and the rights of society with respect to the following legal concepts relevant in nursing and psychiatric nursing: (a) duty to intervene, (b) documentation and charting, and (c) confidentiality.

continued

evolve

For additional resources related to the content of this chapter, visit the Evolve website at
http://evolve.elsevier.com/Varcarolis/essentials.

- Chapter Outline
- Chapter Review Answers

- Concept Map Creator

This chapter introduces you to current legal and ethical issues that may be encountered in the practice of psychiatric nursing. A fundamental goal of psychiatric care is to strike a balance between the rights of the individual patient and the rights of society at large. This chapter is designed to assist you in understanding the implications of ethical or legal issues on the provision of care in a psychiatric setting.

An **ethical dilemma** results when there is a conflict between two or more courses of action, each carrying with them favorable and unfavorable consequences. How we respond to these dilemmas is based partly on our own morals (beliefs of right or wrong) and values. Suppose you are caring for a pregnant woman with schizophrenia who wants to carry the baby to term, but whose family insists she get an abortion. In order to promote fetal safety, her antipsychotic medication will need to be reduced, putting her at risk of exacerbation of the illness. Furthermore, there is a question as to whether she can safely care for the child. If you relied on the ethical principle of autonomy, you may conclude that she has the right to decide. Would other ethical principles be in conflict with autonomy in this case?

At times your values may be in conflict with the value system of the institution. This situation further complicates the decision-making process and necessitates careful consideration of the patient's desires. For example, you may experience a conflict in a setting where older adult patients are routinely tranquilized to a degree with which you don't feel comfortable. Whenever one's value system is challenged, increased stress results.

LEGAL AND ETHICAL CONCEPTS

Ethics is the study of philosophical beliefs about what is considered right or wrong in a society. **Bioethics** is a more specific term that refers to the ethical questions that arise in health care. The five basic principles of bioethics are as follows:

1. **Beneficence**: the duty to act so as to benefit or promote the good of others. Spending extra time to help calm an extremely anxious patient is a beneficent act.
2. **Autonomy**: respecting the rights of others to make their own decisions. Acknowledging the patient's right to refuse medication is an example of promoting autonomy.
3. **Justice**: the duty to distribute resources or care equally, regardless of personal attributes. An example of justice is when an intensive care unit (ICU) nurse devotes equal attention to someone who has attempted suicide as to someone who suffered a brain aneuryism.
4. **Fidelity** (nonmaleficence): maintaining loyalty and commitment to the patient and doing no wrong to the patient. Maintaining expertise in nursing skill through nursing education demonstrates fidelity to patient care.
5. **Veracity**: one's duty to communicate truthfully. Describing the purpose and side effects of psychotropic medications in a truthful and nonmisleading way is an example of veracity.

Law and ethics are closely related because law tends to reflect the ethical values of society. It should be noted that although you may feel obligated to follow ethical guidelines, these guidelines should not override laws. For example, if you are aware of a statute or a specific rule or regulation created by the state board of nursing that prohibits a certain action (e.g., restraining patients against their will) and you feel you have an ethical obligation to protect the patient by engaging in such an action (e.g., using restraints), you would be wise to follow the law.

MENTAL HEALTH LAWS

Laws have been enacted to regulate the care and treatment of the mentally ill. Mental health laws, or statutes, vary from state to state; in order to understand the legal climate of your specific state, you are encouraged to review its code. This can be accomplished by visiting the webpage of your state mental health department or by doing an Internet search using the following keywords "mental + health + statutes + (your state)."

Many of these laws have undergone major revision since 1963, which reflects a shift in emphasis from state or institutional care of the mentally ill to community-based care. This was heralded by the enactment of the Community Mental Health Center Act of 1963 under President John F. Kennedy. Along with this shift in emphasis has come the more widespread use of psychotropic drugs in the treatment of mental illness—which has enabled many people to integrate more readily into the larger community—and an increasing awareness of the need to provide the mentally ill with humane care that respects their civil rights.

Civil Rights

People with mental illness are guaranteed the same rights under federal and state laws as any other citizen. Most states specifically prohibit any person from depriving an individual receiving mental health services of his or her **civil rights**, including the right to vote; the right to civil service ranking; the rights related to granting, forfeit, or denial of a driver's license; the right to make purchases and to enter contractual relationships (unless the patient has lost legal capacity by being incompetent), and the right to press charges against another person. The psychiatric patient's rights include the right to humane care and treatment. The medical, dental, and psychiatric needs of the patient must be met in accordance with the prevailing standards accepted in these professions. The mentally ill in prisons and jails are afforded the same protections. The right to religious freedom and practice, the right to social interaction, and the right to exercise and recreational opportunities are also protected.

ADMISSION AND DISCHARGE PROCEDURES
Due Process in Civil Commitment

The courts have recognized that involuntary civil commitment to a mental hospital is a "massive curtailment of liberty" (*Humphrey v. Cady,* 1972) requiring due process protections in the civil commitment procedure. This right derives from the Fifth Amendment of the U.S. Constitution, which states that "no person shall . . . be deprived of life, liberty, or property without due process of law." The Fourteenth Amendment explicitly prohibits states from depriving citizens of life, liberty, and property without due process of law. State civil commitment statutes, if challenged in the courts on constitutional grounds, must afford minimal due process protections to pass the court's scrutiny (*Zinernon v. Burch,* 1990). In most states, a patient can challenge commitments through a **writ of habeas corpus**, which means a "formal written order" to "free the person." The writ of habeas corpus is the procedural mechanism used to challenge unlawful detention by the government.

The writ of habeas corpus and the **least restrictive alternative doctrine** are two of the most important concepts applicable to civic commitment cases. The least restrictive alternative doctrine mandates that the least drastic means be taken to achieve a specific purpose. For example, if someone can safely be treated for depression on an outpatient basis, hospitalization would be too restrictive and unnecessarily disruptive.

Admission to the Hospital

All students are encouraged to become familiar with the important provisions of the laws in their own states regarding admissions, discharges, patient's rights, and informed consent.

A medical standard or justification for admission should exist. A well-defined psychiatric problem must be established, based on current illness classifications in the *Diagnostic and Statistical Manual of Mental Disorders (DSM-IV-TR)* (APA, 2000). The presenting illness should also be of such a nature that it causes an immediate crisis situation or that other less restrictive alternatives are inadequate or unavailable. There should also be a reasonable expectation that the hospitalization and treatment will improve the presenting problems.

Voluntary Admission
Generally, **voluntary admission** is sought by the patient or the patient's guardian through a written application to the facility. Voluntarily admitted patients have the right to demand and obtain release. However, few states require voluntarily admitted patients to be notified of the rights associated with their status. In addition, many states require that a patient submit a written release notice to the facility staff, who reevaluate the patient's condition for possible conversion to involuntary status according to criteria established by state law.

Involuntary Admission (Commitment)
Involuntary admission is made without the patient's consent. Generally, involuntary admission is necessary when a person is in need of psychiatric treatment, presents a danger to self or others, or is unable to meet his or her own basic needs. Involuntary commitment requires that the patient retain freedom from unreasonable bodily restraints,

the right to informed consent, and the right to refuse medications, including psychotropic or antipsychotic medications.

Three different commitment procedures are commonly available: **judicial determination, administrative determination,** and **agency determination.** In addition, a specified number of physicians must certify that a person's mental health status justifies detention and treatment. Involuntary hospitalization can be further categorized by the nature and purpose of the involuntary admission. It may be emergency, observational or temporary, or long-term or formal commitment, or outpatient commitment.

Emergency Involuntary Hospitalization

Most states provide for emergency involuntary hospitalization or civil **commitment** for a specified period (1 to 10 days on average) to prevent dangerous behavior that is likely to cause harm to self or others. Police officers, physicians, and mental health professionals may be designated by law to authorize the detention of mentally ill individuals who are a danger to themselves or others.

Observational or Temporary Involuntary Hospitalization

Civil commitment for observational or temporary involuntary hospitalization is of longer duration than emergency hospitalization. The primary purpose of this type of hospitalization is observation, diagnosis, and treatment for those who have mental illness or pose a danger to themselves or others. The length of time and procedures vary markedly from state to state. A guardian, family member, physician, or other public health officer may apply for this type of admission. Certification by two or more physicians, a judicial review, or administrative review and order is often required for involuntary admission.

Long-Term or Formal Commitment

Long-term commitment for involuntary hospitalization has as its primary purpose extended care and treatment of the mentally ill. Those who undergo extended involuntary hospitalization are committed through medical certification, judicial, or administrative action. Some states do not require a judicial hearing before commitment, but often provide the patient with an opportunity for a judicial review after commitment procedures. This type of involuntary hospitalization generally lasts 60 to 180 days, but may be for an indeterminate period.

Involuntary Outpatient Commitment

Beginning in the 1990s, states began to pass legislation that permitted outpatient commitment as an alternative to forced inpatient treatment. Recently states are using **involuntary outpatient commitment** as a preventive measure,

allowing a court order before the onset of a psychiatric crisis that would result in an inpatient commitment. The order for involuntary outpatient commitment is usually tied to receipt of goods and services provided by social welfare agencies, including disability benefits and housing. To access these goods and services the patient is mandated to participate in treatment and may face inpatient admission if he or she fails to participate in treatment (Chan, 2003; Monahan et al., 2003; Rainey, 2001). Forced treatment raises ethical dilemmas regarding autonomy versus paternalism, privacy rights, duty to protect, and right to treatment, and has been challenged on constitutional grounds.

Discharge from the Hospital

Release from hospitalization depends on the patient's admission status. Patients who sought informal or voluntary admission, as previously discussed, have the right to request and receive release. Some states, however, do provide for conditional release of voluntary patients, which enables the treating physician or administrator to order continued treatment on an outpatient basis if the clinical needs of the patient warrant further care.

Conditional Release

Conditional release usually requires outpatient treatment for a specified period to determine the patient's adherence with medication protocols, ability to meet basic needs, and ability to reintegrate into the community. Generally a voluntarily hospitalized patient who is conditionally released can only be committed through the usual methods for involuntary hospitalization. However, an involuntarily hospitalized patient who is conditionally released may be reinstitutionalized while the commitment is still in effect without recommencement of formal admission procedures.

Unconditional Release

Unconditional release, or **discharge**, is the termination of a patient-institution relationship. This release may be court ordered or administratively ordered by the institution's officials. Generally, the administrative officer of an institution has the discretion to discharge patients.

Release Against Medical Advice (AMA)

In some cases there is a disagreement between mental health care providers and patients as to whether continued hospitalization is necessary. When treatment seems beneficial, but there is no compelling reason (e.g., danger to self or others) to seek an involuntary continuance of stay, patients may be released against medical advice.

PATIENTS' RIGHTS UNDER THE LAW

Psychiatric facilities usually provide patients with a written list of basic patient rights. These rights are derived from a variety of sources, especially legislation that came out of the 1960s. Since then, they have been modified to some degree, but most lists share commonalities in the following text.

Right to Treatment

With the enactment of the Hospitalization of the Mentally Ill Act in 1964, the federal statutory right to psychiatric treatment in public hospitals was created. The statute requires that medical and psychiatric care and treatment be provided to everyone admitted to a public hospital.

Although state courts and lower federal courts have decided that there may be a federal constitutional right to treatment, the U.S. Supreme Court has never firmly defined the **right to treatment** in a constitutional principle. The evolution of these cases in the courts provides an interesting history of the development and shortcomings of our mental health delivery system. Based on the decisions of a number of early court cases, treatment must meet the following criteria:

- The environment must be humane.
- Staff must be qualified and sufficient to provide adequate treatment.
- The plan of care must be individualized.

The initial cases presenting the psychiatric patient's right to treatment arose in the criminal justice system. An interesting case regarding a person's right to treatment is *O'Connor v. Donaldson* (1975). The Court held that a "state cannot constitutionally confine a nondangerous individual who is capable of surviving safely in freedom by himself or with the help of willing and responsible family members or friends."

Right to Refuse Treatment

A companion to the right to consent to treatment is the right to withhold consent. A patient may also withdraw consent at any time. Retraction of consent previously given must be honored, whether it is verbal or written. However, the mentally ill patient's **right to refuse treatment** with psychotropic drugs has been debated in the courts, based partly on the issue of mental patients' competency to give or withhold consent to treatment and their status under the civil commitment statutes. These early cases, initiated by state hospital patients, considered medical, legal, and ethical considerations, such as basic treatment problems, the doctrine of informed consent, and the bioethical principle of autonomy. For a summary of the evolution of one landmark set of cases regarding the patient's right to refuse treatment, see Table 26-1.

The notion of refusing treatment becomes especially important if we consider medication to be a "chemical restraint." If it is, then the infringement on a person's liberty is at least equal to that with involuntary commitment. In this circumstance, the noninstitutionalized, competent, mentally ill patient has the right, through substituted judgment, to determine whether to be involuntarily committed or to be medicated.

Cases involving the right to refuse psychotropic drug treatment are still evolving. Without clear direction from the Supreme Court, there will be different case outcomes in different jurisdictions.

The numerous cases involving the right to refuse medication have illustrated the complex and difficult task of translating social policy concerns into a clearly articulated legal standard.

Right to Informed Consent

The principle of **informed consent** is based on a person's right to self-determination, as enunciated in the landmark case of *Canterbury v. Spence* (1972):

> The root premise is the concept, fundamental in American jurisprudence, that every human being of adult years and sound mind has a right to determine what shall be done with his own body. . . . True consent to what happens to one's self is the informed exercise of choice, and that entails an opportunity to evaluate knowledgeably the options available and the risks attendant on each (p. 780).

Proper orders for specific therapies and treatments are required and must be documented in the patient's chart. Consent for surgery, electroconvulsive treatment, or the use of experimental drugs or procedures must be obtained. In some state institutions, consent is required for every medication addition or change. Patients have the right to refuse participation in experimental treatments or research and the right to voice grievances and recommend changes in policies or services offered by the facility, without fear of punishment or reprisal.

For consent to be effective legally, it must be informed. Generally, the informed consent of the patient must be obtained by the physician or other health professional to perform the treatment or procedure. Patients must be informed of the nature of their problem or condition, the nature and purpose of a proposed treatment, the risks and benefits of that treatment, the alternative treatment options, the probability that the proposed treatment will be successful, and the risks of not consenting to treatment. It is important for psychiatric nurses to know that the presence

TABLE 26-1	Right to Refuse Treatment: Evolution of Massachusetts Case Law to Present Law	

Case	Court	Decision
Rogers v. Okin, 478 F. Supp. 1342 (D. Mass. 1979)	Federal district court	Ruled that involuntarily hospitalized patients with mental illness are competent and have the right to make treatment decisions. Forcible administration of medication is justified in an emergency if needed to prevent violence and if other alternatives have been ruled out. A guardian may make treatment decisions for an incompetent patient.
Rogers v. Okin, 634 F. 2nd 650 (1st Cir. 1980)	Federal court of appeals	Affirmed that involuntarily hospitalized patients with mental illness are competent and have the right to make treatment decisions. The staff has substantial discretion in an emergency. Forcible medication is also justified to prevent the patient's deterioration. A patient's rights must be protected by judicial determination of competency or incompetency.
Mills v. Rogers, 457 U.S. 291 (1982)	U.S. Supreme Court	Set aside the judgment of the court of appeals with instructions to consider the effect of an intervening state court case.
Rogers v. Commissioner of the Department of Mental Health, 458 N.E.2d 308 (Mass. 1983)	Massachusetts Supreme Judicial Court answering questions certified by federal court of appeals	Ruled that involuntarily hospitalized patients are competent and have the right to make treatment decisions unless they are judicially determined to be incompetent.

of psychotic thinking does not mean that the patient is incompetent or incapable of understanding.

Neither voluntary nor involuntary admission to a mental facility determines whether patients are capable of making informed decisions about the health care they may need. Patients must be considered legally competent until they have been declared incompetent through a legal proceeding. Competency is related to the capacity to understand the consequences of one's decisions. The determination of legal competency is made by the courts. If found incompetent, the court may appoint a legal guardian or representative who is legally responsible for giving or refusing consent for a person the court has found to be incompetent. A court-appointed guardian must always consider the patient's wishes. Guardians are usually selected from among family members. The order of selection is usually (1) spouse, (2) adult children or grandchildren, (3) parents, (4) adult brothers and sisters, and (5) nieces and nephews. In the event that a family member is either unavailable or unwilling to serve as guardian, the court may also appoint a court-trained and court-approved social worker representing the county or state or a member of the community.

Many procedures that nurses perform have an element of implied consent attached. For example, if you approach the patient with a medication in hand and the patient indicates a willingness to receive the medication, **implied consent** has occurred. It should be noted that many institutions, particularly state psychiatric hospitals, have a requirement to obtain informed consent for every medication given. A general rule for you to follow is that the more intrusive or risky the procedure, the higher the likelihood that informed consent must be obtained. The fact that you may not have a legal duty to be the person to inform the patient of the associated risks and benefits of a particular medical procedure does not excuse you from clarifying the procedure to the patient and ensuring his or her expressed or implied consent.

Rights Surrounding Involuntary Commitment and Psychiatric Advance Directives

Patients concerned that they may be subject to involuntary psychiatric commitment can prepare an advance psychiatric directive document that will express their treatment choices. The advance directive for mental health decision making should be followed by health care providers when patients are not competent to make informed decisions for themselves. This document can clarify the patient's choice of a surrogate decision maker and instructions about hospital choices, medications, treatment options, and emergency interventions. Identification of individuals who are to be notified of the patient's hospitalization and who may have visitation rights is especially helpful given the privacy demands of the Health Insurance Portability and Accountability Act (HIPAA) (Bazelon, 2003).

Rights Regarding Restraint and Seclusion

As mentioned, the use of the least restrictive means of restraint for the shortest duration is always the general rule. Verbal interventions or enlisting the cooperation of patients are the first approaches. Typically, medication is considered if verbal interventions fail. Chemical interventions are usually considered less restrictive than mechanical, but can have a greater effect on the patient's ability to relate to the environment. When used judiciously, psychopharmacology is extremely effective and helpful as an alternative to other physical methods of restraint.

The history of mechanical restraint and seclusion is one that is marked by abuses and overuse, and even a tendency to use restraint as punishment. This was especially true before the 1950s, when there were no effective chemical treatments. Legislation has dramatically reduced this problem by mandating strict guidelines. Behavioral restraint and seclusion are authorized as an intervention under the following circumstances:

- When the particular behavior is physically harmful to the patient or a third party
- When alternative or less-restrictive measures are insufficient in protecting the patient or others from harm
- When a decrease in sensory overstimulation (seclusion only) is needed
- When the patient anticipates that a controlled environment would be helpful and requests seclusion

As indicated, most state laws prohibit the use of unnecessary physical restraint or isolation. The use of seclusion and restraint is permitted only under the following circumstances (Simon, 1999):

- On the written order of a physician
- When orders are confined to specific time-limited periods (e.g., 2 to 4 hours)
- When the patient's condition is reviewed and documented regularly (e.g., every 15 minutes)
- When the original order is extended after review and reauthorization (e.g., every 24 hours) and specifies the type of restraint

---

BOX 26-1

Contraindications to Seclusion and Restraint

- Extremely unstable medical and psychiatric conditions*
- Delirium or dementia leading to inability to tolerate decreased stimulation*
- Severe suicidal tendencies*
- Severe drug reactions or overdoses or need for close monitoring of drug dosages*
- Desire for punishment of patient or convenience of staff

*Unless close supervision and direct observation are provided.
From Simon, R.I. (2001). *Concise guide to psychiatry and law for clinicians* (3rd ed., p. 117). Washington, DC: American Psychiatric Press.

In an emergency, the nurse may place a patient in seclusion or restraint and obtain a written or verbal order as soon as possible thereafter. With the exception of a patient-initiated request to be placed in seclusion, federal laws require an emergency situation to exist in which an immediate risk of harm to the patient or others can be documented. While in restraints the patient must be protected from all sources of harm. The behavior leading to restraint or seclusion and the time the patient is placed in and released from restraint must be documented; the patient in restraint must be assessed at regular and frequent intervals (e.g., every 15 to 30 minutes) for physical needs (food, hydration, toileting), safety, and comfort, and these observations also must be documented (every 15 to 30 minutes). The patient must be removed from restraints when safer and quieter behavior is observed.

Recent changes in the law regarding the use of restraint and seclusion agencies have continued to revise their policies and procedures, further limiting these practices. Despite deep-held beliefs among practitioners who have used restraints, most agencies have found no negative effect associated with the reduced use of restraints and seclusion. Alternative methods of therapy and cooperation with the patient have been successful. Nurses also need to know under which circumstances the use of seclusion and restraints is contraindicated (Box 26-1).

MAINTENANCE OF PATIENT CONFIDENTIALITY
Ethical Considerations

Confidentiality of care and treatment is also an important right for all patients, particularly psychiatric patients. Any discussion or consultation involving a patient should be conducted discreetly and only with individuals who have a

BOX 26-2

Code of Ethics for Nurses

The House of Delegates of the American Nurses Association approved these nine provisions at its June 30, 2001, meeting in Washington, D.C. In July 2001, the Congress of Nursing Practice and Economics voted to accept the new language of the interpretive statements, resulting in a fully approved revised *Code of Ethics for Nurses with Interpretive Statements*.

1. The nurse, in all professional relationships, practices with compassion and respect for the inherent dignity, worth, and uniqueness of every individual, unrestricted by considerations of social or economic status, personal attributes or the nature of health problems.
2. The nurse's primary commitment is to the patient, whether an individual, family, group, or community.
3. The nurse promotes, advocates for, and strives to protect the health, safety, and rights of the patient.
4. The nurse is responsible and accountable for individual nursing practice and determines the appropriate delegation of tasks consistent with the nurse's obligation to provide optimum patient care.

5. The nurse owes the same duties to self as to others, including the responsibility to preserve integrity and safety, to maintain competence, and to continue personal and professional growth.
6. The nurse participates in establishing, maintaining, and improving health care environments and conditions of employment conducive to the provision of quality health care and consistent with the values of the profession through individual and collective action.
7. The nurse participates in the advancement of the profession through contributions to practice, education, administration, and knowledge development.
8. The nurse collaborates with other health professionals and the public in promoting community, national, and international efforts to meet health needs.
9. The profession of nursing, as represented by associations and their members, is responsible for articulating nursing values, for maintaining the integrity of the profession and its practice, and for shaping social policy.

From American Nurses Association. (2001). *Code of ethics for nurses with interpretive statements.* Washington, DC: Nursesbooks.org.

need and a right to know this privileged information. The American Nurses Association (ANA) *Code of Ethics for Nurses* (2001) asserts the duty of the nurse to protect confidential patient information (Box 26-2). Failure to provide this protection may harm the nurse-patient relationship, as well as the patient's well-being. However, the code clarifies that this duty is not absolute. In some situations disclosure may be mandated to protect the patient, other people, or the public health.

Legal Considerations

Health Insurance Portability and Accountability Act

The psychiatric patient's right to receive treatment and to have medical records kept confidential is legally protected. The fundamental principle underlying the ANA *Code of Ethics for Nurses* on confidentiality is a person's constitutional **right to privacy**. Generally, your legal duty to maintain confidentiality is to protect the patient's right to privacy. The **Health Insurance Portability and Accountability Act (HIPAA)** became effective on April 14, 2003. Therefore, you may not, without the patient's consent, disclose information obtained from the patient or information in the medical record to anyone except those individuals for whom it is necessary for implementation of the patient's treatment plan. Special protection of notes used

in psychotherapy that are kept separate from the patient's health information was created by this HIPAA rule (2003). Discussions about a patient in public places such as elevators and the cafeteria, even when the patient's name is not mentioned, can lead to disclosures of confidential information and liabilities for you and the hospital.

Patients' Employers

Your release of information to the patient's employer about the patient's condition, without the patient's consent, is a breach of confidentiality that subjects you to liability for the tort of invasion of privacy as well as a HIPAA violation. On the other hand, discussion of a patient's history with other staff members to determine a consistent treatment approach is not a breach of confidentiality.

Generally, for a situation to be created in which information is privileged, a patient-health professional relationship must exist and the information must concern the care and treatment of the patient. The health professional may refuse to disclose information to protect the patient's privacy. However, the right to privacy is the patient's right, and health professionals cannot invoke confidentiality for their own defense or benefit.

Rights After Death

A person's reputation can be damaged even after death. It is therefore important not to divulge information after a person's death that could not have been legally shared before the death. The Dead Man's Statute protects confidential information about people when they are not alive to speak for themselves.

A legal privilege of confidentiality is enacted legislatively and in some states exists to protect the confidentiality of professional communications (e.g., nurse-patient, physician-patient, attorney-patient). The theory behind such privileged communications is that patients will not be comfortable or willing to disclose personal information about themselves if they fear that nurses will repeat their confidential conversations.

In some states in which the legal privilege of confidentiality has not been legislated for nurses, you must respond to a court's inquiries regarding the patient's disclosures even if this information implicates the patient in a crime. In these states the confidentiality of communications cannot be guaranteed. If a duty to report exists, you may be required to divulge private information shared by the patient.

Patient Privilege and Human Immunodeficiency Virus Status

Some states have enacted mandatory or permissive statutes that direct health care providers to warn a spouse if a partner tests positive for human immunodeficiency virus (HIV). Nurses must understand the laws in their jurisdiction of practice regarding privileged communications and warnings of infectious disease exposure.

Exceptions to the Rule

Duty to Warn and Protect Third Parties

The California Supreme Court, in its 1974 landmark decision *Tarasoff v. Regents of University of California*, ruled that a psychotherapist has a **duty to warn** a patient's potential victim of potential harm. A university student who was in counseling at a California university was despondent over being rejected by Tatiana Tarasoff. The psychologist notified police verbally and in writing that the young man may be dangerous to Tarasoff. The police questioned the student, found him to be rational, and secured his promise to stay away from his love interest. The student killed Tarasoff 2 months later. This case created much controversy and confusion in the psychiatric and medical communities over breach of patient confidentiality and its effect on the therapeutic relationship in psychiatric care and over the ability of the psychotherapist to predict when a patient is truly dangerous. This trend continues as other jurisdictions have adopted or modified the California rule despite the objections of the psychiatric community. These jurisdictions view public safety to be more important than privacy in narrowly defined circumstances.

The *Tarasoff* case acknowledged that generally there is no common law duty to aid third parties. An exception is when special relationships exist, and the court found the patient-therapist relationship sufficient to create a duty of the therapist to aid Ms. Tarasoff, the victim. The duty to protect the intended victim from danger arises when the therapist determines—or, pursuant to professional standards, should have determined—that the patient presents a serious danger to another. Any action reasonably necessary under the circumstances, including notification of the potential victim, the victim's family, and the police, discharges the therapist's duty to the potential victim.

In 1976, the California Supreme Court issued a second ruling in the case of *Tarasoff v. Regents of University of California* (now known as *Tarasoff II*). This ruling broadened the earlier ruling, the duty to warn, to include the **duty to protect.**

Most states have similar laws regarding the duty to warn third parties of potential life threats. The duty to warn usually includes the following:

* Assessing and predicting the patient's danger of violence toward another
* Identifying the specific individual(s) being threatened
* Taking appropriate action to protect the identified victims

Nursing Implications. As this trend toward making it the therapist's duty to warn third parties of potential harm continues to gain wider acceptance, it is important for students and nurses to understand its implications for nursing practice. Although none of these cases has dealt with nurses, it is fair to assume that in jurisdictions that have adopted the Tarasoff doctrine, the duty to warn third parties will be applied to advanced-practice psychiatric mental health nurses in private practice who engage in individual therapy.

If, however, a staff nurse who is a member of a team of psychiatrists, psychologists, psychiatric social workers, and other psychiatric nurses does not report patient threats of harm against specified victims or classes of victims to the team of the patient's management psychotherapist for assessment and evaluation, this failure is likely to be considered substandard nursing care.

So, too, the failure to communicate and record relevant information from police, relatives, or the patient's old records might also be deemed negligent. Breach of patient-nurse confidentiality should not pose ethical or legal dilemmas for nurses in these situations, because a team approach to the delivery of psychiatric care presumes communication of pertinent information to other staff members to develop a treatment plan in the patient's best interest.

Child and Elder Abuse Reporting Statutes

Because of their interest in protecting children, all 50 states and the District of Columbia have enacted **child abuse reporting statutes**. Although these statutes differ from state to state, they generally include a definition of child abuse, a list of individuals required or encouraged to report abuse, and the governmental agency designated to receive and investigate the reports. Most statutes include civil penalties for failure to report. Many states specifically require nurses to report cases of suspected abuse.

There is a conflict between federal and state laws with respect to child abuse reporting when the health care professional discovers child abuse or neglect during the suspected abuser's alcohol or drug treatment. Federal laws and regulations governing confidentiality of patient records, which apply to almost all drug abuse and alcohol treatment providers, prohibit any disclosure without a court order. In this case, federal law supersedes state reporting laws, although compliance with the state law may be maintained under the following circumstances:

- If a court order is obtained, pursuant to the regulations
- If a report can be made without identifying the abuser as a patient in an alcohol or drug treatment program
- If the report is made anonymously (some states, to protect the rights of the accused, do not allow anonymous reporting)

As reported incidents of abuse to other persons in society surface, states may require health professionals to report other kinds of abuse. A growing number of states are enacting **elder abuse reporting statutes**, which require registered nurses (RNs) and others to report cases of abuse of older adults. Agencies who receive federal funding (i.e., Medicare or Medicaid) must follow strict guidelines for reporting and preventing elder abuse. Older adults are defined as adults 65 years of age and older. These laws also apply to dependent adults—that is, adults between 18 and 64 years of age whose physical or mental limitations restrict their ability to carry out normal activities or to protect themselves—when the RN has actual knowledge that the person has been the victim of physical abuse.

Under most state laws, a person who is required to report suspected abuse, neglect, or exploitation of a disabled adult and who willfully does not do so is guilty of a misdemeanor crime. Most state statutes declare that anyone who makes a report in good faith is immune from civil liability in connection with the report.

You may also report knowledge of, or reasonable suspicion of, mental abuse or suffering. Dependent adults as well as older adults are protected by the law from purposeful physical or fiduciary neglect or abandonment. **Because** state laws vary, students are encouraged to become familiar with the requirements of their states.

TORT LAW APPLIED TO PSYCHIATRIC SETTINGS

Torts are a category of civil law that commonly applies to health care practice. A **tort** is a civil wrong for which money damages may be collected by the injured party (the plaintiff) from the wrongdoer (the defendant). The injury can be to person, property, or reputation. Because tort law has general applicability to nursing practice, this section may contain a review of material previously covered elsewhere in your nursing curriculum.

Nurses in psychiatric settings may encounter provocative, threatening, or violent behavior. Such behavior may require the use of restraint or seclusion until a patient demonstrates quieter and safer behavior. Accordingly, the nurse in the psychiatric setting should understand the **intentional torts** of **battery**, **assault**, and **false imprisonment** (described in Box 26-3).

Common Liability Issues

Protection of Patients

Legal issues common in psychiatric nursing relate to the failure to protect the safety of patients. If a suicidal patient is left alone with the means to harm himself or herself, the nurse who has a duty to protect the patient will be held responsible for the resultant injuries. Leaving a suicidal patient alone in a room on the sixth floor with an open window is an example of unreasonable judgment on the part of the nurse. Precautions to prevent harm must be taken whenever a patient is restrained. Miscommunications and medication errors are common in all areas of nursing, including psychiatric care. A common area of liability in psychiatry is abuse of the therapist-patient relationship. Issues of sexual misconduct during the therapeutic relationship have become a source of concern in the psychiatric community. Misdiagnosis is also frequently charged in legal suits. See Table 26-2 for common liability issues.

Violence

Violent behavior is not acceptable in our society. Nurses must protect themselves in both institutional and community settings. Employers are not typically held responsible for employee injuries caused by violent patient behavior. Nurses have placed themselves knowingly in the range of danger by agreeing to care for unpredictable patients. It is therefore important for nurses to protect themselves by

BOX 26-3

False Imprisonment and Negligence: *Plumadore v. State of New York* (1980)

Mrs. Plumadore was admitted to Saranac Lake General Hospital for a gallbladder condition. Her medical workup revealed emotional problems stemming from marital difficulties, which had resulted in suicide attempts several years before her admission. After a series of consultations and tests, she was advised by the attending surgeon that she was scheduled to have gallbladder surgery later that day. After the surgeon's visit, a consulting psychiatrist who examined her directed her to dress and pack her belongings because he had arranged to have her admitted to a state hospital at Ogdensburg.

Subsequently, two uniformed state troopers handcuffed her and strapped her into the backseat of a patrol car. She was also accompanied by a female hospital employee and was

transported to the state hospital. On arrival, the admitting psychiatrist recognized that the referring psychiatrist lacked the requisite authority to order her involuntary commitment. He therefore requested that she sign a voluntary admission form, which she refused to do. Despite Mrs. Plumadore's protests regarding her admission to the state hospital, the psychiatrist assigned her to a ward without physical or psychiatric examination and without the opportunity to contact her family or her medical doctor. The record of her admission to the state hospital noted an "informed admission," which is patient-initiated voluntary admission in New York.

The court awarded $40,000 to Mrs. Plumadore for false imprisonment, negligence, and malpractice.

TABLE 26-2   Common Liability Issues

Issue	Examples
Patient safety	Suicide risks
	Restraints
	Miscommunication
	Medication errors
	Boundary violations (e.g., sexual misconduct)
	Misdiagnosis
Defamation of character:	Harms patient's reputation
• Slander (spoken)	Confidential information divulged
• Libel (written)	Truth is a defense
Supervisory liability (vicarious liability)	Inappropriate delegation of duties
	Lack of supervision of those supervising
Intentional torts	Voluntary acts intended to bring a physical or mental consequence
• May carry criminal penalties	Purposeful acts
• **Punitive damages** may be awarded	Carelessness or recklessness
	No patient consent
• Not covered by malpractice insurance	Self-defense or protection of others may serve as a defense to charges of an intentional tort
Negligence or malpractice	Carelessness
	Foreseeability of harm
Assault and battery	Person apprehensive (assault) of harmful or offensive touching (battery)
	Threat to use force (words not enough) with opportunity and ability
	Treatment without patient's consent
False imprisonment	Intent to confine to a specific area
	Indefensible use of seclusion or restraints
	Detain voluntarily admitted patient with no agency or legal policies to support detaining

participating in setting policies that create a safe environment. Good judgment means not placing oneself in a potentially violent situation. Nurses, as citizens, have the same rights as patients not to be threatened or harmed. Appropriate security support should be readily available to the nurse practicing in an institution. When you work in community settings, you must avoid placing yourself unnecessarily in dangerous environments, especially when alone at night. You should use common sense and enlist the support of local law enforcement officers when needed. A violent patient is not being abandoned if placed safely in the hands of the authorities.

The psychiatric mental health nurse must also be aware of the potential for violence in the community when a patient is discharged following a short-term stay. The duty of the nurse to protect the patient as well as others who may be threatened by the violent patient is discussed in the section Duty to Warn and Protect Third Parties earlier in this chapter. The nurse's assessment of the patient's potential for violence must be documented and acted on if there is legitimate concern regarding discharge of a patient who is discussing or exhibiting potentially violent behavior. The psychiatric mental health nurse must communicate his or her observations to the medical staff when discharge decisions are being considered.

Negligence/Malpractice

Negligence or **malpractice** is an act or an omission to act that breaches the duty of due care and results in or is responsible for a person's injuries. The five elements required to prove negligence are (1) duty, (2) breach of duty, (3) cause in fact, (4) proximate cause, and (5) damages. Foreseeability or likelihood of harm is also evaluated.

Duty is measured by a standard of care. When nurses represent themselves as being capable of caring for psychiatric patients and accept employment, a duty of care has been assumed. The duty is owed to psychiatric patients to understand the theory and medications used in the specialty care of these patients. People who represent themselves as possessing superior knowledge and skill, such as psychiatric nurse specialists, are held to a higher standard of care in the practice of their profession. The staff nurse who is assigned to a psychiatric unit must be knowledgeable enough to assume a reasonable or safe duty of care for the patients.

If you are not capable of providing the standard of care that other nurses would be expected to supply under similar circumstances, you have breached the duty of care. **Breach of duty** is the conduct that exposes the patient to an unreasonable risk of harm, through either commission or omission of acts by the nurse. If you do not have the required education and experience to provide certain interventions,

you have breached the duty by neglecting or omitting to provide necessary care. You can also act in such a way that the patient is harmed and can thus be guilty of negligence through acts of commission.

Cause in fact may be evaluated by asking the question, "Except for what the nurse did, would this injury have occurred?" **Proximate cause,** or legal cause, may be evaluated by determining whether there were any intervening actions or individuals that were, in fact, the causes of harm to the patient. **Damages** include actual damages (e.g., loss of earnings, medical expenses, and property damage) as well as pain and suffering. **Foreseeability of harm** evaluates the likelihood of the outcome under the circumstances.

DETERMINATION OF A STANDARD OF CARE

Professional standards of practice determined by professional associations differ from the standards embodied in the minimal qualifications set forth by state licensure for entry into the profession of nursing. The ANA has established standards for psychiatric mental health nursing practice and credentialing for the psychiatric mental health RN and the advanced-practice RN in psychiatric mental health nursing (ANA, 2007).

Standards for psychiatric mental health nursing practice differ markedly from minimal state requirements because the primary purposes for setting these two types of standards are different. The state's qualifications for practice provide consumer protection by ensuring that all practicing nurses have successfully completed an approved nursing program and passed the national licensing examination. The professional association's primary focus is to elevate the practice of its members by setting standards of excellence.

Nurses are held to the standard of care provided by other nurses possessing the same degree of skill or knowledge in the same or similar circumstances. In the past, community standards existed for urban and rural agencies. However, with greater mobility and expanded means of communication, national standards have evolved. Psychiatric patients have the right to the standard of care recognized by professional bodies governing nursing, whether they are in a large or a small, a rural or an urban, facility. Nurses must participate in continuing education courses to stay current with existing standards of care.

Hospital policies and procedures set up institutional criteria for care, and these criteria, such as the frequency of rounds for patients in seclusion, may be introduced to prove a standard that the nurse met or failed to meet. The shortcoming of this method is that the hospital's policy may be substandard. For example, the state licensing laws for institutions might set a minimal requirement for staffing or frequency of rounds for certain patients, and the hospital policy might fall below that minimum. **Substandard institutional policies do not absolve the individual nurse of responsibility to practice on the basis of professional standards of nursing care.**

Like hospital policy and procedures, custom can be used as evidence of a standard of care. For example, in the absence of a written policy on the use of restraint, testimony might be offered regarding the customary use of restraint in emergency situations in which the combative, violent, or confused patient poses a threat of harm to self or others. Using custom to establish a standard of care may result in the same defect as in using hospital policies and procedures: custom may not comply with the laws, recommendations of the accrediting body, or other recognized standards of care. Custom must be carefully and regularly evaluated to ensure that substandard routines have not developed. Substandard customs do not protect you when a psychiatric patient charges that a right has been violated or that harm has been caused by the staff's common practices.

Guidelines for Nurses Who Suspect Negligence

It is not unusual for a student or practicing nurse to suspect negligence on the part of a peer. In most states, as a nurse you have a legal duty to report such risks of harm to the patient. It is also important that you document the evidence clearly and accurately before making serious accusations against a peer. If you question a physician's orders or actions, or those of a fellow nurse, it is wise to communicate these concerns directly to the person involved. If the risky behavior continues, you have an obligation to communicate these concerns to a supervisor, who should then intervene to ensure that the patient's rights and well-being are protected.

If you suspect a peer of being chemically impaired or of practicing irresponsibly, you have an obligation to protect not only the rights of the peer but also the rights of all patients who could be harmed by this impaired peer. If, after you have reported suspected behavior of concern to a supervisor, the danger persists, you have a duty to report the concern to someone at the next level of authority. It is important to follow the channels of communication in an organization, but it is also important to protect the safety of the patients. If the supervisor's actions or inactions do not rectify the dangerous situation, you have a continuing duty to report the behavior of concern to the appropriate authority, such as the state board of nursing.

A useful reference for nurses is the ANA's *Guidelines on Reporting Incompetent, Unethical, or Illegal Practices* (1994).

Duty to Intervene and Duty to Report

The psychiatric mental health nurse has a duty to intervene when the safety or well-being of the patient or another person is obviously at risk. A nurse who follows an order that is known to be incorrect or that the nurse believes will harm the patient is responsible for the harm that results to the patient. **If you have information that leads you to believe that the physician's orders need to be clarified or changed, it is your duty to intervene and protect the patient.** It is important that you communicate with the physician who has ordered the treatment to explain the concern. If the treating physician does not appear willing to consider your concerns, you should carry out the duty to intervene through other appropriate channels.

It is important for you to express your concerns to the supervisor to allow the supervisor to communicate with the appropriate medical staff for intervention in the physician's treatment plan. As the patient's advocate, you have a duty to intervene to protect the patient; at the same time, you do not have the right to interfere with the physician-patient relationship.

It is also important to follow agency policies and procedures for communicating differences of opinion. If you fail to intervene and the patient is injured, you may be partly liable for the injuries that result because of failure to use safe nursing practice and good professional judgment.

The legal concept of **abandonment** may also arise when a nurse does not leave a patient safely back in the hands of another health professional before discontinuing treatment. When the nurse is given an assignment to care for a patient, the nurse must provide the care or ensure that the patient is safely reassigned to another nurse. Abandonment issues arise when accurate, timely, and thorough reporting has not occurred or when follow-through of patient care, on which the patient is relying, has not occurred. The same principles apply for the psychiatric mental health nurse who is working in a community setting. For example, if a suicidal patient refuses to come to the hospital for treatment, you cannot abandon the patient but must take the necessary steps to ensure the patient's safety. These actions may include enlisting the assistance of the law in temporarily involuntarily committing the patient.

The duty to intervene on the patient's behalf poses many legal and ethical dilemmas for nurses in the workplace. Institutions that have a chain-of-command policy or other reporting mechanisms offer some assurance that the proper authorities in the administration are notified. Most patient care issues regarding physicians' orders or treatments can be settled fairly early in the process by the nurse's discussion of the concerns with the physician. If further intervention by the nurse is required to protect the patient, the next step in the chain of command can be followed. Generally, the nurse then notifies the immediate nursing supervisor; the supervisor thereupon discusses the problem with the physician, and then with the chief of staff of a particular service, until a resolution is reached. If there is no time to resolve the issue through the normal process because of the life-threatening nature of the situation, the nurse must act to protect the patient's life.

Unethical or Illegal Practices

The issues become more complex when a professional colleague's conduct, including that of a student nurse, is criminally unlawful. Specific examples include the diversion of drugs from the hospital and sexual misconduct with patients. Increasing media attention and the recognition of substance abuse as an occupational hazard for health professionals have led to the establishment of substance abuse programs for health care workers in many states. These programs provide appropriate treatment for impaired professionals to protect the public from harm and to rehabilitate the professional.

The problem previously discussed—of reporting impaired colleagues—becomes a difficult one, particularly when no direct harm has occurred to the patient. Concern for professional reputations, damaged careers, and personal privacy rather than public protection has generated a code of silence regarding substance abuse among health professionals.

Several states now require reporting of impaired or incompetent colleagues to the professional licensing boards. In the absence of such a legal mandate, the questions of whether to report and to whom to report become ethical ones. You are again urged to use the ANA's *Guidelines on Reporting Incompetent, Unethical, or Illegal Practices* (1994). Chapter 16 deals more fully with issues related to the chemically impaired nurse.

The duty to intervene includes the duty to report known abusive behavior. Most states have enacted statutes to protect children and older adults from abuse and neglect. Psychiatric mental health nurses working in the community may be required by law to report unsafe relationships they discover.

DOCUMENTATION OF CARE
Purpose of Medical Records

The purpose of the medical record is to provide accurate and complete information about the care and treatment of patients and to give health care personnel responsible for that care a means of communicating with each other. The medical record allows for continuity of care. A record's usefulness is determined by evaluating, when the record is read later, how accurately and completely it portrays the patient's behavioral status at the time it was written. The patient has the right to see the chart, but the chart belongs to the institution. The patient must follow appropriate protocol to view his or her records.

For example, if a psychiatric patient describes to a nurse a plan to harm himself or herself or another person and that nurse fails to document the information, including the need to protect the patient or the identified victim, the information will be lost when the nurse leaves work, and the patient's plan may be carried out. The harm caused could be linked directly to the nurse's failure to communicate this important information. Even though documentation takes time away from the patient, the importance of communicating and preserving the nurse's memory through the medical record cannot be overemphasized.

Facility Use of Medical Records

The medical record has many other uses aside from providing information on the course of the patient's care and treatment to health care professionals. A retrospective chart review can provide valuable information to the facility on the quality of care provided and on ways to improve that care. A facility may conduct reviews for risk management purposes to determine areas of potential liability for the facility and to evaluate methods used to reduce the facility's exposure to liability. For example, documentation of the use of restraints and seclusion for psychiatric patients may be reviewed by risk managers. Accordingly, the chart may be used to evaluate care for quality assurance or peer review. Utilization review analysts review the chart to determine appropriate use of hospital and staff resources consistent with reimbursement schedules. Insurance companies and other reimbursement agencies rely on the medical record in determining what payments they will make on the patient's behalf.

Medical Records as Evidence

From a legal perspective, the chart is a recording of data and opinions made in the normal course of the patient's hospital care. It is deemed to be good evidence because it is presumed to be true, honest, and untainted by memory lapses. Accordingly, the medical record finds its way into legal cases for a variety of reasons. Some examples of its use include determining (1) the extent of the patient's damages and pain and suffering in personal injury cases, such as when a psychiatric patient attempts suicide while under the protective care of a hospital; (2) the nature and extent of injuries in child abuse or elder abuse cases; (3) the nature and extent of physical or mental disability in disability cases; and (4) the nature and extent of injury and rehabilitative potential in workers' compensation cases.

Medical records may also be used in police investigations, civil conservatorship proceedings, competency hearings, and commitment procedures. In states that mandate mental health legal services or a patients' rights advocacy program, audits may be performed to determine the facility's compliance with state laws or violation of patients' rights. Finally, medical records may be used in professional and hospital negligence cases.

During the discovery phase of litigation, the medical record is a pivotal source of information for attorneys in determining whether a cause of action exists in a professional negligence or hospital negligence case. Evidence of the nursing care rendered will be found in what the nurse charted.

Nursing Guidelines for Computerized Charting

Accurate, descriptive, and legible nursing notes serve the best interests of the patient, the nurse, and the institution. As computerized charting becomes more widely available, it will also be important for psychiatric mental health nurses to understand how to protect the confidentiality of these records. Institutions must also protect against intrusions into the privacy of the patient record systems.

Concerns for the privacy of the legitimate patient's records have been addressed legally by federal laws that provide guidelines for agencies that use computerized charting. These guidelines include the recommendation that staff be assigned a password for entering patients' records to identify which staff have gained access to patients' confidential information. There are penalties, including grounds for firing the staff, if they enter a record for which they are not authorized to have access. Only those staff who

have a legitimate need to know about the patient are authorized to access a patient's computerized chart.

It is important for you to keep your password private and never to allow someone else to access a record under your password. You are responsible for all entries into records using your password. The various systems used allow specific timeframes within which the nurse must make any necessary corrections if a charting error is made.

Any charting method that improves communication between care providers should be encouraged. Courts assume that nurses and physicians read each other's notes on patient progress. Many courts take the attitude that if care is not documented, it did not occur. Your charting also serves as a valuable memory refresher if the patient sues years after the care is rendered. In providing complete and timely information on the care and treatment of patients, the medical record enhances communication among health professionals. Internal institutional audits of the record can improve the quality of care rendered. Nurses' charting is improved by following the guidelines in Box 5-6. Chapter 5 describes common charting forms and gives examples as well as the pros and cons of each.

FORENSIC NURSING

Forensic nursing is the application of psychiatric nursing or any medical specialty principles of practice when utilized in a court of law to assist the court to utilize this knowledge to reach a decision on a contested issue. The nurse acts as an advocate, educating the court about the science of nursing in this courtroom based practice of forensic nursing. Examples of psychiatric forensic nursing may include cases related to patient competency, fitness to stand trial, and commitment or responsibility for a crime. The application of nursing facts are related and applied to the legal facts. Forensic cases also pertain to personal injury and murder proceedings. A dentist may serve as a forensic dentist in identifying a tooth as it relates to a corpse.

KEY POINTS TO REMEMBER

- States' power to enact laws for public health and safety and for the care of those unable to care for themselves often pits the rights of society against the rights of the individual.
- Psychiatric nurses frequently encounter problems requiring ethical choices.
- The nurse's privilege to practice nursing carries with it the responsibility to practice safely, competently, and in a manner consistent with state and federal laws.

- Knowledge of the law and the ANA *Code of Ethics for Nurses* and ANA Standards of Care from the *Psychiatric–Mental Health Nursing: Scope and Standards of Practice* are essential to provide safe, effective psychiatric nursing care and will serve as a framework for decision making when the nurse is presented with complex problems involving competing interests.

CRITICAL THINKING

1. Two nurses, Joe and Beth, have worked on the psychiatric unit for 2 years. During the past 6 months, Beth has confided to Joe that she has been experiencing a particularly difficult marital situation. Joe has observed that over the 6 months Beth has become increasingly irritable and difficult to work with. He notices that minor tranquilizers are frequently missing from the unit dose cart on the evening shift. He complains to the pharmacy and is informed that the drugs were stocked as ordered. Several patients state that they have not been receiving their usual drugs. Joe finds that Beth has recorded that the drugs have been given as ordered. He also notices that Beth is diverting the drugs.

   A. What action, if any, should Joe take?
   B. Should Joe confront Beth with his suspicions?
   C. If Beth admits that she has been diverting the drugs, should Joe's next step be to report Beth to the supervisor or to the board of nursing?
   D. Should Joe make his concern known to the nursing supervisor directly by identifying Beth, or should he state his concerns in general terms?
   E. Legally, must Joe report his suspicions to the board of nursing?
   F. Does the fact that harm to the patients is limited to increased agitation affect your responses?

2. A 40-year-old man who is admitted to the emergency department for a severe nosebleed has both nares packed. Because of his history of alcoholism and the probability of ensuing delirium tremens, the patient is transferred to the psychiatric unit. He is admitted to a private room, placed in restraints, and checked by a nurse every hour per physician's orders. While unattended, the patient suffocates, apparently by inhaling the nasal packing, which had become dislodged from the nares. On the next 1-hour check, the nurse finds the patient without pulse or respiration. A state statute requires that a restrained patient on a psychiatric unit be assessed by a nurse every hour for safety, comfort, and physical needs.

   A. If standards are not otherwise specified, do statutory requirements set forth minimal or maximal standards?
   B. Does the nurse's compliance with the state statute relieve him or her of liability in the patient's death?
   C. Does the nurse's compliance with the physician's orders relieve him or her of liability in the patient's death?

   D. Was the order for the restraint appropriate for this type of patient?
   E. What factors did you consider in making your determination?
   F. Was the frequency of rounds for assessment of patient needs appropriate in this situation?
   G. Did the nurse's conduct meet the standard of care for psychiatric nurses? Why or why not?
   H. What nursing action should the nurse have taken to protect the patient from harm?

3. Assume that there are no mandatory reporting laws for impaired or incompetent colleagues in the following clinical situation. In a private psychiatric unit in California, a 15-year-old boy is admitted voluntarily at the request of his parents because of violent, explosive behavior that seems to stem from his father's recent remarriage after his parents' divorce. A few days after admission, while in group therapy, he has an explosive reaction to a discussion about weekend passes for Mother's Day. He screams that he has been abandoned and that nobody cares about him. Several weeks later, on the day before his discharge, he elicits from the nurse a promise to keep his plan to kill his mother confidential. Consider the ANA *Code of Ethics for Nurses* on patient confidentiality, the principles of psychiatric nursing, the statutes on privileged communications, and the duty to warn third parties in answering the following questions:

   A. Did the nurse use appropriate judgment in promising confidentiality?
   B. Does the nurse have a legal duty to warn the patient's mother of her son's threat?
   C. Is the duty owed to the patient's father and stepmother?
   D. Would a change in the admission status from voluntary to involuntary protect the patient's mother without violating the patient's confidentiality?
   E. Would your response be different depending on the state in which the incident occurred? Why or why not?
   F. What nursing action, if any, should the nurse take after the disclosure by the patient?

CHAPTER REVIEW

Choose the most appropriate answer.

1. Which resource will provide the least authoritative help for a psychiatric mental health nurse faced with a patient care ethical dilemma?
   1. *Psychiatric–Mental Health Nursing: Scope and Standards of Practice* (ANA)
   2. Federal and state laws
   3. ANA *Code of Ethics for Nurses*
   4. Peer opinion

2. The single most important action nurses can take to protect the rights of a psychiatric patient is to:
   1. be aware of that state's laws regarding care and treatment of the mentally ill.
   2. refuse to participate in imposing restraint or seclusion.
   3. document concerns about unit short staffing.
   4. practice the five principles of bioethics.

3. To provide appropriate care for a patient who has been admitted involuntarily to a psychiatric unit, the nurse must be aware of the fact that the patient has the right to:
   1. refuse psychotropic medications.
   2. be treated by unit staff of his or her choice.
   3. be released within 24 hours of making a written request.
   4. have a consultation with other mental health professionals at the hospital's expense.

4. In which situation might the psychiatric mental health nurse incur liability?
   1. Placing a patient with annoying behavior in seclusion
   2. Reporting the substandard practice of a nurse peer
   3. Reporting threats against a third party to the treatment team
   4. Discussing an unclear medical order with the physician

5. Observing the patient's right to privacy permits the psychiatric mental health nurse to:
   1. freely disclose information in the medical record to the patient's employer.
   2. use information about the patient when preparing a journal article.
   3. discuss observations about the patient with the treatment team.
   4. disclose confidential information after the patient's death.

REFERENCES

American Nurses Association (ANA). (1994). *Guidelines on reporting incompetent, unethical, or illegal practices.* Kansas City, MO: Author.

American Nurses Association (ANA). (2001). *Code of ethics for nurses with interpretive statements.* Washington, DC: Nursesbooks.org.

American Nurses Association (ANA), American Psychiatric Nursing Association, and International Society of Psychiatric Mental Health Nurses (2007). *Psychiatric mental-health nursing. Scope and standards of practice.* Silver Springs, MD: Nursesbooks.org.

American Psychiatric Association (APA). (2000). *Diagnostic and statistical manual of mental disorders (DSM-IV-TR)* (4th ed., text rev.). Washington, DC: Author.

Bazelon, D.L. (2003). *Advance psychiatric directives.* Washington, DC: Bazelon Center for Mental Health Law.

Canterbury v. Spence, 464 F.2d 772 (D.C. Cir. 1972), quoting *Schloendorff v. Society of N.Y. Hosp.,* 211 N.Y. 125, 105 N.E. 92, 93 (1914).

Chan, C. *Mandatory outpatient treatment: Issues to consider.* Paper presented at the 153rd Annual Meeting of the American Psychiatric Association. Chicago. May 17, 2003.

Health Insurance Portability and Accountability Act (HIPAA). U.S.C. 45 C.F.R § 164.501 (2003).

Humphrey v. Cady, 405 U.S. 504 (1972).

Illinois v. Russel, 630 N.E.2d 794 (Ill. Sup. Ct. 1994).

Monahan, J., Swartz, M., & Bonnie, R.J. (2003). Mandated treatment in the community for people with mental disorders. *Health Affairs,* 22(5), 28-38.

O'Connor v. Donaldson, 422 U.S. 563 (1975).

Plumadore v. State of New York, 427 N.Y.S.2d 90 (1980).

Rainey, C.J. *Mandated outpatient treatment resources and data.* Presented at the American Psychiatric Association 53rd Institute on Psychiatric Services. Orlando, FL. October 10-14, 2001.

Simon, R.I. (1999). The law and psychiatry. In R.E. Hales, S.C. Yudofsky, & J.A. Talbott (Eds.), *The American Psychiatric Press textbook of psychiatry* (3rd ed.). Washington, DC: American Psychiatric Press.

Tarasoff v. Regents of University of California, 529 P.2d 553, 118 Cal Rptr 129 (1974).

Tarasoff v. Regents of University of California, 551 P.2d 334, 131 Cal Rptr 14 (1976).

Zinermon v. Burch, 494 U.S. 113, 108 L.Ed.2d 100, 110 S. Ct. 975 (1990).

CHAPTER 27

Settings for Psychiatric Care

Margaret Jordan Halter

Key Terms and Concepts

Objectives

1. Describe the evolution of treatment settings for psychiatric care.
2. Identify the inpatient and outpatient treatment environments in which psychiatric care is provided.
3. Describe the mental health professionals who assist people with mental illness symptoms or mental illnesses.
4. Explain payment methods for psychiatric care.

evolve

For additional resources related to the content of this chapter, visit the Evolve website at http://evolve.elsevier.com/Varcarolis/essentials.

- Chapter Outline
- Chapter Review Answers
- Concept Map Creator

Obtaining traditional health care is pretty straight-forward: diagnoses tend to be based on objective measurements. For example, if you wake up with a sore throat, you know what to do and pretty much what will happen. It is likely that if you feel bad enough, you will go see your primary care provider (PCP), be examined, and maybe get a throat culture to diagnose the problem. If the cause is bacterial, you will probably be prescribed an antibiotic. If you do not improve in a certain length of time, your PCP may order more tests or recommend that you see an ear, nose, and throat specialist.

Compared to obtaining treatment for physical disorders, entry into the mental health care system for the treatment of mental health problems can be a mystery. In fact, although 46% of the population will have a diagnosable mental disorder over the course of a lifetime, and 80% of that population will eventually seek treatment, the delay in treatment is often years or decades (Kessler et al., 2005).

Challenges in accessing and navigating this care system exist for several reasons. One reason is that we just do not have much of a frame of reference. We are unlikely to benefit from the experience of others because having a psychiatric illness is often hidden as a result of embarrassment or concern over the **stigma**, or a sense of responsibility, shame, and being flawed associated with these disorders. You may know that when your grandmother had heart disease, she saw a cardiac specialist and had a coronary artery bypass, but you may be unaware that she was also treated for depression by a psychiatrist.

Seeking treatment for mental health problems is also complicated by the very nature of mental illness. At the most extreme, disorders with a psychotic component may disorganize thoughts and impede a person's ability to recognize the need for care. Even major depression, a common psychiatric disorder, may interfere with motivation to seek care because the illness often brings about feelings of apathy, hopelessness, and anergia.

Mental health symptoms are also confused with other problems. For example, anxiety disorders often manifest in somatic symptoms such as racing heartbeat, sweaty palms, and dizziness, which could be symptoms of cardiac problems. Prudence would dictate ruling out other causes, such as physical illness, particularly because diagnosing psychiatric illness is largely based on symptoms and not on objective measurements like electrocardiograms (ECGs) and blood counts. This necessary process of ruling out other illnesses often results in an often troublesome treatment delay.

Further complicating treatment for mental illness is the unique nature of the system of care, which is rooted in the public as well as private sectors. The purpose of this chapter is to provide an overview of this system, briefly examine the evolution of mental health care, and explore different venues by which people receive treatment for mental health problems. Treatment options are roughly presented in order of acuteness, beginning with those in the **least restrictive environment**—the setting that provides the necessary care while allowing the greatest personal freedom. The chapter also explores how mental health care is funded and the challenges in securing adequate funding.

BACKGROUND

The mental health care system differs from care for most illnesses in that people with financial resources have a variety of treatment options, whereas the state (and in some cases county) governments coordinate a separate care system for uninsured individuals, often with the most serious and persistent illnesses. This separate system of care has it roots in asylums that were created in most existing states before the Civil War, in an environment of optimism about recovery and belief that states had a special responsibility to care for the "insane." Effective treatments were not yet developed and community care was virtually nonexistent. By the early 1950s, there were only two real options for psychiatric care—a private psychiatrist's office or a mental hospital. At that time, there were 550,000 patients in state hospitals. A majority were individuals with disabling conditions who had become "stuck" in the asylums.

The creation of Medicare and especially Medicaid during the 1960s Great Society reform period created new funding and incentives. Medicaid had an especially potent effect because it paid for short-term hospitalization in general hospitals and medical centers, and for long-term care in nursing homes, while not covering care for most patients in psychiatric hospitals. These incentives stimulated development of general hospital psychiatric units, and led states to transfer geriatric patients from 100% state-paid psychiatric hospitals to Medicaid-reimbursed nursing facilities.

These forces combined to lead to the gradual and incomplete creation of state- and county-financed community care systems to complement, and largely replace, functions of the state hospitals. By 2005, the number of state psychiatric hospitals was reduced to about 250 facilities, and the use of those hospitals was reduced even more dramatically to a census of about 50,000 patients daily. Figure 27-1 illustrates the current structure of one state mental health and substance abuse system. In Ohio, two state agencies, the Ohio Department of Mental Health and the Ohio Department of Alcohol and Drug Addiction Services, certify, monitor, and fund agencies that provide services. These agencies may be for profit or nonprofit. A county

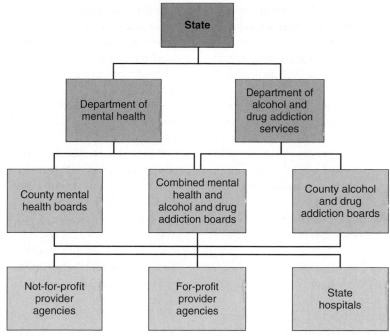

Figure 27-1 ■ An example of a state system of mental health and substance abuse care.

board or county boards (depending on whether the alcohol or substance abuse and mental health boards are combined) provide more local oversight and management of these agencies.

Related to the shift from hospital to community care were the pharmacological breakthroughs in the latter half of the 20th century that led to dramatic changes in the provision of psychiatric care. The introduction of chlorpromazine (Thorazine), the first antipsychotic medication, in the early 1950s, contributed to hospital discharges. Gradually, more psychopharmacological agents were added to treat psychosis, depression, anxiety, and other disorders, and treatment could be provided not only from specialists in psychiatry but also from general practitioners.

Our current system of psychiatric care includes inpatient and outpatient settings. Decisions for level of care tend to be based on the condition being treated and the acuteness of the problem. However, these are not the only criteria. Levels of care may be influenced by such factors as a concurrent psychiatric or substance abuse problem, medical problems, acceptance of treatment, social supports, and disease chronicity or potential for relapse.

OUTPATIENT CARE SETTINGS

Primary care providers (PCPs) are the first choice for most people when they are ill, but what about mental disorders? Imagine that you are feeling depressed, so depressed,

in fact, that you are miserable and can't do the things you normally do. You recall that your friend who was depressed saw a psychiatrist (or was that a psychologist?), but that seems awfully drastic. You do not feel *that* bad, and maybe you are not really even depressed. Perhaps you are coming down with something. After all, you have been tired and you are not eating very well. You may decide to visit your PCP, a general health care provider who may be a doctor, advanced-practice nurse, or physician's assistant in an office, hospital, or clinic.

This is not an unusual course of action. Seeking help for mental health problems from PCPs rather than from mental health specialists is common and similar to seeking help for other medical disorders. In fact, PCPs actually deliver 50% of mental health care in the United States and prescribe 66% of all psychopharmacological drugs (Patterson et al., 2002). Most people treated for psychiatric disorders will not go beyond this level of care and may feel more comfortable being treated in a familiar setting. Furthermore, being treated in primary care rather than in the mental health system may lessen the degree of stigma attached to getting psychiatric care.

Drawbacks to being treated by PCPs include time constraints because a 15-minute appointment is usually inadequate for a mental and physical assessment. Because PCPs typically have limited training in psychiatry, they may lack the expertise in the diagnosis and treatment of psychiatric disorders (Depression and Bipolar Support Alliance, 2006).

Whereas this may be the only source many people use for receiving mental health services, sometimes PCPs refer people into specialty mental health care.

Psychiatric care providers provide treatment for mental health problems in private facilities, in conjunction with other care providers, or in nonprofit service agencies (e.g., Family Services, Catholic Charities, and Jewish Social Services). Mental health professionals are specialists who treat people who have psychiatric disorders. The most well-known group of mental health care providers who prescribe and manage medications is psychiatrists. Prescriptive authority is also held by advanced-practice psychiatric nurses and physicians' assistants in most of the United States, and by psychologists in some states. Social workers, counselors, and pastoral counselors also provide outpatient therapy.

Community mental health centers (CMHCs) grew out of President Kennedy's Community Mental Health Centers Act of 1963, signaling a new policy preference for community care as opposed to institutionalization. Although only about 700 of the anticipated 2800 CMHCs were funded, the legislation marked a change in direction and led to state laws and budgets favoring community care. CMHCs are regulated through state mental health departments and funded by the state. Some areas may provide local funding. Because of this limited government funding, financial support services may be restricted to those whose income and medical expenses make them eligible. Typically, fees are determined using a sliding scale based on income and ability to pay.

Community-based facilities provide comprehensive services to prevent and treat mental illness. These services include assessment, diagnosis, individual and group counseling, case management, medication management, education, rehabilitation, and vocational or employment services. Some centers may provide an array of services across the life span, whereas others may be population specific, such as adult, geriatric, or children.

Psychiatric home care can be provided by any mental health professional, but it is typically nurses with inpatient experience who are able to provide biologically based and psychotherapeutic care while working through agencies such as visiting nurses. Home care may reduce the need for costly and disruptive hospitalizations and may provide a more comfortable and safe alternative to clinical settings. To qualify for reimbursement, patients must have a psychiatric diagnosis, be under the care of a PCP, and be home-bound. The designation of homebound generally is given when patients cannot safely leave home, if leaving home causes undue stress, if the nature of the illness results in a refusal to leave home, or if they cannot leave home unaided. However, Medicare reimbursement does allow for the person to leave home once a week for religious services and once a week for hair care.

Intensive outpatient programs (IOPs) provide structured programs to bridge the gap between inpatient and outpatient treatment for people who require more than outpatient care or who may need a transition from an intensive setting. Treatment includes individual and group therapy and psychosocial education for at least 4 hours per week.

Partial hospitalization programs (PHPs) have been around since the 1960s, and like IOPs, function as an intermediate step between outpatient and inpatient care. They are the most intensive of outpatient options and tend to be 4 to 8 hours per day for up to 5 days a week. Structured programs are provided with nursing and medical supervision, intervention, and treatment. They are located within general hospitals, psychiatric hospitals, and as part of community mental health programs. Patients whose symptoms are under control spend a certain number of hours at the facility each day and at night return to their homes, where they can be supported by family and friends. Additionally, coping strategies that are learned during the program can be applied and practiced in the outside world, and then later explored and discussed. A multidisciplinary team facilitates group therapy, individual therapy, other therapies (e.g., art and occupational), and pharmacological management. Patients who are admitted to PHPs are closely monitored in case of need for readmission to inpatient care.

Role of Nurses in Outpatient Care Settings

Registered nurses who work in outpatient settings provide nursing care for individuals with mental illness, alcoholism, substance abuse, mental retardation, or developmental disabilities, as well as their families or caretakers. Community mental health nurses work to develop and implement a plan of care along with the multidisciplinary treatment team. They may choose to be certified in psychiatric mental health nursing or hold advanced-practice degrees.

Community mental health nurses need to be very knowledgeable about community resources such as shelters for abused women, food banks for people with severe financial limitations, and agencies that provide employment options for people with mental illness. Nurses may also assess the patient and living arrangements in the home, provide teaching, refer to community supports, and supervise unlicensed care staff. An important concept for community mental health nurses is viewing the entire community as a patient. This perspective promotes community interventions such as conducting stress reduction classes and facilitating grief support groups.

TABLE 27-1	Number and Rate of 24-Hour Hospital and Residential Treatment Beds by Type of Mental Health Organization			

Type of Organization	1980	1990	2000
Number of 24-Hour Hospital and Residential Treatment Beds			
All organizations	274,713	272,253	215,221
State and county mental hospitals	156,482	98,789	59,403
Private psychiatric hospitals	17,157	44,871	26,789
Non-federal general hospitals with separate psychiatric services	29,384	53,479	37,692
Veterans Administration (VA) medical centers	33,796	21,712	13,030
Residential treatment centers for emotionally disturbed children	20,197	29,756	33,421
All other organizations*	1,433	23,646	44,886
24-Hour Hospital and Residential Treatment Beds per 100,000 Civilian Population			
All organizations	124.3	111.6	76.8
State and county mental hospitals	70.2	40.5	21.2
Private psychiatric hospitals	7.7	18.4	9.6
Non-federal general hospitals with separate psychiatric services	13.7	21.9	13.4
VA medical centers	15.7	8.9	4.6
Residential treatment centers for emotionally disturbed children	9.1	12.2	11.9
All other organizations*	0.6	9.7	16

*Includes free-standing psychiatric outpatient clinics, partial care organizations, and multiservice mental health organizations. Multiservice mental health organizations were redefined in 1984.

Adapted from the Substance Abuse and Mental Health Services Administration. (2002). *Mental health, United States, 2002.* Retrieved August 20, 2007, from http://mentalhealth.samhsa.gov/publications/allpubs/SMA04-3938/.

INPATIENT CARE SETTINGS

Inpatient care has undergone significant change over the past quarter century (Table 27-1). During the 1980s, inpatient stays were at their peak as private and non-federal general hospitals psychiatric units proliferated. During the mid-1990s, the number of patient days, psychiatric beds, and psychiatric facilities dipped sharply. This decline was caused by improvements brought about by managed care, tougher limitations of covered days by insurance plans, and alternatives to inpatient hospitalization such as partial hospitalization programs and residential facilities.

Inpatient facilities provide 24-hour nursing care in a safe and structured setting for people who are in need of this most restrictive environment. Such a setting is essential to caring for those who are in need of protection from suicidal ideation, aggressive impulses, medication adjustment and monitoring, crisis stabilization, substance abuse detoxification, and behavior modification. Referrals for inpatient treatment may come from a PCP or mental health provider, agencies, another hospital unit, emergency facilities, or nursing homes. Hospital admissions are made under the services of a psychiatrist, although a PCP also may have admitting privileges.

Patients may be admitted voluntarily or involuntarily (see Chapter 26). Units may be unlocked or locked. Locked units provide privacy and prevent **elopement**—leaving before being discharged (also referred to as being "away without leave" or AWOL). There may also be psychiatric intensive care units (PICUs) within the general psychiatric units to provide better monitoring of those who display an increased risk for danger to self or others.

The **therapeutic milieu** is essential to successful inpatient treatment. Milieu refers to the environment in which holistic treatment occurs and includes all members of the treatment team (Box 27-1), a positive physical setting, interactions between those who are hospitalized, and activities that promote recovery. Inpatient care provides structure in which patients eat meals, receive medication (if necessary), attend activities, and participate in individual and group therapies on a schedule. For those younger than the age of 18, school attendance is required. Patients are active participants in their plans of care and have the right to refuse treatments as long as they have not been declared incompetent. Advocates are usually available to provide advice and counsel for people who have doubts, and most facilities distribute a patient's bill of rights on admission or have it clearly posted. Box 27-2 provides a sample list of patient's rights.

BOX 27-1

Members of the Treatment Team

- **Psychiatric nurse generalists** are licensed registered nurses whose focus is on mental health and illness. They may or may not have certification in psychiatric mental health nursing.
- **Advanced-practice psychiatric nurses** have post-baccalaureate degrees and work as either clinical nurse specialists (CNSs) or nurse practitioners (NPs) and have state certification. Both assess health and psychiatric disorders, provide psychotherapy, and prescribe medications. CNSs tend to focus more on leadership, program development, education, and psychotherapy, whereas NPs focus on differential diagnosis, treatment, medication management, and psychotherapy.
- **Psychiatrists** are medical doctors who have additional specialized training in diagnosing and treating psychiatric disorders. Medication is the dominant treatment used by psychiatrists, although psychotherapy and other psychosocial interventions continue to be used.
- **Psychologists** practice under state regulations and hold doctor of philosophy in psychology degrees (which differ from doctor of medicine). Their expertise lies in evaluation, psychological testing, psychotherapy, and counseling. Some states may allow prescriptive authority for psychologists.
- **Social workers** are licensed by the state and enter general practice with a bachelor's degree in social work, or pursue advanced practice with a master's in social work. They may provide counseling and plan for supportive services such as housing, health care, and treatment after the patient is returned to the community.
- **Counselors** possess a master's degree in psychology, counseling, or a related field and are licensed by the state. They are trained to diagnose and provide individual and group counseling.

- **Occupational therapists** are usually state regulated and are prepared at the bachelor's, master's, or doctoral level. They assist individuals to develop or regain independent living skills, activities of daily living, and role performance that have been affected by mental disorders.
- **Physical therapists** possess master's or doctoral degrees and are accredited by the state. Their role is to rehabilitate individuals with physical disabilities that may be present concurrent with psychiatric disabilities.
- **Art therapists** are prepared at the master's level in art therapy and registered through a professional association. They use art to help people understand their problems, enhance healthy development, and reduce the effects of their illnesses.
- **Recreation therapists** are typically bachelor's prepared and may be licensed by the state or be nationally certified. Recreational activities are used to improve emotional, physical, cognitive, and social well-being.
- **Pharmacists** are state licensed and are prepared through six years of secondary education for a Doctor of Pharmacy (PharmD). They provide distribution and centralized monitoring of drug regimens.
- **Medical personnel** are physicians whose focus is the provision of nonpsychiatric care for comorbid conditions.
- **Mental health workers** or psychiatric aides are nonprofessional staff who may be state certified. They have extensive contact with patients while assisting with hygiene and meals and while participating in unit activities. Mental health workers communicate important information concerning the patient's condition to professional staff.
- **Pastoral counselors** are clergy who have clinical pastoral education and are certified through a the American Association of Pastoral Counselors. They provide individual and group counseling.

Inpatient rooms are usually less institutional looking than other hospital rooms and tend to resemble hotel rooms. Showers may be in the individual rooms or dorm-style, with one or two per hallway. Rooms are private, semiprivate, or occasionally, wards. Units may be made up solely of males or of females, or may be coed. Rooms are designed with safety in mind. Hanging is the most common method of inpatient suicide, therefore strict measures are taken to prevent it. Closet rods and hooks, towel bars, and shower rods are constructed to break if subjected to more than a minimal amount of weight. Sprinkler and shower heads tend to be flush mounted, and utility pipes are enclosed. Other safety measures include locked windows, platform beds rather than mechanical hospital beds to prevent possible crushing, and furniture with rounded corners to reduce intentional injury. Furniture for inpatient rooms tends to be heavy and durable so that it cannot be thrown or dismantled and used as a weapon.

Inpatient care begins with a medical assessment to rule out or consider **comorbid conditions**. Comprehensive assessments are conducted by a multidisciplinary team, and a plan of care is developed, monitored, evaluated, and refined. Crisis intervention and stabilization and keeping the patient safe are goals of inpatient care. Psychotropic medication evaluation, prescription, and management are usually part of the plan of care, as is individual therapy. Electroconvulsive therapy (ECT) may be ordered for certain conditions, particularly people with depression who have been unresponsive to antidepressants.

Typical Items Included in Hospital Statements of a Patient's Rights

- Right to be treated with dignity
- Right to be involved in treatment planning and decisions
- Right to refuse treatment, including medications
- Right to request to leave the hospital, even against medical advice
- Right to be protected against the possible impulse to harm oneself or others that might occur as a result of a mental disorder
- Right to the benefit of the legally prescribed process of an evaluation occurring within a limited period (in most states, 72 hours) in the event of a request for discharge against medical advice that may lead to harm to self or others
- Right to legal counsel
- Right to vote
- Right to communicate privately by telephone and in person

- Right to informed consent
- Right to confidentiality regarding one's disorder and treatment
- Right to choose or refuse visitors
- Right to be informed of research and to refuse to participate
- Right to the least restrictive means of treatment
- Right to send and receive mail and to be present during any inspection of packages received
- Right to keep personal belongings unless they are dangerous
- Right to lodge a complaint through a plainly publicized procedure
- Right to participate in religious worship

Group therapy is an important facet of inpatient care. Coping skills are taught and enhanced through cognitive-behavioral groups that focus on symptom management. Occupational therapy provides an opportunity to practice life skills that have been delayed, hampered, or eroded. Psychoeducational groups focus on specific psychiatric disorders, medication, goal-setting, life planning, and recovery.

Length of stay varies depending on the severity of the illness and symptoms. For example, a patient admitted to the hospital on an emergency basis (PEC) typically stays about 14 days, whereas a person admitted for detoxification usually stays for 3 to 5 days. Therapeutic passes may be helpful so that the patient may go home for limited periods. In some cases, especially with children and people with severe mental illness, privileges and rewards, such as recreational outings, walks on the hospital grounds, and tokens to buy items from a unit "store" may be earned in order to reinforce adaptive behaviors.

Discharge planning begins on the first day of admission based on the patient's unique needs. Case management and collaboration with the patient's outpatient clinician, PCP, family, and community agencies such as the visiting nurse agency facilitate an integrated approach and establish comprehensive transition plans from inpatient to the community setting. This allows the patient to live effectively and safely in the community. Effective case management and collaboration also reduce recidivism.

At discharge, patients should be stabilized. Discharge instructions include follow-up appointments, medication directions, education and prescriptions, and, if necessary,

assistance with living arrangements that may include a private residence, shelter, halfway house, or group home.

Crisis care is provided in emergency departments of general hospitals or in community-based *crisis intervention centers*. Crisis care may be initiated by the individual, friends, family, health care provider, or law enforcement personnel. Some patients are involuntarily committed. Psychiatric emergencies may include suicidal (or homicidal) ideation, acute psychosis, or behavioral responses to drugs. The stay in such facilities tends to be short, usually less than 24 hours. At that point the patient may be discharged to home, referred for inpatient care, or transferred to another community facility such as a shelter.

Residential treatment programs are structured short- or long-term living environments in which individuals are provided with varying levels of supervision and support. The residents also learn to access community support as an alternative to hospitalization and are encouraged to achieve maximal independence.

State Acute Care System

Today's state-operated psychiatric hospitals are an extension of what remains of the old system, although the quality of care in state hospitals has improved dramatically. The clinical role of state hospitals is to serve the most seriously ill patients, but this role varies widely, depending on available levels of community care and on payments by state Medicaid programs. In some states, state hospitals primarily provide intermediate treatment for patients unable to be stabilized in short-term general hospital units, and long-term care for individuals judged too ill for community care. In other states the emphasis is on acute care that is reflective of gaps in the private sector, especially for the uninsured or for those who have exhausted limited insurance benefits.

In most states the state hospitals provide forensic (court-related) care and monitoring as part of their function for those found not guilty by reason of insanity (NGRI). The state or county system also advises the courts as to defendants' sanity who may be judged to have been so ill when they committed the criminal act that they cannot be held responsible, but require treatment instead. One tragic example is that of Andrea Yates, the Texas woman who drowned her five young children under the delusional belief she was saving them. She was found NGRI and was committed to a Texas state psychiatric facility.

General Hospital Psychiatric Units and Private Psychiatric Hospital Acute Care

Acute-care general hospital psychiatric units tend to be housed on a floor or floors of a general hospital. Private psychiatric hospitals are free-standing facilities. As noted, the dramatic growth of acute care psychiatric hospitals and hospital units is the result of a shift away from institutionalization in state-run hospitals. Since that time, reduced reimbursement, managed care, enhanced outpatient options, and expanded availability of outpatient and partial hospitalization programs have resulted in the steady decline of these facilities (Garritson, 1999). Average length of stay has been steadily declining to about 9.5 days (National Association of Psychiatric Health Systems, 2006).

Role of Psychiatric Nurses in Inpatient Care Settings

As the 24-hour-a-day, 7-days-a-week professional care component, nurses are at the center of any acute care inpatient facility. Management of these units, ideally, is by nurses with backgrounds in psychiatric mental health nursing, preferably with advanced-practice degrees. Staff nurses tend to be nurse generalists, that is, nurses who have basic training as registered nurses, and some may have achieved national certification in psychiatric mental health nursing. The staff psychiatric registered nurse carries out the following nursing responsibilities:

- Completion of comprehensive data collection that includes the patient, family, and other health care workers

- Developing, implementing, and evaluating plans of care
- Assisting or supervising mental health care workers (nursing assistants with or without additional training in working with people who have mental illnesses)
- Maintaining a safe environment and therapeutic environment
- Facilitating health promotion through teaching
- Monitoring behavior, affect, and mood
- Oversight of restraint and seclusion
- Coordination of care by the treatment team

Medication management is an essential skill for psychiatric nurses. In this specialty area nurses often exert a strong influence on medication decisions because continual observation of the expected, interactive effects, and adverse effects of medications provide the data necessary for medication adjustment. For example, feedback about a patient's excessive sedation or increased agitation will lead to a decision to decrease or increase the dosage of an antipsychotic medication.

A common misperception regarding psychiatric nurses in acute care settings is that because they "just talk" they lose their skills, including physical tasks such as starting and maintaining intravenous (IV) lines and changing dressings. First, therapeutic communication itself is a skill that people are not born with and must learn. Second, patients on the psychiatric unit are not limited to *DSM-IV-TR* diagnoses and often have complex health care needs. For example, an older adult male with brittle diabetes and a recent foot amputation may become actively suicidal. In this case, it is likely he will be transferred to the psychiatric unit, where his blood sugar will be monitored and wound care completed.

SPECIALTY TREATMENT SETTINGS

Treatment options are available that provide specialized care for specific groups of people. These options include inpatient, outpatient, and residential care.

Pediatric Psychiatric Care

Children with mental illnesses have the same range of treatment options as do adults but receive them apart from adults in pediatric settings. Inpatient care may be necessary if the child's symptoms become severe. Parental or guardian—including Department of Children and Families—involvement in the plan of care is integral so that they understand the illness, treatment, and the family's role in supporting the child. Additionally, hospitalized children, if able, attend school several hours a day.

Geriatric Psychiatric Care

The older adult population may be treated in specialized mental health settings that take into account the effects of aging on psychiatric symptoms. Physical illness and loss of independence can be strong precipitants in the development of depression and anxiety. Dementia is a particularly common problem encountered in geriatric psychiatry. Treatment is aimed at careful evaluation of the interaction of mind and body and providing care that optimizes strengths, promotes independence, and focuses on safety.

Veterans Administration Centers

Active military personnel and veterans who were not dishonorably discharged may receive federally funded inpatient or outpatient care and medication for psychiatric and alcohol or substance abuse. Mental health services are especially important to veterans who have undergone the stress of combat because research suggests they have about twice the incidence of generalized anxiety disorder, panic disorder, and posttraumatic stress disorder compared with veterans who were not deployed (Black et al., 2004).

Forensic Psychiatric Care

Incarcerated populations, both adult and juvenile, have higher than average incidences of mental disorders or substance abuse. Researchers estimate that nearly 24% of the prison population has a severe mental illness (Lamb & Weinberger, 2005). Treatment may be provided within the prison system, where inmates are often separated from the general prison population. State hospitals also treat forensic patients. Most facilities provide psychotherapy, group counseling, medication management, and assistance with transition to the community.

Alcohol and Drug Abuse Treatment

All the mental health settings that were previously described may provide treatment for alcohol and substance abuse, although specialized treatment centers exist apart from the mental health care system. Alcohol treatment is provided to more than 700,000 Americans each day (National Institute on Alcohol Abuse and Alcoholism, 2000). This treatment is typically outpatient and includes counseling, education, medication management, and 12-step programs. Because alcohol detoxification can be life-threatening, inpatient care may be required for medical management. Drug rehabilitation facilities provide inpatient care for detoxification of drugs, including opiates and chemicals, and offer all levels of outpatient care.

Self-Help Options

Getting a good night's sleep, meditating, eating right, exercising, abstaining from smoking, and limiting the use of alcohol are healthy responses to a variety of illnesses such as diabetes and hypertension. As with other medical conditions, lifestyle choices and self-help responses can have a profound influence on the quality of life and the course, progression, and outcome of psychiatric disorders. If we accept the notion that psychiatric disorders are usually a combination of chemistry, genetics, and environment, then it stands to reason that by providing a healthy living situation, we are likely to fare better. If, for example, a person has a family history of anxiety who has demonstrated symptoms of anxiety, then a good first step (or an adjunct to psychiatric treatment) could be to take up yoga and balance the amounts of life's obligations with relaxation.

A voluntary network of self-help groups operates outside the formal mental health care system to provide education, contacts, and support. Since the introduction of Alcoholics Anonymous in the early 20th century, self-help groups have multiplied and have proven to be effective in the treatment and support of psychiatric problems. Groups specific to anxiety, depression, loss, caretakers' issues, bipolar disorder, posttraumatic stress disorder, and most every other psychiatric issue are widely available in most communities.

Consumers, people who use mental health services, and their family members have successfully joined together to shape the delivery of mental health care. Nonprofit organizations such as the National Alliance on Mental Illness (NAMI) encourage self-help and promote the concept of **recovery,** or the self-management of mental illness. These grassroots groups also confront social stigma, influence policies, and support the rights of people experiencing mental illness.

PAYING FOR MENTAL HEALTH CARE

Most Americans are covered by private insurance that pays varying amounts for mental health care. Standard policies allow people to choose their providers, seek treatment, and provide some portion of reimbursement. Managed care plans stipulate which providers members may visit and then may cover the entire costs or require copays from the members. Low-income Medicaid and Medicare recipients may also be enrolled in managed care plans. Both standard policies and managed care plans provide coverage for mental health care, although it is often not at the same rate as is coverage for physical care.

Limits in health insurance are problematic in terms of coverage for mental illnesses. Because most health insurance is employer based and because serious mental illness can lead to job loss, many individuals with serious mental illness have no coverage. State systems exist, in part, as a "safety net" for the limits in health insurance. Furthermore, most private insurance plans (along with Medicare) have had coverage limits that are more restrictive for treatment of mental illness than other illnesses with annual or lifetime caps on days of care or on total expenses.

In 1996, the federal government enacted a **mental health parity** law that made it illegal for companies with more than 50 employees to limit annual or lifetime mental health benefits unless they also limited benefits for physical illnesses. Although this federal legislation was a good start, problems remain. One problem is that reimbursement does not include substance abuse or chemical dependency treatment. Another is that insurers and employers have gotten around the law by limiting the number of treatment sessions, and by charging higher copayments and deductibles. Mental health advocates and providers have responded by pushing for state legislation to shore up the gaps in the federal bill. By 2008, 5 states had adopted parity laws that prohibited exemptions or limitations under private insurance plans for mental health and substance abuse disorders, 33 states had at least limited parity laws, and 13 states had no mental health parity laws (Mental Health America, 2008).

In addition to the state systems of care, public assistance is available for mental health care and costs of living. Four assistance programs are Medicare, Medicaid, Social Security, and the Veterans Administration (VA). Medicare is a national program that provides benefits to those who are 65 years of age or older and to those who have become totally disabled. In the case of mental illness, benefits are limited and coverage may be 50% for outpatient care compared with 80% for non-mental health outpatient care. Medicaid operates under federal guidelines and state regulations and pays mental health care costs for people who have extreme financial need.

States vary widely in how they fund mental health care, but all states must provide benefits for inpatient care, PCP services, and treatment for those younger than age 21. Social Security has two federal programs designed to help people with disabilities. Social Security Disability Insurance (SSDI) may be awarded to individuals who have worked a required length of time, have paid into Social Security, and are disabled for 12 months or more. Supplemental Security Income (SSI) provides benefits based on economic need (Social Security Administration, 2002). More than 60% of children and more than 50% of adults on SSI have brain disorders (mental illness, disability, or both) and the cost of providing disability benefits is projected to escalate rapidly during the next 20 years (Depression and Bipolar Support Alliance, 2006).

A VISION FOR MENTAL HEALTH CARE IN AMERICA

Despite the availability and variety of community psychiatric treatments in the United States, many patients in this country in need of services are not receiving them. In addition to stigma, there are geographic, financial, and systems factors that impede access to psychiatric care. For example, mental health services are scarce in some rural areas, and many American families cannot afford health insurance even if they are working. The President's New Freedom Commission on Mental Health was charged with studying the mental health system and issuing recommendations for its transformation (2003). It is likely that their recommendations will influence the direction of mental health care for the next two decades. Their final report identifies that in a transformed mental health care system:

- Americans understand that mental health is essential to overall health.
- Mental health care is consumer and family driven.
- Disparities in mental health services are eliminated.
- Early mental health screening, assessment, and referral to services are common practice.
- Excellent mental health care is delivered and research is accelerated.
- Technology is used to access mental health care and information.

Psychiatric registered nurses are uniquely qualified to address each of the aforementioned goals by virtue of an integrated educational background that includes biology, psychology, and the social sciences. Nurses specializing in this area will increasingly be in demand. As the population ages, more geropsychiatric nurses will be needed to work with older adult psychiatric patients with complex health problems (Hedelin & Svensson, 1999). Advanced-practice psychiatric nurses may collaborate more with primary health care practitioners or in independent practice to fill the gap in existing community services (Walker et al., 2000). Psychiatric nurses can help make the vision statement from the President's New Freedom Commission on Mental Health (2003) a reality:

We envision a future when everyone with a mental illness will recover, a future when mental illnesses can be prevented or cured, a future when mental illnesses are detected early, and a future when everyone with a mental illness at any stage of life has access to effective treatment supports—essentials for living, working, learning, and participating fully in the community.

KEY POINTS TO REMEMBER

- As compared to seeking care for physical disorders, finding care for psychiatric disorders can be complicated by a two-tiered system of care provided in the private and public sectors.
- Nonspecialist primary care providers treat a significant portion of psychiatric disorders.
- Psychiatric care providers are specialists who are licensed to prescribe medication and conduct therapy. They include psychiatrists, advanced-practice psychiatric nurses, physicians' assistants, and in some states, psychologists.
- Community mental health centers are state-regulated and state-funded facilities that are staffed by a variety of mental health care professionals.
- Other outpatient settings include psychiatric home care, intensive outpatient programs, and partial hospitalization programs.

- Inpatient care is used when less restrictive outpatient options are insufficient in dealing with symptoms. It can be provided in general medical centers, private psychiatric centers, crisis units, and state hospitals.
- Nurses provide the basis for inpatient care and are part of the overall unit milieu that emphasizes the role of the total environment in providing support and treatment.
- Specific populations such as children, veterans, geriatrics, and forensics benefit from treatment geared to their unique needs.
- Financing psychiatric care has been complicated by lack of parity, or equal payment for physical as compared to psychiatric disorders. Legislation has been proposed and passed to improve mental health parity.

CRITICAL THINKING

1. You are a community psychiatric mental health nurse working at a local mental health center. You are doing an assessment interview with a single male patient who is 45 years old. He reports that he has not been sleeping and that his thoughts seem to be "all tangled up." He informs you that he hopes you can help him today because he does not know how much longer he can go on. He does not make any direct reference to suicidal intent. He is disheveled and has been sleeping at shelters. He has little contact with his family and starts to become agitated when you suggest that it might be helpful for you to contact them. He refuses to sign any release of information forms. He admits to recent hospitalization at the local veterans' hospital and reports previous treatment at a dual-diagnosis facility even though he denies substance abuse. In addition to his mental health problems,

he says that he has tested positive for human immunodeficiency virus and takes multiple medications that he cannot name.
   A. What are your biopsychosocial and spiritual concerns about this patient?
   B. What is the highest-priority problem to address before he leaves the clinic today?
   C. Do you feel that you need to consult with any other members of the multidisciplinary team today about this patient?
   D. In your role as case manager, what systems of care will you need to coordinate to provide quality care for this patient?
   E. How will you start to develop trust with the patient to gain his cooperation with the treatment plan?

CHAPTER REVIEW

Choose the most appropriate answer(s).

1. The presence of which symptom will exert the greatest pressure to admit an individual to an inpatient psychiatric unit?
   1. Suicidal ideation
   2. Moderate anxiety
   3. Feelings of sadness
   4. Auditory hallucinations
2. A significant influence allowing psychiatric treatment to move from the hospital to the community was:
   1. television.
   2. the development of psychotropic medication.
   3. identification of external causes of mental illness.

   4. the use of a collaborative approach by patients and staff focusing on rehabilitation.
3. Which of the following is a benefit for patients being treated for mental health problems by a primary care physician rather than a psychiatrist?
   1. A high level of expertise in the diagnosis of psychiatric disorders
   2. Extended time in the physician's office for a thorough psychiatric assessment
   3. Feeling that there is less stigma attached to treatment
   4. A high level of expertise in the management of psychopharmacological medications for psychiatric illnesses

CHAPTER REVIEW—cont'd

4. Of the following services, which are routinely provided by community mental health centers? Select all that apply.
   1. Assessment and diagnosis
   2. Medication management
   3. Vocational and employment services
   4. Emergency community disaster relief

5. A community mental health student nurse is asked by her supervisor to develop a stress reduction class for the residents in the surrounding community. The student nurse resists, saying that her responsibilities are to her patient caseload. The supervisor explains to the student why this assignment is appropriate for her role. Which is the most suitable rationale that the supervisor can provide to the student nurse?
   1. Stress reduction is important to a patient's mental health.
   2. Funding sources will support the class only if it is developed by a nurse.
   3. An important concept for community health nursing is to view the entire community as a patient.
   4. Research has demonstrated that stress reduction reduces hypertension in mental health patients.

REFERENCES

Black, D.W., Carney, C.P., Peloso, P.M., et al. (2004). Gulf War veterans with anxiety: Prevalence, comorbidity, and risk factors. *Epidemiology, 15,* 135-142.

Depression and Bipolar Support Alliance. (2006). *The state of depression in America.* Chicago: Author.

Garritson, S.H. (1999). Availability and performance of psychiatric acute care facilities in California from 1992-1996. *Psychiatric Services, 50,* 1453-1460.

Hedelin, B., & Svensson, P.G. (1999). Psychiatric nursing for promotion of mental health and prevention of depression in the elderly: A case study. *Journal of psychiatric and mental health nursing, 6*(2), 115-124.

Kessler, R.C., Berglund, P., Demler, O., et al. (2005). Lifetime prevalence and age-of-onset distributions of *DSM-IV* disorders in the national comorbidity survey replication. *Archives of General Psychiatry, 62,* 593-602.

Lamb, H.R., & Weinberger, L.E. (2005). The shift of psychiatric inpatient care from hospitals to jails and prisons. *Journal of the American Academy of Psychiatric Law, 33,* 529-534.

Mental Health America (2008). *What have states done to ensure insurance parity?* Retrieved February 18, 2008, from www.mentalhealthamerica.net/go/parity/states.

National Association of Psychiatric Health Systems. (2006, April 12). News release: *New NAPHS Annual Survey tracks behavioral treatment trends.* Retrieved February 18, 2008, from www.naphs.org/News/documents/Annualsurvey2005.pdf.

National Institute on Alcohol Abuse and Alcoholism. (2000). *10th special report to the U.S. Congress on alcohol and health* (NIH Pub No. 00-1583). Bethesda, MD: Author.

Patterson, J., Peek, C.J., Heinrich, R.L., et al. (2002). *Mental health professionals in medical settings: A primer.* New York: Norton.

President's New Freedom Commission on Mental Health. (2003). *Achieving the promise: Transforming mental health care in America.* Retrieved February 18, 2008, from www.mentalhealthcommission.gov/reports/FinalReport/toc.html.

Social Security Administration. (2002). *Benefits for people with disabilities.* Retrieved October 16, 2007, from www.ssa.gov/disability.

Walker, L., Barker, P., & Pearson, P. (2000). The required role of the psychiatric-mental health nurse in primary healthcare: An augmented Delphi study. *Nursing Inquiry, 7*(2), 91-102.

DSM-IV-TR Classification

NOS, Not Otherwise Specified.

An *x* appearing in a diagnostic code indicates that a specific code number is required.

Ellipses (. . .) are used in the names of certain disorders to indicate that the name of a specific mental disorder or general medical condition should be inserted when recording the name (e.g., 293.0 Delirium Due to Hypothyroidism).

If criteria are currently met, one of the following severity specifiers may be noted after the diagnosis:
Mild
Moderate
Severe

If criteria are no longer met, one of the following specifiers may be noted:
In Partial Remission
In Full Remission
Prior History

DISORDERS USUALLY FIRST DIAGNOSED IN INFANCY, CHILDHOOD, OR ADOLESCENCE

Mental Retardation

NOTE: These are coded on Axis II.

317   Mild Mental Retardation

From American Psychiatric Association. (2000). *Diagnostic and statistical manual of mental disorders, Fourth Edition, Text Revision (DSM-IV-TR)*. Washington, DC: Author.

318.0   Moderate Mental Retardation
318.1   Severe Mental Retardation
318.2   Profound Mental Retardation
319   Mental Retardation, Severity Unspecified

Learning Disorders

315.00 Reading Disorder
315.1   Mathematics Disorder
315.2   Disorder of Written Expression
315.9   Learning Disorder NOS

Motor Skills Disorder

315.4   Developmental Coordination Disorder

Communication Disorders

315.31 Expressive Language Disorder
315.32 Mixed Receptive-Expressive Language Disorder
315.39 Phonologic Disorder
307.0   Stuttering
307.9   Communication Disorder NOS

Pervasive Developmental Disorders

299.00 Autistic Disorder
299.80 Rett's Disorder
299.10 Childhood Disintegrative Disorder
299.80 Asperger's Disorder
299.80 Pervasive Developmental Disorder NOS

Attention-Deficit and Disruptive Behavior Disorders

314.xx   Attention-Deficit/Hyperactivity Disorder
.01   Combined Type
.00   Predominantly Inattentive Type
.01   Predominantly Hyperactive-Impulsive Type
314.9   Attention-Deficit/Hyperactivity Disorder NOS
312.xx   Conduct Disorder
.81   Childhood-Onset Type
.82   Adolescent-Onset Type
.89   Unspecified Onset
313.81   Oppositional Defiant Disorder
312.9   Disruptive Behavior Disorder NOS

Feeding and Eating Disorders of Infancy or Early Childhood

307.52   Pica
307.53   Rumination Disorder
307.59   Feeding Disorder of Infancy or Early Childhood

Tic Disorders

307.23   Tourette's Disorder
307.22   Chronic Motor or Vocal Tic Disorder
307.21   Transient Tic Disorder
         Specify if: Single Episode/Recurrent
307.20   Tic Disorder NOS

Elimination Disorders

___._   Encopresis
787.6   With Constipation and Overflow Incontinence
307.7   Without Constipation and Overflow Incontinence
307.6   Enuresis (Not Due to a General Medical Condition)
         Specify type: Nocturnal Only/Diurnal Only/Nocturnal and Diurnal

Other Disorders of Infancy, Childhood, or Adolescence

309.21   Separation Anxiety Disorder
         Specify if: Early Onset
313.23   Selective Mutism
313.89   Reactive Attachment Disorder of Infancy or Early Childhood
         Specify type: Inhibited Type/Disinhibited Type
307.3   Stereotypic Movement Disorder
         Specify if: With Self-Injurious Behavior

313.9   Disorder of Infancy, Childhood, or Adolescence NOS

DELIRIUM, DEMENTIA, AND AMNESTIC AND OTHER COGNITIVE DISORDERS
Delirium

293.0   Delirium Due to . . . *[Indicate the General Medical Condition]*
___._   Substance Intoxication Delirium *(refer to Substance-Related Disorders for substance-specific codes)*
___._   Substance Withdrawal Delirium *(refer to Substance-Related Disorders for substance-specific codes)*
___._   Delirium Due to Multiple Etiologies *(code each of the specific etiologies)*
780.09   Delirium NOS

Dementia

294.xx   Dementia of the Alzheimer's Type, With Early Onset *(also code 331.0 Alzheimer's disease on Axis III)*
.10   Without Behavioral Disturbance
.11   With Behavioral Disturbance
294.xx   Dementia of the Alzheimer's Type, With Late Onset *(also code 331.0 Alzheimer's disease on Axis III)*
.10   Without Behavioral Disturbance
.11   With Behavioral Disturbance
290.xx   Vascular Dementia
.40   Uncomplicated
.41   With Delirium
.42   With Delusions
.43   With Depressed Mood
         Specify if: With Behavioral Disturbance
Code presence or absence of a behavioral disturbance in the fifth digit for Dementia Due to a General Medical Condition:
0 =   Without Behavioral Disturbance
1 =   With Behavioral Disturbance
294.1x   Dementia Due to HIV Disease *(also code 042 HIV on Axis III)*
294.1x   Dementia Due to Head Trauma *(also code 854.00 head injury on Axis III)*
294.1x   Dementia Due to Parkinson's Disease *(also code 332.0 Parkinson's disease on Axis III)*
294.1x   Dementia Due to Huntington's Disease *(also code 333.4 Huntington's disease on Axis III)*

294.1x   Dementia Due to Pick's Disease *(also code 331.1 Pick's disease on Axis III)*

294.1x   Dementia Due to Creutzfeldt-Jakob Disease *(also code 046.1 Creutzfeldt-Jakob disease on Axis III)*

294.1x   Dementia Due to . . . *[Indicate the General Medical Condition not listed above] (also code the general medical condition on Axis III)*

___.__   Substance-Induced Persisting Dementia *(refer to Substance-Related Disorders for substance-specific codes)*

___.__   Dementia Due to Multiple Etiologies *(code each of the specific etiologies)*

294.8   Dementia NOS

Amnestic Disorders

294.0   Amnestic Disorder Due to . . . *[Indicate the General Medical Condition]*
        Specify if: Transient/Chronic

___.__   Substance-Induced Persisting Amnestic Disorder *(refer to Substance-Related Disorders for substance-specific codes)*

294.8   Amnestic Disorder NOS

Other Cognitive Disorders

294.9   Cognitive Disorder NOS

MENTAL DISORDERS DUE TO A GENERAL MEDICAL CONDITION NOT ELSEWHERE CLASSIFIED

293.89   Catatonic Disorder Due to . . . *[Indicate the General Medical Condition]*

310.1   Personality Change Due to . . . *[Indicate the General Medical Condition]*
        Specify type: Labile Type/Disinhibited Type/Aggressive Type/Apathetic Type/Paranoid Type/Other Type/Combined Type/Unspecified Type

293.9   Mental Disorder NOS Due to . . . *[Indicate the General Medical Condition]*

SUBSTANCE-RELATED DISORDERS

The following specifiers may be applied to Substance Dependence as noted:
   [a]With Physiologic Dependence/Without Physiologic Dependence

[b]Early Full Remission/Early Partial Remission/Sustained Full Remission/Sustained Partial Remission
[c]In a Controlled Environment
[d]On Agonist Therapy
The following specifiers apply to Substance-Induced Disorders as noted:
   [I]With Onset During Intoxication/[W]With Onset During Withdrawal

Alcohol-Related Disorders

Alcohol Use Disorders
303.90   Alcohol Dependence[a,b,c]
305.00   Alcohol Abuse

Alcohol-Induced Disorders
303.00   Alcohol Intoxication
291.81   Alcohol Withdrawal
         Specify if: With Perceptual Disturbances
291.0   Alcohol Intoxication Delirium
291.0   Alcohol Withdrawal Delirium
291.2   Alcohol-Induced Persisting Dementia
291.1   Alcohol-Induced Persisting Amnestic Disorder
291.x   Alcohol-Induced Psychotic Disorder
   .5   With Delusions[I,W]
   .3   With Hallucinations[I,W]
291.89   Alcohol-Induced Mood Disorder[I,W]
291.89   Alcohol-Induced Anxiety Disorder[I,W]
291.89   Alcohol-Induced Sexual Dysfunction[I]
291.89   Alcohol-Induced Sleep Disorder[I,W]
291.9   Alcohol-Related Disorder NOS

Amphetamine (or Amphetamine-Like)–Related Disorders

Amphetamine Use Disorders
304.40   Amphetamine Dependence[a,b,c]
305.70   Amphetamine Abuse

Amphetamine-Induced Disorders
292.89   Amphetamine Intoxication
         Specify if: With Perceptual Disturbances
292.0   Amphetamine Withdrawal
292.81   Amphetamine Intoxication Delirium
292.xx   Amphetamine-Induced Psychotic Disorder
   .11   With Delusions[I]
   .12   With Hallucinations[I]
292.84   Amphetamine-Induced Mood Disorder[I,W]
292.89   Amphetamine-Induced Anxiety Disorder[I]

292.89   Amphetamine-Induced Sexual Dysfunction[I]
292.89   Amphetamine-Induced Sleep Disorder[I,W]
292.9   Amphetamine-Related Disorder NOS

Caffeine-Related Disorders

Caffeine-Induced Disorders

305.90   Caffeine Intoxication
292.89   Caffeine-Induced Anxiety Disorder[I]
292.89   Caffeine-Induced Sleep Disorder[I]
292.9   Caffeine-Related Disorder NOS

Cannabis-Related Disorders

Cannabis Use Disorders

304.30   Cannabis Dependence[a,b,c]
305.20   Cannabis Abuse

Cannabis-Induced Disorders

292.89   Cannabis Intoxication
         Specify if: With Perceptual Disturbances
292.81   Cannabis Intoxication Delirium
292.xx   Cannabis-Induced Psychotic Disorder
   .11   With Delusions[I]
   .12   With Hallucinations[I]
292.89   Cannabis-Induced Anxiety Disorder[I]
292.9   Cannabis-Related Disorder NOS

Cocaine-Related Disorders

Cocaine Use Disorders

304.20   Cocaine Dependence[a,b,c]
305.60   Cocaine Abuse

Cocaine-Induced Disorders

292.89   Cocaine Intoxication
         Specify if: With Perceptual Disturbances
292.0   Cocaine Withdrawal
292.81   Cocaine Intoxication Delirium
292.xx   Cocaine-Induced Psychotic Disorder
   .11   With Delusions[I]
   .12   With Hallucinations[I]
292.84   Cocaine-Induced Mood Disorder[I,W]
292.89   Cocaine-Induced Anxiety Disorder[I,W]
292.89   Cocaine-Induced Sexual Dysfunction[I]
292.89   Cocaine-Induced Sleep Disorder[I,W]
292.9   Cocaine-Related Disorder NOS

Hallucinogen-Related Disorders

Hallucinogen Use Disorders

304.50   Hallucinogen Dependence[b,c]
305.30   Hallucinogen Abuse

Hallucinogen-Induced Disorders

292.89   Hallucinogen Intoxication
292.89   Hallucinogen Persisting Perception Disorder
         (Flashbacks)
292.81   Hallucinogen Intoxication Delirium
292.xx   Hallucinogen-Induced Psychotic Disorder
   .11   With Delusions[I]
   .12   With Hallucinations[I]
292.84   Hallucinogen-Induced Mood Disorder[I]
292.89   Hallucinogen-Induced Anxiety Disorder[I]
292.9   Hallucinogen-Related Disorder NOS

Inhalant-Related Disorders

Inhalant Use Disorders

304.60   Inhalant Dependence[b,c]
305.90   Inhalant Abuse

Inhalant-Induced Disorders

292.89   Inhalant Intoxication
292.81   Inhalant Intoxication Delirium
292.82   Inhalant-Induced Persisting Dementia
292.xx   Inhalant-Induced Psychotic Disorder
   .11   With Delusions[I]
   .12   With Hallucinations[I]
292.84   Inhalant-Induced Mood Disorder[I]
292.89   Inhalant-Induced Anxiety Disorder[I]
292.9   Inhalant-Related Disorder NOS

Nicotine-Related Disorders

Nicotine Use Disorder

305.1   Nicotine Dependence[a,b]

Nicotine-Induced Disorder

292.0   Nicotine Withdrawal
292.9   Nicotine-Related Disorder NOS

Opioid-Related Disorders

Opioid Use Disorders

304.00   Opioid Dependence[a,b,c,d]
305.50   Opioid Abuse

Opioid-Induced Disorders

292.89   Opioid Intoxication
         Specify if: With Perceptual Disturbances

292.0	Opioid Withdrawal	
292.81	Opioid Intoxication Delirium	
292.xx	Opioid-Induced Psychotic Disorder	
.11	With Delusions[I]	
.12	With Hallucinations[I]	
292.84	Opioid-Induced Mood Disorder[I]	
292.89	Opioid-Induced Sexual Dysfunction[I]	
292.89	Opioid-Induced Sleep Disorder[I,W]	
292.9	Opioid-Related Disorder NOS	

Phencyclidine (or Phencyclidine-Like)–Related Disorders

Phencyclidine Use Disorders

304.60   Phencyclidine Dependence[b,c]
305.90   Phencyclidine Abuse

Phencyclidine-Induced Disorders

292.89   Phencyclidine Intoxication
         Specify if: With Perceptual Disturbances
292.81   Phencyclidine Intoxication Delirium
292.xx   Phencyclidine-Induced Psychotic Disorder
   .11   With Delusions[I]
   .12   With Hallucinations[I]
292.84   Phencyclidine-Induced Mood Disorder[I]
292.89   Phencyclidine-Induced Anxiety Disorder[I]
292.9   Phencyclidine-Related Disorder NOS

Sedative-, Hypnotic-, or Anxiolytic-Related Disorders

Sedative, Hypnotic, or Anxiolytic Use Disorders

304.10   Sedative, Hypnotic, or Anxiolytic Dependence[a,b,c]
305.40   Sedative, Hypnotic, or Anxiolytic Abuse

Sedative-, Hypnotic-, or Anxiolytic-Induced Disorders

292.89   Sedative, Hypnotic, or Anxiolytic Intoxication
292.0   Sedative, Hypnotic, or Anxiolytic Withdrawal
         Specify if: With Perceptual Disturbances
292.81   Sedative, Hypnotic, or Anxiolytic Intoxication Delirium
292.81   Sedative, Hypnotic, or Anxiolytic Withdrawal Delirium
292.82   Sedative-, Hypnotic-, or Anxiolytic-Induced Persisting Dementia
292.83   Sedative-, Hypnotic-, or Anxiolytic-Induced Persisting Amnestic Disorder
292.xx   Sedative-, Hypnotic-, or Anxiolytic-Induced Psychotic Disorder

   .11   With Delusions[I,W]
   .12   With Hallucinations[I,W]
292.84   Sedative-, Hypnotic-, or Anxiolytic-Induced Mood Disorder[I,W]
292.89   Sedative-, Hypnotic-, or Anxiolytic-Induced Anxiety Disorder[W]
292.89   Sedative-, Hypnotic-, or Anxiolytic-Induced Sexual Dysfunction[I]
292.89   Sedative-, Hypnotic-, or Anxiolytic-Induced Sleep Disorder[I,W]
292.9   Sedative-, Hypnotic-, or Anxiolytic-Related Disorder NOS

Polysubstance-Related Disorder

304.80   Polysubstance Dependence[a,b,c,d]

Other (or Unknown) Substance–Related Disorders

Other (or Unknown) Substance Use Disorders

304.90   Other (or Unknown) Substance Dependence[a,b,c,d]
305.90   Other (or Unknown) Substance Abuse

Other (or Unknown) Substance–Induced Disorders

292.89   Other (or Unknown) Substance Intoxication
         Specify if: With Perceptual Disturbances
292.0   Other (or Unknown) Substance Withdrawal
         Specify if: With Perceptual Disturbances
292.81   Other (or Unknown) Substance–Induced Delirium
292.82   Other (or Unknown) Substance–Induced Persisting Dementia
292.83   Other (or Unknown) Substance–Induced Persisting Amnestic Disorder
292.xx   Other (or Unknown) Substance–Induced Psychotic Disorder
   .11   With Delusions[I,W]
   .12   With Hallucinations[I,W]
292.84   Other (or Unknown) Substance–Induced Mood Disorder[I,W]
292.89   Other (or Unknown) Substance–Induced Anxiety Disorder[I,W]
292.89   Other (or Unknown) Substance–Induced Sexual Dysfunction[I]
292.89   Other (or Unknown) Substance–Induced Sleep Disorder[I,W]
292.9   Other (or Unknown) Substance–Related Disorder NOS

SCHIZOPHRENIA AND OTHER PSYCHOTIC DISORDERS

295.xx   Schizophrenia

The following Classification of Longitudinal Course applies to all subtypes of Schizophrenia:

Episodic With Interepisode Residual Symptoms (*specify if:* With Prominent Negative Symptoms)/Episodic With No Interepisode Residual Symptoms

Continuous (*specify if:* With Prominent Negative Symptoms)

Single Episode in Partial Remission (*specify if:* With Prominent Negative Symptoms)/Single Episode in Full Remission

Other or Unspecified Pattern

.30   Paranoid Type

.10   Disorganized Type

.20   Catatonic Type

.90   Undifferentiated Type

.60   Residual Type

295.40   Schizophreniform Disorder
Specify if: Without Good Prognostic Features/With Good Prognostic Features

295.70   Schizoaffective Disorder
Specify type: Bipolar Type/Depressive Type

297.1   Delusional Disorder
Specify type: Erotomanic Type/Grandiose Type/Jealous Type/Persecutory Type/Somatic Type/Mixed Type/Unspecified Type

298.8   Brief Psychotic Disorder
Specify if: With Marked Stressor(s)/Without Marked Stressor(s)/With Postpartum Onset

297.3   Shared Psychotic Disorder

293.xx   Psychotic Disorder Due to . . . *[Indicate the General Medical Condition]*

.81   With Delusions

.82   With Hallucinations

___.__   Substance-Induced Psychotic Disorder *(refer to Substance-Related Disorders for substance-specific codes)*
Specify if: With Onset During Intoxication/With Onset During Withdrawal

298.9   Psychotic Disorder NOS

MOOD DISORDERS

Code current state of Major Depressive Disorder or Bipolar I Disorder in fifth digit:

1 = Mild

2 = Moderate

3 = Severe Without Psychotic Features

4 = Severe With Psychotic Features
Specify: Mood-Congruent Psychotic Features/Mood-Incongruent Psychotic Features

5 = In Partial Remission

6 = In Full Remission

0 = Unspecified

The following specifiers apply (for current or most recent episode) to Mood Disorders as noted:

[a]Severity/Psychotic/Remission Specifiers

[b]Chronic

[c]With Catatonic Features

[d]With Melancholic Features

[e]With Atypical Features

[f]With Postpartum Onset

The following specifiers apply to Mood Disorders as noted:

[g]With or Without Full Interepisode Recovery

[h]With Seasonal Pattern

[i]With Rapid Cycling

Depressive Disorders

296.xx   Major Depressive Disorder

.2x   Single Episode[a,b,c,d,e,f]

.3x   Recurrent[a,b,c,d,e,f,g,h]

300.4   Dysthymic Disorder
Specify if: Early Onset/Late Onset
Specify: With Atypical Features

311   Depressive Disorder NOS

Bipolar Disorders

296.xx   Bipolar I Disorder

.0x   Single Manic Episode[a,c,f]
Specify if: Mixed

.40   Most Recent Episode Hypomanic[g,h,i]

.4x   Most Recent Episode Manic[a,c,f,g,h,i]

.6x   Most Recent Episode Mixed[a,c,f,g,h,i]

.5x   Most Recent Episode Depressed[a,b,c,d,e,f,g,h,i]

.7   Most Recent Episode Unspecified[g,h,i]

296.89   Bipolar II Disorder[a,b,c,d,e,f,g,h,i]
Specify (current or most recent episode): Hypomanic/Depressed

301.13   Cyclothymic Disorder

296.80   Bipolar Disorder NOS

293.83   Mood Disorder Due to . . . *[Indicate the General Medical Condition]*
Specify type: With Depressive Features/With Major Depressive-Like Episode/With Manic Features/With Mixed Features

___.__   Substance-Induced Mood Disorder *(refer to Substance-Related Disorders for substance-specific codes)*

Specify type: With Depressive Features/With Manic Features/With Mixed Features
Specify if: With Onset During Intoxication/With Onset During Withdrawal

296.90 Mood Disorder NOS

ANXIETY DISORDERS

300.01 Panic Disorder Without Agoraphobia
300.21 Panic Disorder With Agoraphobia
300.22 Agoraphobia Without History of Panic Disorder
300.29 Specific Phobia
Specify type: Animal Type/Natural Environment Type/Blood-Injection-Injury Type/Situational Type/Other Type
300.23 Social Phobia
Specify if: Generalized
300.3 Obsessive-Compulsive Disorder
Specify if: With Poor Insight
309.81 Posttraumatic Stress Disorder
Specify if: Acute/Chronic
Specify if: With Delayed Onset
308.3 Acute Stress Disorder
300.02 Generalized Anxiety Disorder
293.84 Anxiety Disorder Due to . . . *[Indicate the General Medical Condition]*
Specify if: With Generalized Anxiety/With Panic Attacks/With Obsessive-Compulsive Symptoms
___.___ Substance-Induced Anxiety Disorder *(refer to Substance-Related Disorders for substance-specific codes)*
Specify if: With Generalized Anxiety/With Panic Attacks/With Obsessive-Compulsive Symptoms/With Phobic Symptoms
Specify if: With Onset During Intoxication/With Onset During Withdrawal
300.00 Anxiety Disorder NOS

SOMATOFORM DISORDERS

300.81 Somatization Disorder
300.82 Undifferentiated Somatoform Disorder
300.11 Conversion Disorder
Specify type: With Motor Symptom or Deficit/With Sensory Symptom or Deficit/With Seizures or Convulsions/With Mixed Presentation
307.xx Pain Disorder
.80 Associated With Psychologic Factors
.89 Associated With Both Psychologic Factors and a General Medical Condition
Specify if: Acute/Chronic

300.7 Hypochondriasis
Specify if: With Poor Insight
300.7 Body Dysmorphic Disorder
300.82 Somatoform Disorder NOS

FACTITIOUS DISORDERS

300.xx Factitious Disorder
.16 With Predominantly Psychological Signs and Symptoms
.19 With Predominantly Physical Signs and Symptoms
.19 With Combined Psychological and Physical Signs and Symptoms
300.19 Factitious Disorder NOS

DISSOCIATIVE DISORDERS

300.12 Dissociative Amnesia
300.13 Dissociative Fugue
300.14 Dissociative Identity Disorder
300.6 Depersonalization Disorder
300.15 Dissociative Disorder NOS

SEXUAL AND GENDER IDENTITY DISORDERS
Sexual Dysfunctions

The following specifiers apply to all primary Sexual Dysfunctions:
Lifelong Type/Acquired Type
Generalized Type/Situational Type
Due to Psychologic Factors/Due to Combined Factors

Sexual Desire Disorders

302.71 Hypoactive Sexual Desire Disorder
302.79 Sexual Aversion Disorder

Sexual Arousal Disorders

302.72 Female Sexual Arousal Disorder
302.72 Male Erectile Disorder

Orgasmic Disorders

302.73 Female Orgasmic Disorder
302.74 Male Orgasmic Disorder
302.75 Premature Ejaculation

Sexual Pain Disorders

302.76 Dyspareunia (Not Due to a General Medical Condition)

306.51 Vaginismus (Not Due to a General Medical Condition)

Sexual Dysfunction Due to a General Medical Condition

625.8   Female Hypoactive Sexual Desire Disorder Due to . . . *[Indicate the General Medical Condition]*

608.89 Male Hypoactive Sexual Desire Disorder Due to . . . *[Indicate the General Medical Condition]*

607.84 Male Erectile Disorder Due to . . . *[Indicate the General Medical Condition]*

625.0   Female Dyspareunia Due to . . . *[Indicate the General Medical Condition]*

608.89 Male Dyspareunia Due to . . . *[Indicate the General Medical Condition]*

625.8   Other Female Sexual Dysfunction Due to . . . *[Indicate the General Medical Condition]*

608.89 Other Male Sexual Dysfunction Due to . . . *[Indicate the General Medical Condition]*

___.__ Substance-Induced Sexual Dysfunction *(refer to Substance-Related Disorders for substance-specific codes)*
        Specify if: With Impaired Desire/With Impaired Arousal/With Impaired Orgasm/With Sexual Pain
        Specify if: With Onset During Intoxication

302.70 Sexual Dysfunction NOS

Paraphilias

302.4   Exhibitionism

302.81 Fetishism

302.89 Frotteurism

302.2   Pedophilia
        Specify if: Sexually Attracted to Males/Sexually Attracted to Females/Sexually Attracted to Both
        Specify if: Limited to Incest
        Specify type: Exclusive Type/Nonexclusive Type

302.83 Sexual Masochism

302.84 Sexual Sadism

302.3   Transvestic Fetishism
        Specify if: With Gender Dysphoria

302.82 Voyeurism

302.9   Paraphilia NOS

Gender Identity Disorders

302.xx Gender Identity Disorder
    .6   In Children
    .85   In Adolescents or Adults
            Specify if: Sexually Attracted to Males/Sexually Attracted to Females/Sexually Attracted to Both/Sexually Attracted to Neither

302.6   Gender Identity Disorder NOS

302.9   Sexual Disorder NOS

EATING DISORDERS

307.1   Anorexia Nervosa
        Specify type: Restricting Type; Binge-Eating/Purging Type

307.51 Bulimia Nervosa
        Specify type: Purging Type/Nonpurging Type

307.50 Eating Disorder NOS

SLEEP DISORDERS
Primary Sleep Disorders

Dyssomnias

307.42 Primary Insomnia

307.44 Primary Hypersomnia
        Specify if: Recurrent

347   Narcolepsy

780.59 Breathing-Related Sleep Disorder

307.45 Circadian Rhythm Sleep Disorder
        Specify type: Delayed Sleep Phase Type/Jet Lag Type/Shift Work Type/Unspecified Type

307.47 Dyssomnia NOS

Parasomnias

307.47 Nightmare Disorder

307.46 Sleep Terror Disorder

307.46 Sleepwalking Disorder

307.47 Parasomnia NOS

Sleep Disorders Related to Another Mental Disorder

307.42 Insomnia Related to . . . *[Indicate the Axis I or Axis II Disorder]*

307.44 Hypersomnia Related to . . . *[Indicate the Axis I or Axis II Disorder]*

Other Sleep Disorders

780.xx   Sleep Disorder Due to . . . *[Indicate the General Medical Condition]*
.52   Insomnia Type
.54   Hypersomnia Type
.59   Parasomnia Type
.59   Mixed Type
___.__   Substance-Induced Sleep Disorder *(refer to Substance-Related Disorders for substance-specific codes)*
              Specify type: Insomnia Type/Hypersomnia Type/ Parasomnia Type/Mixed Type
              Specify if: With Onset During Intoxication/With Onset During Withdrawal

IMPULSE-CONTROL DISORDERS NOT ELSEWHERE CLASSIFIED

312.34   Intermittent Explosive Disorder
312.32   Kleptomania
312.33   Pyromania
312.31   Pathologic Gambling
312.39   Trichotillomania
312.30   Impulse-Control Disorder NOS

ADJUSTMENT DISORDERS

309.xx   Adjustment Disorder
.0   With Depressed Mood
.24   With Anxiety
.28   With Mixed Anxiety and Depressed Mood
.3   With Disturbance of Conduct
.4   With Mixed Disturbance of Emotions and Conduct
.9   Unspecified
              Specify if: Acute/Chronic

PERSONALITY DISORDERS

NOTE: These are coded on Axis II.
301.0   Paranoid Personality Disorder
301.20   Schizoid Personality Disorder
301.22   Schizotypal Personality Disorder
301.7   Antisocial Personality Disorder
301.83   Borderline Personality Disorder
301.50   Histrionic Personality Disorder
301.81   Narcissistic Personality Disorder
301.82   Avoidant Personality Disorder
301.6   Dependent Personality Disorder
301.4   Obsessive-Compulsive Personality Disorder
301.9   Personality Disorder NOS

OTHER CONDITIONS THAT MAY BE A FOCUS OF CLINICAL ATTENTION

Psychological Factors Affecting Medical Condition

316   . . . *[Specified Psychological Factor] Affecting . . . [Indicate the General Medical Condition]*
Choose name based on nature of factors:
   Mental Disorder Affecting Medical Condition
   Psychological Symptoms Affecting Medical Condition
   Personality Traits or Coping Style Affecting Medical Condition
   Maladaptive Health Behaviors Affecting Medical Condition
   Stress-Related Physiological Response Affecting Medical Condition
   Other or Unspecified Psychological Factors Affecting Medical Condition

Medication-Induced Movement Disorders

332.1   Neuroleptic-Induced Parkinsonism
333.92   Neuroleptic Malignant Syndrome
333.7   Neuroleptic-Induced Acute Dystonia
333.99   Neuroleptic-Induced Acute Akathisia
333.82   Neuroleptic-Induced Tardive Dyskinesia
333.1   Medication-Induced Postural Tremor
333.90   Medication-Induced Movement Disorder NOS

Other Medication-Induced Disorder

995.2   Adverse Effects of Medication NOS

Relational Problems

V61.9   Relational Problem Related to a Mental Disorder or General Medical Condition
V61.20   Parent-Child Relational Problem
V61.10   Partner Relational Problem
V61.8   Sibling Relational Problem
V62.81   Relational Problem NOS

Problems Related to Abuse or Neglect

V61.21   Physical Abuse of Child *(code 995.5 if focus of attention is on victim)*

V61.21 Sexual Abuse of Child (*code 995.5 if focus of attention is on victim*)

V61.21 Neglect of Child (*code 995.5 if focus of attention is on victim*)

___.___ Physical Abuse of Adult

V61.12 (if by partner)

V62.83 (if by person other than partner) (*code 995.81 if focus of attention is on victim*)

___.___ Sexual Abuse of Adult

V61.12 (if by partner)

V62.83 (if by person other than partner) (*code 995.83 if focus of attention is on victim*)

Additional Conditions That May Be a Focus of Clinical Attention

V15.81 Noncompliance With Treatment

V65.2   Malingering

V71.01 Adult Antisocial Behavior

V71.02 Child or Adolescent Antisocial Behavior

V62.89 Borderline Intellectual Functioning
        NOTE: *This is coded on Axis II.*

780.9   Age-Related Cognitive Decline

V62.82 Bereavement

V62.3   Academic Problem

V62.2   Occupational Problem

313.82 Identity Problem

V62.89 Religious or Spiritual Problem

V62.4   Acculturation Problem

V62.89 Phase of Life Problem

ADDITIONAL CODES

300.9   Unspecified Mental Disorder (nonpsychotic)

V71.09 No Diagnosis or Condition on Axis I

799.9   Diagnosis or Condition Deferred on Axis I

V71.09 No Diagnosis on Axis II

799.9   Diagnosis Deferred on Axis II

NANDA-International–Approved Nursing Diagnoses

Activity intolerance
Activity intolerance, risk for
Airway clearance, ineffective
Allergy response, latex
Allergy response, risk for latex
Anxiety
Anxiety, death
Aspiration, risk for
Attachment, risk for impaired parent/child
Autonomic dysreflexia
Autonomic dysreflexia, risk for

Behavior, risk-prone health
Body image, disturbed
Body temperature, risk for imbalanced
Bowel incontinence
Breastfeeding, effective
Breastfeeding, ineffective
Breastfeeding, interrupted
Breathing pattern, ineffective

Cardiac output, decreased
Caregiver role strain
Caregiver role strain, risk for
Comfort, readiness for enhanced
Communication, impaired verbal
Communication, readiness for enhanced
Conflict, decisional
Conflict, parental role

Confusion, acute
Confusion, chronic
Confusion, risk for acute
Constipation
Constipation, perceived
Constipation, risk for
Contamination
Contamination, risk for
Coping, compromised family
Coping, defensive
Coping, disabled family
Coping, ineffective
Coping, ineffective community
Coping, readiness for enhanced
Coping, readiness for enhanced community
Coping, readiness for enhanced family

Death syndrome, risk for sudden infant
Decision making, readiness for enhanced
Denial, ineffective
Dentition, impaired
Development, risk for delayed
Diarrhea
Dignity, risk for compromised human
Distress, moral
Disuse syndrome, risk for
Diversional activity, deficient

Energy field, disturbed
Environmental interpretation syndrome, impaired

Failure to thrive, adult
Falls, risk for
Family processes: alcoholism, dysfunctional

From NANDA-International. (2007). *NANDA-I nursing diagnosis: Definitions and classification 2007-2008*, Philadelphia: Author.

Family processes, interrupted
Family processes, readiness for enhanced
Fatigue
Fear
Fluid balance, readiness for enhanced
Fluid volume, deficient
Fluid volume, excess
Fluid volume, risk for deficient
Fluid volume, risk for imbalanced

Gas exchange, impaired
Glucose, risk for unstable blood
Grieving
Grieving, complicated
Grieving, risk for complicated
Growth, risk for disproportionate
Growth and development, delayed

Health maintenance, ineffective
Health-seeking behaviors
Home maintenance, impaired
Hope, readiness for enhanced
Hopelessness
Hyperthermia
Hypothermia

Identity, disturbed personal
Immunization status, readiness for enhanced
Incontinence, functional urinary
Incontinence, overflow urinary
Incontinence, reflex urinary
Incontinence, stress urinary
Incontinence, total urinary
Incontinence, urge urinary
Incontinence, risk for urge urinary
Infant behavior, disorganized
Infant behavior, risk for disorganized
Infant behavior, readiness for enhanced organized
Infant feeding pattern, ineffective
Infection, risk for
Injury, risk for
Injury, risk for perioperative-positioning
Insomnia
Intracranial adaptive capacity, decreased

Knowledge, deficient
Knowledge, readiness for enhanced

Lifestyle, sedentary
Liver function, risk for impaired
Loneliness, risk for

Memory, impaired
Mobility, impaired bed
Mobility, impaired physical
Mobility, impaired wheelchair

Nausea
Neglect, unilateral
Noncompliance
Nutrition, readiness for enhanced
Nutrition: less than body requirements, imbalanced
Nutrition: more than body requirements, imbalanced
Nutrition: more than body requirements, risk for imbalanced

Oral mucous membrane, impaired

Pain, acute
Pain, chronic
Parenting, impaired
Parenting, readiness for enhanced
Parenting, risk for impaired
Peripheral neurovascular dysfunction, risk for
Poisoning, risk for
Post-trauma syndrome
Post-trauma syndrome, risk for
Power, readiness for enhanced
Powerlessness
Powerlessness, risk for
Protection, ineffective

Rape-trauma syndrome
Rape-trauma syndrome, compound reaction
Rape-trauma syndrome, silent reaction
Religiosity, impaired
Religiosity, readiness for enhanced
Religiosity, risk for impaired
Relocation stress syndrome
Relocation stress syndrome, risk for
Role performance, ineffective

Self-care, readiness for enhanced
Self-care deficit, bathing/hygiene
Self-care deficit, dressing/grooming
Self-care deficit, feeding
Self-care deficit, toileting
Self-concept, readiness for enhanced
Self-esteem, chronic low
Self-esteem, situational low
Self-esteem, risk for situational low
Self-mutilation
Self-mutilation, risk for

Sensory perception, disturbed

Sexual dysfunction

Sexuality pattern, ineffective

Skin integrity, impaired

Skin integrity, risk for impaired

Sleep deprivation

Sleep, readiness for enhanced

Social interaction, impaired

Social isolation

Sorrow, chronic

Spiritual distress

Spiritual distress, risk for

Spiritual well-being, readiness for enhanced

Stress overload

Suffocation, risk for

Suicide, risk for

Surgical recovery, delayed

Swallowing, impaired

Therapeutic regimen management, effective

Therapeutic regimen management, ineffective

Therapeutic regimen management, ineffective community

Therapeutic regimen management, ineffective family

Therapeutic regimen management, readiness for enhanced

Thermoregulation, ineffective

Thought processes, disturbed

Tissue integrity, impaired

Tissue perfusion, ineffective

Transfer ability, impaired

Trauma, risk for

Urinary elimination, impaired

Urinary elimination, readiness for enhanced

Urinary retention

Ventilation, impaired spontaneous

Ventilatory weaning response, dysfunctional

Violence, risk for other-directed

Violence, risk for self-directed

Walking, impaired

Wandering

APPENDIX C

Answers to Chapter Review Questions

evolve Visit the Evolve website at **http://evolve.elsevier.com/Varcarolis/essentials** for rationales and text page references.

Chapter 1
1. 1, 2, 4
2. 2
3. 3
4. 1
5. 2

Chapter 2
1. 3
2. 4
3. 3
4. 2
5. 4

Chapter 3
1. 1
2. 3
3. 1
4. 3
5. 1

Chapter 4
1. 1
2. 3
3. 1
4. 2
5. 1, 2, 4

Chapter 5
1. 2
2. 1
3. 2
4. 1
5. 3

Chapter 6
1. 1
2. 3
3. 1
4. 1

Chapter 7
1. 1
2. 3
3. 4
4. 3
5. 4

Chapter 8
1. 3
2. 2
3. 3
4. 4
5. 4

Chapter 9
1. 2
2. 3
3. 4
4. 1, 2, 3, 4
5. 2

Chapter 10
1. 4
2. 2
3. 4
4. 2
5. 1, 2, 3, 4

Chapter 11
1. 1
2. 3
3. 2
4. 1
5. 1

Chapter 12
1. 2
2. 4
3. 1
4. 3
5. 2

Chapter 13
1. 1
2. 2
3. 1
4. 2
5. 2

Chapter 14
1. 4
2. 4
3. 1
4. 1
5. 3

Chapter 15
1. 1
2. 4
3. 1
4. 1
5. 1

Chapter 16
1. 3
2. 1
3. 4
4. 1
5. 1

Chapter 17
1. 1
2. 3
3. 1
4. 1
5. 3

Chapter 18
1. 1
2. 4
3. 2
4. 1
5. 4

Chapter 19
1. 1
2. 4
3. 1, 4
4. 4

Chapter 20
1. 4
2. 4
3. 4
4. 3

Chapter 21
1. 3
2. 1
3. 1
4. 4
5. 3

Chapter 22
1. 1
2. 2
3. 4
4. 3
5. 1, 2, 3, 4

Chapter 23
1. 1
2. 1
3. 1, 2
4. 4
5. 4

Chapter 24
1. 2, 3
2. 4
3. 1, 3
4. 3
5. 1

Chapter 25
1. 1
2. 1
3. 2
4. 4
5. 1

Chapter 26
1. 4
2. 1
3. 1
4. 1
5. 3

Chapter 27
1. 1
2. 2
3. 3
4. 1, 2, 3
5. 3

Glossary

A

abstract thinking The ability to conceptualize ideas (e.g., finding meaning in proverbs).

abuse An act of misuse, deceit, or exploitation; wrong or improper use of or action toward another, resulting in injury, damage, maltreatment, or corruption.

accommodation The ability to change one's way of thinking to introduce new ideas, objects, or experiences.

acrophobia Fear of high places.

acting-out behaviors Behaviors that originate on an unconscious level to reduce anxiety and tension. Anxiety is displaced from one situation to another in the form of observable responses (e.g., anger, crying, or violence).

activities of daily living For a person with a chronic mental illness, the activities necessary to live independently as an adult.

acute anxiety Anxiety that is precipitated by an imminent loss or a change that threatens an individual's sense of security.

addiction Loss of control with respect to use of a drug (e.g., alcohol), use of the drug despite the presence of related problems, and a tendency to relapse after stopping use. Addiction may also refer to nonchemical dependencies.

Adult Children of Alcoholics (ACOA) A support group for adult children of alcoholics, who often experience similar difficulties and problems in their adult lives as a result of having an alcoholic parent or parents.

adventitious crisis A crisis that is not part of everyday life but involves an event that is unplanned and accidental. Adventitious crises include natural disasters and crimes of violence such as rapes or muggings.

affect The external manifestation of feeling or emotion that can be assessed by a nurse by observing facial expression, tone of voice, and body language. For example, a patient may be said to have a flat affect, meaning that there is an absence or a near absence of facial expression. Some people, however, use the term loosely to mean a feeling, emotion, or mood.

ageism A system of destructive, erroneous beliefs about older adults; a bias against older people based solely on their age.

aggression Any verbal or nonverbal (actual or attempted, conscious or unconscious) forceful means of harm or abuse of another person or object.

agnosia Loss of the ability to recognize familiar objects. For example, a person may be unable to identify familiar sounds, such as the ringing of a doorbell (auditory agnosia), or familiar objects, such as a toothbrush or keys (visual agnosia).

agoraphobia Anxiety/panicky feelings about being in places or situations in which escape might be difficult or embarrassing or in which help may not be available should an anxiety attack occur. For some individuals these feelings occur at home, in crowded supermarkets, in places of worship—places that clearly are not open. People with agoraphobia actively avoid places or situations associated with anxiety. For some, life becomes increasingly constricted until, in the most severe cases, they may not be able to leave the home.

agraphia Loss of a previous ability to write resulting from brain injury or brain disease.

akathisia Regular rhythmic movements, usually of the lower limbs; constant pacing may also be seen; often noticed in people taking antipsychotic medication.

562

akinesia Absence or diminution of voluntary motion. Akinesia is usually accompanied by a parallel reduction in mental activity.

Al-Anon A support group for spouses and friends of alcoholics.

Alateen A nationwide network for children more than 10 years of age who have alcoholic parents.

alcohol withdrawal delirium An organic mental disorder that occurs 40 to 48 hours after cessation or reduction of long-term heavy alcohol intake and that is considered a medical emergency; often referred to by the older term *delirium tremens* (DTs).

alcoholic hallucinations Visual and tactile hallucinations reported to occur in alcohol-dependent patients suffering from alcohol withdrawal delirium.

Alcoholics Anonymous (AA) A self-help group for recovering alcoholics that provides support and encouragement to those involved in continuing recovery.

alcoholism The end stage of the continuum that includes addiction to and dependence on the drug alcohol.

Alzheimer's disease A primary cognitive impairment disorder characterized by progressive deterioration of cognitive functioning, with the end result that the person may not recognize once-familiar people, places, and things. The ability to walk and talk is absent in the final stages.

ambivalence The holding, at the same time, of two opposing emotions, attitudes, ideas, or wishes toward the same person, situation, or object.

amnesia Loss of memory for events within a specific period of time; may be temporary or permanent.

anergia Lack of energy; passivity.

anger An emotional response to the perception of frustration of desires or threat to one's needs.

anhedonia The inability to experience pleasure.

anorexia A medical term that signifies a loss of appetite. A person with anorexia nervosa, however, may not have any loss of appetite and often is preoccupied with food and eating. A person with this disorder may suppress the desire for food in order to control his or her eating.

Antabuse (disulfiram) A drug given to alcoholics that produces nausea, vomiting, dizziness, flushing, and tachycardia if alcohol is consumed.

anticholinergic side effects Side effects caused by the use of some medications (e.g., neuroleptics and tricyclic antidepressants). Symptoms include dry mouth, constipation, urinary retention, blurred vision, and dry mucous membranes.

anticipatory grief Grief that occurs before an actual loss. During this time, painful feelings may be partially resolved.

antidepressants Drugs predominantly used to elevate mood in people who are depressed.

antimanic drugs Drugs used in the treatment of a manic state to lower an elevated and unstable mood and to reduce irritability and aggressiveness.

antipsychotic drugs (neuroleptics, major tranquilizers) Drugs that have the ability to decrease psychotic, paranoid, and disorganized thinking and positively alter bizarre behaviors; they are thought to reduce the effects of the neurotransmitter dopamine by blocking the dopamine receptors.

antisocial (sociopathic, psychopathic) Terms often used interchangeably to refer to a syndrome in which a person lacks the capacity to relate to others. These people do not experience discomfort in inflicting pain on or observing pain in others, and they constantly manipulate others for personal gain. Common characteristics and behaviors seen in people with this disorder include crimes against society, aggressiveness, inability to feel remorse, untruthfulness and insincerity, unreliability, and failure to follow any life plan.

anxiety A state of feeling apprehension, uneasiness, uncertainty, or dread resulting from a real or perceived threat whose actual source is unknown or unrecognized.

anxiolytics (antianxiety drugs, minor tranquilizers) Drugs prescribed, usually on a short-term basis, to reduce anxiety.

apathy A state of indifference.

aphasia Difficulty in the formulation of words; loss of language ability. In extreme cases, a person may be limited to a few words, may babble, or may become mute.

apraxia Loss of ability to perform purposeful movements. For example, a person may be unable to shave, dress, or perform other once-familiar and purposeful tasks.

assault An intentional act that is designed to make the victim fearful and that produces reasonable apprehension of harm.

assertiveness Asking for what one wants or acting to get what one wants in a way that respects the rights and feelings of other people.

assertiveness training Instruction in communication skills that help people ask directly in appropriate (nondemanding, nonthreatening, and nondemeaning) ways for what they want.

assimilation The incorporation of new ideas, objects, and experiences into the framework of one's thoughts.

associative looseness A disturbance of thinking in which ideas shift from one subject to another in an oblique or unrelated manner. When this condition is severe, speech may be incoherent.

attention deficit hyperactivity disorder A behavioral disorder usually manifested before the age of 7 years that includes overactivity, chronic inattention, and difficulty dealing with multiple stimuli.

autistic thinking Thoughts, ideas, or desires derived from internal, private stimuli or perceptions that often are incongruent with reality.

automatic obedience The performance of all simple commands in a robot-like fashion; may be present in catatonia.

aversion therapy A behavioral technique that uses negative reinforcement or conditioning to alter or eliminate an unwanted or negative behavior.

avolition Lack of motivation.

axon The part of the neuron that conveys electrical impulses away from the cell body.

B

basal ganglia Pockets of integrating gray matter deep within the cerebrum that are involved in the regulation of movement, emotions, and basic drives.

battering Physical attack, such as hitting, kicking, biting, throwing, and burning.

battery The harmful or offensive touching of another person.

behavior modification A treatment modality that focuses on modifying and changing specific observable dysfunctional patterns of behavior by means of stimulus-and-response conditioning. Examples of behavioral therapy techniques include operant conditioning, token economy, systematic desensitization, aversion therapy, and flooding.

binge-purge cycle An episodic, uncontrolled, rapid ingestion of large quantities of food over a short period, followed by purging (vomiting; overexercising; misusing laxatives, diuretics, or other medications); seen in people with bulimia nervosa.

biofeedback A technique for gaining conscious control over unconscious body functions, such as blood pressure and heartbeat, to achieve relaxation or the relief of stress-related physical symptoms; involves the use of self-monitoring equipment.

bipolar disorders Mood disorders that include one or more manic episodes and usually one or more depressive episodes.

bisexuality Sexual attraction toward both males and females, which may be acted on by engaging in both heterosexual and homosexual activities.

blocking A sudden obstruction or interruption in the spontaneous flow of thinking or speaking that is perceived as an absence or deprivation of thought.

blurred or diffuse boundaries A blending together of roles, thoughts, and feelings of individuals so that clear distinctions among family members (or others) fail to emerge.

body image One's internalized sense of the physical self.

borderline personality disorder A disorder characterized by disordered images of self, impulsive and unpredictable behavior, marked shifts in mood, and instability in relationships with others.

boundaries Those functions that maintain a clear distinction among individuals within a family or group and between family members and the outside world. Boundaries may be clear, diffuse, rigid, or inconsistent.

bulimia Episodes of excessive and uncontrollable intake of large amounts of food (binges), usually alternating with compensatory activities such as self-induced vomiting, use of cathartics and/or diuretics, and self-starvation. These alternating behaviors characterize the eating disorder bulimia nervosa.

C

case management Duties of a health care worker (e.g., a nurse) that involve assuming responsibility for a patient or group of patients—arranging assessments of need, formulating a comprehensive plan of care, arranging for delivery of services to address individual patient needs, and assessing and monitoring the services delivered.

catatonia A state of psychologically induced immobilization at times interrupted by episodes of extreme agitation.

catecholamines A group of biogenic amines that are derived from phenylalanine and contain catechol as the aromatic portion. Certain of these amines, such as epinephrine, norepinephrine, and dopamine, are neurotransmitters and exert an important influence on peripheral and central nervous system activity.

cathexis A psychoanalytical term used to describe the emotional attachment or bond to an idea, an object, or, most commonly, a person.

character The sum of a person's relatively fixed personality traits and habitual modes of response.

chemical restraint A drug given for the specific purpose of inhibiting a certain behavior or movement.

child abuse—battering Physical assault of a child such as hitting, kicking, biting, throwing, and burning.

child abuse—neglect A type of child abuse that can be physical (e.g., failure to provide medical care), developmental (e.g., failure to provide emotional nurturing and cognitive stimulation), educational (failure to provide educational opportunities to the child in accordance with the state's education laws), or a combination of these.

child abuse—physical endangerment Reckless behaviors toward a child that could lead to the child's serious physical injury, such as leaving a young child alone or placing the child in a hazardous environment.

child abuse—sexual Sexual maltreatment of a child, which can take many forms. Essentially it is those acts designed to stimulate the child sexually or to use a child for sexual stimulation, either of the perpetrator or of another person.

chronic anxiety Anxiety that a person has lived with for a long time. Chronic anxiety may take the form of chronic fatigue, insomnia, discomfort in daily activities, or discomfort in personal relationships.

chronic illness An illness that has persisted over a long period and generally involving progressive deterioration, with a resulting increase in functional impairment, symptoms, and disability.

chronic pain Pain that a patient has had for longer than 6 months.

circadian rhythm A 24-hour biological rhythm that influences specific regulatory functions such as the sleep-wake cycle, body temperature, and hormonal and neurotransmitter secretions. The 24-hour biological rhythm is controlled by a "pacemaker" in the brain that sends messages to various systems in the body such as those mentioned.

circumstantial speech A pattern of speech characterized by indirectness and delay before the person gets to the point or answers a question; the person gets caught up in countless details and explanations.

clang association The meaningless rhyming of words, often in a forceful manner.

clinical (or critical) pathway A written plan or "map" identifying predetermined times that specific nursing and medical interventions (e.g., diagnostic studies, treatments, activities, medications, teaching, discharge teaching) will be implemented (e.g., day 1 or day 2 for hospital settings, or week 1 or month 2 for community-based settings).

codependent A term used to describe coping behaviors that prevent individuals from taking care of their own needs and have as their core a preoccupation with the thoughts and feelings of another or others. It usually refers to the dependence of one person on another person who is addicted in one form or another.

cognition The act, process, or result of knowing, learning, or understanding.

cognitive impairment syndrome/disorder A disturbance in orientation, memory, intellect, judgment, and affect caused by physiological changes in the brain. Delirium and dementia are two examples of cognitive impairment syndromes. An older term is *chronic mental disorder.*

cognitive rehearsal A technique in which a patient imagines each successive step in the sequence leading to the completion of a task, identifying potential "roadblocks" (cognitive, behavioral, or environmental) and planning strategies to deal with them before they produce an unwanted failure experience.

cognitive therapy A treatment method (particularly useful for depressive disorders) that emphasizes the revision of a person's maladaptive thought processes, perceptions, and attitudes.

community nursing center (CNC) A nurse-managed center that provides direct access to professional nurses who offer holistic patient-centered health services for reimbursement.

compensation Making up for deficits in one area by excelling in another area in order to raise or maintain self-esteem.

compulsion Repetitive, seemingly purposeless behaviors performed according to certain rules known to the patient to temporarily reduce escalating anxiety.

concrete thinking Thinking grounded in immediate experience rather than abstraction. There is an overemphasis on specific detail as opposed to general and abstract concepts.

confabulation The filling in of a memory gap with a detailed fantasy believed by the teller. The purpose is to maintain self-esteem. It is seen in organic conditions such as Korsakoff's psychosis.

confidentiality The ethical responsibility of a health care professional that prohibits the disclosure of privileged information without the patient's informed consent.

conscious Denoting experiences that are within a person's awareness.

consensual validation The reality checking of thoughts, feelings, and actions with others. If a child grows up in an environment in which the chance to validate thoughts, feelings, and behaviors is decreased, the child's ability to perceive reality is greatly impaired.

conversion An unconscious defense mechanism in which anxiety is expressed as a physical symptom that has no organic cause.

coping mechanism A way of adjusting to environmental stress without altering one's goals or purposes. A coping mechanism may be either conscious or unconscious.

cotherapist A therapist who shares responsibility for therapeutic work, usually work done with groups or families.

countertransference   The tendency of the nurse (therapist, social worker) to displace onto the patient feelings that are a response to people in the nurse's past. Strong positive or strong negative reactions to a patient may indicate countertransference.

crisis   A temporary state of disequilibrium (high anxiety) in which a person's usual coping mechanisms or problem-solving methods fail. Crisis can result in personality growth or disorganization.

crisis intervention   A brief, active, and collaborative therapy that draws on an individual's personal coping abilities and resources within the family, health care setting, or community.

culture   The total lifestyle of a given people, the social legacy the individual acquires from his or her group, or the environment that is the creation of humankind.

cunnilingus   Oral sexual contact with the female sex organs.

cyclothymia   A chronic mood disturbance (of a least 2 years' duration) involving both hypomanic and dysthymic mood swings. Delusions are never present, and these mood swings usually do not warrant hospitalization or grossly impair a person's social, occupational, or interpersonal functioning.

D

decode   Interpret the meaning of autistic communications, such as those characterized by looseness of associations.

defense mechanism   An unconscious intrapsychic process used to ward off anxiety by preventing conscious awareness of threatening feelings. Defense mechanisms can be used in a healthy or a not-so-healthy manner. Examples are repression, projection, sublimation, denial, and regression.

delayed grief   A dysfunctional reaction to grief in which a person may not experience the pain of loss; however, the pain is manifested as chronic depression, intense preoccupation with body functioning (hypochondriasis), phobic reactions, or acute insomnia.

delirium   An acute, usually reversible alteration in consciousness typically accompanied by disturbances in thinking, memory, attention, and perception; the syndrome has multiple causes.

delirium tremens (DTs)   See *alcohol withdrawal delirium.*

delusion   A false belief held to be true even with evidence to the contrary (e.g., the false belief that one is being singled out for harm by others).

dementia   A progressive and usually irreversible deterioration of cognitive and intellectual functions and memory without impairment in consciousness.

dendrite   The part of the neuron that conveys electrical impulses toward the cell body.

denial   Escaping of unpleasant realities by ignoring their existence.

depersonalization   A phenomenon whereby a person experiences a sense of unreality of or estrangement from the self. For example, one may feel that one's extremities have changed, that one is seeing oneself from a distance, or that one is in a dream.

depressive mood syndrome   Defined by the American Psychiatric Association as a depressed mood or loss of interest that lasts at least 2 weeks and is accompanied by symptoms such as weight loss and difficulty concentrating.

derealization   The false perception by a person that his or her environment has changed. For example, everything seems bigger or smaller, or familiar objects appear strange and unfamiliar.

desensitization   The reduction of intense reactions to a stimulus (as in a phobia) by repeated exposure to the stimulus in a weaker or milder form.

detachment   An interpersonal and intrapersonal dissociation from affective expression. Therefore, the individual appears cold, aloof, and distant. This behavior is thought to be learned and is viewed as defensive.

Diagnostic and Statistical Manual of Mental Disorders, Fourth Edition, Text Revision (DSM-IV-TR)   A classification of mental disorders that includes descriptions of diagnostic categories. The *DSM-IV-TR* is the most widely accepted system of classifying abnormal behaviors used in the United States today.

diffuse boundaries   See *blurred* or *diffuse boundaries.*

disorientation   Confusion and impaired ability to identify time, place, and person.

displacement   Transfer of emotions associated with a particular person, object, or situation to another person, object, or situation that is nonthreatening.

dissociation   An unconscious defense mechanism that allows blocking of overwhelming anxiety stemming from disintegration of functions of consciousness, memory, identity, or perception of environment.

dissociative disorders   Disorders reflecting a disturbance in the normally well-integrated continuum of consciousness, memory, identity, and perception.

distractibility   Inability to maintain attention; tendency to shift from one area or topic to another with minimal provocation.

double-bind message   A communication that contains two contradictory messages given by the same person at the same time, to which the receiver is expected to respond. Constant double-bind situations result in feelings of helplessness, fear, and anxiety in the recipient of such messages.

drug abuse Defined by the American Psychiatric Association as the maladaptive and consistent use of a drug despite the presence of social, occupational, psychological, or physical problems exacerbated by such drug use; or recurrent use in situations that are physically hazardous, such as driving while intoxicated.

drug dependence Impaired control of drug use despite adverse consequences, the development of tolerance to the drug, and the occurrence of withdrawal symptoms when drug intake is reduced or stopped.

drug interaction The reciprocal action between two or more drugs taken simultaneously, which produces an effect different from the usual effects of either drug taken alone. The interacting drugs may be potentiating or inhibitory, and serious side effects may result.

drug tolerance A need for higher and higher dosages of a drug to achieve intoxication or the desired effect.

dual diagnosis The coexistence of a psychiatric disease with substance abuse. A person with a dual diagnosis is chronically dependent on a drug or alcohol and also has another psychiatric disorder such as a depressive or personality disorder.

dyskinesia Involuntary muscular activity, such as tic, spasm, or myoclonus.

dyspareunia Persistent genital pain in either a male or a female before, during, or after sex.

dysthymia A mild to moderate mood disturbance characterized by a chronic depressive syndrome that is usually present for many years. The depressive mood disturbance is hard to distinguish from the person's usual pattern of functioning, and the person has minimal social or occupational impairment.

dystonia Abnormal muscle tonicity resulting in impaired voluntary movement. May occur as an acute side effect of neuroleptic (antipsychotic) medication, in which it manifests as muscle spasms of the face, head, neck, and back.

E

echolalia Mimicry or imitation of the speech of another person.

echopraxia Mimicry or imitation of the movements of another person.

ego One of three psychological processes that make up the Freudian system of personality (id, ego, superego). The ego is one's sense of self and provides such functions as problem solving, mobilization of defense mechanisms, reality testing, and the capability of functioning inde-

pendently. The ego is said to be the mediator between one's primitive drives (the id) and internalized parental and social prohibitions (the superego).

ego boundaries The individual's perception of the boundaries between himself or herself and the external environment.

ego-alien/ego-dystonic Synonymous terms used to describe symptoms that are unacceptable to the person who has them and are not compatible with the person's view of himself or herself (e.g., fear of cats).

ego-syntonic A term used to describe symptomatic behaviors or beliefs that do not seem to bother the person or that seem right to the person. For example, a very paranoid person who wrongly believes that the government is out to get him or her truly believes this thought, and it is consistent with the way this person experiences life.

egocentric Self-centered.

electroconvulsive therapy (ECT) An effective treatment for depression in which a grand mal seizure is induced by passing an electrical current through electrodes that are applied to the temples. The administration of a muscle relaxant minimizes seizure activity and prevents damage to long bones and cervical vertebrae.

elopement Escape.

emotional abuse Essentially, depriving an individual of a nurturing atmosphere in which he or she can thrive, learn, and develop. Emotional abuse takes many forms (e.g., terrorizing, demeaning, consistently belittling, withholding warmth).

empathy The ability of one person to get inside another's world and see things from the other person's perspective and to communicate this understanding to the other person.

enabling Helping a chemically dependent individual avoid experiencing the consequences of his or her drinking or drug use. It is one behavioral component of a codependency role.

endorphins Naturally produced chemicals (peptides) with morphine-like action. They are usually found in the brain and are associated with reduction of pain and feelings of well-being.

enmeshed boundaries See *blurred or diffuse boundaries*.

enuresis Nocturnal and/or daytime involuntary discharge of urine.

epinephrine (adrenaline) A catecholamine secreted by the adrenal gland and by fibers of the sympathetic nervous system. It is responsible for many of the physical manifestations of fear and anxiety.

ethics The discipline concerned with standards of values, behaviors, or beliefs adhered to by individuals or groups.

eustress   A positive type of stress that reflects a person's confidence in the ability to successfully master given demands or tasks.

euthymia   A normal mood state.

extrapyramidal side effects   A variety of signs and symptoms that are often side effects of the use of certain psychotropic drugs, particularly the phenothiazines. Three reversible extrapyramidal side effects are acute dystonia, akathisia, and pseudoparkinsonism. A fourth, tardive dyskinesia, is the most serious and is not reversible.

F

family system   Those individuals who make up the family unit and contribute to the functional state of the family as a unit.

family therapy   A treatment modality that focuses on the relationships within the family system.

family triangle   A dysfunctional phenomenon in which a third person is brought into a two-person relationship to help relieve anxiety or stress between two family members. Triangles are dysfunctional because the lowering of anxiety comes from diversion from the conflict rather than from resolution of the conflict between the two members.

fantasy   Mental imagery that is unrestrained by reality and represents an attempt to solve problems in a private world. One difference between a healthy person and a schizophrenic, for example, is that a schizophrenic may not know where fantasy ends and reality begins.

fear   A reaction to a specific danger.

feedback   Communication of one person's impressions of and reactions to another person's actions or verbalizations.

fellatio   Oral sexual contact with the penis.

fetish   An object or part of the body to which sexual significance or meaning is attached.

fight-or-flight response (sympathetic response)   The body's physiological response to fear or rage that triggers the sympathetic branch of the autonomic nervous system as well as the endocrine system. This response is useful in emergencies; however, a sustained response can result in pathophysiological changes such as high blood pressure, ulcers, and cardiac problems.

flight of ideas   A continuous flow of speech in which the person jumps rapidly from one topic to another. Sometimes the listener can keep up with the changes; at other times it is necessary to listen for themes in the incessant talking. Themes often include grandiose and fantasized evaluation of personal sexual prowess, business ability, artistic talents, and so forth.

formication   A tactile hallucination or illusion involving the sensation of insects crawling on the body or under the skin.

frustration   The curtailment of personal goals, satisfaction, or security by conditions of external reality or by internal controls.

fugue   An altered state of consciousness involving both memory loss (as in psychogenic amnesia) and travel away from home or from one's usual work locale; that is, fugue involves flight as well as forgetfulness. Often called *psychogenic* or *dissociative fugue*.

G

general adaptation syndrome (GAS)   The body's organized response to stress, as elucidated by Hans Selye. It progresses through three stages: (1) the stage of alarm, (2) the stage of resistance, and (3) the stage of exhaustion.

genogram   A systematic diagram of the three-generational relationships within a family system.

grandiosity   Exaggerated belief in or claims about one's importance or identity.

grief   The subjective feelings and affect that are precipitated by a loss.

group   Two or more individuals who have a relationship with one another, are interdependent, and may share some norms.

group dynamics   The interactions and interrelations among members of a therapy group and between members and the therapist. The effective use of group dynamics is essential in group treatment.

group process   The interaction continually taking place among members of a group.

group therapy   Psychotherapy based on the examination of group interaction with a view toward understanding and eventually changing the ways in which patients interact with others.

H

hallucination   A sense perception (seeing, hearing, tasting, smelling, or touching) for which no external stimulus exists (e.g., hearing voices when none are present).

health maintenance organization (HMO)   An organization that contracts with a group or individuals to offer designated health care services to plan members for a fixed, prepaid premium (an example of a managed care program).

histrionics   A dramatic presentation of oneself with pervasive and excessive emotionality in order to seek attention, love, and admiration.

homelessness—chronic   Long-term lack of a home or permanent residence. It represents the final stage in a lifelong series of crises and missed opportunities and is the culmination of a gradual disengagement from supportive relationships and institutions.

homosexuality　Sexual attraction to or preference for a person of the same sex.

hopelessness　The belief of a person that no one can help him or her; extreme pessimism about the future.

hospice philosophy　A philosophy characterized by the acceptance of death as a natural conclusion to life and the belief that patients rather than health care providers should make the end-of-life decisions regarding how they want to live and die.

hostility　Anger that is destructive in nature and purpose.

hotline　A telephone crisis counseling service often used in crisis intervention centers to provide immediate contact between a person in crisis and a counselor.

hypermetamorphosis　The desire to touch everything in sight.

hyperorality　The desire to taste everything, chew everything, and put everything into one's mouth.

hypersomnia　The spending of increased time in sleep, possibly to escape from painful feelings; however, the increased sleep is not experienced as restful or refreshing.

hypochondriasis　Excessive preoccupation with one's physical health in the absence of any organic pathology.

hypomania　An elevated mood with symptoms less severe than those of mania. A person in hypomania does not experience impairment in reality testing, nor do the symptoms markedly impair the person's social, occupational, or interpersonal functions.

hysterical personality disorder　A disorder characterized by dramatic, emotionally intense, unstable behavior.

I

id　One of three psychological processes that make up the Freudian system of personality (id, ego, and superego). The id is the source of all primitive drives and instincts and is considered to be the reservoir of all psychic energy.

idea of reference　The false impression that outside events have special meaning for oneself.

identification　Unconscious assumption of the thoughts, mannerisms, or behaviors of a person or group in order to decrease anxiety.

identity　The sense of self based on experience, memories, perceptions, and emotions.

illusion　An error in the perception of a sensory stimulus. For example, a person may mistake polka dots on a pillow for hairy spiders.

impotence　The inability to achieve or maintain a penile erection of sufficient quality to engage in successful sexual intercourse.

impulsiveness　The tendency to engage in actions that are abrupt, unplanned, and directed toward immediate gratification.

incest　A sexual relationship between close biological relatives.

insight　Understanding and awareness of the reasons for and meaning behind one's motives and behavior.

insomnia　Inability to fall asleep or to stay asleep, early morning awakening, or both.

intellectualization　The excessive use of reasoning, logic, or words to avoid confronting undesirable impulses, emotions, and interpersonal situations.

intimacy　Emotional closeness.

intoxication　Maladaptive behavioral or psychological changes caused by excessive use of a drug or alcohol.

intrapsychic　Within the self.

introjection　The process by which a person incorporates or takes into his or her own personality qualities or values of another person or group with whom intense emotional ties exist.

intuition　Knowledge or insight gained without conscious rational thinking.

isolation　The separation of thought, ideas, or actions from their emotional aspects.

J

judgment　The ability to make logical, rational decisions.

L

la belle indifférence　An affect or attitude of unconcern about a symptom that is seen when the symptom is unconsciously used to lower anxiety. The lack of concern is thought to be a sign that the primary goal has been achieved.

labile　Characterized by rapid shifts; unstable.

lesbian　A female homosexual.

libido　Sexual drive.

limbic system　The part of the brain that is related to emotions and is referred to by some as the "emotional brain." It is involved in the mediation of fear and anxiety; anger and aggression; love, joy, and hope; and sexuality and social behavior.

limit setting　The reasonable and rational setting of parameters for patient behavior that provide control and safety.

lithium carbonate　Known as an antimanic drug because it can stabilize the manic phase of a bipolar disorder. When effective, it can modify future manic episodes and protect against future depressive episodes.

living will　An expression by a person, while competent, of his or her preference that life-sustaining treatment be continued, withheld, or withdrawn if he or she becomes terminally ill and is no longer able to make health care decisions.

looseness of association   A pattern of thinking that is haphazard, illogical, and confused, and in which connections in thought are interrupted; it is seen primarily in schizophrenic disorders.

M

magical thinking   The belief that thinking something can make it happen; it is seen in children and psychotic patients.

malingering   A conscious effort to deceive others, often for financial gain, by pretending to have physical symptoms.

managed care   A term referring to an organized system that integrates cost management and provision of health care. Health maintenance organizations (HMOs), preferred provider organizations (PPOs), and managed care options offered by government and private indemnity health insurance plans are the basic types of managed care organization.

mania   An unstable elevated mood in which delusion, poor judgment, and other signs of impaired reality testing are evident. During a manic episode, patients have marked impairment of social, occupational, and interpersonal functioning.

manipulation   Purposeful behavior directed at getting one's needs met, sometimes without regard for the needs, goals, and feelings of others.

masochism   The deriving of unconscious or conscious gratification from the experience of mental or physical pain; often used to refer to deviant sexual behaviors.

maturational crisis   A normal state in growth and development in which a specific maturational task must be learned but old coping mechanisms are no longer adequate or acceptable.

mental status examination   A formal assessment of cognitive functions such as intelligence, thought processes, and capacity for insight.

milieu   The physical and social environment of an individual.

milieu therapy   Therapy that focuses on manipulation of the environment (both physical and social) to effect positive change.

mnemonic disturbance   Loss of memory.

modeling   A technique in which desired behaviors are demonstrated. The patient learns to imitate these behaviors in appropriate situations.

mood   Defined by the American Psychiatric Association as a pervasive and sustained emotion that, when extreme, can markedly color the way the individual perceives the world.

mood syndrome   An alteration in mood with associated symptoms that occurs for a minimal period.

mourning   The process by which grief is resolved.

multiple personality disorder   A severe dissociative disorder in which one or more distinct subpersonalities exist within an individual, each of which may be dominant at different times. Each subpersonality is a complex unit with its own memories, behavioral patterns, and social relationships, which may be very different from those of the primary personality.

N

narcissism (narcism)   Self-involvement with lack of empathy for others; the narcissistic person is very self-centered and self-important; narcissism is normal in children but pathological when it occurs in adults to the same degree.

narcissistic personality disorder   A disorder characterized by a pervasive pattern of grandiosity, need for admiration, and lack of empathy for others.

National Alliance for the Mentally Ill (NAMI)   A national support group for families of the mental ill with many local and state affiliates; provides educational programs and political action.

negativism   Opposition or resistance, either covert or overt, to outside suggestions or advice.

negligence   An act, or failure to act, that breaches the duty of due care and results in or is responsible for another person's injuries.

neologism   A word a person makes up that has meaning only for that person; often part of a delusional system.

neuroleptic malignant syndrome   A rare and sometimes fatal reaction to high-potency neuroleptic drugs. Symptoms include muscle rigidity, fever, and elevated white blood cell count. It is thought to result from dopamine blockage at the basal ganglia and hypothalamus.

neuron   A specialized cell in the central nervous system. Each neuron has a cell body, an axon, and dendrites.

neurotransmitter   A chemical substance that functions as a neural messenger. Neurotransmitters are released from the axon terminal of the presynaptic neuron when stimulated by an electrical impulse.

nihilism   A delusion that the self or part of the self does not exist.

no-suicide contract   A contract made between a nurse or counselor and a patient, outlined in clear and simple language, in which the patient states that her or she will not attempt self-harm and in which specific alternatives are given for the person instead.

nonverbal communication   Communication without words, such as body language, facial expressions, or gestures.

nursing The diagnosis and treatment of human responses to actual or potential health problems.

O

obesity A condition characterized by a body weight that is at least 20% higher than the acceptable standard or ideal weight.

obsession An idea, impulse, or emotion that a person cannot put out of his or her consciousness; the condition can be mild or severe.

organic mental disorder As defined by the American Psychiatric Association, a specific brain syndrome for which a cause is known; for example, alcohol withdrawal delirium or Alzheimer's disease.

orientation The ability to relate the self correctly to time, place, and person.

overt anxiety Anxiety in which the attendant physical, physiological, and cognitive symptoms are evident and may be assessed.

P

panic Sudden, overwhelming anxiety of such intensity that it produces disorganization of the personality, loss of rational thought, and inability to communicate, along with specific physiological changes.

paranoia A state characterized by the presence of intense and strongly defended irrational suspicions. These ideas cannot be corrected by experience and cannot be modified by facts or reality.

passive-aggressive behavior Behavior that represents an indirect expression of anger or aggressive feelings. Behavior may seem passive but is motivated by unconscious anger and often triggers anger and frustration in others. Examples of passive-aggressive behavior are being late, forgetting, making "mistakes," and acting obtuse.

peer review Review of clinical practice with peers, supervisors, or consultants.

perception The mental process by which intellectual, sensory, and emotional data are organized logically or meaningfully.

perseveration The involuntary repetition of the same thought, phrase, or motor response (e.g., brushing teeth, walking); it is associated with brain damage.

personality Deeply ingrained personal patterns of behavior, traits, and thoughts that evolve, both consciously and unconsciously, as a person's style and way of adapting to the environment.

phobia An intense irrational fear of an object, situation, or place. The fear persists even though the object of the fear is harmless and the person is aware of the irrationality.

physical restraint Any manual method or mechanical device, material, or equipment that inhibits free movement.

play therapy An intervention that allows a child to symbolically express feelings such as aggression, self-doubt, anxiety, and sadness through the medium of play.

pleasure principle A tendency to seek immediate gratification of impulses and tension reduction; the id operates according to the pleasure principle.

polydrug abuse The pathological use of more than one drug.

polypharmacy The taking of more than one drug at any given time.

postvention Therapeutic interventions with the significant others of an individual who has committed suicide.

poverty of speech A speech pattern characterized by brevity and uncommunicativeness.

pressure of speech A speech pattern characterized by forceful energy manifested in frantic, jumbled speech as when a manic individual struggles to keep pace with racing thoughts.

primary anxiety Anxiety that is a result of intrapersonal or intrapsychic causes, such as a phobia.

primary depression Defined by the American Psychiatric Association as a depressive mood episode that is not caused by known organic factors and is not part of another psychotic disorder, such as schizophrenia.

primary gain The anxiety relief resulting from the use of defense mechanisms or symptom formation such as somatization (e.g., getting a headache instead of feeling angry).

primary process In psychoanalytic theory, a primitive and unconscious psychological activity in which the id attempts to reduce tension by forming an image of or hallucinating the object that would satisfy its need.

projection The unconscious attributing of one's own intolerable wishes, emotions, or motivations to another person.

projective identification A primitive form of projection used to externalize aggressive feelings. Once projection has occurred, fear of the person who is the object of the projection is coupled with a desire to control the person.

prolonged grief A dysfunctional grief reaction in which the bereaved remains intensely preoccupied with memories of the deceased many years after the person has died.

psychiatric liaison nurse A nurse with a master's degree and a background in psychiatric and medical-surgical nursing. The liaison nurse functions as a nursing consultant in addressing psychosocial concerns and as a clinician in helping the patient deal more effectively with physical and emotional problems.

psychiatry The science of treating disorders of the psyche. It is the medical specialty involved in the study, diagnosis, treatment, and prevention of mental disorders.

psychoeducational therapy A strategy of teaching patients and their families about disorders, treatments, coping techniques, and resources. It helps empower patients and families by having them become more involved and prepares them to participate in their own care once they have the requisite knowledge.

psychogenic Denoting a physical condition caused by psychological factors.

psychogenic amnesia The loss of memory for an event or period of time that is associated with overwhelming anxiety and pain. The loss of memory is related to psychological stress.

psychomotor agitation Constant involvement in some tension-relieving activity, such as constantly pacing, biting one's nails, smoking, or tapping one's fingers on a tabletop.

psychomotor retardation Extreme slowness of and difficulty in movements that in the extreme can entail complete inactivity and incontinence.

psychosexual development Emotional and sexual growth from birth to adulthood.

psychosis An extreme response to psychological or physical stressors that leads to pronounced distortion or disorganization of affective response, psychomotor function, and behavior. Reality testing is impaired, as evidenced by hallucinations or delusions.

psychosocial rehabilitation The development of the skills necessary for a person with chronic mental illness to live independently.

psychosomatic An older term describing the interaction of the mind (psyche) and the body (soma). The term was used in reference to certain disease thought to be caused by psychological factors. Referred to in the first edition of the *Diagnostic and Statistical Manual of Mental Disorders*.

psychotherapy A treatment modality based on the development of a trusting relationship between the patient and therapist for the purpose of exploring and modifying the patient's behavior in a positive direction.

psychotropic Affecting the mind.

psychotropic drugs Drugs that have an effect on psychic function, behavior, or experience.

R

racism A belief that inherent differences between races determine people's achievement and that one's own race is superior.

rape See *sexual assault/rape*.

rape-trauma syndrome A syndrome characterized by an acute phase and a long-term reorganization process that occurs after an actual or attempted sexual assault. Each phase has separate symptoms.

rationalization Justification of illogical or unreasonable ideas, actions, or feelings by the development of acceptable explanations that satisfy the teller as well as the listener.

reaction-formation (overcompensation) The process of keeping unacceptable feelings or behaviors out of awareness by developing the opposite emotion or behavior.

reality principle The ability to delay immediate gratification and modify desires in accordance with the demands of society and external reality. The ego operates according to the reality principle.

receptor A protein molecule located within or on the outer membrane of cells of various tissues, such as neurons, muscle, and blood vessels. A receptor receives chemical stimulation that causes a chemical reaction resulting in either stimulation or inhibition of the activity of the cell.

reframing A technique of changing the viewpoint of a situation and replacing it with another viewpoint that fits the facts equally well but alters the entire meaning.

regression In the face of overwhelming anxiety, the return to an earlier, more comforting (although less mature) way of behaving.

relapse A recurrence of the manifestations of a disease after a period of improvement; in a substance use disorder, the process of becoming dysfunctional in sobriety that ends in a return to chemical use.

relaxation response A set of physiological changes that result in decreased activity of the sympathetic part of the autonomic nervous system and a shift to the parasympathetic mode, which induces a state of relaxation. It is the opposite of the fight-or-flight response and has a stabilizing effect on the nervous system.

repression The exclusion of unpleasant or unwanted experiences, emotions, or ideas from conscious awareness; considered the first line of psychological defense.

respite care Temporary supervision and care of a patient who lives with his or her family. The purpose of respite care is to provide the family with some relief from the demands of the patient's need for continuous care.

restraint See *physical restraint* and *chemical restraint*.

reuptake The return of neurotransmitters to the presynaptic cell after communication with receptors on the postsynaptic cell.

rigid or disengaged boundaries Adherence to the "rules and roles" within a family no matter what the situation.

Rigid boundaries prevent family members from trying out new roles or taking on more mature functions.

ritual   A repetitive action that a person must execute over and over until he or she is exhausted or anxiety is decreased; it is often performed to lessen the anxiety triggered by an obsession.

role playing   A technique used in individual, group, or family therapy in which the therapist or a group member acts out the behavior of another member to increase that individual's ability to see a situation from another point of view. It is also a useful tool that therapists, teachers, and others use to help people practice skills in a safe environment before they try them in real-life situations, such as practicing asking for a raise, discussing a crucial topic with a person in authority, or saying no to someone without becoming defensive or angry.

S

sadism   The deriving of sexual pleasure and erotic gratification from the infliction of pain, abuse, or humiliation on another.

scapegoat   A member of a group or family who becomes the target of others' aggression but who may not be the actual cause of their hostility or frustration.

schizoaffective disorder   A disorder that includes a mixture of schizophrenic and affective symptoms (i.e., alterations in mood as well as disturbances in thought); it is considered by some to be a severe form of bipolar disorder.

schizoid personality disorder   A personality disorder in which there is a serious defect in interpersonal relationships. Characteristics include lack of warmth, aloofness, and indifference to the feelings of others.

schizophrenia   A group of mental disorders characterized by severe disturbance of thought and associative looseness, impaired reality testing (hallucinations, delusions), and limited socialization.

seasonal affective disorder (SAD)   A recently studied syndrome that appears to affect mostly women and is characterized by hypersomnia, fatigue, weight gain, irritability, and interpersonal difficulties during the winter months. It has been successfully managed with daily treatments of 2 to 3 hours of bright light.

seclusion   The last step in a process to maximize the safety of a patient and others in which the patient is placed alone in a specially designed room for protection and close observation.

secondary anxiety   Anxiety that is a result of physiological abnormalities such as certain medical disorders (e.g., neurological, endocrine, or circulatory) or is secondary to a pervasive psychiatric disorder such as depression.

secondary dementia   Dementia that is a result of an underlying disease process, such as a metabolic, nutritional, or neurological disorder. Dementia related to acquired immunodeficiency syndrome is an example.

secondary depression   A depressive mood syndrome that is caused by a physical illness or another psychiatric disorder or is part of an organic mental disorder; essentially, it is depression secondary to other causes.

secondary gain   Those advantages a person realizes from whatever symptoms or relief behaviors he or she uses. These advantages include increased attention from others, avoidance of expected responsibilities, financial gain, and the ability to manipulate others in the environment.

secondary process   In psychoanalytical theory, a process consistent with the reality principle; that is, realistic thinking.

selective inattention   The failure to notice or attend to an almost infinite number of more-or-less meaningful details of one's own living that might cause anxiety. A concept articulated by H. S. Sullivan.

selective serotonin reuptake inhibitors (SSRIs)   First-line antidepressants that block the reuptake of serotonin, permitting serotonin to act for an extended period at the synaptic binding sites in the brain.

self-concept   A person's image of the self.

self-esteem   The individual's feeling that he or she has worth or value.

self-help group   A group of people with similar problems or concerns who meet to receive peer support and encouragement and work together using their strengths to gain control over their lives.

self-mutilation   The act of self-induced pain or injury without the intent to kill oneself.

sexual assault/rape   Forced and violent vaginal, anal, or oral penetration against the victim's will and without the victim's consent. Legal definitions vary from state to state.

situational crisis   A crisis arising from an external as opposed to an internal source. Most people experience situational crises to some extent during the course of their lives (e.g., the death of a loved one, marriage, divorce, or a change in health status).

social phobia   A phobia of an interpersonal nature, such as fear of public speaking, fear of eating in front of others, or fear of writing or performing in public.

social skills training   Training that uses the principles of guidance, demonstration, practice, and feedback to enhance a patient's skills in community living. Training focuses on skills such as introducing oneself, starting and ending a conversation, asking for assistance, and other simple yet essential social interactions; it is often helpful in combating the negative symptoms of schizophrenia.

somatic therapy Treatment that involves the body, such as the use of medications or electroconvulsive therapy.

somatization The expression of psychological stress through physical symptoms.

specific phobia Fear and avoidance of a single object, situation, or activity. Specific phobias are very common in the general population.

spirituality The devotion or receptiveness to religious or moral values. Spirituality includes a search for meaning and purpose; a relationship with a higher being; and adherence to transcendent values such as hope, love, and forgiveness. It is frequently experienced through a formal faith tradition.

splitting A primitive defense mechanism in which the person sees self or others as all good or all bad, failing to integrate the positive and negative qualities of the self and others into a cohesive whole.

spouse abuse The intentional physical or emotional injury of one's spouse.

stereotype The assumption that all people in a similar cultural, racial, or ethnic group think and act alike.

stereotyped behavior A motor pattern that originally had meaning to the person (e.g., sweeping the floor or washing windows) but has become mechanical and lacks purpose.

stress The body's arousal response to any demand, change, or perceived threat.

stupor A state in which a person is dazed and awareness of his or her environment appears deadened. For example, a person may sit motionless for long periods and in extreme cases may appear to be in a coma.

subconscious Experiences, thoughts, feelings, and desires that are not in immediate awareness but can be recalled to consciousness; often called the *preconscious*. The subconscious mind helps repress unpleasant thoughts or feelings.

sublimation The unconscious process of substituting constructive and socially acceptable activities for strong impulses that are not acceptable in their original form, such as strong aggressive or sexual drives.

suicidal ideation Thoughts a person has regarding killing himself or herself.

suicide The ultimate act of self-destruction in which a person purposefully ends his or her own life.

suicide attempt Any willful, self-inflicted, life-threatening attempt at suicide that did not lead to death.

suicide gesture A suicide attempt that is planned to be discovered and is made for the purpose of influencing or manipulating others.

sundown syndrome Increasing destabilization of cognitive abilities (e.g., confusion) and lability of mood during the late afternoon, early evening, or night. Seen in people with cognitive disorders.

superego One of three psychological processes that make up the Freudian system of personality (id, ego, and superego). The superego is the internal representative of the values, ideals, and moral standards of society. The superego is said to be the moral arm of the personality.

support group A group that uses a variety of modalities to help people cope with overwhelming situations or alter unwanted behaviors during stressful periods.

suppression The conscious removal from awareness of disturbing situations or feelings; the only defense mechanism that operates on a conscious level.

symbolization The process by which one object or idea comes to represent another. For example, the nurse's keys on a locked unit may represent power and autonomy, or a fancy house may represent prestige and power.

synapse The gap between the membrane of one neuron and the membrane of another neuron. The synapse is the point at which the transmission of the nerve impulse occurs.

synesthesia A condition in which the stimulation of one sense also gives rise to a subjective sensation in another sense, such as hearing colors or seeing sounds; the phenomenon may be experienced by people taking hallucinogenic drugs.

T

tangentiality A disturbance in associative thinking in which the speaker goes off the topic. When it happens frequently and the speaker does not return to the topic, interpersonal communication is destroyed.

Tarasoff **decision** A California court decision that imposes a duty on the therapist to warn the appropriate person or persons when the therapist becomes aware that a patient presents a risk of harm to a specific person or persons.

tardive dyskinesia A serious and irreversible side effect of the phenothiazines and related drugs that consists of involuntary tonic muscle spasms typically involving the tongue, fingers, toes, neck, trunk, or pelvis.

therapeutic encounter A brief, informal meeting between nurse and patient in which the relationship is useful and important for the patient.

therapeutic nurse-patient relationship A therapeutic relationship requiring that the nurse maximize his or her communication skills, understanding of human behaviors, and personal strengths in order to enhance personal growth in the patient. This relationship occurs in all clinical settings, not just those on a psychiatric unit.

time-out   The removal or disengagement of an individual (especially a child) from a situation so that the person can regain self-control.

token economy   A behavioral approach to eliciting desired behaviors that involves application of the principles and procedures of operant conditioning; it is generally used in the management of a social setting such as a ward, classroom, or halfway house. Targeted behaviors are awarded tokens that can be exchanged for desired goods or privileges.

tort   A civil wrong for which money damages (or other relief) may be obtained by the injured party (plaintiff) from the wrongdoer (defendant).

transference   The experiencing of thoughts and feelings toward a person (often the therapist) that were originally held toward a significant person in one's past. Transference is a valuable tool used by therapists in psychoanalytical psychotherapy.

transsexual   A person who has an early and persistent feeling that he or she is trapped in a body with the wrong genitals. The individual believes that he or she is, and was always meant to be, of the opposite sex.

triangle   See *family triangle*.

U

unconscious   The repressed memories, feelings, thoughts, or wishes that are not available to the conscious mind. Usually these unconscious memories, feelings, thoughts, or wishes are associated with intense anxiety and can greatly affect an individual's behavior.

undoing   An act or behavior unconsciously designed to make up for or negate a previous act or behavior (e.g., bringing the boss a present after talking about the boss unfavorably to co-workers).

V

validate   See *consensual validation*.

values clarification   A process of self-discovery in which a person explores and determines his or her personal values and identifies what priority these values hold in personal decision making. This process can lead to increased awareness of why the person behaves in certain ways.

vegetative signs of depression   Significant changes from normal functioning in those activities necessary to support physical life and growth, such as eating, sleeping, elimination, and sex, during a depressive episode.

W

waxy flexibility   Excessive maintenance of posture; for example, after the arms or legs are placed in a certain position, the individual holds that same position for hours.

withdrawal symptoms   The negative physiological and psychological reactions that occur when a drug taken for a long time is reduced in dosage or no longer taken.

word salad   A mixture of words meaningless to the listener and to the speaker as well.

Index

Brief Guide to Cultural Assessment

A. Language
1. What is your primary spoken language?
2. How would you rate your fluency in English?
3. Would you like an interpreter?

B. Communication style
1. *Observe nonverbal communication (gesture, posture, eye movement).*
2. What are your feelings about touch?
3. *Observe how much eye contact the patient is comfortable with.*
4. How much or little do people make eye contact in your culture?

C. Family group
1. Describe the members of your family.
2. Who makes the decisions in your family?
3. Which family member can you confide in?

D. Social supports
1. Are there people outside the family (friends, meighbors) that you are close to and feel free to confide in?
2. Is there a place where you can go for support (church, school, work, club)?

E. Religious beliefs and practices
1. How important are religious or spiritual practices in your life?
2. Does your faith help in times of stress?
3. Who do you seek when you are medically ill? Mentally upset?
4. Are there any restrictions on diet or medical interventions within your religious, spiritual, or cultural beliefs?
5. To whom can the patient talk to in times of stress or sickness?

F. Health and illness beliefs
1. When you become ill what it the first thing you do to take care of the illness?
2. How is this condition (medical or mental) viewed by your culture?
3. Are there special health care practices within your culture that address your medical/mental problem?
4. What are the attitudes of mental illness in your culture?